MW00837357

LEEDS BEC
Leeds Metropolitan University
17 0445862 7

STUDIES ON NEUROPSYCHOLOGY, DEVELOPMENT, AND COGNITION
Series Editor:

Linas Bieliauskas, Ph.D.
University of Michigan, Ann Arbor, MI, USA

TRAUMATIC BRAIN INJURY IN SPORTS

AN INTERNATIONAL NEUROPSYCHOLOGICAL PERSPECTIVE

Edited by

Mark R. Lovell[1]
Ruben J. Echemendia[2]
Jeffrey T. Barth[3]
Michael W. Collins[1]

[1]University of Pittsburgh Medical Center
[2]Pennsylvania State University
[3]University of Virginia

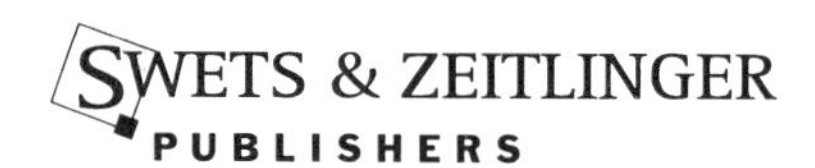

LISSE ABINGDON EXTON (PA) TOKYO

Library of Congress Cataloging-in-Publication Data

A Catalogue record for the book is available from the Library of Congress.

Copyright © 2004 Swets & Zeitlinger B.V., Lisse, The Netherlands

All rights reserved. No part of this publication or the information contained herein may be reproduced, stored in a retrieval system, or transmitted in any form or by any means, electronic, mechanical, by photocopying, recording or otherwise, without written prior permission from the publishers.

Although all care is taken to ensure the integrity and quality of this publication and the information herein, no responsibility is assumed by the publishers nor the author for any damage to property or persons as a result of operation or use of this publication and/or the information contained herein.

Published by: Swets & Zeitlinger Publishers
www.szp.swets.nl

ISBN 90 265 1961 3

Contents

SECTION II MODELS OF NEUROPSYCHOLOGICAL ASSESSMENT
Edited by Mark R. Lovell

SECTION III METHODOLOGICAL ISSUES
Edited by Jeffrey T. Barth

From the Series Editor

I am most happy to introduce *Traumatic Brain Injury in Sports: A Neuropsychological and International Perspective* as the next volume in our series. This text, edited by and including contributions from many of the most prominent researchers in the field, provides a comprehensive review of neuropsychological studies in an international range of sports, ranging from South African rugby to equestrian sports, as well as professional American football, hockey, and boxing. In addition, the text addresses the necessary methodological issues and practical considerations which need to be considered in studies and evaluations in this field, as well as neuroimaging findings, biomechanics, and pathophysiology, and even the potential for relationships of sports injury to the genetic context. One will find here a ready reference to the range of neuropsychological issues that needs to be addressed in the context of clinical evaluations as well as study design. Ethical and age-related caveats are treated as well. I trust that the reader will be satisfied with this addition to our continuing focus on the interface between empirical research and its useful clinical consideration.

Linas A. Bieliauskas
Ann Arbor, July 2003

Introduction

Like all fledgling disciplines, Sports Neuropsychology is undergoing very rapid development. This book represents a compilation of contemporary thought and published research in the field. In addition to serving as a comprehensive review of neuropsychological approaches to the management of mild traumatic brain injury (concussion), this book has also been designed to provide an international perspective on the subject of concussion in sports. This perspective was adopted to highlight both similarities and differences between assessment and treatment strategies throughout the world and to advance the overall state of knowledge internationally.

Traumatic Brain Injury in Sports: an International Neuropsychological Perspective has been structured to cover four core areas of interest. *Section 1* begins with a historical view of application of neuropsychological assessment in sports. A chapter that provides an epidemiological perspective follows this chapter. Next, the focus of the book moves to a discussion of the biomechanical, neurometabolic and neuroanatomical aspects of concussion (Chapters 3, 4 and 5). These chapters are designed to provide the reader with a state-of- of the-art understanding of the forces that lead to concussion as well as the acute and more chronic changes in brain function and structure that can occur, even following seemingly mild injury. The section concludes with a review of the potential genetic contributions to injury vulnerability and recovery. In addition to reviewing the specific topics listed above, *Section I* attempts to meld current research gleaned form both animals and human subjects into a more coherent understanding of the neurophysiological recovery process following concussion. The question of when brain metabolism returns to normal is not just an issue of academic interest but, as illustrated throughout this book, may have a direct impact on long-term brain function and individual psychological, social, and academic adjustment.

Section II is structured to provide a review of current Neuropsychological assessment programs throughout the world that have been designed to help sports-medicine personnel make more informed decisions regarding the return to play within specific sports environments. This section provides a panoramic view of the spectrum of sports-related concussion throughout both amateur and professional sports. Specifically, the sports of ice hockey, American football, soccer, boxing, Australian rules football, rugby and equestrian events are discussed in some detail, highlighting both differences and similarities between sports and discussing sports specific clinical approaches to concussion management. Differences between amateur and professional sports are specifically discussed as these environments differ substantially regarding the design of neuropsychological assessment programs, their implementation and how return to play decisions are made following injury.

In contrast to the largely clinical perspective presented in *Section II*, *Section III* provides a comprehensive review of technical and methodological issues germane to the use of neuropsychological assessment strategies in sports. Following an initial discussion of basic approaches to neuropsychological research within the context of sports, the important issues of reliability and validity in sports neuropsychology are discussed in detail. In addition to a basic discussion of reliability and validity issues, this section also provides a discussion regarding the implementation of new statistical techniques for the assessment of meaningful clinical change following injury. Finally, this section provides a thorough discussion of computer-based neuropsychological assessment procedures and their potential use in sporting environments. Computer-based neuropsychological assessment techniques represent an important advance that has led to the widespread implementation of neuropsychological testing procedures internationally.

The fourth and final section of this book is structured to review a variety of important topics that are highly relevant to the management of sports-related concussions. For instance, strategies for consultation with sports organizations are discussed in Chapter 21, with specific reference to work with high school, collegiate and professional sports organizations. Chapter 22 presents a discussion of current psychotherapeutic approaches to working with brain-injured athletes. Cultural issues in the neuropsychological assessment of athletes are discussed in Chapter 23 with an emphasis on the appreciation of how cultural factors can affect neuropsychological assessment results and the clinical interpretation of test results. Chapter 24 provides a comprehensive review of potential gender differences in response to brain injury and recovery. Chapter 25 reviews potential ethical conflicts and the resolution of these conflicts is discussed in this chapter. Finally, Chapter 26 provides a specific framework for making return-to-play decisions following concussion with consideration of neurological, neuropsychological, individual, and family issues.

References

Aubry, M., Cantu, R., Dvorak, J., Graf-Baumann. T., Johnston, K.M., Kelly, J. et al. Summary and agreement statement of the 1ste International Symposium on Concussion in Sport, Vienna, 2001. *Clinical Journal of Sports Medicine, 12*, 6–11.

SECTION I

BASIC CONCEPTS

EDITED BY

MICHAEL W. COLLINS

Chapter 1

HISTORICAL PERSPECTIVES

Scott D. Bender[1]
Jeffrey T. Barth[2, 3]
James Irby[2]

[1]Department of Neurology, University of Virginia Medical School
[2]Department of Psychiatric Medicine, University of Virginia Medical School
[3]Department of Neurological Surgery, University of Virginia Medical School

The forced retirements of high-profile professional athletes such as Troy Aikman, Brett Lindros, and Steve Young have heightened the public's awareness of concussion in sports. Researchers have now demonstrated that concussion is a common health problem with appreciable risk of sequelae, including persistent disability (Malec, 1999).

For years scientists and health care professionals have relied on neuropsychological tests for clinical evidence of very mild traumatic brain injury (mTBI). However, only relatively recently have these tests been used to assess mTBI and concussion in sports. In this time, neuropsychology has played a vital role in developing a definition of concussion, injury severity ratings, and return to play criteria. It also has improved outcome prediction based on neurocognitive functioning. Sports neuropsychology has emerged as an important area both for research in clinical neuropsychology (e.g., to describe neurocognitive effects of mild head injury in general) and for the protection of players (e.g., to document sports-related deficits and to predict recovery). This chapter provides an historical perspective, an introduction to the epidemiology and pathophysiology of mTBI, and a review of the current status of assessment and classification in sports neuropsychology. Subsequent chapters provide more comprehensive discussions of these topics.

Historical Perspectives

Though the term "cerebral concussion" likely was not used with regularity until the Renaissance, references to what were probably concussions were made in ancient history. For example Hippocrates (460-370 BC) described in his writings a concussive-like syndrome involving head trauma, aphasia, and temporary unconsciousness. Galen (129-216 AD) appears to have made the first mention of sports-related brain injury in his writings on the gladiatorial games of the Roman Empire (McCrory & Berkovic, 2001).

In modern American history, very few safety regulations existed before President Theodore Roosevelt established the Intercollegiate Athletic Association of the United States (IAAUS) in 1906 (officially termed the National Collegiate Athletic Association [NCAA] in 1910). In 1904 alone, 19 players were killed or paralyzed playing football (Kelly, 1999), and the sport appeared to be growing in brutality. In response, leaders from Harvard, Yale and Princeton decided to change the rules to ban mass formations and gang tackling, and to include the forward pass. Approximately 70 years later, the rules of football again were changed to ban "spearing," and the importance of protective gear received greater attention.

Prior to the 1980s mild brain injuries (whether sports-related or not) received relatively little attention, while moderate to severe brain injuries predominated the neurological and neuropsychological literature. Patients with mild brain injuries were thought to recover quickly and completely in the vast majority if not all cases. In fact, Miller (1961) proposed that those who were slow to recover from mTBI were experiencing "accident neurosis" (or "compensation neurosis") and would recover once they had received remuneration for their injuries. Similar lines of thought pervaded the health community despite the work of Symonds (1962) and Oppenheimer (1968), who each cogently argued that the effects of mTBI were considerable and at times irreversible. Psychological weakness, psychiatric disturbance, or secondary gain (e.g., malingering) were considered to be more likely etiologies for poor recovery from mild brain injury.

Two lines of research shed more light on the observations of Symonds (1962) and Oppenheimer (1968) and opened the door to later rigorous study of mTBI. In animals, research by Gennarelli, Adams, and Graham (1981) revealed shear-strain injury to axonal fibers in the brainstems of mildly concussed primates. In humans, Gronwall and Wrightson (1974) reported slowed processing speed, impaired attention/concentration, and delayed return to work in mildly brain-injured patients. A few years later, Rimel, Giordani, Barth, Boll, and Jane (1981) found that 55% of all closed head injuries were classified as mTBI. Follow up study at 3 months post injury showed that 34% had not returned to their previous level of employment. Numerous investigations have since documented neurocognitive deficits (Barth, Macciocchi, Boll, Giordani, & Rimel, 1983; Leininger, Gramling, Ferrel, Kreutzer, & Peck, 1990; Ruff et al., 1989) and occasionally parenchymal lesions (on MRI; e.g., Levin, Amparo et al., 1987) in mild brain-injured patients.

Despite the indications that mTBI might be more prevalent and serious than previously thought, disagreement continued regarding the definition, expected course, role of psychological factors, and pathophysiological mechanisms of mTBI (Barth, Diamond, & Errico, 1996). With respect to the definition of concussion, Wills and Leathem (2001) recently reviewed several studies of rugby injuries and found that only one investigator provided an operational definition of concussion. They suggest that there has been an over-reliance on loss of consciousness (LOC) as an indicator of concussion and that "true estimates [of concussion] are vastly underreported" (p. 647). The varied criteria for concussion and mTBI, inconsistent use of the terms "concussion" and "mTBI," broad use of "minor" and "mild," and confusion regarding the differences between "head" and "brain" injury appear to have created methodological confounds that limit the utility and generalizability of mTBI research.

Criticism regarding mild brain injury research methodology began at the outset. Early studies were criticized for (1) lacking generalizability to humans and (2) not adequately accounting for the effects of premorbid factors, such as prior head injury, substance abuse, pending litigation, or prior intellectual level. Research to address the latter criticism has reaffirmed findings of neurocognitive deficits in samples of mild brain-injured patients, especially those in the early stages of recovery (Dikmen, McLean, & Temkin, 1986; Levin, Mattis et al., 1987; McLean, Temkin, Dikmen, & Wyler, 1983). These studies were instrumental in changing the perception that mTBI was invariably an inconsequential ailment.

The Sports Arena as Clinical Neuropsychology Lab

The problems of finding adequate controls and accounting for the effects of premorbid functioning concerned clinical researchers for years. Barth et al. (1989) found a solution to these problems by using a test-retest design to assess collegiate football players before and after mild brain injury. The football arena offered a large number of potential participants who were likely to experience mild deceleration head trauma.

Barth et al.'s (1989) seminal study involving ten universities (n = 2350) found that those players who sustained a mild brain injury showed neurocognitive deficits at 24-hours post concussion and 5 days later, but recovered to better than preseason baseline and in line with controls by the 10th day. Consistent with other studies (e.g., Dikmen et al., 1986; Macciocchi, Barth,

Alves, Rimel, & Jane, 1996; McLean et al., 1983), these well motivated, young adults recovered rapidly from mild brain injuries. Largely because of the Barth et al. (1989) study, the sports arena was quickly recognized as a unique, relatively well-controlled laboratory for assessing mTBI. This study also set the methodological standard for baseline and serial neuropsychological testing, since then the study of athletes has proven to be a rich source of data regarding the effects of mTBI sustained on and off the field. The technique of using athletics as a model for understanding brain injury in general was termed, the Sports as a Laboratory Assessment Model (SLAM; Barth, Freeman, & Broshek, 2002).

Epidemiology of mTBI

Epidemiological studies indicate that 1 to 2 million new cases of mTBI are reported each year in the United Stated alone (Jennett & Frankowski, 1990; Thurman & Guerrero, 1997) and many more never come to the attention of health care professionals. Segalowitz and Lawson (1995) found that 30-37% of their sample of high school and university students sustained a mild brain injury. Subtle symptoms likely associated with concussion, such as sleep disturbance, social problems, and a variety of psychiatric diagnoses (e.g., attention deficits, depression, and reading, speech, and language disorders) were common. Given that millions of high school students participate in athletics each year, it is perhaps not surprising that approximately 300,000 of these mild brain injuries, or concussions, occur in sporting events. Gerberich, Priest, Boen, Staub, and Maxwell (1983) estimated that 200,000 concussions occur in high school football games each season. That would mean that 20% of all high school football players sustain at least one concussion each year. Almost half of the collegiate football players surveyed in 1989 reported having had a concussion by the time they reached college (e.g., Barth et al., 1989).

Studies often underestimate the incidence of mTBI because many patients do not present to hospitals or to health care professional after suffering a mild concussion. Athletes in particular seem prone to underreporting their injuries in efforts to stay in the game; about 50% of cases of concussion across sports result in a referral to a health care professional (Powell & Barber-Foss, 1999). In football (63% of all sports-related injuries), tackling and being tackled appear to cause the most injuries (about 60%). Most sports show an increased risk of injury during games versus practice (wrestling is an exception) probably due to heightened intensity and motivation to win. There is evidence to suggest that the frequency of concussions is on the rise (Dick, 1997). The increase in size and speed of athletes and the consequent increase in force when making contact are likely contributors, but improved reporting methods may also help explain the rise.

Mechanisms of Mild Traumatic Brain Injury and Concussion

Mild concussion in sports usually occurs from rapid deceleration due to impact with stationary or opposing forces, which is translated on the brain as linear and/or rotational force. Newtonian physics can be used to describe these forces. Barth, Varney, Ruchinskas, and Francis (1999) point out that, based on a formula originally used by Varney and Varney (1995), a football player running at 10 ft/sec will decelerate at a rate of 9.3 g after making contact with another player and stopping within 2 inches (formula: $a = [v^2 - v_o^2]/2sg$). Thus, assuming his head stops within a similar distance, the forces acting on his brain are 9.3 times that of its resting weight. An interaction of several factors including mass, weight, velocity, hardness and surface area of the impacting object predicts the extent of neuronal damage. Naunheim, Standeven, Richter, and Lewis (2000) used helmet-mounted accelerometers to measure the forces associated with contact to the head in soccer, football, and ice hockey. It appears that peak accelerations were greatest for soccer, but no recorded impact exceeded the acceleration level considered likely to produce significant neurocognitive sequelae.

The aforementioned forces may result in diffuse pathophysiological changes to the brain. Diffuse brain injury includes white matter and axonal stretching and shearing (termed Diffuse Axonal Injury, DAI), particularly when rotational forces are present. Axonal stretching in mTBI can result in swollen, beaded, and varicose fibers, which render neurons dysfunctional but not destroyed (Echemendia & Lovell, 2000). Like concussion, the severity of DAI is often graded from least severe (Grade I) to most severe (Grade III). In addition, parenchymal cytoarchitecture, particularly in the brainstem, can be disrupted by linear, tensile, or compressive strains. Though in rare cases of concussion axonal shearing can result in hemorrhage and subsequent coma, the vast majority of concussions fail to yield identifiable changes on CT or MRI. Thus, health care professionals tend to rely on neuropsychological assessment to identify brain dysfunction in these cases.

Neurochemical changes to the brain accompany the above mechanical changes immediately following mTBI (Wojtys et al., 1999). A commonly held view is that a neurochemical cascade creates cells that are vulnerable to dysfunction. In brief, an increased demand for glucose occurs with a concomitant reduction in cerebral blood flow (CBF). Excess glutamate is released and subsequent influxes of extracellular potassium inhibit the action potential (which likely accounts for the alterations of consciousness). A state of *hyper*glycolysis leads to rapid glucose loss, followed by decreased CBF and *hypo*glycolysis, which in turn leaves cells vulnerable or damaged. Interestingly, potassium might not reach suprathreshold levels for several seconds, which may explain the fact that some athletes make it to the sideline before collapsing from their injury (Maroon et al., 2000). The duration of decreased CBF seems to be critical in determining neurological outcome, as even brief interruptions in CBF can lead to ischemia and neurocognitive deficits.

Cholinergic pathways may also be at risk from concussion, as has been demonstrated in boxing (Jordan et al., 1997). The susceptibility to dysfunction of the hippocampus and related circuitry due to disruption of cholinergic pathways is well documented (Schmidt & Grady, 1995). Genetic factors are also likely involved. For example, Kutner, Erlanger, Tsai, Jordan, and Relkin (2000) found that older professional football players who possessed the APOE 4 allele scored lower on cognitive tests than did those without the allele. However, neurochemical outcome is likely predicated on a combination of factors such as age, APOE genotype, and/or cumulative exposure.

Definition of Concussion and Injury Severity

Initial definitions of concussion were so broad that they were not useful. In 1980, the definition was simplified to say that concussion was characterized by "immediate and transient post-traumatic impairment in neural function, such as alteration of consciousness, disturbance of vision, equilibrium, etc., due to brainstem involvement" (Maroon et al., 2000, p. 661). The authors proposed 3 grades of severity: Grade I- mild concussion with no LOC, Grade II- moderate concussion with LOC and recovery within 5 minutes, and Grade III- severe concussion with LOC lasting greater than 5 minutes.

In 1986, Cantu added post-traumatic amnesia to the list of mental changes in the definition of concussion. By 1991, Kelly et al. had developed what would become the Colorado Guidelines for the Management of Cerebral Concussion (CGMCC). The CGMCC criteria highlighted confusion in Grade I concussion and emphasized both confusion and post traumatic amnesia (PTA) in Grade II concussion. The latest American Academy of Neurology (AAN) definition and gradation system evolved from these guidelines and reflects the shift of LOC as a component of Grade II to LOC being the hallmark of Grade III concussion. Though consensus has not been forthcoming, concussion is now defined as any traumatically induced alteration in mental status that may or may not involve LOC (Quality Standards Subcommittee, AAN, 1997). Definitions and criteria continue to evolve as our understanding of concussion improves. Cantu is in the process of revising his guidelines based on the accumulated data (see Chapter 26 in this volume). The current gradations, emphasizing the presence of confusion and amnesia, are used to determine when a player is eligible to return to competition. Table 1.1 displays two common definitions of concussion and Table 1.2 displays the AAN's return to play criteria.

It is clear that differing opinions about the relative importance of various diagnostic criteria still exist; at least 27 gradation systems have been proposed. The McGill group recently contended that because more than 75% of concussions incurred in sports do not involve LOC, a new grading system with 3 subdivisions of Grade I concussion is warranted. (Leclerc et al., 2001). Hinton-Bayre and Geffen (2002) found no relationship between the grade

Table 1.1. Two common definitions of concussion by gradation.

Author	Definitions	
Cantu	Grade 1	no LOC; PTA < 30 min
	Grade 2	LOC < 5 min; PTA > 30 min & < 24-h
	Grade 3	LOC > 5 min or PTA > 24-h
AAN	Grade 1	transient confusion, no LOC, symptoms resolve in < 15 min
	Grade 2	transient confusion, no LOC, symptoms last > 15 min
	Grade 3	LOC of any duration

AAN = American Academy of Neurology; LOC = loss of consciousness; PTA = post-traumatic amnesia

Table 1.2. AAN recommendations for return to play based on grade of concussion.

Grade of Concussion		
1	2	3
Return same day if asymptomatic within 15 min of concussion	Remove athlete from contest; return in 1 week if asymptomatic on exertion that week	Remove athlete from contest; return after asymptomatic 1 week (for brief LOC) or 2 weeks (for prolonged LOC)

AAN = American Academy of Neurology; LOC = loss of consciousness

of concussion (according to 3 commonly used grading systems) and level of neurocognitive impairment in rugby players. Such findings, coupled with the fact that none of the guidelines have been based on scientific data regarding the process of recovery, has lead some researchers to believe that current concussion management guidelines are inadequate for making return to play decisions (Collins, Lovell, & McKeag, 1999).

Player Protection and Return to Play Criteria

It has been almost a century since Theodore Roosevelt implemented important rule changes in football to protect players. Subsequent changes in tackling technique, and improvements in helmet design and padding likely have reduced the number and severity of injuries, but direct comparison is difficult. The speed and weight of football players have steadily increased, ostensibly raising the likelihood of injury. Though clinical neuroscience has had some difficulty keeping up with this pace, a large body of knowledge regarding severity of brain injury, criteria for return to play, second impact syndrome, and sideline assessment has accumulated in the sports concussion literature. As a result, new injury prevention techniques (e.g., rule changes and better sport-specific equipment, education, and focus on skill acquisition) are being discussed and tested.

Determining if and when a player can return to competition is a critical decision with significant and perhaps catastrophic consequences. If a skilled player is held from play unnecessarily, his team may lose. More importantly, if he is allowed to return prematurely, he may suffer serious and possibly irreversible injury (see Second Impact Syndrome, this and subsequent chapters). While the importance of maintaining safety is obvious, many would argue that the pressure to win (and to return to play as soon as possible) is greater than it has ever been. Social and professional pressures and lack of controlled research have militated against the development and implementation of reliable methods for determining whether a player is ready to return to play. Despite this impediment, sports medicine researchers and team physicians have developed return to play criteria based on professional opinion and some level of consensus. Though the original attempts lacked uniformity and were based on little scientific evidence, most clinicians consider severity assessment the critical component of return to play criteria (Polin, Alves, & Jane, 1996).

Table 1.3. Cantu's guidelines for return to play following concussion based on number andseverity of concussions.

	Number of Concussions		
Severity	1st Concussion	2nd Concussion	3rd Concussion
Grade I	Return if asymptomatic at exertion	Return in 2 weeks if asymptomatic for the past week	Terminate season; return next season if asymptomatic
Grade II	Return after asymptomatic for 7 days	Must sit out at least 30 days; may return if asymptomatic for 7 days; consider terminating season	Terminate season; return next season if asymptomatic
Grade III	Must sit out at least 30 days; then return when asymptomatic for 7 days	Terminate season; return next season if asymptomatic	

Practical guidelines for return to play have been provided by Cantu (1986; 1991), Kelly et al., (1991) and the American Academy of Neurology (Quality Standards Subcomittee, 1997), among others. Each includes recommendations for return following one, two, or three successive injuries in a single season contingent upon the injury severity rating. For example, Cantu (1991) recommends that an athlete terminate participation for the season after three Grade I or two Grade III injuries (see Table 1.3). This is an outgrowth of Quigley's Rule (Schneider, 1973), which stated that athletes should discontinue participation in sports following three cerebral concussions. The current criteria for safe return to same day play are (1) neurologic signs and symptoms clear within 15 minutes at rest and exertion, (2) neurologic exam is normal, and (3) no loss of consciousness (Cantu, 2001).

Multiple Concussions and Second Impact Syndrome

Recent evidence suggests that a history of concussion both increases the risk of sustaining a more severe concussion and decreases the threshold for sustaining a concussion of any severity in the future (Collins et al., 2002). This is significant because many athletes are at risk for concussion due to the nature of the sport, and their return to competition is often contingent on the number of concussions they have suffered.

The main reason that athletes must meet the aforementioned return to play criteria before returning to competition is that the brain appears to be incrementally vulnerable to subsequent trauma. The apparently rare but potentially devastating effect of successive mild concussions with resultant severe brain injury is termed, Second Impact Syndrome (SIS) and was first described by Schneider in 1973. The syndrome is said to occur when a second concussion is sustained before the signs and symptoms of the first have resolved. The circumstances surrounding the second concussion differ from the first only in its end result, which usually involves coma. Cantu and Voy (1995) estimate that SIS occurs in football one to two times per year but also occurs in other contact sports. Twenty-six SIS-related deaths have been confirmed since 1984 (Maroon et al., 2000). The mere possibility of SIS underscores the importance of reliable return to play criteria and neurocognitive assessment to be certain that full recovery has taken place.

Though the exact pathophysiology of SIS is poorly understood, available evidence suggests that the first impact results in subclinical edema and increased intracranial pressure (ICP), which make the brain susceptible to further injury. Significant ICP following the second impact impairs blood flow and causes severe tissue damage ("malignant cerebral edema"). Recent studies suggest that the reduction in blood flow is due to autoregulatory dysfunction and consequent vascular congestion (Alves & Polin, 1996). It appears that the vasoconstriction associated with Ca^{2+} influx near the site of injury is specifically responsible for the reduced blood flow (Wojtys et al., 1999).

Age may influence this change in brain physiology. Prins, Lee, Cheng, Becker, and Hovda (1996) found that immature rodents subjected to fluid percussion brain injury suffered more morphological and physiological damage than mature mice. However, there appears to be a critical maturational period during which the developing brain is most vulnerable. Insults before or after this period may yield relatively less damage. Though this time frame is unclear in humans, it may be that the period of vulnerability predisposes the brain to catastrophic injury when subjected to repeated concussions. This might explain the apparent increased risk of SIS in adolescent young adults.

SIS remains an indistinct and poorly understood diagnostic entity and some researchers question its existence. For example, at least one attempt to provide diagnostic criteria (Definite, Probable, or Possible SIS) based on clinicopathophysiologic features failed to identify any of 17 cases as Definite SIS (McCrory & Berkovic, 1998). In 12 of the cases, even the possibility of SIS was ruled out. More can be found on this intriguing issue in subsequent chapters of this volume.

Sideline Assessment of Concussion

Quick and accurate evaluation of mental status on the field and on the sideline is one of the most challenging problems faced by team physicians and trainers. Interruptions, distractions, confined space, and a very limited time frame are just some of the problems faced by the player and the examiner. The highly heterogeneous nature of concussion further complicates assessment and diagnosis. The assessments require a well-formulated plan that can be implemented quickly and routinely in order to be effective.

On the field, the injured player undergoes "ABC assessment" (patent Airway, regular Breathing, normal blood Circulation/pulse) and a brief mental status exam. Questions such as those proposed by Maddocks, Dicker, and Saling (1995) appear to discriminate concussed from non-concussed players better than standard orientation questions, and can be started on the field. Once off the field of play, the player undergoes a more comprehensive evaluation, including a neuropsychological exam. The Standardized Assessment of Concussion (SAC; McCrea et al., 1998) is the first very brief, yet systematic empirically based, and validated assessment tool for sideline evaluations. It includes brief tests of orientation, attention, and memory and is used in conjunction with a brief neurologic exam or neurologic checklist (e.g., Sideline Concussion Checklist, Kutner & Barth, 1998) to determine the extent of neurologic/cognitive compromise (as a gross screening), the need to cease competition, and the necessity of further monitoring. The SAC now has 3 equivalent alternate forms (McCrea, 2001) and despite its vulnerability to practice and ceiling effects, it is clearly the best sideline assessment available at this time.

Neuropsychological Evaluation of the Athlete

Barth et al. (1989) are credited with establishing the standard for assessment of amateur athletes. The beginnings of neurocognitive assessment in the professional ranks are less clear but appear to have begun in boxing. Researchers looked to boxing as a model of brain injury because it is the only major sport in which the goal is to "inflict brain damage, cause a concussion or render the opponent unconscious" (Jordan et al., 1997, p. 453). Since Martland's (1928) paper on the "punch drunk" syndrome, a body of literature has accumulated on the effects of the multiple relatively low-energy blows characteristic of some boxing injuries. Neurological and neuropsychological investigations have documented acute and persistent deficits in boxers who have experienced knockouts or subsequent blows to the head (Casson et al., 1984; Jordan et al., 1997; McLatchie et al. 1987; Roberts, 1969). Although the literature suggests that impairment is fairly prominent, the results of many of the investigations have been inconsistent, primarily due to methodological problems (e.g., small sample sizes, inappropriate controls, etc.).

Mark Lovell recognized that similar injuries were likely to occur in the National Football League (NFL). With the Pittsburgh Steelers, he established the first clinically oriented program aimed at facilitating decision-making for return to play following a concussion. A brief yet broad-ranging battery is administered to each player at preseason and again in the event of a concussion.

Several league-wide neuropsychological testing programs have now been established at both the collegiate and professional levels. Lovell's work with the Pittsburgh Steelers Organization has expanded to involve neuropsychological assessment of over 1,500 professional football players representing numerous National Football League teams. Ruben Echemendia developed a multi-sport neuropsychological testing program at Penn State University involving hundreds of athletes from football, men's and women's soccer, men's ice hockey, men's and women's basketball, wrestling, and women's lacrosse. Lovell and Echemendia have also established a similar league-wide neuropsychological testing program with the National Hockey League. A network of neuropsychologists across North America allows players to be evaluated in any city in which they play.

In addition to other innovative neuropsychological studies with football players (e.g., Collins, Grindel et al. 1999; Lovell & Collins, 1998; Olesniewicz, Sallis, Jones, & Copp, 1997), neuropsychological investigations have been conducted in amateur and professional soccer (Abreau, Templer, Schuyler, & Hutchison, 1990; Matser, Kessels, Lezak, Jordan, & Troost, 1999), rugby, (Hinton-Bayre, Geffen, & McFarland, 1997), ice hockey, (Lovell & Collins, 2001; Tegner & Lorentzon, 1991), and equestrian sports (Bailes, 1999; for a current review see Broshek, this volume). Epidemiological data regarding concussion and brain injury are available for cycling (Noakes, 1995), winter sports (Prall, Winston, & Brennan, 1995), and golf

(McGuffie, Fitzpatrick, & Hall, 1998). Formal study of concussion in these sports is forthcoming.

Soccer has received increased media attention in large part due to reports of risk of injury when heading the ball (Babbs, 2000; Matser, Kessels, Lezak, Jordan & Troost, 1999). It is critical to note that important factors such as the frequency of heading another player's head, hitting the goal post, making contact with the ground, and body-to-body contact were seldom controlled in early studies. Grote and Donders (2000) add that many studies were poorly controlled demographically (e.g., some participants were heavy alcohol users) and in some cases conventional testing procedures were not used. Nevertheless, concussions do occur in soccer. Delaney, Lacroix, Leclerc, and Johnston (2002) found that nearly 63% of soccer players in their one-season survey reported symptoms of concussion. To date, the evidence for frank neurocognitive impairment from heading alone is equivocal and well-controlled research on this matter is still required to draw appropriate conclusions.

Social Forces in Sports Neuropsychology

Professional sports is a multibillion dollar industry. College sports often generate more money for their academic institutions than any other single branch of the school. Shulman and Bowen (2001) describe three factors that account for the rising interest in sports in this country. The first of these is the growth of the United States' entertainment-driven economy and the commercialization of athletics, which has resulted in huge financial incentives for athletic organizations to produce winning teams. This has been especially transforming for collegiate athletics departments, which have become increasingly influential within academic institutions.

The second factor involves the heightened competitiveness of college admissions. Career advancement in our knowledge-based economy has amplified the importance of a college education, particularly from institutions with impressive reputations. As a result, admissions offices have become more interested in candidates with distinctive qualifications and talents and thus "...introduced onto the college campus a group of athletes who are as specialized in their own ways as the most intensely focused computer scientists." (Shulman & Bowen, 2001, p. 23). Third, the increased competence and specialization of pre-college athletic talent coupled with the firm institutionalization of sports at the collegiate level, has raised the bar for pre-collegiate athletic competition, with a focus on greater specialization at younger and younger ages. The World Health Organization, and the International Federation of Sports Medicine, have shown concern about these trends, stating in 1998 that, "There is growing evidence that excessive...and intensive training may increase the rate of [player] overuse and catastrophic injuries." (p. 446).

Computerized Assessment in Sports Neuropsychology

It appears that much of neuropsychology's future promise lies with computerized assessment. Computerized testing allows the examiner to assess common sequelae of concussion, including subtle changes in processing speed to the millisecond. Computers also reduce the impact of practice effects by providing multiple equivalent forms of the test. The Automated Neuropsychological Assessment Metrics (ANAM) was introduced to address this issue. The number of alternate forms is almost infinite and it can be configured to assess a specific neurocognitive domain or several domains (Koffler, 1999). Early data on the ANAM indicate that it measures constructs also measured by common traditional neuropsychological tests that are sensitive to brain injury: Cognitive processing speed, resistance to interference, and working memory (Bleiberg, Kane, Reeves, Garmoe, & Halpern, 2000).

At least two other computer-administered measures are being validated in this country. First, the Immediate Measurement of Performance and Cognitive Testing (IMPACT; Maroon et al., 2000) was recently developed for athletes in particular. Cognitive domains including reaction time and a range of attentional and memory skills are assessed. There are three forms, and like the ANAM, the alternate forms can be combined in many ways to reduce practice effects. A post-concussion scale is included to provide self-report data regarding common signs and symptoms of concussion (e.g., headache, nausea, drowsiness, etc.).

Second, the Concussion Resolution Index (CRI, Headminder), an internet-based measure of cognitive functioning, was developed by David Erlanger and colleagues (2001) to help determine when a player can return to play. It records both simple and complex reaction time, attention, memory, and cognitive processing speed. The initial validation showed (1) that the CRI is very sensitive to reduced cognitive efficiency following concussion (88% of concussed athletes were detected) and (2) that the cognitive tests of the CRI improve detection of symptoms over self-report by 25% at the second follow-up (Erlanger et al., 2001). Because it is web-based, the CRI is accessible to health care officials in remote locations (e.g., when traveling to "away" games), which is particularly appealing for teams who travel regularly. Other important advances in computerized assessment are discussed in the Special Issues section of this volume.

Future Directions of Sports Neuropsychology

Sports neuropsychology also seems well positioned to take advantage of advances in biotechnology. The potential benefit of using a mouthpiece to reduce translational forces in head injury has already been discussed (Barth, Freeman, & Winters, 2000; Winters, 2001). It may be possible in the near future to transmit specific telemetry data to the sideline to help determine the forces that occur in head trauma at the moment of impact. Advances in helmet composition, shape, and padding are also being made. Accelerometers have shown promise in helmet design and development by documenting forces and levels of dissipation based on helmet shape. Mechanical limits on the degree to which the head is free to move (e.g., neck braces) are also under investigation.

Use of laboratory tests on the sideline is promising. For example, assessment of blood oxygen levels could provide immediate information regarding oxygen saturation and glucose utilization. The continued investigation of genetic testing is also needed to clarify the relationship between APOE4 and concussion and dementia. Other genes involved in neurodegenerative processes will likely require attention as well.

Further explication of the symptom constellation of concussion as well as the particular combinations of clinical features that best predict injury severity are warranted. It is not unusual for players to complain of persistent headache or "being in a fog," yet perform at or above baseline levels on neuropsychological tests. Moreover, concussions present in numerous ways despite apparently highly similar injury characteristics. This suggests that there may be more than one type of concussion, that some individuals are at increased risk premorbidly, and that different batteries of tests may be needed. The roles of such factors as age, education, learning disability, history of concussion, intellectual level, psychosocial functioning, and general physical health in recovery from concussion require further examination (Barth, Diamond, & Errico, 1996; Collins et al., 1999).

More research like that of McCrea et al. (2002) documenting the slope of early recovery from concussion is needed, as it will likely have important implications for return to play decisions. Researchers must also find ways to streamline existing measures while maintaining the clinical utility.

Finally, special attention to education and prevention of concussion in all sports is warranted. Although not yet proven, it is reasonable to expect that children experience more severe DAI (shearing from rotational forces) and coup-contracoup injuries, given their immature frames and musculature. This underscores the importance of education in youth sports. Education can also help athletes of all ages be more forthcoming about their injuries. Currently, it is still considered a sign of toughness to "stick it out" despite injury and this message is conveyed to young athletes. This may be especially common for concussion because it can be less obvious to observers.

Summary and Recommendations

The commercialization of athletics and the resultant increase in media attention given to famous athletes, including those who have sustained multiple concussions, has generated increased awareness of the potential seriousness of mild brain injury. Physicians and athletic trainers in sports medicine have turned to the clinical and scientific literature for guidance regarding sideline medical assessment, whether children should "head" soccer balls, or when an athletic career should be retired after multiple concussions. The realm of athletic competition facilitates access to an at-risk population, baseline testing and testing shortly after injury, and straightforward follow up (McCrea et al., 2002). Because of our increasing awareness and research in sports concussion, significant rule changes have been made, particularly in football. However, continued change is necessary. Proper techniques should be taught by coaches at all levels. Cantu and Mueller (2000) recommend that emphasis be put on conditioning and fitness of the head and neck on proper fitting equipment, and on properly trained on-field personnel in case of catastrophic injury. The primary goal is to ensure player safety during athletic competition. By using the playing field as a lab, neuropsychology has helped formulate return to play criteria, severity ratings, recovery curves, and other tactics. As a discipline, it is ideally suited to continue advancing this goal.

References

Abreau, F., Templer, D.I., Schuyler, B.A., & Hutchison, H.T. (1990). Neuropsychological assessment of soccer players. *Neuropsychology, 4,* 175–181.

Alves, W.M., & Polin, R.S. (1996). Sports-related head injury. In R.K. Narayan, J.E. Wilberger, & J.T. Povlishock (Eds.), *Neurotrauma.* New York: McGraw-Hill.

Babbs, C.F. (2000). Brain injury in amateur soccer players. *Journal of the American Medical Association, 283*(7), 882–883.

Bailes, J.E. (1999). Organized and recreational sports. In J.E. Bailes, M.R. Lovell, & J.C. Maroon (Eds.), *Sports-Related Concussion* (pp. 91–101). St. Louis, MO: Quality Medical Publishing.

Barth, J.T., Alves, W.M., Ryan, T.V., Macciocchi, S.N., Rimel, R.W., Jane, J.A. et al. (1989). Mild head injury in sports: Neuropsychological sequelae and recovery of function. In H.S., Levin, H.S. Eisenberg, & A.L. Benton (Eds.), *Mild Head Injury* (pp. 257–275). New York: Oxford University Press.

Barth, J.T., Freeman, J.R., & Broshek, D.K. (2002). Mild head injury. In V.S. Ramachandran (Ed.), *Encyclopedia of the human brain: Vol. 3* (pp. 81–92). San Diego, CA: Academic Press.

Barth J.T., Diamond R., & Errico, A. (1996). Mild head injury and post concussionsyndrome: does anyone really suffer? *Clinical Electroencephalography, 27*(4),183–186.

Barth, J.T., Freeman J.R., & Winters J.E. (2000). Management of sports-related concussions. *Dental Clinics of North America, 44*(1), 67–83.

Barth, J.T., Macciocchi, S.N., Boll, T.J., Giordani, B., & Rimel, R.W. (1983). Neuropsychological sequelae of minor head injury. *Neurosurgery, 13,* 529–533.

Barth, J.T., Varney, R.N., Ruchinskas, R.A., & Francis, J.P. (1999). Mild head injury: The new frontier in sports medicine. In N. Varney & R. Roberts (Eds.), *The Evaluation and Treatment of Mild Traumatic Brain Injury.* Mahwah, NJ: Lawrence Erlbaum.

Bleiberg, J., Kane, L., Reeves, D.L., Garmoe, W.S., & Halpern, E. (2000). Factor analysis of computerized and traditional tests used in mild brain injury research. *Clinical Neuropsychologist, 14(3),* 287–94.

Cantu, R.C. (1986). Guidelines for return to contact sports after cerebral concussion. *Physician Sports Medicine, 14*, 755–783.

Cantu, R.C. (1991). Criteria for return to competition after a closed head injury. In J.S. Torg, (Ed.), *Athletic Injuries to the Head Neck and Face* (pp. 323–330). St. Louis, MO: Mosby Year Book.

Cantu, R.C. (2001). Classification and clinical management of concussion. In J.E. Bailes, & A.L. Day (Eds.), *Neurological Sports Medicine*. Rolling Meadows, Illinois: American Association of Neurological Surgeons.

Cantu, R., & Voy, R. (1995). Second Impact Syndrome: A risk in any contact sport. *The Physician and Sports Medicine, 23*(6), 114.

Cantu, R.C., & Mueller, F.O. (2000). Catastrophic football injuries. *Neurosurgery, 47*(3), 673–675.

Casson, J.R., Siegel, O., Sham, R., Campbell, E.Q., Tarlau, M., & DiDomenico, A. (1984). Brain damage in modern boxers. *Journal of the American Medical Association, 251*, 2663–2667.

Collins, M.W., Lovell, M., Iverson, G., Cantu, R.C., Maroon, J.C., & Field, M. (2002). Cumulative effects of concussion in high school athletes. *Neurosurgery, 51*(5), 1175–1181.

Collins, M.W., Grindel, S.H., Lovell, M.R., Dede, D., Moser, D., Phalin, B. et al. (1999). Relationship between concussion and neuropsychological performance in college football players. *Journal of the American Medical Association, 282*(10), 964–970.

Collins, M.W., Lovell, M.R., & McKeag, D.B. (1999. Current issues in managing sports-related concussion. *Journal of the American Medical Association, 282*(10), 2283–2285.

Delaney, J.S., Lacroix, V.J., Leclerc, S., & Johnston, K.M. (2002). Concussion among university football and soccer players. *Clinical Journal of Sports Medicine, 12*, 331–338.

Diamond, P.T., & Gayle, S.D. (2001). Head injuries in men's and women's lacrosse: A 10 year analysis of the NEISS database. *Brain Injury, 15*(6), 537–544.

Dick, R.W. (1997). A summary of head and neck injuries in collegiate athletics using the NCAA Injury Surveillance System. In E.F. Hoerner (Ed.), *Head and Neck Injuries in Sports*. Philadelphia: American Society for Testing and Materials.

Dikmen, S., McLean, A., & Temkin, N. (1986). Neuropsychological and psychological consequences of minor head injury. *Neurosurgery, 48*, 1227–1232.

Echemendia, R.J, & Lovell, M.R. (2000). Neuropsychological evaluation of mild traumatic brain injury in sports. *Paper presented at the annual meeting of the National Association of Neuropsychology.*

Erlanger, D.M., Saliba, E., Barth, J.T., Almquist, J., Webright, W., & Freeman, J. (2001). Monitoring resolution of postconcussion symptoms in athletes: Preliminary results of a web-based neuropsychological test protocol. *Journal of Athletic Training, 36*(3), 280–287.

FIMS/WHO Ad Hoc Committee on sports and children. (1998). *Bulletin of the World Health Organization, 76*(5), 445-447.

Gennarelli, T.A., Adams, G.H., & Graham, D.I. (1981). Acceleration induced head injury in the monkey: The model, its mechanism, and physiological correlate. *Acta Neuropathologia, 7(suppl.)*, 23–25.

Gerberich, S.G., Priest, J.D., Boen, J.R., Staub, C.P., & Maxwell, R.E. (1983). Concussion incidences and severity in secondary school varsity football players. *American Journal of Public Health, 73*, 1370–1375.

Gronwall, D., & Wrightson, P. (1974). Delayed recovery of intellectual function after minor head injury. *Lancet, 2*, 604-609.

Grote, C., & Donders, J. (2000). Brain injury in amateur soccer players. *Journal of the American Medical Association, 283*(7), 882–883.

Hinton-Bayre, A.D., &, Geffen, G. (2002). Severity of sports-related concussion and neuropsychological test performance. *Neurology, 59,* 1068–1070.

Hinton-Bayre, A.D., Geffen, G., & McFarland, K. (1997). Mild head injury and speed of information processing: A prospective study of professional rugby league players. *Journal of Experimental and Clinical Neuropsychology, 19*(2), 275–289.

Jennett, B., & Frankowski, R.F. (1990). Epidemiology of head injury. In R. Brinkman (Ed.), *Handbook of Clinical Neurology,* (pp. 1–16). New York: Elsevier.

Jordan, B., Relkin, N.R., Ravdin, L.D., Jacobs, A.R., Bennett, A., & Gandy, S. (1997). Apolipoprotein E4 associated with chronic traumatic brain injury in boxing. *The Journal of the American Medical Association, 278,* 136–140.

Kelly, J.P. (1999). Traumatic brain injury and concussion in sports. *Journal of the American Medical Association, 282*(10), 989–991.

Kelly, J.P., Nichols, J.S., Filley, C., Lillehei, K.O., Rubinstein, D., Kleinschmidt-DeMasters, B.K. (1991). Concussion in sports: Guidelines for the prevention of catastrophic outcome. *The Journal of the American Medical Association, 266,* 2867–2869.

Koffler, S.P. (1999). Computerized testing. In J.E. Bailes, M.R. Lovell., & J.C. Maroon (Eds.), *Sports-Related Concussion.* St. Louis, Missouri: Quality Medical Publishing.

Kutner, K.C., & Barth, J.T. (1998). Sideline Concussion Checklist-B. In K. Kutner & J. Barth (Eds.), Sports-Related Head Injury, *The National Academy of Neuropsychology Bulletin, 14,* 19–23.

Kutner, K.C., Erlanger, D.M., Tsai, J., Jordan, B., & Relkin, N.R. (2000). Lower cognitive performance of older football players possessing apolipoprotein E4. *Neurosurgery, 47*(3), 651–657.

Leclerc, S., Lassonde, M., Delaney, S., Lacroix, V., & Johnston, K. (2001). Recommendations for grading concussions in athletes. *Sports Medicine, 31*(8), 629–636.

Leininger, B.E., Gamling, S.E., Ferrel, A.D., Kreutzer, J.S., & Peck, E.A. (1990). Neuropsychological deficits in symptomatic minor head injury patients after concussion and mild concussion. *Journal of Neurology, Neurosurgery, and Psychiatry, 53,* 293–296.

Levin, H.S., Amparo, E.G., Eisenberg, H.M., Williams, D.H., High, W.M., McArdle, C.B., &Weiner, R.L. (1987). Magnetic resonance imaging and computerized tomography in relation to neurobehavioral sequelae of mild and moderate head injuries. *Journal of Neurosurgery, 66*(5), 706–713.

Levin, H.S., Mattis, S., Ruff, R., Eisenberg, H.M., Marshall., L.F., Tabaddor, K., High, W.M., Frankowski, R.F. (1987). Neurobehavioral outcome following minor head injury: A three-case center study. *Journal of Neurosurgery, 66*(2), 234–243.

Lovell, M.R., & Collins, M.W. (1998). Neuropsychological assessment of the college football player. *Journal of Head Trauma and Rehabilitation, 13*(2), 9–26.

Lovell, M.R., & Collins, M.W. (2001). Neuropsychological assessment of the head-injured professional athlete. In J.E. Bailes, & A.L. Day (Eds.), *Neurological Sports Medicine.* Rolling Meadows, Illinois: American Association of Neurological Surgeons.

Macciocchi, S.N., Barth, J.T., Alves, W., Rimel, R.W., & Jane, J.A. (1996). Neuropsychological functioning and recovery following mild head injury in collegiate athletes. *Neurosurgery, 39*(3), 510–514.

Maddocks, D.L., Dicker, G.D., & Saling, M.M. (1995). The assessment of orientation following concussion in athletes. *Clinical Journal of Sports Medicine, 5,* 32–35.

Malec, J.F. (1999). Mild Traumatic Brain Injury: The Scope of the Problem. In N. Varney & R. Roberts (Eds.), *The Evaluation and Treatment of Mild Traumatic Brain Injury*. Mahwah, NJ: Lawrence Erlbaum.

Maroon, J.C., Lovell, M.R., Norwig, J., Podell, K., Powell, J.W., & Hartl, R. (2000). Cerebral concussion in athletes: Evaluation and neuropsychological testing. *Neurosurgery, 47*(3), 659–669.

Martland, H. S. (1928). Punch-drunk. *Journal of American Medical Association, 19,* 1103-1107.

Matser, E. Kessels, A., Lezak, M., Jordan, B., & Troost, J. (1999). Neuropsychological impairment in amateur soccer players. *Journal of the American Medical Association, 282*, 971–973.

McCrea, M., Kelly, J.P., Randolph, C., Cisler, R., & Berger, L. (2002). Immediate neurocognitive effects of concussion. *Neurosurgery, 50*(5), 1032–1042.

McCrea, M. (2001). Sideline assessment of concussion. In J.E. Bailes, & A.L. Day (Eds.), *Neurological Sports Medicine*. Rolling Meadows, Illinois: American Association of Neurological Surgeons.

McCrea, M., Kelly, J., Randolph, C., Kluge, J., Bartolic, E., Finn, G., & Baxter, B. (1998). Standardized Assessment of Concussion (SAC): On-site mental status evaluation of the athlete. *Journal of Head Trauma Rehabilitation, 13*(2), 27–35.

McCrory, P.R., & Berkovic, S.F. (2001). The history of clinical and pathophysiological concepts and misconceptions. *Neurology, 57*, 2283–2289.

McCrory, P.R., & Berkovic, S.F. (1998). Second Impact Syndrome. *Neurology, 50*, 677–683.

McGuffie, A.C., & Fitzpatrick, M.O. (1998). Golf-related head injuries in children: The little tigers. *Scottish Medical journal, 43*, 139.

McLatchie, G., Brooks, N., Galbraith, S., Hutchinson, J.S., Wilson, L., Melville, I., & Teasdale, E. (1987). Clinical neurological examination, neuropsychology, electroencephalography and computed tomographic head scanning in active amateur boxers. *Journal of Neurology, Neurosurgery, and Psychiatry, 50,* 96–99.

McLean A., Temkin, N.R., Dikmen S., & Wyler A.R. (1983). The behavioral sequelae of head injury. *Journal of Clinical Neuropsychology, 5*(4), 361–376.

Miller, H. (1961). Accident neurosis. *British Medical Journal, 1*, 919–925.

Naunheim R.S., Standeven J., Richter C., & Lewis, L.M. (2000). Comparison of impact data in hockey, football, and soccer. *Journal of Trauma-Injury Infection & Critical Care, 48*(5), 938–944.

Noakes, T.D. (1995). Fatal cycling injuries. *Sports Medicine, 20*, 348–362.

Olesniewicz, M.H., Sallis, R.E., Jones, K., & Copp, N. (1997). *The neuropsychological changes that occur from head concussions in football at the NCAA Division III Level.* Paper presented at the Sports Related Concussion and Nervious System Injuries Conference, Orlando, FL.

Oppenheimer, R.D. (1968). Microscopic lesions in the brain following head injury. *Journal of Neurology, Neurosurgery, and Psychiatry, 31*, 299–306.

Polin, R.S., Alves, W.M., & Jane, J.A. (1996). Spots and head injuries. In R.W. Evans (Ed.), *Neurology and Trauma* (pp. 166–185). Philadelphia: W.B. Saunders.

Powell, J.W., & Barber-Foss, K.D. (1999). Traumatic brain injury in high school athletes. *The Journal of the American Medical Association, 282*(10), 958–963.

Prall, J.A., Winston, K.R., & Brennan, R. (1995). Severe snowboarding injuries (abstract). *Injury, 26*, 539–542.

Prins, M.L., Lee, S.M., Cheng, C.Y., Becker, D.P., & Hovda, D.A. (1996). Fluid percussion brain injury in the developing and adult rat: A comparative study of mortality, morphology, intracranial pressure, and mean arterial blood pressure. *Developmental Brain Research, 95*, 272–282.

Quality Standards Subcommittee, American Academy of Neurology. (1997). Practice Parameter: The management of concussion in sports (summary statement). *Neurology, 48*, 581–585.

Rimel, R.W., Giordani, M.A., Barth, J.T., Boll, T.J., & Jane, J.A. (1981). Disability caused by minor head injury. *Neurosurgery, 9*, 221–228.

Roberts, A.H. (1969). *Brain Damage in Boxers. A Study of the Prevalence of Traumatic Brain Encephalopathy among Ex-professional Boxers.* London: Pitman Medical and Scientific.

Ruff, R.M., Levin, H.S., Mattis, S., High, W.M., Marshall, L., Eisenberg, H.M., & Tabaddor, K. (1989). Recovery of memory after mild head injury: A three center study. In H.S. Levin & A.L. Benton (Eds.), *Mild Head Injury* (pp. 176–188). New York: Oxford Press.

Schmidt, R.H., & Grady, M.S. (1995). Loss of forebrain cholinergic neurons following mild and moderate brain injury. *Journal of Neurosurgery, 83*, 496–502.

Schneider, R.C. (1973). *Head and neck injuries in football: Mechanisms, treatment, and prevention.* Baltimore, MD: Williams & Wilkens.

Segalowitz, S.J., & Lawson, S. (1995). Subtle symptoms associated with self-reported mild head injury. *Journal of Learning Disabilities, 28*, 309–319.

Shulman, J.L., & Bowen, W.G. (2001). The institutionalization and regulation of college sports in historical perspective. In J.L. Shulman & W.G. Bowen (Eds.), *The Game of Life: College Sports and Education Values.* Princeton University Press.

Symonds, C. (1962). Concussion and its sequelae. *Lancet, 1*, 1–5.

Tegner, Y., & Lorentzon, R. (1991). Ice hockey injuries: Incidence, nature, and causes. *British Journal of Sports Medicine, 25*, 87–89.

Thurman D., & Guerrero J. (1997). Trends in hospitalization associated with traumatic brain injury. *Journal of the American Medical Association, 282*(10), 954–757.

Varney, N.R., & Varney, R.N. (1995). Brain injury without head injury: Some physics of automobile collisions with particular reference to brain injuries occurring without physical head trauma. *Applied Neuropsychology, 2*, 47–62.

Wills, S.M., & Leathem, M., (2001). Sports-related brain injury research: Methodological difficulties associated with ambiguous terminology. *Brain Injury, 15*(7), 645–648.

Wojtys, E.M., Hovda, D., Landry, G., Boland, A., Lovell, M. McCrea, M., & Minkoff, J. (1999). Concussion in sports. *The American Journal of Sports Medicine, 27*(5), 676–687.

Winters, J.E. (2001). Commentary: Role of properly fitted mouthguards in prevention of sports-related concussion. *Journal of Athletic Training, 36*(3), 339–341.

Chapter 2

DIAGNOSIS, MANAGEMENT, AND PREVENTION

John W. Powell
Michigan State University

Background

Throughout the United States there are millions of people of all ages that participate in a wide variety of sports and recreational activities. Inherent in each of these activities is the potential for injury. Among the most common occurrences are injuries to the soft tissue and bone, e.g., contusions, lacerations, sprains, strains and fractures. In general, these injuries, when provided with appropriate medical care, recover fully and result in the participant's full return to the activity. In addition to the more common injuries, there are the less common and more serious cases that result in permanent disability. Within the wide range of injuries that are possible in sports there is one type of injury that, for the most part, has little affect on the participant, yet may also produce long term or permanent disability. This injury category is most often represented by traumatic injuries to the brain. Traditionally, the less severe episodes of brain injury are referred to as concussions and the more serious occurrences are referred to as traumatic brain injuries. The frequency and severity of these injuries is a predominate topic of discussion among groups that sponsor sports and recreational activities, the medical professionals that are concerned with managing the care of the injury and the individual participants. In order to provide perspective for a discussion of the relative importance of concussions associated with sports, it is important to have a clear definition of the injury. Once the operational definition is set, we can consider the relative risk of the injury within the context of the sport, the mechanisms and circumstances that result in injury, the proper identification of the injury, procedures for managing the care of the injured and procedures that minimize the risk of brain injury.

What is a Concussion?

Historically, an injury to the head that resulted from some type of impact was identified as a concussion. The identification of a concussion included a wide range of signs and symptoms exhibited by the patient and recorded by the physician. As far back as 1966, a working definition of a concussion was published by the Committee on Head Injury Nomenclature of the Congress of Neurological Surgeons as "a clinical syndrome characterized by immediate and transient post-traumatic impairment of neural function, such as alteration of consciousness, disturbance of vision, equilibrium, etc. due to brain stem involvement."(Committee on Head Injury, 1966) According to Kelly et al. (1991) the concussion has been defined as a trauma-induced alteration in mental status that may or may not involve a loss of consciousness (Kelly et al., 1991). Over the past several years, a great deal of discussion has flourished among members of the sports medicine and neuroscience community regarding the appropriate description of concussion, the classification of concussion, the management of persons that suffered concussion and guidelines for the return to competition following concussion (Kelly et al., 1991, Cantu, 1986, Cantu, 1991, Gronwall, 1986, Wrightson, 1989, Quality Standards Subcommittee, 1997, Kay, 1993). These on-going discussions have produced more than ten different classification systems for concussion, each of which takes a slightly different position (Sturmi, Smith, & Lombardo 1998). In general, most agree that the signs and symptoms, along with neuro-cognitive deficits and the presence of a loss of consciousness are integrated in order to describe a concussion. The management guidelines associated with these classification systems differ in their specifics, but are similar in their recommendation that no player should return to competition until the signs, symptoms and cognition have returned to normal.

In much of the current literature, the most popular description of a concussion is similar to the one offered by Kelly et al. (1991). The definition of concussion that we will consider for the remainder of the discussion identifies an injury that results from an impact to the head that creates some mental alteration in which the person may or may not show cognitive deficits; may show or report any number of signs and symptoms; and may or may not experience a loss of consciousness. This definition includes the idea that the presence of a wide variety of signs, symptoms and cognitive deficiencies are more important features of the concussion than the loss of consciousness. While unconsciousness is an important sign for a head injury, its use as a definitive indicator of injury severity and decision making regarding a player's return to play is limited. (Lovell, Iverson, Collins, McKeag, & Maroon, 1999).

Until the early 90s, the size and scope of the problem of concussion in sports was not clearly identified. It was at this time that the issue of sports concussions exploded in the daily newspapers when several professional athletes retired from their game and cited a history of concussions and post concussion syndrome as the reason for their retirement. The media attention generated by these high profile cases produced a heightened awareness of concussion among the media and the fans. As the public learned more about these athletes, the medical community was increasing its efforts to identify and manage concussions so as to minimize the risk of disability. Specific concerns arose regarding the effects of multiple concussions, the time necessary for full recovery and the importance of the time interval between subsequent concussions (Executive Summary, 1991). As a result of these concerns, the research community increased its efforts regarding the accurate identification and the management of concussions as well as the long-term effects of concussion on the individual player. These continuing research efforts are adding new and exciting information to the professional body of knowledge in order to begin reducing the risk of injury.

Potential for Injury

People participate in sports for a wide variety of reasons. The professional athlete uses sports as a livelihood. College athletes receive scholarships and prepare for entry into the professional levels. High school participants work toward the possibility of college scholarships and kids participate for fun. The risk of injury in all levels of play is derived primarily from the nature of the sport and the specific activities associated with game. For example, collision sports like football and ice hockey will characteristically have more acute injuries than sports like swimming and track. Boxing will have more head related trauma because of the focus of the sport. Within each sport there is a general injury pattern as well as a pattern of specific types of injury that is unique to the sport. For example a cauliflower ear is most often associated with wrestling while shoulder inflammation is more common in baseball players than in soccer players. One injury often associated with collision sports is the concussion or, as noted is some of the more recent literature, the mild traumatic brain injury (MTBI) (Powell & Barber-Foss, 1999). This injury results from a direct blow to the head or from an acceleration/deceleration force, both linear and rotational, to the tissue of the brain. In sports, the direct blow to the head is generally considered the mechanism most often associated with the concussion. This direct blow to the head may produce focal damage at the site of the impact, damage opposite to the site of impact (counter coup) or damage to the individual axons in the brain known a diffuse axonal injury (DAI). The severity of the injury is a function of the magnitude and direction of these linear and rotational forces both separately and in combination with each other. Another component of the brain that influences the extent of the tissue damage is related to the brain's ability to manage the internal stress and strain placed on the tissue as a result of the injury forces. While it would seem that the amount of force at the time of collision would be the determining factor for injury frequency and severity, there are cases in which the forces appear to be high enough to result in injury and no injury occurs. On the other hand, there are cases where serious injury has resulted from what may seem to be a relative low force (Cantu, 1996). All of these factors, when combined at the moment of injury, make the concussion a very unique injury and an injury that requires special attention regarding its management during recovery.

The head injury forces that may act on the brain during a practice or game session can originate and be associated with a variety of different scenarios. Head impact may result from a collision between players and be either incidental (unintentional) or intentional (fighting) acts. There may be collisions with objects either carried by the players (sticks) or associated with the participation environments i.e., playing surfaces, boundary obstructions, or game operations equipment. The impact may be considered as a part of the game as in football or very unusual as in volleyball. In sports where the perceived risk of head injury is high, as in boxing, football, ice hockey and men's lacrosse, the governance bodies for the sport have mandated head protection in the form of helmets. Even with the head protected by a helmet, concussions continue to occur. The important consideration is that the concussion can occur in any activity regardless of the nature of the activity and that when the concussion occurs it has a potential for long term impairment for the player.

As we consider the risk of injury, it is important to note that only a small percentage of the head collisions that occur within the context of the sport produce an identifiable concussion. To demonstrate this point, consider the number of head impacts estimated for one season of high school football. A small study of high school football collisions has identified, as a conservative estimate, at least 354 million head impacts occurring during a typical fall season of practices and games (Powell, 1999). This estimate is based on the number of clearly identifiable head impacts between players and/or playing surfaces recorded by high school football coaches as they reviewed 10 game films. Collisions among players that were thought to occur but were not clearly evident in the game films were not recorded as head impacts. The coaches documented collisions from 1193 football plays and produced 7835 clearly identified head impacts. The National Federation of State High School Association's information regarding football participation identifies more than 14,000 high schools that play football. For the purposes of the study, it was assumed that there are 15,000 high schools that play football and each school played at least 15 games (includes varsity and subvarsity games). These totals were multiplied by the number of plays per game (119) and the average head impacts per play (6.6). This produces approximately 177 million game impacts. The study suggested that there was at least as many impacts in the practice conditions. The combination of games and practices result in the estimate of 354 million sport-related head impacts. While the study examined ten game films, it can serve as an operational estimate of the frequency of head collisions during a typical high school football season (Powell, 1999).

In a 3-year study (1995-1997) of high school football injuries conducted by the National Athletic Trainers' Association, it was estimated that 39,566 mild traumatic brain injuries occur during an average high school football season. (Powell & Barber-Foss, 1999). The certified athletic trainers on-site at the schools that participated in the study recorded injuries from both practices and games. Among the reported injuries 78% missed less than 8 days of participation due to their injury, 18% lost from 8-21 days and 4% lost more than 21 days. If we combine the annual estimated frequency of MTBI (39,566) in the NATA study with head collision frequency estimates (354,000,000), it would appear that one concussion occurs in approximately 9,000 clearly visible head impacts and one concussion that misses more than 21 days occurs in every 2.4 million impacts. While these study figures provide only hypothetical estimates, they serve well in describing the nature of the risk of concussion. There is more than an ample number of opportunities for head impacts to produce concussions, yet the number of concussions that actually occur is relatively small.

It is clear from this simple exercise that there is more than an ample opportunity for head impacts in high school football to produce concussions and that not all head impacts produce concussions. If the concussions in high school football are relatively infrequent and the severity of the ones that do occur is low, then why worry about concussions? The answer is that any concussion, regardless of how it may appear at the time of injury, has the potential for becoming more serious over time and therefore must be identified and properly managed by the medical community at its initial onset and throughout its recovery.

Concussion Management

The most challenging issues facing medical and paramedical professionals' focuses on the accurate identification of the concussion and once identified, the care and management of the patient and his/her return to participation. One of the considerations in identification is the variety of signs and symptoms that may or may not be present. The concussion may be present with headache, dizziness, and nausea and/or memory alterations. The injury may result in short or long term unconsciousness or no loss of consciousness. The signs and symptoms present at the time of injury may disappear very quickly or they may linger for hours, days, weeks or months. In some rare cases the initial signs and symptoms may disappear and then reappear with dramatic consequences. The player may demonstrate cognitive effects of the concussion or may have no cognitive deficits. It is important to consider that the signs and symptoms reported by the patient may be the result of a variety of specific injuries. For example, headache, nausea and dizziness may be the result of an injury to the brain or a disruption of the vestibular canals. If the injury was to the cortical area of the brain, then cognitive deficits would be expected. If the injury was a vestibular problem, then cognitive findings may be normal. It is unclear at this time how all of these different factors integrate in the injury event and therefore it becomes extremely important that the injury is accurately documented and repeatedly evaluated during the recovery period. In addition to the clinical findings regarding the concussion, it is important for clinicians to involve the player's friends and family in the follow-up process. There are instances where a player reports no signs or symptoms, yet, if asked, the people around the player would indicate a variation in the player's behavior away from the field of play. These behavioral changes may be indicative of residual effects of the concussion.

Once the concussion has been identified and appropriate medical care has been made available, the question of return to participation becomes as an important decision. How long should the person wait to return to collision sports? How long should the person wait to return to non-collision sports? What is the potential for the player to sustain a second concussion? And, does this second injury create more significant damage than the first one? How can the player be sure that the brain has truly "returned to normal?" One of the most important ways to support these difficult decisions is to use the documentation of the case, including signs, symptoms, neuro-cognitive baselines, and player behavior as decision-making tools. The neuroscience and sports medicine community have identified all of these areas as issues for research.

Injury Prevention

Injury prevention, regardless of the type of injuries or type of activity includes two separate levels of concern. The first is to do everything possible in managing the players and the environment to prevent injuries. For example, the pre-participation activities applied to a knee injury include pre-participation physicals, conditioning programs, teaching programs and protective equipment (when applicable). It is important to note that when all has been done to prevent injuries, the efforts will not be 100% successful; some participants will sustain injury. The second aspect of complete injury prevention program is to have a strategy to prevent the original injury from being re-injured. To do this, the clinician uses a variety of clinical tests (Lachman's, etc), diagnostic technology (MRI, etc.) and on-the-field performance measures to determine the readiness of the player to return to participation. The player is continually monitored for pain, strength, range of motion, and functional performance. When these parameters have returned to normal, the player may be cleared to return to participation. Given the fact that injuries will continue to occur, even under the blanket of a strong injury prevention program, the realistic goal of the program is to minimize the risk of injury.

Concussion prevention

An injury prevention program for concussions follows the same strategy as a prevention program for any other injury. Preventing the initial concussion should include informing the players regarding the risk of head injury, pre-participation evaluation for any history of concussion, instruction in techniques to minimize their risk of concussion and a documentation of the player's neuro-cognitive function. Variation between knee injury and concussion prevention occurs in the second level of injury prevention when the clinician must determine the player's readiness to return to participation as a factor in preventing re-injury. To do this, the clinician must rely on the player's report of signs and symptoms, the return to normal of neuro-cognitive function and a subjective assessment of the player's behavior. The problem arises when the player reports signs and symptoms are normal, the diagnostic technology shows normal findings and neuro-cognitive function has returned to normal, is the player really ready to return? The answer lies in the clinician's ability to integrate subjective evaluations of a player's behaviors and the objective findings of the clinical evaluations into the decision to return to participation. There are still many unanswered questions regarding the time needed to fully recover from concussion; how many concussions are too many; and how much time between concussions is required to minimize the risk of re-injury. The areas will be addressed throughout the sections of the remainder of this text.

Continuing with the concern for preventing concussion, the following discussion addresses the issue in three sections; consideration for pre-participation, procedures at the time of participation, and procedures for post injury management.

Concussion pre-participation prevention

The pre-participation section of injury prevention emphasizes things that are done ahead of time to minimize the number of concussions. Consider a two point approach; programs that monitor the participation conditions, and information regarding the player's medical history and physical readiness to participate.

Pre-event (playing conditions)

1) Teaching the player about protecting the head during participation. This is especially true for sports that wear helmets.
2) Players should be informed as to the nature of concussion and the importance it has regarding their health.
3) Emphasis on the players to report any signs or symptoms of concussion.
4) For sports that require helmets,
   - Players should be informed of the warnings regarding the use of the protective helmets.
   - Players must be taught that the helmet cannot protect them from all head injuries.

- The protection afforded by the helmet is based on its proper use and proper maintenance.
- Players must realize the importance of examining their helmet daily in order to identify potential areas that require maintenance.

5) For sports that do not require helmets but use sticks, e.g., women's lacrosse and field hockey, the players must be taught to respect the potential for concussion as a result of impact with the stick.
6) Establish procedures for handling the concussion, when and if it occurs
   - Develop and implement an Emergency Action Plan
   - Establish procedures for on the field management
   - Develop decision-making protocols regarding return to play following a concussion.

Pre-event (player information)

1) Establishing the presence of a history of brain injury for each participant.
   - Sport related as well as non-sport related
   - Number of events
   - Time since the last event
   - Time between events
2) Establish neuro-cognitive baseline for participants.

Prevention at the time of participation

The prevention of injury during this phase focuses on the association between the injury and the conditions that exist at the time the injury occurs, e.g., games or practices. Like the pre-participation section, the protective equipment being worn is essential for protection and should be monitored during participation for any defects. It is important to continually evaluate and monitor the participation rules that are designed to protect the head. For example, the referees must enforce the rules regarding the use of the head as the initial point of contact in football, i.e., spearing. In other sports, rule infractions stemming from fighting or illegal use of player implements, e.g., high-sticking in ice hockey must be enforced.

In addition to the protective equipment worn by the player, it is important to examine the general participation facility (playing field or arena) for potential hazards. For example, are the corners of the scorer's table that is next to the basketball court padded? Are there objects close to the sidelines of the soccer field that present a hazard? It is important that fields and courts where participation takes place are evaluated and continually monitored for the existence or appearance of potential hazards for participants. It is important that the risk of concussion from competition not increase because of poor playing conditions or the presence of foreseeable hazards.

An important feature in concussion management is an accurate and thorough assessment of the injured player's condition. If a player sustains a knee injury, the physicians and athletic trainers have a cadre of clinical tests

(Lachman's Test, Pivot-Shift Test, etc) and diagnostic procedures (X-ray, MRI, etc) to identify the injury and its severity. Unfortunately, the same level of sophistication in the methods of identifying and evaluating the severity of a concussion is not on a par. Until more research is completed regarding the specific nature of the tissue damage associated with concussion, it is paramount that clinicians use a variety of tools to assist in identifying and managing the injury. Traditionally, concussions were identified based on the signs and symptoms present and reported by the player at the time of injury. Recent efforts within the sports medicine and research communities have produced protocols for evaluating concussions on the sideline. Specific areas of interest include, but are not limited to, balance and postural sway, neurocognitive baseline and follow-up evaluations (McCrea, Kelly, Kluge, Ackley, & Randolph, 1997; Lovell & Collins, 2001; Guskiewicz, Riemann, Perrin & Nashner, 1997; Lovell & Collins, 1998). Research is continuing regarding the use of technology to evaluate the concussion and in the future we may have the consistency of tools to evaluate and manage concussions that are on par with other sports injuries.

Post event prevention

Once the concussion has been clearly identified, the player must be continually monitored regarding the presence of signs, symptoms and neuro-cognitive functioning. The clinician supervising the player's recovery must include information regarding the patient's interactions with family and friends to support decisions during recovery. While the athlete may report with no lingering symptoms, the patient's behavior away from the clinical or sports setting may provide valuable information regarding the player's recovery from concussion.

Regardless of the quality of the pre-participation and participation phases of the prevention program, concussions will still occur. When they occur there must be a management program to evaluate and refer players to the proper medical professionals. As the player recovers from the concussion, the decisions regarding the players return to participation must be individualized for each case. The challenge of the medical profession is to be able to return the player to competition with a minimum of risk for a second injury. The research being done in the area of baseline neuropsychological testing, standardized sideline evaluation and formal monitoring and evaluation procedures represent a positive step forward in offering objective information for use in the return to play decision.

The Injury Prevention Team

Establishing and maintaining injury prevention programs for sports injuries including concussions, is a process that requires input from numerous areas. The best programs integrate the planning and implementation of injury prevention procedures that have included support from the program sponsors, the medical supervisors, the coaches, the community and the participants. Each of these groups contributes significantly to the best program.

The sponsors, for example, have specific challenges to face. They must be the driving force behind the injury prevention program. They must take into consideration the nature of the sport and the activities of the players as they make decisions that will affect the injury risk pattern. Specific areas that require attention are facilities and equipment, player protective equipment and competitive rules and regulations.

The medical community, including physicians and athletic trainers, become the key people for the implementation of program features. They must be prepared to identify and manage the injuries that occur and to implement rehabilitation and recovery protocols that will minimize the risk of re-injury.

The coaches are responsible to see that players are prepared for the rigors of the game. Player's must be instructed in methods to maximize performance and minimize the risk of injury, specifically concussion. The coaches on the practice field and on the game field must enforce the rules regarding safety. In addition to coaches, referees are charged with the responsibility for enforcing the rules of the game and therefore play a pivotal role in the protection of participants.

The community, especially the parents and families of the participants, need to understand the importance of their role in injury prevention. They are in the best position to monitor the player's aches and pains off the field and out of site of the coaches and medical personnel. They need to be willing to provide information to the medical team in order to maintain the highest standards for the care and management of injuries.

It is especially important that the participants take an active role in preventing injuries. Players must learn the proper protective measures associated with their sport to minimize injury. They must monitor their personal playing equipment for defects and report any deficiencies for immediate repair. They must report any injuries to the athletic trainer or physician. The little injuries that occur daily, when reported and managed properly, are less likely to become a time loss injury. Early recognition of injury, like the early recognition of disease, is essential if the effect of the injury on the player and the player's participation are to be minimized.

When all is said and done, the player's safety is a function of the combined knowledge and expertise of people from medicine, the school, the athletic programs and the program participants. The best way to prevent injuries, including concussions, in sports is to be sure that players participate under the umbrella of well-designed injury prevention program based on the combined input of an interdisciplinary injury prevention team.

References

Cantu, R.C. (1986). Guidelines for return to contact sports after a cerebral concussion. *Physician and Sports Medicine, 14*(10), 75–83.

Cantu, R.C. (1991). Minor head injuries in sports. *Adolescent Medicine.* State of the Art Reviews, 2, 141–148.

Cantu, R.C. (1996). Head injuries in sport. *British Journal of Sports Medicine, 30*(4), 289–296.

Committee on Head Injury Nomenclature of the Congress of Neurological Surgeons. Glossary of head injury, including some definitions of injury to the cervical spine. (1966). *Clinical Neurosurgery, 12,* 386–394.

Executive Summary. (1991). *In Proceedings of the Mild Brain Injury. National Athletic Trainers Association Research and Education Foundation, April 16–18, 1991.*

Gronwall, D. (1986). Rehabilitation programs for patients with mild head injury: components, problems, and evaluation. *Journal of Head Trauma Rehabilitation, 1,* 53–62.

Guskiewicz, K.M., Riemann, B.L., Perrin, D.H., & Nashner, L.M. (1997). Alternative approaches to the assessment of mild head injury in athletes. *Medicine Science in Sports and Exercise.* 7(Supplement): s213-s221.

Kay, T. (1993). Neuropsychological treatment of mild traumatic brain injury. *Journal of Head Trauma Rehabilitation, 8*(3), 74–85.

Kelly, J.P., Nichols, J.S., Filley, C.M., Lillehei, K.O., Rubinstein, D., Kleinschmidt-DeMasters, B.K. (1991). Concussion in sports: guidelines for the prevention of catastrophic outcome. *Journal of the American Medical Association, 226,* 2867–2869.

Lovell, M.R., & Collins, M.W. (1998). Neuropsychological assessment of the college football player, *Journal of Head Trauma Rehabilitation, 13*(2), 9–26.

Lovell, M.R., & Collins, M.W. (2001). Neuropsychological assessment of the head-injured professional athlete. In J.E. Bailes & A.L. Day (Eds.*), Neurological Sports Medicine: A Guide for Physicians and Athletic Trainers* (pp. 169–179). American Association of Neurological Surgeons.

Lovell, M.R., Iverson, G.L., Collins, M.W., McKeag, D., & Maroon J.C. (1999). Does loss of consciousness predict neuropsychological decrements after concussion? *Clinical Journal of Sports Medicine, 9*(4), 193–198.

McCrea, M., Kelly, J.P., Kluge, J., Ackley, B., & Randolph, C. (1997). Standardized assessment of concussion in football players. *Neurology, 48,* 586–588.

Powell, J.W. (1999). Injury patterns in selected high school sports. In: J.E. Bailes, M. Lovell, J.C. Maroon (Eds.), *Sports Related Concussions* (pp. 75–90). St. Louis Mo: Quality Medical Publishing Inc.

Powell, J.W., & Barber-Foss, K.D. (1999). Traumatic brain injuries in high school athletes, *Journal of the American Medical Association, 282,* 958–963.

Quality Standards Subcommittee. (1997). American Academy of Neurology. Practice parameter: the management of concussion in sports. *Neurobiology, 48,*1– 5.

Sturmi, J.E., Smith, C., & Lombardo, J.A. (1998). Mild brain trauma in sports. Diagnosis and treatment guidelines. *Sports Medicine, 25*(6), 351–358.

Wrightson, P. (1989). Management of disability and rehabilitation services after mild head injury. In: H.S. Levin, H.M. Eisenberg, A.L. Benton, (Eds.), *Mild Head Injury* (pp. 245–256). New York, NY: Oxford University Press.

Chapter 3

BIOMECHANICS OF BRAIN INJURY IN ATHLETES

James A. Newman
Biokinetcs and Associates LTD. Ottawa, Canada

Introduction

Biomechanics is simply the application of the principles of mechanics to biological systems – most often the human system. **Mechanics** is that branch of physics dealing with the relationship between forces and movement. It encompasses related fields called s**tatics, dynamics** and **kinematics.** The head injury of interest here is that which occurs as a result of impact. Hence the biomechanics of head injury involves the study of the relationship between the forces that are developed or applied and the way the head moves during impact that are associated with head injury.

Biomechanical Principles

There are many types of head injuries that occur as a result of head impact. Among these are scalp injuries, fractures of the skull, and various kinds of brain injuries. We shall consider here only brain injuries. In fact, we shall consider only those brain injuries that occur when the skull is not significantly deformed – let alone fractured. Given that the skull is deformable, this excludes some brain injury mechanisms including, subdural and/or epidural hematoma that are directly associated with local skull in-bending, ballistic type injuries, and low-speed crushing mechanisms. However, there are a great number of injuries that can occur solely as a result of head motion. These include simple concussion, subdural hematoma due to shearing action at the skull brain interface, as well as diffuse axonal injury and coma. The non-deformable skull assumption is valid when the impact is not of exceptionally high velocity, or when the force developed during impact is well distributed over a large area of the skull. This latter requirement is often met when a helmet is worn, or if impact is with a yielding surface such as a boxing glove, an airbag or a soft surface like sand.

A second principle we shall invoke is that the brain is injured because it is deformed (within the non-deformable skull) to an extent beyond that which can be tolerated. This deformation can lead to rupture of blood vessels or nerves or simple stretching of neural or vascular tissue. It is hypothesized further that it is the motion of the skull that causes the motion of the brain within the skull and that the degree or probability of brain injury is directly related somehow to the nature of the skull movement.

One of the principle objectives of the study of biomechanics of head trauma is the development of better head protection. The main problem in this regard is of course, how do you tell if in fact one design is better than another. If someone is trying to promote, for example, a "better" hockey helmet, how can you verify this improved performance? Well, you could put it on someone's head and compare it to some other design when that individual is whacked on the head, or you could introduce the product into the game of hockey and wait and see if the expected improvements materialize. Neither of these approaches is of course viable. You cannot subject any individual to a potentially injurious head impact without some independent knowledge of how the head will react to impact. That of course is where head protection performance standards come in. The next part of the discussion may appear somewhat tedious, but stay with it for a while because it really is quite important.

Head Protection Standards

Standards for head protection cannot rely upon how a living human being will respond to impact. They must rely upon some human surrogate, i.e., a mechanical dummy. Now since you cannot injury a dummy, i.e. it cannot be concussed or killed, we need some other measure of how the dummy responds and this must be somehow correlated to the likelihood of head injury in a real human being. We have not yet reached the stage where we can correlate the response of the dummy to specific neuropsychological responses of an injured human being.[1] At the very best, the field has developed only to the point that dummy responses can be correlated to brain injury *severity*.

The second aspect of such a standard is that the impact to be delivered to the dummy must somehow reflect the environment in which the head protection is to perform. Nearly everyone is familiar with the kind of crash testing done on automobiles. The driver and passenger dummy are seated in the test vehicle that is crashed into a standard barrier. The effectiveness of the airbags is judged by examining the way the dummies' heads respond during

[1] With the possible exception of loss of consciousness.

the crash. This response is monitored by way of instruments imbedded in the dummy heads. These instruments monitor how a dummy head moves – that is all they do.

The same sort of approach is used with helmet standards except the impact is more typical of that which would occur in the specific application. In hockey for example, the impacts that are delivered to a helmeted headform represent the hazards associated with skates and goalposts. In football, the impacting surface typically characterizes the ground surface or another player's helmet. In equestrian activities, a fallen rider may well be exposed to a horse's hoof and this too is reflected in the particular standard. Usually, helmet standards involve dropping a helmeted headform from some predetermined height (to achieve a typical velocity) onto a specified anvil (typical of the particular application).

Regardless of the differences in the various activities, be it athletics, automotive, industrial, military or whatever, the head being protected is the same head. Establishing tolerance limits for the head is essentially independent of the particular activity. In keeping with our hypothesis above, regardless of the application, it is the *motion* of the test headform that established the degree or probability of a brain injury occurring under those impact circumstances.

Put simply, our theoretical analogy to the human head is that of a rigid container within which is a deformable substance whose physical properties are similar to brain matter. The biomechanical head injury assessment functions to be reviewed here are all based upon the *motion* of the container. That is, it is the detailed characteristics of the way the skull moves that determine the probability that a head injury will occur. The motion of the test headform will, if the headform is biofidelic,[2] indicate the likelihood of head injury to a human.

Kinematics

Kinematics is the science of motion. Readers who are versed in these matters might wish to proceed directly to the next section. Our discussions here of the biomechanics of head injury will be confined to discussion of head motion alone.[3]

In engineering systems, motion is analyzed by employing an orthogonal three-dimensional coordinate system. Essentially they are

- Anterior – posterior. x axis. Fore-aft
- Lateral left – right. y axis. Transverse
- Superior – inferior. z axis. Up-down

[2] Biofidelity in this instance means that the headform dynamically reacts to impact the same way that a human head would if impacted under the same conditions. Test headforms employed today are reasonably biofidelic (Foster et al., 1977).

[3] Thus we are talking about the **biokinematics** of head injury.

Motion of any magnitude in any direction can be resolved into three component parts each aligned with each of the three axes or dimensions.

There are basically 12 different forms of motion that can be described using this system. Six are linear forms of motion and six are angular. When a body moves in a linear fashion, it is said to translate. When a body's angular orientation changes, it is said to rotate.

The six linear forms are simply
1. positive x – forward
2. negative x – backwards
3. positive y – to the right
4. negative y – to the left
5. positive z – downward
6. negative z – upward

The six angular types correspond to positive or negative rotation about each of the three orthogonal axes.[4] Complete rigid body motion (no matter how complex) can be fully described by describing the individual component motions relative to each of the three axes. For example,
- A bullet from a rifle translates along a single x-axis and at the same time rotates (spins) about the x-axis.
- A soccer ball when kicked travels upward (-z) then downward (+z) while spinning (rotating) about its transverse, y-axis.
- A Ferris wheel rotates about a transverse axis. The cars on the Ferris wheel do not rotate but translate (or move linearly) but on a circular path.
- The head of a football player that is struck by an opposing player will translate and rotate about all three axes during the impact.

Motion (or movement) is described in terms of how the **position** of a body changes as a function of time. A few more definitions...
- **Displacement** is the net change of position. A football player who runs back a kick off from his own goal line will be displaced 100 yards. Note that he may run further than a hundred yards as his direction changes. This is the difference between displacement and **distance**; the former being "as the crow flies".
- **Velocity** is the time rate of change of displacement. If it takes 25 seconds to complete the run, his *average* velocity would have been 4 yards/second. His instantaneous **speed** (i.e. his rate of change of distance traveled) as he changes direction may be considerably higher.
- **Acceleration** is the time rate of change of velocity. If the player goes from a stationary position when he first catches the ball to a velocity of 10

4 The system is often said to have six degrees of freedom since only six types f motion (three linear and three angular) can occur at the same time. (One can't be going backward and forward at the same time).

yards/sec during the first 2 seconds he has the ball, his *average* acceleration during this time would have been 5yds/sec/sec.[5]

As the reader will observe, the units of acceleration can be somewhat confusing. In the field of biomechanics, the unit of acceleration is usually the G.

One fundamental and unchanging aspect of our planet is the acceleration due to gravity. It equals approximately 32.2 feet/sec/sec and is the rate at which the velocity of any body (stone or a feather) changes in freefall (in a vacuum). It is given its own unit called a G. A Formula 1 racecar can accelerate in a straight line at over 2Gs. A jet pilot can experience 7 to 10Gs during high-speed maneuvers. When the head of a football player is impacted by another player, or by the ground, his head may experience linear acceleration higher than 100Gs.

When any part of the human body is subjected to high levels of acceleration, certain physiological responses occur. These can include loss of consciousness.[6] Both linear and angular accelerations usually occur in head impact. Both forms of motion can cause the brain to be deformed within the (assumed rigid) skull. Historically, brain injury criteria have been expressed in Gs. In fact however, it is currently regarded that rotational motion of the skull is more likely to result in brain motion than will pure linear motion.[7] Be that as it may, it is important not to conclude that acceleration (of either kind) *causes* brain injury. The movement of the head when subjected to an impact, and the injury which may or may not be sustained, are both responses to that impact. The question that the field of biomechanics tries to address is; are there any correlations between these responses? That is, does the observed/measured movement of the head relate to the type or severity of the injury that the brain may sustain?

For completeness, a couple more relationships may be helpful.

- **Kinetic energy** is proportional to the square of the velocity change. Given there are two types of velocity, linear and angular, it exists in both linear and rotational forms.
- **Power** is the time rate of change of energy. It too is associated with linear and angular motion.

---

5 To further confuse the issue consider the following. A person gets in his car at his house at 1pm. Accelerates the car to 30 mph. Maintains that velocity for an hour arriving back home at 2pm after decelerating[6] back to 0 mph. Regardless of the distance he traveled (about 30 miles) his displacement is zero. Regardless of what speed he may have achieved his average velocity was zero. And though he accelerated and decelerated during the run, his average acceleration during the hour was zero.

6 The tolerance of the head to impact is not the same for all axes. For example, it is generally felt that the head can sustain higher acceleration in the fore-aft direction than laterally. Similarly, different tolerances are associated with the different rotational modes.

7 There is no angular equivalent to the G.

With this background, it is now possible to review the development of some of the various biomechanical (biokinematic) head injury assessment functions that have evolved over the past 40 years.

Kinematic Head Injury Assessment Functions

In practice, any relationship between the manner by which the human head moves during impact and the injury that may occur is of little value, since we do not generally know how the head moves under impact. That is, a head that is impacted and injured is not usually observed, let alone instrumented with devices that could measure its complex kinematic response. In fact, all of the functions described below are usually applied to test headforms.[8]

Dummy headforms are typically instrumented with electronic transducers that generate a signal proportional to acceleration. As many as three linear and three angular accelerometers may be employed.

The simplest and one of the still most widely used criteria is that of maximum linear acceleration.

$$A_{max} < N$$

This function takes no account of possible different directional sensitivities. N is simply the maximum permissible value of the resultant linear acceleration of the headform during impact. Any rotational features are not incorporated or it is assumed that they are somehow accounted for in the linear measurement. It has been and continues to be employed in most helmet standards throughout the world (Snell, 1995 for example). The value that N is set to is determined essentially by the severity of injury that one is trying to deal with. To prevent concussion, the limiting value would be around 80G. To prevent a fatal head injury, N might be set as high as 400Gs.

Other investigators have suggested that though peak acceleration may be a necessary criterion, it is not sufficient. It is evident that higher speed impacts will more likely result in head injury. Hence those impacts that result in a high velocity change are more dangerous even though the acceleration peak is the same. A measure of the velocity change is the duration of the acceleration pulse or the width of the acceleration trace when plotted on a time scale. To handle this, the concept of "dwell times" was introduced. Dwell times basically limit the shape of the acceleration pulse by fixing the maximum permissible time at various acceleration levels. Maximum linear acceleration with dwell times is employed by the NHTSA for the US motorcycle helmet standard. (FMVSS Standard 218, 1997).

---

[8] Some have been used to examine the response of cadaver specimens and animals in experimental research (Hodgson & Thomas, 1971).

$$a_m < 400G$$
$$\text{time at } 200G < 2\text{msec}$$
$$\text{time at } 150G < 4\text{msec}$$

This particular head injury assessment function, indeed the concept of dwell times, has never been verified with actual biomechanical data. Again, no measure of directional sensitivity is included.

A third approach is to use the average resultant linear acceleration and the time duration of the entire impact event itself. The most widely known relationship employing this approach is that associated with the Wayne State University concussion tolerance curve (Gurdjian et al., 1964). It is of the form

$$\bar{a}^{2.5} T < 1{,}000$$

where T is the total time duration of the impact event expressed in seconds.[9] It too basically says the lower the acceleration the longer it can be sustained.[10] Historically, the equation provides a boundary between a "safe' and "unsafe" headform response. It has never actually been used in any performance test but is the basis for the Severity Index SI (Gadd, 1966). It is of the form

$$SI = \int_T a^{2.5} dt < N$$

where a is the time dependent resultant linear acceleration of the center of gravity of the head. With acceleration expressed in Gs, the SI is set to a limiting value of 1200 in the current NOCSAE standard for football helmets (NOCSAE, 1997).

$$[1/(t_2 - t_1) \int_{t_1}^{t_2} a\,(t)dt]^{2.5}\,(t_2 - t_1) < 1.000$$

A more complex but mathematically more appropriate expression of the above is the Head Injury Criterion HIC. It is of the form.

It was first employed as part of the US Department of Transportation safety standard for car occupant protection (FMVSS 208, 1999), and is now the most widely referenced head injury assessment function. Recent analyses of all available experimental cadaver data have been conducted (Mertz et al., 1996). This has led to the conclusion that HIC = 1000 corresponds to a 20% probability of a serious head injury. It is this criterion that is used to judge the effectiveness of crash protection in modern cars.

The above three functions all suffer from at least one serious theoretical flaw. With acceleration expressed in G units, the functions all have units of

---

9 Note that since a is dimensionless, this expression has the units of time (seconds).

10 Expressed differently, higher acceleration can be tolerated with lower velocity change.

seconds. Time alone cannot be a measure of impact severity. If acceleration is expressed properly as ft/sec/sec., the units of the above are $ft^{2.5}/sec^4$. This too is nonsensical. The reason they work at all is that each contains the value of the maximum acceleration (the first of our criteria).

Let us now turn our attention to angular motion. The only guidance here comes from the pioneering work of Ommaya and coworkers (Ommaya, 1984). For severities in the range where concussion might be expected, they had proposed the following limits.

AIS[11]	Acceleration, rad/s^2	Velocity Change, rad/s
0	<4500	<30
1	<1700	>30

The suggestion here is that fairly high rotational acceleration can be sustained if the angular velocity change is not too high. If the velocity change is high, much lower acceleration is tolerable. These criteria are not frequently referenced since they consider rotational motion alone without regard for the linear motion that will accompany any head impact.

Few attempts have been made to examine the combined effects of both forms of motion. One is that developed by the author (Newman 1986). The Generalized Model for Brain Injury Tolerance GAMBIT is of the form

$$G_{max}(t) = \left[\left(\frac{a_{res}(t)}{250}\right)^2 + \left(\frac{\alpha_{res}(t)}{25000}\right)^2\right]^{\frac{1}{2}}$$

It is a non-dimensional measure of impact severity. With a expressed in Gs and α in rad/sec^2, G = 1 was set to correspond to a 50% probability of AIS>3. The function is a weighted sum that acknowledges that as higher linear accelerations are experienced, the tolerable rotational acceleration is lower (and vice versa). Though it correlated well with the then existing biomechanical data, the function has not been widely employed, as it does not include a separate measure of impact duration(velocity change). The function has been expressed in terms of the component directions but in its current form, does not include any directional sensitivity.

Recent studies of mild traumatic brain injury MTBI in professional football in the United States, has yielded yet another criterion function (Newman et al., 2000). This seems to be the first significant change in these matters in recent years. The new function correlates well to historical databases and includes directional sensitivity for both forms of motion. Time duration is also included as an implicit variable. It is has been validated with actual concussion events that have occurred in football that have been reconstructed with crash test dummies. The model is based upon the rather simple premise that, head injury probability/severity depends on the rate of change of kinetic

[11] Abbreviated Injury Scale (AAAM, 1990).

energy of the head during impact. The rate of change of kinetic energy is what is more commonly known as **power**. An equation describing the rate of change of energy of the head, for both forms of motion is of the form

$$HIP = ma_x\, a_x dt + ma_y\, a_y dt + ma_z\, a_z dt + I_x\alpha_x\, \alpha_x dt + I_y\alpha_y\, \alpha_y dt + I_z\alpha_z\, \alpha_z dt$$

where HIP is the head impact power, m is the mass of the head and the Is are the mass moments of inertia of the head about the respective axes. The probability of concussion as a function of HIP has been determined. On the basis of this data, a 50% chance of a concussion occurs if the change of kinetic energy of the head reaches about 12.7kW. A concussion is almost a certainty if the power level reaches 25kW.

Currently, additional MTBI data are being collected and it is anticipated that the HIP will be extended to become a MTBI Index. The Power Index will take a form similar to that above but will include coefficients that both non-dimensionalize the function and include parameters that directly reflect the differences in brain injury tolerance associated with skull movement in different directions.

Summary

Head injury tolerances to impact have been described in terms of the motion of a rigid headform representing the human head. Various functional relationships between the head acceleration and head injury severity have been reviewed. None of the measures relates to a specific injury mechanism or type. They relate only to the severity of closed brain injury associated with rigid skull motion. Research continues to seek a functional relationship between the severity or probability of such brain injury and the detailed manner by which the head moves upon impact.

References

Association for the Advancement of Automotive Medicine. (1990). The abbreviated injury scale.

Federal Motor Vehicle Safety Standard (FMVSS). (1999). 208, Title 49 Code of Federal Regulations (CFR), Department of Transport, National Highway Traffic Safety Administration.

Federal Motor Vehicle Safety Standard (FMVSS). (1997). 218, National Highway Traffic Safety Administration, Department of Transportation, Motorcycle Helmets.

Foster, J.K., Kortage, J.O., & Wolanin, M.J. (1977). Hybrid III – A biomechanically based crash test dummy. *Proceedings of the 21st Stapp Car Crash Conference*, 973–1014.

Gadd, C.W. (1966). Use of a weighted-impulse criterion for estimating injury hazard. *Proceedings of the Tenth Stapp Car Crash Conference*, 164–174.

Gurdjian, E.E., Roberts, V.L., & Thomas, L.M. (1964). Tolerance curves of acceleration and intracranial pressure and protective index in experimental head injury. *Journal of Trauma, 600.*

Hodgson, V.R. & Thomas, L.M. (1971). Comparison of head acceleration injury indices in cadaver skull fracture. *Proceedings of the 15th Stapp Car Crash Conference,* 190–206.

Mertz, H.J., Prasad, P., & Nusholtz, G. (1996). Head injury risk assessment for forehead impacts. *SAE Paper No. 960099.*

National Operating Committee on Standards for Athletic Equipment (NOCSAE). (1977). doc. 002–96, Standard Performance Specification for Newly Manufactured Football Helmets.

Newman, J.A. (1986). A generalized model for brain injury threshold (GAMBIT). *Presented at the International IRCOBI Conference on the Biomechanics of Impact,* 121–131.

Newman, J.A., Shewchenko, N. & Welbourne, N. (2000). A proposed new biomechanical head injury assessment function – the maximum power index" Presented at the 44th Stapp Conference, 215–247.

Ommaya, A.K. (1984). Head injury biomechanics. George G. Snively Memorial Lecture, *Association for the Advancement of Automotive Medicine.*

Snell Standard B95 for Protective Headgear for Use with Bicycles, 1995.

Chapter 4

THE PATHOPHYSIOLOGY OF TRAUMATIC BRAIN INJURY

Christopher C. Giza[1,2]
David A. Hovda[1,3]
[1]Division of Neurosurgery and [2]Pediatric Neurology, and
[3]Department of Medical and Molecular Pharmacology, David Geffen School of Medicine at UCLA, Los Angeles, CA

Traumatic brain injury (TBI) is a leading cause of death and disability in young people (Conroy & Kraus 1988; Tepas, DiScala, Ramenofsky, & Barlow 1990) occurring with a peak incidence of 200-400/100,000 in adolescents, an earlier peak of 120-280/100,000 in children under 5 years of age and a late peak in the elderly (150-250/100,000) (Kraus & McArthur, 2000). Concussion is the most common type of TBI (Kraus, McArthur, Silverman, & Jayaraman, 1996) and is defined as any traumatically induced cerebral dysfunction, with or without loss of consciousness. One of the hallmarks of concussion is the relative paucity of gross structural change in the brain with transient or persistent motor, cognitive or behavioral impairment. That is, the brain is rendered dysfunctional without prominent physical damage.

If the concussed brain is not physically disrupted, then what is the underlying etiology of this cerebral dysfunction? Several mechanisms have been implicated, including ionic shifts, abnormal energy metabolism, altered vascular reactivity and impaired neurotransmission. Brain concussion triggers a multi-layered neurometabolic cascade of physiologic changes that has important implications for cerebral vulnerability, cell death, plasticity and persistent neurocognitive deficits. Our chapter will describe this cascade and its time course in an experimental animal model of concussion. Concussion-induced physiologic derangements will then be discussed in greater detail, from the initial neurotransmitter release and ionic shifts to later alterations of cerebral glucose metabolism and blood flow and ultimately, to chronic impairment of cognition and behavior. The final sections are dedicated to topics of particular interest for sports-related concussion, including the post-concussive window of vulnerability, consequences of multiple successive brain injuries, overuse injury, and developmental brain injury.

The Post-Concussive Neurometabolic Cascade

Traumatic brain injury (TBI) triggers a complex and interwoven sequence of ionic and metabolic events from which damaged cells may eventually recover or, in certain circumstances, degenerate and die (Fig. 4.1). After concussion, there is a significant K^+ efflux from cells, due to mechanical membrane disruption, axonal stretch, and opening of voltage-dependent K^+ channels. Nonspecific depolarization of neurons leads to release of the excitatory neurotransmitter glutamate, which compounds the K^+ flux by activating N-methyl D-aspartate (NMDA) and d-amino-3-hydroxy-5-methyl-4-isoxazole-propionic acid (AMPA) receptors. In an attempt to restore the membrane potential, the Na^+-K^+ ATPase works overtime, consuming increasing amounts of ATP. To meet these elevated ATP requirements, there is a marked upregulation of

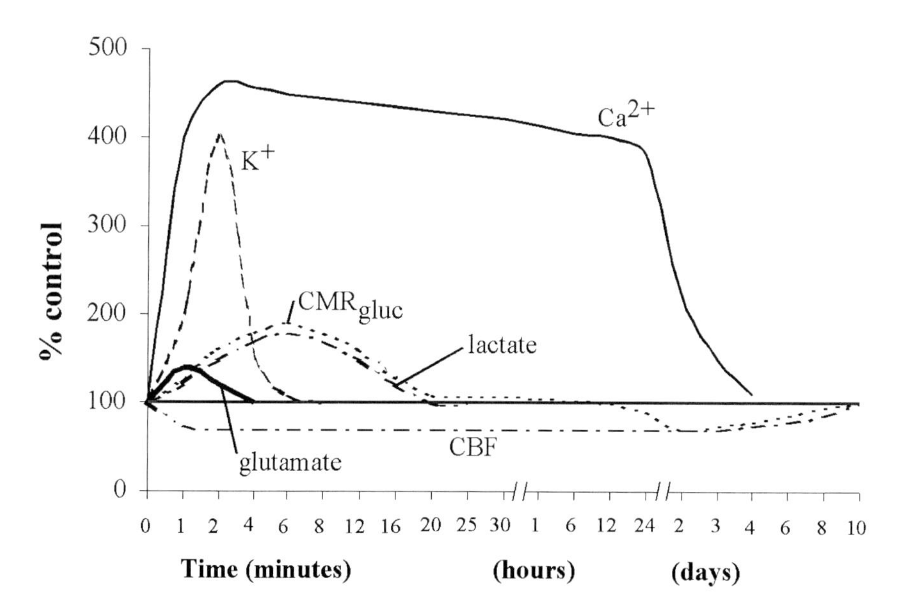

Figure 4.1. Neurometabolic cascade following experimental brain injury in rat.

cellular glycolysis that occurs within minutes after TBI. However, ATP production via oxidative phosphorylation is impaired following TBI. Thus, ATP demand increases at a time when ATP production is deficient, triggering an energy crisis in the traumatized brain. During this period of hyperglycolysis, there is also a commensurate increase in lactate production.

In addition to K^+ efflux, NMDA receptor activation permits a rapid and sustained influx of Ca^{2+}. Elevated intracellular Ca^{2+} can be sequestered in mitochondria, eventually leading to dysfunction of oxidative metabolism and further increasing the cell's dependence on glycolysis-generated ATP. Calcium accumulation may also activate proteases that eventually lead to cell damage or death, and, in axons, excess Ca^{2+} can lead to dysfunction and breakdown of neurofilaments and microtubules.

These ionic shifts and acute alterations in cellular energy metabolism occur in a post-traumatic setting where cerebral blood flow (CBF) is diminished, although not to ischemic levels. Rather, it is the mismatch between glucose delivery and glucose consumption that may predispose to secondary injury. CBF may remain depressed for several days after TBI, possibly limiting the ability of the brain to respond adequately to subsequent perturbations in energy demand.

After the initial period of profound post-injury ionic disturbance and resultant increase in glucose metabolism, the local cerebral metabolic rate for glucose ($lCMR_{gluc}$) decreases significantly below baseline, as does oxidative metabolism. In the rat, this period of diminished glucose metabolism is seen in the cerebral cortex ipsilateral to injury as early as 6 hours after fluid percussion and does not normalize until between 5 and 10 days later. Ipsilateral hypometabolism may also been seen in regions of the hippocampus at 6 hours post-injury, generally normalizing by 24 hours. The precise mechanism of this phenomenon is as yet unknown but it likely involves intracellular calcium accumulation and impaired mitochondrial oxidative metabolism. It is currently uncertain as to whether this period of diminished cerebral metabolism is protective or whether it represents a second potential period of vulnerability.

Early Post-Concussive Pathophysiology (Minutes To Hours)

Acute potassium efflux

Following TBI, the initial ionic response is an abrupt, marked elevation of extracellular potassium (Takahashi, Manaka, & Sano, 1981; Hubschmann & Kornhauser, 1983). Several mechanisms have been proposed to account for this efflux (Fig. 4.2). First, nonspecific breakdown of the plasma membrane may lead to K^+ leakage, particularly in the vicinity of contusions or hemorrhage (Takahashi et al., 1981; Hubschmann & Kornhauser, 1983). However, significant elevations of K^+ occur after concussive brain injury even in the absence of gross pathological change (Takahashi et al., 1981; Katayama, Becker, Tamura, & Hovda, 1990). This may be attributed to the

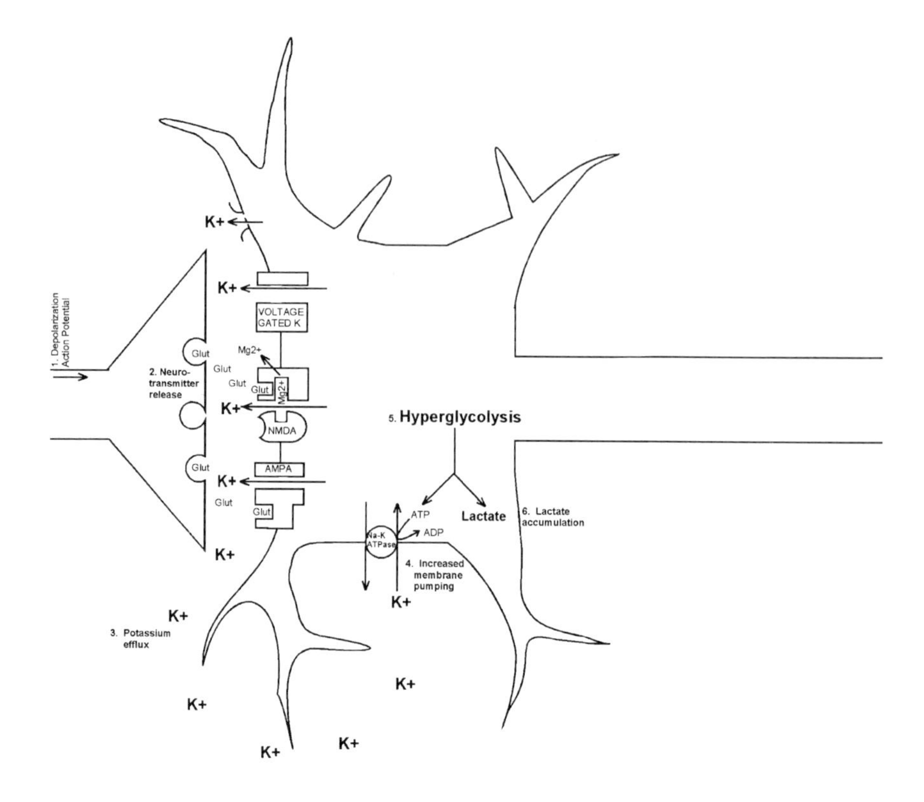

Figure 4.2. Post-traumatic potassium cascade.

diffuse mechanical force associated with brain trauma; indeed, deformation alone may induce depolarization and neuronal firing (Julian & Goldman 1962). Some of this K^+ flux also seems to occur via voltage-gated K^+ channels (Katayama et al., 1990).

Another mechanism for post-traumatic increases in K^+ is through ligand-gated ion channels opened by indiscriminate release of excitatory neurotransmitters, particularly glutamate (Katayama et al., 1990). Activation of kainate and AMPA receptors by excitatory amino acids (EAAs) allows the flow of both sodium and potassium ions across the cell membrane. EAAs also trigger NMDA receptors, which open channels permeable to Ca^{2+} in addition to Na^+ and K^+. Increased post-injury glutamate levels have been shown to correlate with increased K^+ levels, and treatment with the EAA blocker kynurenic acid greatly attenuates this post-traumatic elevation of K^+ (Katayama et al., 1990).

In the normal brain, excess extracellular K^+ is subject to reuptake by surrounding glial cells (Ballanyi, Grafe, & Bruggencate, 1987; Kuffler, 1967; Paulson & Newman, 1987). This compensatory mechanism can maintain physiologic extracellular K^+ levels even after mild concussion or ongoing seizure activity (Moody, Futamachi, & Prince, 1974; Sypert & Ward, 1974) but is overcome by more severe brain trauma (D'Ambrosio, Maris, Grady, Winn, & Janigro, 1999) or ischemia (Astrup, Rehncrona, & Siesjo, 1980; Hansen, 1977; Hanson, 1988). Initially there is a slow rise in extracellular K^+, followed by an abrupt increase as the physiologic ceiling for K^+ balance is overcome. This triggers neuronal depolarization, release of EAAs, and further massive K^+ flux through EAA/ligand-gated ion channels. In the wake of this wave of excitation is a subsequent wave of hyperpolarization and relative suppression of neuronal activity (Nicholson & Kraig, 1981; Prince, Lux, & Neher, 1973; Sugaya, Takato, & Noda, 1975; Van Harreveld, 1978; Somjen & Giacchino, 1985), a phenomenon termed "spreading depression". One important difference between classic "spreading depression" and post-concussive K^+ release is that TBI affects wide areas of the brain simultaneously. Thus, loss of consciousness, amnesia and cognitive impairment may be clinical correlations to post-TBI K^+ release and a "spreading depression-like" state.

Hyperglycolysis and lactate production

In response to perturbations of transmembrane ionic gradients, cells respond with an activation of energy-requiring ionic pumps (Bull & Cummins, 1973; Mayevsky & Chance, 1974; Rosenthal, LaManna, Yamada, Younts, & Somjen, 1979) (to attempt to restore the normal membrane potential. This results in an increase in glucose utilization. It is now well established that concussive injury to the brain also triggers dramatic increases in the $lCMR_{gluc}$ (Shah & West, 1983; Sunami et al., 1989; Yoshino, Hovda, Kawamata, Katayama, & Becker, 1991). Using 2-deoxyglucose autoradiography in rats, $lCMR_{gluc}$ rose up to 81% in cortex ipsilateral to injury. These elevations are seen immediately and persist up to 30 minutes after fluid percussion injury (Yoshino et al.), and up to 4 hours after cortical contusion injury (in areas distant from the actual contusion core) (Samii & Hovda, 1998). Increases in $lCMR_{gluc}$ are also seen over the same time course in ipsilateral hippocampus. Given that cerebral oxidative metabolism normally runs near maximal capacity, it follows that acute increases in energy demand would necessarily require increases in glycolysis (Ackerman & Lear, 1989; Lear & Ackerman, 1989).

Lactate accumulation in the brain occurs after injuries leading to neuronal damage such as ischemia (32-34) (Corbett, Laptook, Nunnally, Hassan, & Jackson, 1988; Biros & Dimlich, 1987; Richards et al., 1987), and also after insults which do not cause overt morphologic change such as concussion (Nilsson & Ponten, 1977; Yang, DeWitt, Becker & Hayes, 1985; DeWitt et al., 1986; Meyer, Kondo, Nomura, Sakamoto, & Teraura, 1970; Nelson, Lowry, & Passonneau, 1966; Nilsson & Nordstrom, 1977). Lactate levels may increase either due to decreased metabolism or increased production. Following concussive brain injury, there is convincing evidence of an acute hyperglycolytic state (Shah & West, 1983; Sunami et al., 1989; Yoshino et al., 1991) as well as an impairment of oxidative metabolism (Verweij et al., 1997; Xiong, Peterson, Muizelaar, & Lee, 1997; Xiong et al., 1998). This increase in glycolysis may be due to both increased demand to drive ionic pumps as well as a decrease in ATP production due to diminished mitochondrial function. In ischemia, oxidative phosphorylation is impaired, and increases in lactate are primarily due to decreased metabolism. However, the accumulation of lactate after concussive injury results from both increased glycolysis and diminished oxidative metabolism, and is therefore fundamentally different than that seen in ischemia.

Elevated lactate has been implicated in neuronal dysfunction by inducing acidosis, membrane damage, altered blood brain barrier permeability and cerebral edema (Friede & Van Houten, 1961; Gardiner, Smith, Kagstrom, Shohami, & Siesjo, 1982; Kalimo, Rehncrona, Soderfeldt, Olsson, & Siesjo, 1981; Kalimo, Rehncrona, & Soderfeldt, 1981; Myers 1979; Siemkowicz & Hansen, 1978). In TBI models, excess lactate appears to leave the affected cells more vulnerable to secondary ischemic injury (Becker & Jenkins, 1987). It remains to be seen whether this relationship holds in the setting of repeated TBI. An alternative hypothesis proposed by Tsacopoulos and Magistretti holds that following injury, glia increase production of lactate, which is then transported into neurons as an alternate fuel source during the period of energy crisis (Tsacopoulos & Magistretti, 1996).

Uncoupling of cerebral blood flow and glucose metabolism

Cerebral blood flow (CBF) changes have also been well documented in acute head trauma. Experimentally, fluid percussion injury may precipitate an almost immediate reduction of up to 50% in cerebral blood flow (Yuan, Prough, Smith, & DeWitt, 1988; Yamakami & McIntosh, 1989; Velarde, Fisher, & Hovda, 1992; Doberstein, Velarde, Badie, & Hovda, 1992), however, this reduction does *not* approach the levels associated with frank ischemia (85% reduction) (Ginsberg, Zhao, Alonso, Loor-Estades, Dietrich, & Busto, 1997). Clinically, human brain injury may also demonstrate decreases in CBF; however, ischemia is not a major component of isolated concussive brain injury in humans.

Normally, cerebral blood flow is tightly coupled to cerebral glucose metabolism. Although post-traumatic decreases in CBF do not lead to overt ischemia, the injured brain may dramatically increase ATP utilization, requiring increased delivery of substrate to power cellular recovery mechanisms. In this setting of greater demand (hyperglycolysis), impaired supply of metabolites may become an important factor in delayed injury or increased vulnerability to further insults.

Intermediate Post-Concussive Pathophysiology (Hours to Days)

Persistent calcium influx and impaired oxidative metabolism

In the hours following experimental TBI, there is a rapid and sustained influx of Ca^{2+} (Cortez, McIntosh, & Noble, 1989; Fineman, Hovda, Smith,

Yoshino, & Becker, 1993; McIntosh, 1993; Osteen, Moore, Prins, & Hovda, 2001). Neuronal depolarization and nonspecific membrane disruption after trauma lead to release of EAAs that, in turn, activate NMDA receptors. The activated NMDA receptor creates an open channel through which Ca^{2+} can enter the cell (Fig. 4.3). Calcium has been shown to accumulate in cerebral ischemia (Choi, 1988; Dienel, 1984; Kato, Kogure, & Nakano, 1989; Sakamoto, Kogure, Kato, & Ohtomo, 1986; Rappaport, Young, & Flamm, 1987; Deshpande, Siesjo, & Wieloch, 1987), spinal cord contusion (Stokes, Fox, & Hollinden, 1983; Young, Ven, & Blight, 1982; Young & Koreh, 1986; Happel et al., 1981), or concussive brain injury (Fineman et al., 1993; Osteen et al., 2001). The time course of calcium flux after fluid percussion injury has been well characterized, with an immediate increase in radiolabeled $^{45}Ca^{2+}$ accumulation particularly in the cerebral cortex, dorsal hippocampus and striatum ipsilateral to the injury. This elevation persists for at least 48 hours without resulting in significant morphological damage, returning to normal by 4 days. Administration of an N-type Ca^{2+} channel blocker diminishes the level and duration of post-traumatic $^{45}Ca^{2+}$ accumulation (Badie, Prins, & Hovda, 1993; Hovda et al., 1994).

When faced with excessive increases of intracellular Ca^{2+}, the cell may sequester calcium in mitochondria (Verweij et al. 1997; Xiong, Gu, Peter-

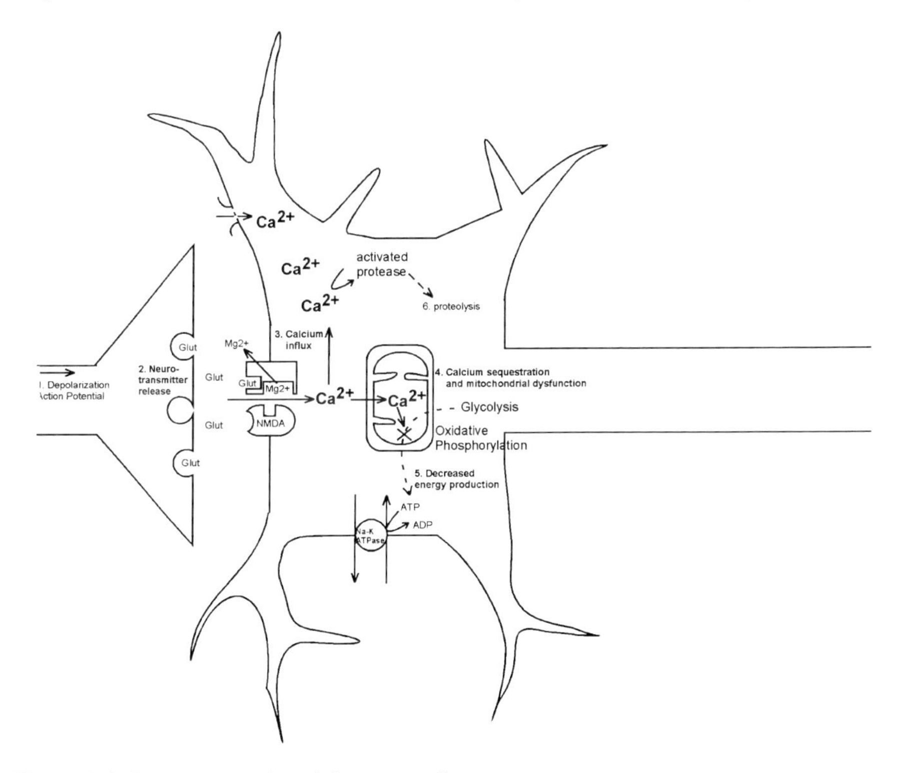

Figure 4.3. Post-traumatic calcium cascade.

son, Muizelaar, & Lee, 1997). Increases in mitochondrial Ca^{2+} can lead to metabolic dysfunction and eventually, energy failure. Cytochrome oxidase (CO) histochemistry has been used to detect long-term changes in oxidative metabolism in many brain injury models (Hovda, Yoshino, Kawamata, Katayama, & Becker, 1991). In ipsilateral cerebral cortex, relative reductions in CO activity were detected 1 day after fluid percussion injury. This reduction in oxidative metabolism recovered on day 2 and was reinstated on day 3, becoming most pronounced 5 days after injury. By 10 days, cortical CO activity recovered to normal levels. Lesser but more persistent changes were seen in ipsilateral hippocampus, with decreased CO activity evident up to 10 days in some regions. Other injury models in which diminished oxidative metabolism is seen include cortical contusion and ablation.

This reduction of oxidative metabolism occurs in the setting of a delayed post-traumatic decline in glycolysis, which is first evident 24 hours after experimental FPI in the rat (Fig. 4.1). Diffuse post-injury impairment of glucose metabolism measured by 2-deoxyglucose autoradiography has also been reported after ischemia (Nedergaard, Jakobsen, & Diemer, 1988; Kushner et al., 1984; Shiraishi, Sharp, & Simon, 1989), cortical freezing lesions (Pappius, 1982; Colle, Holmes, & Pappius, 1986), tumors (Kushner et al., 1984; Patronas et al., 1984) and neocortical ablations (Feeney, Sutton, & Boyeson, 1985; Sutton, Hovda, & Chugani, 1989). In humans, these post-traumatic changes in glucose metabolism may last significantly longer (Bergsneider et al., 2000). Overall decreased cerebral glucose metabolism may account for post-TBI impairments in consciousness, memory and cognition. What is not clear is whether this hypometabolism is somehow protecting the injured brain from the detrimental effects of acute CBF/glucose metabolism mismatch or whether this represents a period during which the brain is metabolically unable to rise to the challenge of increased ATP demands. If the latter is true, this would be important for two reasons. One would be that a second ionic derangement, such as a second concussion, would be less rapidly compensated due to insufficient energy to drive increases in Na^{+}/K^{+} ATPase activity. The second consequence of an obligatory period of post-TBI metabolic depression might be that the brain is less able to be activated in response to stimuli, which has already been demonstrated experimentally in animals (Dietrich, Alonso, Busto, & Ginsberg, 1994; D'Ambrosio, Maris, Grady, Winn, & Janigro, 1998). In an athlete, an impairment of cerebral activation in response to stimuli might manifest as decreased performance, which in some sports would predispose the individual to a greater risk for a second injury. Similarly, the acquisition of new skills could be impaired during this period of metabolic depression. A final consideration would be that forced attempts to activate hypometabolic cortex may actually be damaging, a form of secondary injury.

Post-concussive decreases in magnesium

After experimental traumatic brain injury, intracellular levels of Mg^{2+} have been shown to decrease significantly and remain depressed for up to 4 days

(Vink, McIntosh, Demediuk, Faden 1987; Vink, McIntosh, Weiner, & Faden, 1987; Vink, Faden, & McIntosh, 1988; Vink & McIntosh, 1990). This decrease in Mg^{2+} has been correlated with post-traumatic neurological deficits in rats (McIntosh, Faden, Yamakami, & Vink, 1988). Using $MgCl_2$ or $MgSO_4$, the post-injury depression of Mg^{2+} has been partially alleviated, with concomitant improvements in neurologic motor performance.

There are many postulated mechanisms as to how decreased Mg^{2+} leads to neuronal dysfunction after brain injury. Magnesium is so tightly woven into the fabric of cellular energy metabolism that a decrease in intracellular Mg^{2+} may have a multitude of detrimental effects (Garfinkel & Garfinkel, 1985; Ebel & Gunther, 1980; Aikawa 1981). Generation of ATP is impaired in both glycolysis and oxidative phosphorylation when magnesium levels are low. Magnesium is also necessary for initiation of protein synthesis and maintenance of the cellular membrane potential.

In addition, the voltage-gate of the NMDA receptor ionophore is dependent on the presence of Mg^{2+}. At rest, a Mg^{2+} ion obstructs the channel and is only dislodged by depolarization; in a state of Mg^{2+} depletion, this voltage block may be overcome more easily, leading to greater influx of Ca^{2+} and its myriad of potentially dangerous intracellular sequelae.

White matter damage and axonal dysfunction

Acutely, stretch injury to axons leads to altered membrane potential and even depolarization. Changes in membrane permeability may be demonstrated up to 6 hours post-injury by horseradish peroxidase techniques (Pettus, Christman, Giebel, & Povlishock, 1996; Povlishock & Pettus, 1996). This increased axolemmal permeability appears to lead to axonal Ca^{2+} influx and mitochondrial swelling (Fig. 4.4), which has been seen after primary axotomy following crush injury (Mata, Staple, & Fink, 1986) and has more recently been reported after stretch injury without primary axotomy (Maxwell, McCreath, Graham, & Gennarelli, 1995).

Axonal microtubules may be affected by Ca^{2+} influx in several ways. One subtype of microtubule, dubbed cold-labile, is exquisitely sensitive to Ca^{2+}, and rapidly broken down in the presence of elevated Ca^{2+}. Cold-stable microtubules, on the other hand, are more resistant to Ca^{2+}; however, when Ca^{2+} interacts with calmodulin, they too may undergo disassembly. Loss of microtubules appears most pronounced at the nodes of Ranvier, and may occur 6-24 hours after initial axonal injury, depending on the model (Pettus & Povlishock, 1996; Maxwell & Graham, 1997).

Neurofilaments also undergo structural changes after axonal tensile injury. Starting as early as 5 minutes and lasting up to 6 hours after injury, neurofilaments may undergo compaction (Maxwell & Graham, 1997). This decrease in interneurofilament distance is hypothesized to be due to alterations in neurofilament sidearms, possibly by collapse or cleavage. Changes in phosphorylation may affect neurofilament structural stability or conformation (Sternberger & Sternberger, 1983; Nakamura et al., 1990; Nixon, 1993).

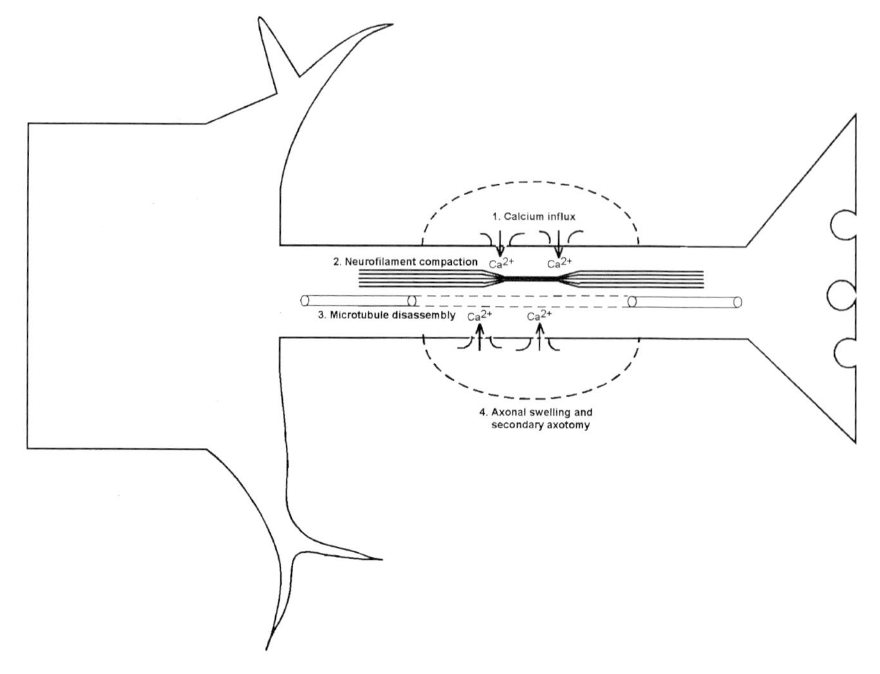

Figure 4.4. Mechanisms of diffuse axonal injury

Alternately, activation of calpain may lead to sidearm proteolysis and neurofilament collapse (Johnson, Greenwood, Costello, & Troncoso, 1991).

Late Changes Following Concussion (Days, Weeks or Longer)

Delayed calcium accumulation and cell death

Intracellular accumulation of Ca^{2+} is of great importance given the well described role of Ca^{2+} in secondary cell death (Schanne, Kane, Young, & Farber, 1979; Choi, 1987); however, the presence of increased Ca^{2+} post-concussion does not inevitably lead to detectable levels of neuronal loss. After mild and moderate experimental concussive injuries, Ca^{2+} accumulation peaks in 2 days and resolves, without significant cell loss, in 4 days (Fineman et al., 1993; Osteen et al., 2001). In animals sustaining more severe injuries and demonstrating morphological damage, the elevation of $^{45}Ca^{2+}$ at the injury site persists beyond 4 days (Fineman, Hovda et al.; Osteen et al.). This suggests that there is a threshold of injury or Ca^{2+} accumulation, beyond which anatomic changes can be seen after concussive brain injury. However, these findings may also mean that there is a window of intervention for the reduction of post-TBI Ca^{2+} influx that may be neuroprotective. Not surprisingly, there are also specific patterns of Ca^{2+} accumulation seen after comparable injuries at different developmental ages (Fig. 4.5)(Osteen et al., 2001).

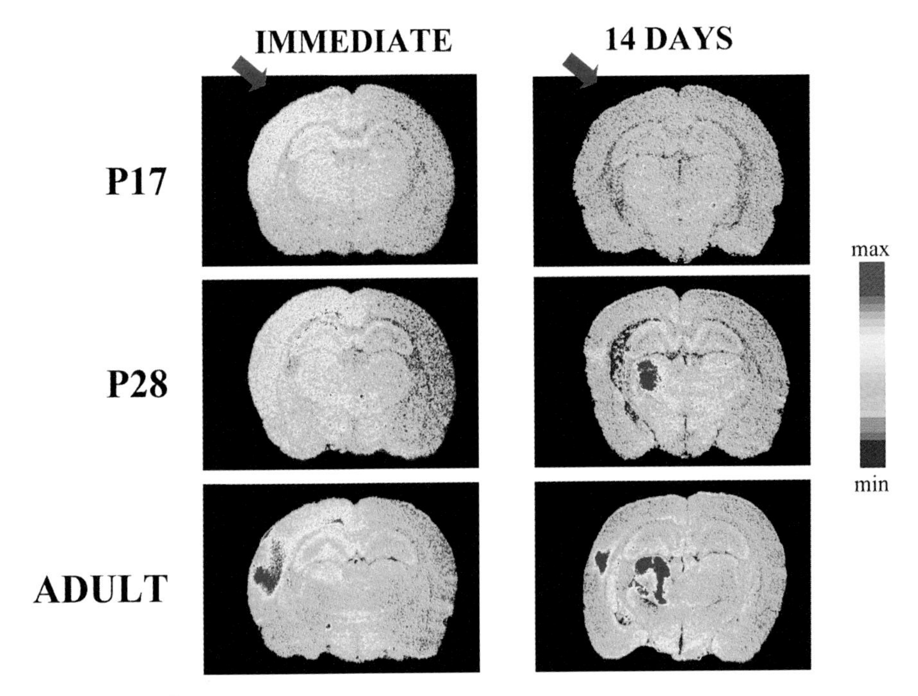

Figure 4.5. Ca^{2+} autoradiographs.

Secondary axotomy

Acutely after injury, structural changes in axonal microtubules and neurofilaments are seen, possibly in response to injury-induced Ca^{2+} influx. These disruptions lead to foci of impaired axonal transport, which continues to function in intact axonal segments. Thus, membranous organelles moving along the axon will accumulate in areas of cytoskeletal abnormality, leading to focal axonal swelling (Maxwell & Graham, 1997). Over time, neurofilament compaction worsens, axolemmal-myelin connections are disrupted, and evidence of a constriction appears in the center of the area of axonal swelling (Povlishock & Christman, 1995). This constriction ultimately leads to secondary axotomy with resultant formation of axonal bulbs. The earliest signs of secondary axonal disconnection are seen beginning 4 hours post-injury, but may continue to evolve over many days or even weeks in humans (Blumbergs et al., 1994).

Neurotransmitter alterations

Post-injury derangements in neurotransmission are another potential mechanism by which concussion can lead to long term deficits. A number of studies have implicated brain injury with subacute changes in glutamatergic (Miller et al., 1990; Giza, Lee, Kremen, & Hovda, 2000; Osteen, Giza, & Hovda, 2000; Sihver et al., 2001), adrenergic (Feeney et al., 1985; Pappius, 1988), and cholinergic (Gorman, Fu, Hovda, Murray, & Traystman, 1996; Dixon et al.,

1999; Sihver et al., 2001) neurotransmission. A consequence of brain injury is the eventual downregulation of excitatory neurotransmitter receptor function, which can last for days to months, depending on the receptor and the severity of injury. Diminished excitatory neurotransmission has been associated with cognitive deficits such as impaired attention, learning and memory.

Inhibitory neurotransmission also appears to be altered after TBI (Sihver et al., 2001). Studies have demonstrated a loss of GABAergic inhibitory neurons after experimental brain injury and suggest a relationship between loss of inhibition and subsequent development of seizures (Lee, Smith, Hovda, & Becker, 1995). The balance of excitatory and inhibitory inputs in specific brain regions is perturbed following TBI, and these changes may lead to lasting problems.

Post-concussive Vulnerability and Repeated Concussion

Concussive brain injury has been shown to elicit a neurometabolic cascade of acute ionic changes, metabolic perturbations and axonal dysfunction. Longer-term derangements that follow brain trauma include calcium accumulation, elevations in lactate, decreased glucose metabolism, decreased cerebral blood flow, axonal disconnection and neurotransmitter disturbances. It is during this post-injury period, when energy metabolism may already be stretched to its limits, that the cell is most vulnerable to further insults (Jenkins, Marmarou, Lewelt, & Becker, 1986). Clinically, much of the management of the head-injured patient focuses on preventing delayed neuronal damage by maintaining cerebral perfusion, restoring electrolyte balance, providing adequate oxygenation and minimizing excessive cerebral metabolic demands.

Metabolic periods of potential post-traumatic vulnerability to a second concussion

One practical issue concerning athletic head injury is the appropriate time to refrain from sporting activity after a concussion. Understanding post-injury metabolic changes in a model of experimental concussive brain injury may suggest a time frame for increased vulnerability to repeated brain concussion.

First, the period of glucose metabolism-cerebral blood flow uncoupling may represent a time of increased danger for the injured brain. In the rat cortex, this period begins immediately after concussion and appears to last for at least 30 minutes (Yoshino et al., 1991). At a time of metabolic stress (increased glucose need and decreased delivery), the brain may be less tolerant of further increases in metabolic demand in response to a second injury. Thus, neurons that are transiently dysfunctional after an initial injury may become irreversibly damaged after a recurrent injury.

Secondly, the accumulation of intracellular Ca^{2+} that occurs post-injury may leave cells in a perilous situation when faced with repeated Ca^{2+} influx. High levels of intracellular Ca^{2+} lead to mitochondrial dysfunction, impairing metabolism at a time when the cell can least tolerate it. Increased Ca^{2+} may also activate proteases that begin the cascade leading to cell death. In rats, the period of post-traumatic Ca^{2+} accumulation appears to last from 2-4 days (Fineman et al., 1993; Osteen et al., 2001).

Lastly, changes in neurotransmission may signal a period of vulnerability. Impaired excitatory neurotransmission may occur for days after concussion in immature rats (Giza et al., 2000). A second injury during this period may trigger further diminution of receptor activity, leading to more severe or longer duration neurocognitive problems. Particularly in sports, where a player may be "back in the game" before full functional recovery, subtle impairments in cognition will likely place the individual at greater risk for recurrent injury.

Alternatively, decreases in inhibitory GABAergic neurons following TBI in adult rats may leave them more vulnerable to uncontrolled excitatory input such as the massive post-concussive K+ efflux and glutamate release. Excessive excitation can result in seizure activity, increased energy demand and even cell death.

Each of these trauma-induced physiologic changes (hyperglycolysis, Ca^{2+} accumulation, neurotransmitter dysfunction) has its own particular time frame. Preliminary studies with a double concussion model demonstrate comparable increases in morphologic injury and prolonged metabolic depression when the two concussions were separated by 1, 2, or 5 hours (Fu, Smith, Thomas, & Hovda, 1992). In another study, double-concussed rats (1-2 hours between injuries) showed significantly increased glial fibrillary acidic protein (GFAP; a marker for gliosis/scarring) immunostaining and evidence of cell loss when compared with rats receiving only a single fluid percussion injury (Badie, Hovda, & Becker, 1992). In rats, therefore, it appears the time period of vulnerability to second concussion is at least 5 hours. It remains to be seen how this translates into the human condition. In general, the time frame for events in rats is significantly shorter than analogous periods in humans, so it would not be surprising if the duration of increased vulnerability in humans is actually much longer than in rat experimental models. Interestingly, when multiple mild experimental concussions precede a more severe one by 3-5 days, a recent study in rats suggests that the early injuries precondition the brain for an improved functional outcome (Allen, Gerami, & Esser, 2000), although the anatomic injury appears unchanged. However, other studies show that repeated mild head injuries can lead to long-term cognitive dysfunction, even in the absence of overt structural damage (DeFord et al., 2002). Obviously, mechanism and severity of injury clearly has effects on the magnitude and duration of post-concussive metabolic dysfunction, and are likely other important variables to consider when developing back-to-play guidelines.

Other considerations with repeat concussive injury

Second impact syndrome is a very rare but catastrophic occurrence where a relatively minor second trauma superimposed on a brain recovering from an initial injury leads to rapid neurologic deterioration, cerebral edema and death (Cantu 1995). While diagnostic criteria for the syndrome are still undergoing debate, initial reports suggest a strong predilection for children and adolescents (Pickles, 1950; Bruce et al., 1981; Bruce, 1984; Aldrich et al., 1992; MMWR, 1997). Children and adults respond to brain injury differently, with children seemingly more vulnerable to cerebral swelling and subdural hematomas after mild injury. One proposed mechanism for second impact syndrome suggests impaired autoregulation in the traumatized developing brain leads to hyperemia and edema (Lobato et al., 1991; Snoek, Minderhoud, & Wilmink, 1984).

Another important issue is the possibility of permanent brain dysfunction or damage after multiple concussions. It may well be that the window of vulnerability to a second brain injury has two components. First, there may be an acute period where the brain is more susceptible to ionic and metabolic derangements that can lead to cell death, and second, a more chronic phase where recovering neurotransmitter systems are at risk for developing permanent dysfunction through aberrant connections, with or without cell loss.

Overuse Injury

After many sports-related injuries, there is often significant pressure for the athlete to return to practice and/or competition as soon as physically possible. In general, there is an increasing awareness about the potential danger for rapid return to competitive play after cerebral concussion, particularly in regards to vulnerability to a second brain injury. On the other hand, return to vigorous practice might appear to be a safe alternative and a reasonable method for maintaining physical performance and conditioning until the athlete is ready to return to play.

Experimental studies with unilateral rat cortical injury have demonstrated the importance of limb use in restoration of function after brain lesioning (Schallert, Kozlowski, Humm, & Cocke, 1997). After unilateral forelimb somatosensory cortex lesions, there is an overgrowth of dendrites in the homotypic cortical region of the uninjured hemisphere that is dependent on continued use of the uninjured forelimb. In unilaterally injured rats, immobilization of the intact forelimb not only impaired cortical dendritic growth but also resulted in more severe and long-lasting behavioral deficits. Perhaps even more concerning was the finding that this immobilization, and, hence, overuse of the injured limb, led to a marked increase in the lesion size in the injured cortex (Kozlowski, James, & Schallert, 1996). This suggests that increased functional demand placed upon the damaged cortex acutely may actually exacerbate the deficit, both anatomically and behaviorally. While there is no doubt that rehabilitative efforts are beneficial after brain injury, these findings would seem to indicate that, at least shortly after brain injury, it is possible to get "too much of a good thing".

A follow-up to the forced overuse study above demonstrated that when immobilization of the intact forelimb occurred within the first 7 days after cortical injury, there was both an impairment of functional recovery and a greater loss of brain tissue at the injury site. If the forced overuse was initiated longer than a week after cortical injury, there was still a delay in functional recovery, but the increase in the lesion size was not seen (Humm, Kozlowski, James, Gotts, & Schallert, 1998). Thus, there appear to be post-brain injury windows of vulnerability, not only to a second injury as described in the previous section, but also possibly to excessive behavioral stimulation in the immediate post-injury period. It is not clear whether this post-injury sensitivity to overuse occurs in humans and if so, what its duration may be. At the very least, further studies are warranted in this area, and it may be prudent to limit extreme post-TBI behavioral rehabilitation or return to practice to a time period somewhat after the acute injury, particularly after severe concussion or repeated concussions.

Concussion in the Developing Brain

Athletic brain injury is of particular concern in children, who tend to participate in sports putting them at risk for head trauma and in whom neurological development is ongoing. Positron emission tomography (PET) studies of cerebral glucose metabolism in children up to age 15 years demonstrate clear differences in levels of $lCMR_{gluc}$ when compared with adults (Chugani, Phelps, & Mazziotta, 1987). It is not unreasonable to assume that a diffuse injury might have lasting effects upon the complex neurochemical and anatomic events that occur during brain development. It is also important to realize that, although signs of overt neurologic dysfunction may not necessarily be prominent after juvenile brain injury, it is difficult to assess the possibility of lost cognitive potential, which may only be demonstrable at a later developmental period or under specific circumstances. Conversely, not all developmental difficulties that arise in a child post-injury are necessarily a result of the injury, as many brain-injured children have pre-existing neurological or behavioral abnormalities.

Age-specific vulnerability

Clinical experience suggests that, in general, the young brain may recover more rapidly and more completely from injury than the mature brain. This improvement in outcome has been attributed to greater plasticity in the developing brain. Immature rats subjected to moderate lateral fluid percussion injury show no evidence of neurological or pathological deficits post-trauma (Prins, Lee, Cheng, Becker, & Hovda, 1996; Prins & Hovda, 1998; Fineman, Giza, Nahed, Lee, & Hovda, 2000). In a weight drop model, post-traumatic deficits are only seen at levels of injury where mortality in unventilated rats approaches 75% (Adelson, Dixon, Robichaud, & Kochanek, 1997). Spatial learning as assessed by Morris Water Maze performance is impaired by moderate concussive injury in adult rats, but not in postnatal day 17 rat pups (Prins & Hovda, 1998). Post-traumatic hyperglycolysis is also seen in immature rats, with levels of glucose utilization generally higher than that seen in adults after injury. Delayed hypometabolism of glucose is evident bilaterally 1 day after concussion, is milder than in adults, and resolves completely by 3 days (Thomas, Prins, Samii, & Hovda, 2000).

However, there is also sufficient evidence to suggest that there are periods of developmental vulnerability when the immature brain is more sensitive to injury. Mortality after pediatric brain injury is higher in young children when compared with adolescents. Some series report an increased incidence of severe cerebral edema in head injured young children as a possible factor for this higher mortality (Aldrich et al., 1992). In an experimental model of developmental fluid percussion injury, immature rats became hypotensive after concussion of all severities and tended to have longer apnea times than adults after mild injuries; in addition, mortality among immature rats subjected to severe levels of fluid percussion approached 100% (Prins, Lee et al., 1996).

Developmental plasticity and traumatic brain injury

Developmental deficits after childhood brain trauma are difficult to assess due to variations in injury severity, location, and disruption of normal childhood activities resulting from hospitalization and corresponding rehabilitation. Long-term follow-up studies demonstrate persistent neurocognitive deficits in 23.7% of brain-injured children at 5 years (Klonoff, Low, & Clark, 1977). In a study of visual and verbal memory function one year after closed head injury in 3 pediatric age ranges, injury severity was related to severity of post-traumatic visual memory deficits in all groups, consistent with the fact that visual memory functions were already well established in even the earliest age group. Verbal memory, which was rapidly expanding in adolescents but not well developed in younger children, demonstrated a relationship with injury severity only in adolescents. This is one example of how injury at a particular developmental time point may manifest age-dependent sequelae (Levin, Eisenberg, Wigg, & Kobayashi, 1982).

Environment enrichment is an experimental model of developmental plasticity wherein rats reared as a group in a cage with multiple objects, toys and tunnels demonstrate neuroanatomic changes and improved cognitive performance. Characteristic anatomic features of enrichment include increased cortical thickness and cortical weight, due to increased neuronal size, more elaborate dendritic arborization, more synapses and more glial cells (Rosenzweig & Bennett, 1996; Bennett, Diamond, Krech, & Rosenzweig, 1964; Greenough, Volkmar, & Juraska, 1973). When tested for spatial learning capacity with the Morris Water Maze, rats reared in the enriched environment consistently outperform their littermates reared in standard laboratory cages (Tees, Buhrman, & Hanley, 1990). Although enrichment may occur at

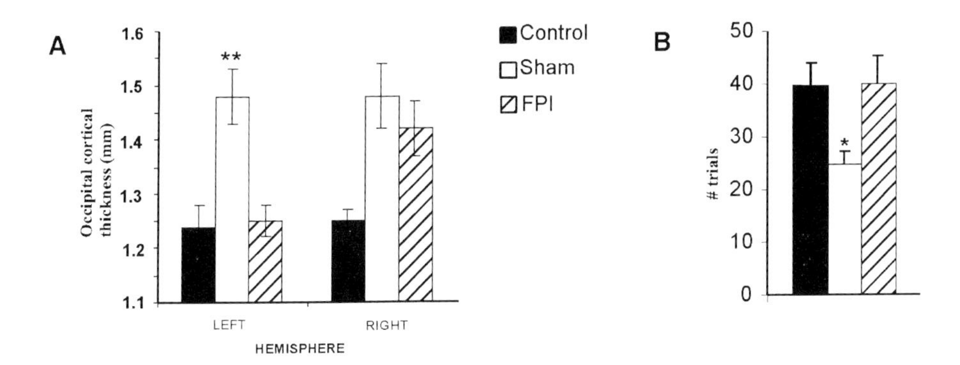

Figuur 4.6. Effects of FPI on enriched environment-induced plasticity.

any age, it is usually most robust in young preweanling rats (Venable et al., 2000), becoming more difficult to elicit with increasing age.

When postnatal day 20 rat pups were subjected to moderate lateral fluid percussion injury, they demonstrated no overt neurological deficits or alterations in open field activity. Morris Water Maze testing showed no difference between injured and uninjured rat pups, and histologic evaluation revealed no structural lesions or cell loss. However, when these brain-injured young rats were reared in an enriched environment, they failed to develop the typical anatomic changes described above, and their performance in the Morris Water Maze was equivalent to unenriched rats (Fig. 4.6; (Fineman et al., 2000)).

Thus, in this model, brain concussion led to a defect in developmental plasticity in the absence of detectable baseline morphologic and behavioral abnormalities. Recently, other studies in the immature brain have substantiated this idea of a trauma-induced developmental disability, by demonstrating impairment of experience-dependent dendritic arborization (Ip, Giza, Griesbach, & Hovda, 2002) and aberrant synaptic architecture (Prins, Povlishock, & Phillips, 2003) after experimental concussion. It remains to be seen whether this impairment of normal development is permanent or if there is a window of dysfunction after which the animal may regain the ability for neural reorganization.

Summary

Even in the absence of significant degenerative change, concussive brain injury induces a complex pathophysiological cascade that begins with immediate disturbances of ionic flux, neurotransmitter release, glucose metabolism and cerebral blood flow. In an animal experimental model, acute increases in glucose utilization give way to diminished glycolysis and oxidative metabolism which may persist a week or longer. Calcium influx occurs early and recovers more rapidly, usually over several days. Axonal injury may be immediate, but delayed secondary axotomy has been reported weeks after injury in humans. Persistent dysfunction in excitatory and inhibitory neurotransmission is a potential mechanism for chronic cognitive and neurobehavioral symptoms following brain concussion. Current guidelines for return to play only upon resolution of all neurocognitive deficits are a good starting point, but more precise time-windows may be elucidated with increasing understanding of and improved ability to monitor specific derangements such as cerebral glucose metabolism, regional brain activation, and neurotransmitter levels.

Repeated injury may magnify reversible neurometabolic abnormalities to the point of permanent cellular degeneration. In some cases, repeated injury may consist of premature activation of injured neurons in the absence of trauma. Also, cerebral responsiveness may be diminished in the post-injury period, raising the risk of an early return to normal play by increasing the likelihood of injury recurrence.

Finally, traumatic injury to the immature brain should be taken seriously, despite the apparent resiliency of youth. Diffuse biomechanical cerebral injury may disrupt normal developmental neural pathways and impair experience-dependent plasticity, with a resultant loss of cognitive potential. Additionally, the developing brain may be uniquely vulnerable to alterations in metabolism, connectivity and neurotransmission but may only manifest deficits with time; therefore, injured children should be closely monitored for the later appearance of behavioral and intellectual difficulties.

Acknowledgements

Special thanks to G.G. Heintz-Jacobs for her assistance in preparation of this manuscript.

Figures 4.1–4.4 are reprinted from R.C. Canta, *Neurologic Athlete Head and Spine Injuries*, 2000, with permission from Elsevier.

Figures 4.5 and 4.6 are taken from Osteen et al., *Journal of Neurotrauma*, 2001, and Fineman et al., *Journal of Neurotrauma*, 2000, respectively, with permission from Mary Ann Liebert Publishing.

References

Ackermann, R.F., Lear, J.L. (1989). Glycolysis-induced discordance between glucose metabolic rates measured with radiolabeled fluorodeoxyglucose and glucose. *Journal of Cerebral Blood Flow Metabolism, 9*(6), 774–785.

Adelson, P.D., Dixon, C.E., Robichaud, P., & Kochanek, P.M. (1997). Motor and cognitive functional deficits following diffuse traumatic brain injury in the immature rat. *Journal of Neurotrauma, 14*(2), 99–108.

Aikawa, J,.K. (1981). *Magnesium: Its Biologic Significance*. Boca Raton, FL: CRC Press.

Aldrich, E.F., Eisenberg, H.M., Saydjari, C., Luerssen, T.G., Foulkes, M.A., Jane, J.A. et al. (1992). Diffuse brain swelling in severely head-injured children. A report from the NIH Traumatic Coma Data Bank. *Journal of Neurosurgery, 76*(3), 450–454.

Allen, G.V., Gerami, D., & Esser, M.J. (2000). Conditioning effects of repetitive mild neurotrauma on motor function in an animal model of focal brain injury. *Neuroscience, 99*(1), 93–105.

Astrup, J., Rehncrona, S., & Siesjo, B.K. (1980). The increase in extracellular potassium concentration in the ischemic brain in relation to the preischemic functional activity and cerebral metabolic rate. *Brain Research, 199*(1), 161–174.

Badie, H., Hovda, D.A., & Becker, D.P. (1992). Glial fibrillary acidic protein (GFAP) expression following concussive brain injury: A quantitative study of the effects of a second insult [abstract]. *Journal of Neurotrauma, 9*, 56.

Badie, H., Prins, M.L., & Hovda, D.A. (1993). Omega-conopeptide reduces the extent of calcium accumulation following traumatic brain injury [Abstract]. *Society for Neuroscience, 19*, 1485.

Ballanyi, K., Grafe, P., & ten Bruggencate, G. (1987). Ion activities and potassium uptake mechanisms of glial cells in guinea-pig olfactory cortex slices. *Journal of Physiology* (London), *382*, 159–174.

Becker, D.P. & Jenkins, L.W. (1987). The pathophysiology of head trauma. In T.A. Miller, B. Rowlands (Eds.), *The Physiological Basis of Modern Surgical Care* (pp. 763–788). St. Louis: Mosby.

Bennett, E.L., Diamond, M.C., Krech, D., & Rosenzweig, M.R. (1964). Chemical and anatomical plasticity of brain. *Science, 164*, 610–619.

Bergsneider, M., Hovda, D.A., Lee, S.M., Kelly, D.F., McArthur, D.L., Vespa, P.M. et al. (2000). Dissociation of cerebral glucose metabolism and level of consciousness during the period of metabolic depression following human traumatic brain injury. *Journal of Neurotrauma, 17*(5), 389–401.

Biros, M.H. & Dimlich, R.V. (1987). Brain lactate during partial global ischemia and reperfusion: effect of pretreatment with dichloroacetate in a rat model. *American Journal of Emergency Medicine, 5*(4), 271–277.

Blumbergs, P.C., Scott, G., Manavis, J., Wainwright, H., Simpson, D.A., & McLean, A.J. (1994). Staining of amyloid precursor protein to study axonal damage in mild head injury. *Lancet, 344*(8929), 1055–1056.

Bruce, D.A., Alavi, A., Bilaniuk, L., Dolinskas, C., Obrist, W., & Uzzell, B. (1981). Diffuse cerebral swelling following head injuries in children: the syndrome of "malignant brain edema". *Journal of Neurosurgery, 54*(2), 170–178.

Bruce, D.A. (1984). Delayed deterioration of consciousness after trivial head injury in childhood [editorial]. *British Medial Journal (Clinical Research Ed), 289*(6447), 715–716.

Bull, R.J., & Cummins, J.T. (1973). Influence of potassium on the steady-state redox potential of the electron transport chain in slices of rat cerebral cortex and the effect of ouabain. *Journal of Neurochemistry, 21*(4), 923–937.

Cantu, R.C. (1995). Second impact syndrome: A risk in any contact sport. *Physician Sports Medicine, 23*, 27–34.

Choi, D.W. (1987). Ionic dependence of glutamate neurotoxicity. *Journal of Neuroscience, 7*(2), 369–379.

Choi, D.W. (1988). Calcium-mediated neurotoxicity: relationship to specific channel types and role in ischemic damage. *Trends Neuroscience, 11*(10), 465–469.

Chugani, H.T., Phelps, M.E., Mazziotta, J.C. (1987). Positron emission tomography study of human brain functional development. *Annals of Neurology, 22*(4), 487–497.

Colle, L.M., Holmes, L.J., & Pappius, H.M. (1986). Correlation between behavioral status and cerebral glucose utilization in rats following freezing lesion. *Brain Research, 397*(1), 27-36.

Conroy, C. & Kraus, J.F. (1988). Survival after brain injury. Cause of death, length of survival, and prognostic variables in a cohort of brain-injured people. *Neuroepidemiology, 7*(1), 13–22.

Corbett, R.J., Laptook, A.R., Nunnally, R.L., Hassan, A., & Jackson, J. (1988). Intracellular pH, lactate, and energy metabolism in neonatal brain during partial ischemia measured in vivo by 31P and 1H nuclear magnetic resonance spectroscopy. *Journal of Neurochemistry, 51*(5), 1501–1509.

Cortez, S.C., McIntosh, T.K., & Noble, L.J. (1989). Experimental fluid percussion brain injury: vascular disruption and neuronal and glial alterations. *Brain Research, 482*(2), 271–282.

D'Ambrosio, R., Maris, D.O., Grady, M.S., Winn, H.R., & Janigro, D. (1999). Impaired K(+) homeostasis and altered electrophysiological properties of post-traumatic hippocampal glia. *Journal of Neuroscience, 19*(18), 8152–8162.

D'Ambrosio, R., Maris, D.O., Grady, M.S., Winn, H.R., & Janigro, D. (1998). Selective loss of hippocampal long-term potentiation, but not depression, following fluid percussion injury. *Brain Research, 786*(1–2), 64–79.

DeFord, S.M., Wilson, M.S., Rice, A.C., Clausen, T., Rice, L.K., Barabnova, A., Bullock, R., & Hamm, R.J. (2002). Repeated mild brain injuries result in cognitive impairment in B6C3F1 mice. *Journal of Neurotrauma, 19*(4), 427–438.

Deshpande, J.K., Siesjo, B.K., & Wieloch, T. (1987). Calcium accumulation and neuronal damage in the rat hippocampus following cerebral ischemia. *Journal of Cerebral Blood Flow and Metabolism, 7*(1), 89–95.

DeWitt, D.S., Jenkins, L.W., Wei, E.P., Lutz, H., Becker, D.P., & Kontos, H.A. (1986). Effects of fluid-percussion brain injury on regional cerebral blood flow and pial arteriolar diameter. *Journal of Neurosurgery, 64*(5), 787–794.

Dienel, G.A. (1984). Regional accumulation of calcium in postischemic rat brain. *Journal of Neurochemistry, 43*(4), 913–925.

Dietrich, W.D., Alonso, O., Busto, R., & Ginsberg, M.D. (1994). Widespread metabolic depression and reduced somatosensory circuit activation following traumatic brain injury in rats. *Journal of Neurotrauma, 11*(6), 629–640.

Dixon, C.E., Kochanek, P.M., Yan, H.Q., Schiding, J.K., Griffith, R.G., Baum, E., Marion, D.W., & DeKosky, S.T. (1999). One-year study of spatial memory performance, brain morphology, and cholinergic markers after moderate controlled cortical impact in rats. *Journal of Neurotrauma, 16*(2), 109–122.

Doberstein, C., Velarde, F., Badie, H., & Hovda, D.A. (1992). Changes in local cerebral blood flow following concussive brain injury [Abstract]. *Society for Neuroscience, 18*, 175.

Ebel, H. & Gunther, T. (1980). Magnesium metabolism: a review. *Journal of Clinical Chemistry and Clinical Biochemistry, 18*(5), 257–270.

Feeney, D.M., Sutton, R.L., & Boyeson, M.G. (1985). The locus coeruleus and cerebral metabolism: Recovery of function after cortical injury. *Physiological Psychology, 13*, 197–203.

Fineman, I., Giza, C.C., Nahed, B.V., Lee, S.M., & Hovda, D.A. (2000). Inhibition of neocortical plasticity during development by a moderate concussive brain injury. *Journal of Neurotrauma, 17*(9), 739–749.

Fineman, I., Hovda, D.A., Smith, M., Yoshino, A., & Becker, D.P. (1993). Concussive brain injury is associated with a prolonged accumulation of calcium: A 45Ca autoradiographic study. *Brain Research, 624*(1–2), 94–102.

Friede, R.L. & Van Houten, W.H. (1961). Relations between post mortem alterations and glycolytic metabolism in the brain. *Experimental Neurology, 4*, 197–204.

Fu, K., Smith, M.L., Thomas, S., & Hovda, D.A. (1992). Cerebral concussion produces a state of vulnerability lasting for as long as 5 hours [Abstract]. *Journal of Neurotrauma, 9*, 59.

Gardiner, M., Smith, M.L., Kagstrom, E., Shohami, E., & Siesjo, B.K. (1982). Influence of blood glucose concentration on brain lactate accumulation during severe hypoxia and subsequent recovery of brain energy metabolism. *Journal of Cerebral Blood Flow and Metabolism, 2*(4), 429–438.

Garfinkel, L. & Garfinkel, D. (1985). Magnesium regulation of the glycolytic pathway, and the enzymes involved. *Magnesium, 4*(2–3), 60–72.

Ginsberg, M.D., Zhao, W., Alonso, O.F., Loor-Estades, J.Y., Dietrich, W.D., & Busto, R. (1997). Uncoupling of local cerebral glucose metabolism and blood flow after acute fluid-percussion injury in rats. *American Journal of Physiology, 272*(6 Pt 2), H2859–H2868.

Giza, C.C., Lee, S.M., Kremen, T.J., & Hovda, D.A. (2000). Decreased N-Methyl D-Aspartate receptor (NMDAR) activity after developmental fluid percussion injury (FPI) demonstrated by changes in subunit composition [Abstract]. *Restorative Neurology and Neuroscience, 16*[3–4], 170.

Giza, C.C. & Hovda, D.A. (2000). Ionic and Metabolic Consequences of Concussion. In R.C. Cantu (Ed.), *Neurologic Athletic Head and Spine Injuries* (pp. 80–100). St. Louis: W.B. Saunders Company.

Gorman, L.K., Fu, K., Hovda, D.A., Murray, M., & Traystman, R.J. (1996). Effects of traumatic brain injury on the cholinergic system in the rat. *Journal of Neurotrauma, 13*(8), 457–463.

Greenough, W.T., Volkmar, F.R., & Juraska, J.M. (1973). Effects of rearing complexity on dendritic branching in frontolateral and temporal cortex of the rat. *Experimental Neurology, 41*(2), 371–378.

Hansen, A.J. (1977). Extracellular potassium concentration in juvenile and adult rat brain cortex during anoxia. *Acta Physiologica Scandinavica, 99*(4), 412–420.

Hansen, A.J. (1978). The extracellular potassium concentration in brain cortex following ischemia in hypo- and hyperglycemic rats. *Acta Physiologica Scandinavica, 102*(3), 324–329.

Happel, R.D., Smith, K.P., Banik, N.L., Powers, J.M., Hogan, E.L., & Balentine, J.D. (1981). Ca2+-accumulation in experimental spinal cord trauma. *Brain Research, 211*(2), 476–479.

Hovda, D.A., Fu, K., Badie, H., Samii, A., Pinanong, P., & Becker, D.P. (1994). Administration of an omega-conopeptide one hour following traumatic brain injury reduces 45calcium accumulation. *Acta Neurochirurgica.* Supplementum (Wien), *60*, 521–523.

Hovda, D.A., Yoshino, A., Kawamata, T., Katayama, Y., & Becker, D.P. (1991). Diffuse prolonged depression of cerebral oxidative metabolism following concussive brain injury in the rat: A cytochrome oxidase histochemistry study. *Brain Research, 567*(1), 1–10.

Hubschmann, O.R. & Kornhauser, D. (1983). Effects of intraparenchymal hemorrhage on extracellular cortical potassium in experimental head trauma. *Journal of Neurosurgery, 59*(2), 289–293.

Humm, J.L., Kozlowski, D.A., James, D.C., Gotts, J.E., & Schallert, T. (1998). Use-dependent exacerbation of brain damage occurs during an early post- lesion vulnerable period. *Brain Research, 783*(2), 286–292.

Ip, E.Y., Giza, C.C., Griesbach, G.S., & Hovda, D.A. (2002). Effects of enriched environment and fluid percussion injury on dendritic arborization within the cerebral cortex of the developing rat. *Journal of Neurotrauma, 19*(5), 573–585.

Jenkins, L.W., Marmarou, A., Lewelt, W., & Becker, D.P. (1986). Increased vulnerability of the traumatized brain to early ischemia. In A. Baethmann & G.K. Go (Eds.), *Mechanisms of Secondary Brain Damage* (pp. 273–282). New York: Plenum Press.

Johnson, G.V., Greenwood, J.A., Costello, A.C., & Troncoso, J.C. (1991). The regulatory role of calmodulin in the proteolysis of individual neurofilament proteins by calpain. *Neurochemical Research, 16*(8), 869–873.

Julian, F. & Goldman, D. (1962). The effects of mechanical stimulation on some electrical properties of axons. *The Journal of General Physiology, 46*, 297–313.

Kalimo, H., Rehncrona, S., Soderfeldt, B., Olsson, Y., & Siesjo, B.K. (1981). Brain lactic acidosis and ischemic cell damage: 2. Histopathology. *Journal of Cerebral Blood Flow and Metabolism, 1*(3), 313–327.

Kalimo, H., Rehncrona, S., & Soderfeldt, B. (1981). The role of lactic acidosis in the ischemic nerve cell injury. *Acta Neuropathology*. Supplementum (Berl), 7, 20–22.

Katayama, Y., Becker, D.P., Tamura, T., & Hovda, D.A. (1990). Massive increases in extracellular potassium and the indiscriminate release of glutamate following concussive brain injury. *Journal of Neurosurgery, 73*(6), 889–900.

Kato, H., Kogure, K., & Nakano, S. (1989). Neuronal damage following repeated brief ischemia in the gerbil. *Brain Research, 479*(2), 366–370.

Klonoff, H., Low, M.D., & Clark, C. (1977). Head injuries in children: A prospective five-year follow-up. *Journal of Neurology, Neurosurgery, and Psychiatry, 40*(12), 1211–1219.

Kozlowski, D.A., James, D.C,. & Schallert, T. (1996). Use-dependent exaggeration of neuronal injury after unilateral sensorimotor cortex lesions. *Journal of Neuroscience, 16*(15), 4776–4786.

Kraus, J.F. & McArthur, D.L. (2000). Epidemiology of Head Injury. In P.R. Cooper & J.G. Golfinos (Eds.), *Head Injury* (pp. 1–25). San Francisco: McGraw-Hill.

Kraus, J.F., McArthur, D.L., Silverman, T.A., & Jayaraman, M. (1996). Epidemiology of Brain Injury. In R.K. Narayan, J.E. Wilberger & J.T. Povlishock (Eds.), *Neurotrauma* (pp. 13–30). San Francisco: McGraw-Hill.

Kuffler, S.W. (1967). Neuroglial cells: Physiological properties and a potassium mediated effect of neuronal activity on the glial membrane potential. Proceedings of the Royal Society of London. Series B. *Biological Sciences, 168*(10), 1–21.

Kushner, M., Alavi, A., Reivich, M., Dann, R., Burke, A., & Robinson, G. (1984). Contralateral cerebellar hypometabolism following cerebral insult: a positron emission tomographic study. *Annals Neurology, 15*(5), 425–434.

Lear, J.L. & Ackermann, R.F. (1989). Why the deoxyglucose method has proven so useful in cerebral activation studies: the unappreciated prevalence of stimulation-induced glycolysis. *Journal of Cerebral Blood Flow and Metabolism, 9*(6), 911–913.

Lee, S.M., Smith, M.L., Hovda, D.A., & Becker, D.P. (1995). Concussive brain injury results in chronic vulnerability of post-traumatic seizures [Abstract]. *Society for Neuroscience, 21*, 762.

Levin, H.S., Eisenberg, H.M., Wigg, N.R., & Kobayashi, K. (1982). Memory and intellectual ability after head injury in children and adolescents. *Neurosurgery, 11*(5), 668–673.

Lobato, R.D., Rivas, J.J., Gomez, P.A., Castaneda, M., Canizal, J.M., Sarabia, R. et al. (1991). Head-injured patients who talk and deteriorate into coma. Analysis of 211 cases studied with computerized tomography [see comments]. *Journal of Neurosurgery, 75*(2), 256–261.

Mata, M., Staple, J., & Fink, D.J. (1986). Changes in intra-axonal calcium distribution following nerve crush. *Journal of Neurobiology, 17*(5), 449–467.

Maxwell, W.L., McCreath, B.J., Graham, D.I., & Gennarelli, T.A. (1995). Cytochemical evidence for redistribution of membrane pump calcium- ATPase and ecto-Ca-ATPase activity, and calcium influx in myelinated nerve fibres of the optic nerve after stretch injury. *Journal of Neurocytology, 24*(12), 925–942.

Maxwell, W.L. & Graham, D.I. (1997). Loss of axonal microtubules and neurofilaments after stretch-injury to guinea pig optic nerve fibers. *Journal of Neurotrauma, 14*(9), 603–614.

Mayevsky, A. & Chance, B. (1974). Repetitive patterns of metabolic changes during cortical spreading depression of the awake rat. *Brain Research, 65*(3), 529–533.
McIntosh, T.K. (1993). Novel pharmacologic therapies in the treatment of experimental traumatic brain injury: a review. *Journal of Neurotrauma, 10*(3), 215–261.
McIntosh, T.K., Faden, A.I., Yamakami, I., & Vink, R. (1988). Magnesium deficiency exacerbates and pretreatment improves outcome following traumatic brain injury in rats: 31P magnetic resonance spectroscopy and behavioral studies. *Journal of Neurotrauma, 5*(1), 17–31.
Meyer, J.S., Kondo, A., Nomura, F., Sakamoto, K., & Teraura, T. (1970). Cerebral hemodynamics and metabolism following experimental head injury. *Journal of Neurosurgery, 32*(3), 304–319.
Miller, L.P., Lyeth, B.G., Jenkins, L.W., Oleniak, L., Panchision, D., Hamm, R.J. et al. (1990). Excitatory amino acid receptor subtype binding following traumatic brain injury. *Brain Research, 526*(1), 103–107.
Morbidity Mortality Weekly Report (MMWR). (1997). Sports related recurrent brain injuries-United States. 224–227.
Moody, W.J., Futamachi, K.J., & Prince, D.A. (1974). Extracellular potassium activity during epileptogenesis. *Experimental Neurology, 42*(2), 248–263.
Myers, R,E. (1979). A unitary theory of causation of anoxic and hypoxic brain pathology. *Advances in Neurology, 26*, 195–213.
Nakamura, Y., Takeda, M., Angelides, K.J., Tanaka, T., Tada, K., & Nishimura, T. (1990). Effect of phosphorylation on 68 KDa neurofilament subunit protein assembly by the cyclic AMP dependent protein kinase in vitro. *Biochemical and Biophysical Research Communications, 169*(2), 744–750.
Nedergaard, M., Jakobsen, J., & Diemer, N.H. (1988). Autoradiographic determination of cerebral glucose content, blood flow, and glucose utilization in focal ischemia of the rat brain: influence of the plasma glucose concentration. *Journal of Cerebral Blood Flow and Metabolism, 8*(1), 100–108.
Nelson, S.R., Lowry, O.H., & Passonneau, J.V. (1966). Changes in energy reserves in mouse brain associated with compressive head injury. In W.F. Caveness & A.E. Walker (Eds.), *Head Injury* (pp. 444–447). Philadelphia: JB Lippincott.
Nicholson, C. & Kraig, R.P. (1981). The Behavior of Extracellular Ions During Spreading Depression. In T. Zeuthen (Ed.), *The Application of Ion-Selective Electrodes* (pp. 217–238). New York: Elsevier, North-Holland.
Nilsson, B. & Nordstrom, C.H. (1977). Rate of cerebral energy consumption in concussive head injury in the rat. *Journal of Neurosurgery, 47*(2), 274–281.
Nilsson, B. & Ponten, U. (1977). Exerimental head injury in the rat. Part 2: Regional brain energy metabolism in concussive trauma. *Journal of Neurosurgery, 47*(2), 252–261.
Nixon, R.A. (1993). The regulation of neurofilament protein dynamics by phosphorylation: clues to neurofibrillary pathobiology. *Brain Pathology, 3*(1), 29–38.
Osteen, C.L., Giza, C.C., & Hovda, D.A. (2000). Changes in N-Methyl D-Aspartate Receptor (NMDAR) number and subunit composition after fluid percussion (FP) injury appear to prepare the hippocampus for neuroplasticity in adult rats [Abstract]. *Restorative Neurology and Neuroscience, 16*[3–4], 210.
Osteen, C.L., Moore, A.H., Prins, M.L., & Hovda, D.A. (2001). Age-Dependency of 45Calcium Accumulation Following Lateral Fluid Percussion: Acute and Delayed Patterns. *Journal of Neurotrauma, 18*(2), 141–62.
Pappius, H.M. (1982). Dexamethasone and local cerebral glucose utilization in freeze-traumatized rat brain. *Annals Neurology, 12*(2), 157–162.
Pappius, H.M. (1988). Significance of biogenic amines in functional disturbances resulting from brain injury. *Metabolic Brain Disease, 3*(4), 303–310.

Patronas, N.J., Di Chiro, G., Smith, B.H., De La, P.R., Brooks, R.A., Milam, H.L. et al. (1984). Depressed cerebellar glucose metabolism in supratentorial tumors. *Brain Research, 291*(1), 93–101.

Paulson, O.B. & Newman, E.A. (1987). Does the release of potassium from astrocyte endfeet regulate cerebral blood flow? *Science, 237*(4817), 896–898.

Pettus, E.H., Christman, C.W., Giebel, M.L., & Povlishock, J.T. (1994). Traumatically induced altered membrane permeability: its relationship to traumatically induced reactive axonal change. *Journal of Neurotrauma, 11*(5), 507–522.

Pettus, E.H. & Povlishock, J.T. (1996). Characterization of a distinct set of intra-axonal ultrastructural changes associated with traumatically induced alteration in axolemmal permeability. *Brain Research, 722*(1-2), 1–11.

Pickles, W. (1950). Acute general edema of the brain in children with head injuries. *New England Journal of Medicine, 242*, 607–611.

Povlishock, J.T. & Pettus, E.H. (1996). Traumatically induced axonal damage: Evidence for enduring changes in axolemmal permeability with associated cytoskeletal change. *Acta Neurochirurgica.* Supplementum (Wien), *66*, 81–86.

Povlishock, J.T. & Christman, C.W. (1995). The pathobiology of traumatically induced axonal injury in animals and humans: A review of current thoughts. *Journal of Neurotrauma, 12*(4), 555–564.

Prince, D.A., Lux, H.D., & Neher, E. (1973). Measurement of extracellular potassium activity in cat cortex. *Brain Research, 50*(2), 489–495.

Prins, M.L. & Hovda, D.A. (1998). Traumatic brain injury in the developing rat: effects of maturation on Morris water maze acquisition. *Journal of Neurotrauma, 15*(10), 799–811.

Prins, M.L., Lee, S.M., Cheng, C.L., Becker, D.P., & Hovda, D.A. (1996). Fluid percussion brain injury in the developing and adult rat: A comparative study of mortality, morphology, intracranial pressure and mean arterial blood pressure. Brain Research. *Developmental Brain Research, 95*(2), 272–282.

Prins, M.L., Povlishock, J.T., & Phillips, L.L. (2003). The effects of combined fluid percussion traumatic brain injury and unilateral entorhinal deafferentation on the juvenile rat brain. *Developmental Brain Research, 140*(1), 93–104.

Rappaport, Z.H., Young, W., & Flamm, E.S. (1987). Regional brain calcium changes in the rat middle cerebral artery occlusion model of ischemia. *Stroke, 18*(4), 760–764.

Richards, T.L., Keniry, M.A., Weinstein, P.R., Pereira, B.M., Andrews, B.T., Murphy, E.J. et al. (1987). Measurement of lactate accumulation by in vivo proton NMR spectroscopy during global cerebral ischemia in rats. *Magnetic Resonance in Medicine, 5*(4), 353–357.

Rosenthal, M., LaManna, J., Yamada, S., Younts, W., & Somjen, G. (1979). Oxidative metabolism, extracellular potassium and sustained potential shifts in cat spinal cord in situ. *Brain Research, 162*(1), 113–127.

Rosenzweig, M.R. & Bennett, E.L. (1996). Psychobiology of plasticity: Effects of training and experience on brain and behavior. *Behavioral Brain Research, 78*(1), 57–65.

Sakamoto, N., Kogure, K., Kato, H., & Ohtomo, H. (1986). Disturbed Ca2+ homeostasis in the gerbil hippocampus following brief transient ischemia. *Brain Research, 364*(2), 372–376.

Samii, A. & Hovda, D.A. (1998). Delayed increases in glucose utilization following cortical impact injury [Abstract]. *Society for Neuroscience, 24*, 738.

Schallert, T., Kozlowski, D.A., Humm, J.L., & Cocke, R.R. (1997). Use-dependent structural events in recovery of function. *Advances in Neurology, 73*, 229–238.

Schanne, F.A., Kane, A.B., Young, E.E., & Farber, J.L. (1979). Calcium dependence of toxic cell death: A final common pathway. *Science, 206*(4419), 700–702.

Shah, K.R. & West, M. (1983). The effect of concussion on cerebral uptake of 2-deoxy-D-glucose in rat. *NeuroscienceLetters, 40*(3), 287–291.

Shiraishi, K., Sharp, F.R., & Simon, R.P. (1989). Sequential metabolic changes in rat brain following middle cerebral artery occlusion: A 2-deoxyglucose study. *Journal of Cerebral Blood Flow and Metabolism, 9*(6), 765–773.

Siemkowicz, E. & Hansen, A.J. (1978). Clinical restitution following cerebral ischemia in hypo-, normo- and hyperglycemic rats. *Acta Neurologica Scandinavica, 58*(1), 1–8.

Sihver, S., Marklund, N., Hillered, L., Langstrom, B., Watanabe, Y., & Bergstrom, M. (2001). Changes in mACh, NMDA and GABA(A) receptor binding after lateral fluid- percussion injury: in vitro autoradiography of rat brain frozen sections. *Journal of Neurochemistry, 78*(3), 417–423.

Snoek, J.W., Minderhoud, J.M., & Wilmink, J.T. (1984). Delayed deterioration following mild head injury in children. *Brain, 107* (Pt 1), 15-36.

Somjen, G.G. & Giacchino, J.L. (1985). Potassium and calcium concentrations in interstitial fluid of hippocampal formation during paroxysmal responses. *Journal of Neurophysiology, 53*(4), 1098-1108.

Sternberger, L.A. & Sternberger, N.H. (1983). Monoclonal antibodies distinguish phosphorylated and nonphosphorylated forms of neurofilaments in situ. *Proceedings of the National Academy of Sciences of the United States of America, 80(19),* 6126–6130.

Stokes, B.T., Fox, P., & Hollinden, G. (1983). Extracellular calcium activity in the injured spinal cord. *Experimental Neurology, 80*(3), 561–572.

Sugaya, E., Takato, M., & Noda, Y. (1975). Neuronal and glial activity during spreading depression in cerebral cortex of cat. *Journal of Neurophysiology, 38*(4), 822–841.

Sunami, K., Nakamura, T., Ozawa, Y., Kubota, M., Namba, H., & Yamaura, A. (1989). Hypermetabolic state following experimental head injury. *Neurosurgical Review*, Supplementum 1, *12*, 400–411.

Sutton, R.L., Hovda, D.A., & Chugani, H.T. (1989). Time course of local cerebral glucose utilization (LCGU) alteration after motor cortex ablation in the rat [Abstract]. *Society for Neuroscience, 15*, 128.

Sypert, G.W. & Ward, A.A. Jr. (1974). Changes in extracellular potassium activity during neocortical propagated seizures. *Experimental Neurology, 45*(1), 19–41.

Takahashi, H., Manaka, S., & Sano, K. (1981). Changes in extracellular potassium concentration in cortex and brain stem during the acute phase of experimental closed head injury. *Journal of Neurosurgery, 55*(5), 708–717.

Tepas, J.J., III, DiScala, C., Ramenofsky, M.L., & Barlow, B. (1990). Mortality and head injury: the pediatric perspective. *Journal of Pediatric Surgery, 25*(1), 92–95.

Tees, R.C., Buhrmann, K., & Hanley, J. (1990). The effect of early experience on water maze spatial learning and memory in rats. *Developmental Psychobiology, 23(5*), 427–439.

Thomas, S., Prins, M.L., Samii, M., & Hovda, D.A. (2000). Cerebral metabolic response to traumatic brain injury sustained early in development: A 2-deoxy-D-glucose autoradiographic study. *Journal of Neurotrauma, 17*(8), 649–665.

Tsacopoulos, M., & Magistretti, P.J. (1996). Metabolic coupling between glia and neurons. *Journal of Neuroscience, 16*(3), 877–885.

Van Harreveld, A. (1978). Two mechanisms for spreading depression in the chicken retina. *Journal of Neurobiology, 9*(6), 419–431.

Velarde, F., Fisher, D.T., & Hovda, D.A. (1992). Fluid percussion injury induces prolonged changes in cerebral blood flow [Abstract]. *Journal of Neurotrauma, 9*, 402.

Venable, N., Pinto-Hamuy, T., Arraztoa, J.A., Contador, M.T., Chellew, A., Peran, C. et al. (1988). Greater efficacy of preweaning than postweaning environmental enrichment on maze learning in adult rats. *Behavioral Brain Research, 31*(1), 89–92.

Verweij, B.H., Muizelaar, J.P., Vinas, F.C., Peterson, P.L., Xiong, Y., & Lee, C.P. (1997). Mitochondrial dysfunction after experimental and human brain injury and its possible reversal with a selective N-type calcium channel antagonist (SNX-111). *Neurological Research, 19*(3), 334–339.

Vink, R., McIntosh, T.K., Demediuk, P., & Faden, A.I. (1987). Decrease in total and free magnesium concentration following traumatic brain injury in rats. *Biochemical and Biophysical Research Communications, 149*(2), 594–599.

Vink, R., McIntosh, T.K., Weiner, M.W., & Faden, A.I. (1987). Effects of traumatic brain injury on cerebral high-energy phosphates and pH: A 31P magnetic resonance spectroscopy study. *Journal of Cerebral Blood Flow and Metabolism, 7*(5), 563–571.

Vink, R., Faden, A.I., & McIntosh, T.K. (1988). Changes in cellular bioenergetic state following graded traumatic brain injury in rats: Determination by phosphorus 31 magnetic resonance spectroscopy. *Journal of Neurotrauma, 5*(4), 315–330.

Vink, R. & McIntosh, T.K. (1990). Pharmacological and physiological effects of magnesium on experimental traumatic brain injury. *Magnesium Research, 3*(3), 163–169.

Xiong, Y., Peterson, P.L., Muizelaar, J.P., & Lee C.P. (1997). Amelioration of mitochondrial function by a novel antioxidant U-101033E following traumatic brain injury in rats. *Journal of Neurotrauma, 14*(12), 907–917.

Xiong, Y., Peterson, P.L., Verweij, B.H., Vinas, F.C., Muizelaar, J.P., & Lee, C.P. (1998). Mitochondrial dysfunction after experimental traumatic brain injury: combined efficacy of SNX-111 and U-101033E. *Journal of Neurotrauma, 15*(7), 531–544.

Xiong, Y., Gu, Q., Peterson, P.L., Muizelaar, J.P., & Lee, C.P. (1997). Mitochondrial dysfunction and calcium perturbation induced by traumatic brain injury. *Journal of Neurotrauma, 14*(1), 23–34.

Yamakami, I. & McIntosh, T.K. (1989). Effects of traumatic brain injury on regional cerebral blood flow in rats as measured with radiolabeled microspheres. *Journal of Cerebral Blood Flow and Metabolism, 9*(1), 117–124.

Yang, M.S., DeWitt, D.S., Becker, D.P., & Hayes, R.L. (1985). Regional brain metabolite levels following mild experimental head injury in the cat. *Journal of Neurosurgery, 63*(4), 617–621.

Yoshino, A., Hovda, D.A., Kawamata, T., Katayama, Y., & Becker, D.P. (1991). Dynamic changes in local cerebral glucose utilization following cerebral conclusion in rats: evidence of a hyper- and subsequent hypometabolic state. *Brain Research, 561*(1), 106–119.

Young, W. & Koreh, I. (1986). Potassium and calcium changes in injured spinal cords. *Brain Research, 365*(1), 42–53.

Young, W., Yen, V., & Blight, A. (1982). Extracellular calcium ionic activity in experimental spinal cord contusion. *Brain Research, 253*(1-2), 105–113.

Yuan, X.Q., Prough, D.S., Smith, T.L., & DeWitt, D.S. (1988). The effects of traumatic brain injury on regional cerebral blood flow in rats. *Journal of Neurotrauma, 5*(4), 289–301.

Chapter 5

NEUROIMAGING IN SPORTS-RELATED BRAIN INJURY

Erin D. Bigler[1]
William W. Orrison, Jr.[2,3]
[1]Brigham Young University, LDS Hospital Salt Lake City, Utah, University of Utah
[2]University of Utah School of Medicine Brigham Young University
[3]Academic Medical Institute of Nevada

Although there are numerous ways that a sports-related brain injury can occur, the majority of these injuries are relatively mild (Benson et al., 1999; Collins, Lovell & McKeag, 1999; Kelly & Rosenberg 1997; McCrea et al., 1997). Therefore, the important neuroimaging characteristics, when such abnormalities are present, are those typically observed in the "mild" type of injury (Alexander, 1995; Stuss, 1995; Weight, 1998). Since most research on neuroimaging of mild traumatic brain injury (TBI) has been performed on cases of injury from motor vehicle accidents (MVA), much of the information available for review incorporates literature from MVA related mild TBI (Glasgow Coma Scale [GCS] ≥ 13; Bigler 1999a, b, c). Understanding the nature and clinical significance of neuroimaging findings in TBI is important in rehabilitation (Consensus Panel, 1999) and long-term outcome (Colantonio, Dawson & McLellan, 1998). Therefore, it is important to provide objective guidelines for the interpretation of neuroimaging findings in the context of assessing and treating mild TBI (Bigler, 1999b, 2001b).

In the mildest form of sports-related head injury, neuroimaging of any type is typically not performed, rather medical decisions are made by the athlete's clinical presentation. For example, a momentary loss of consciousness followed by a quick recovery period with no persisting symptoms typically does not warrant any neuroimaging. In contrast, more significant mild head injury (i.e., longer duration of unconsciousness or confusion [see Chapter 1, this volume] or the persistence of neurocognitive symptoms) typically will require some neuroimaging studies, most often computerized tomography (CT), magnetic resonance (MR) imaging or both. However, CT and routine MR provide only structural information about anatomy, which may be insensitive to some of the pathophysiological changes characteristic of mild TBI. Typically, the reason that neuroimaging studies are done acutely in sports-

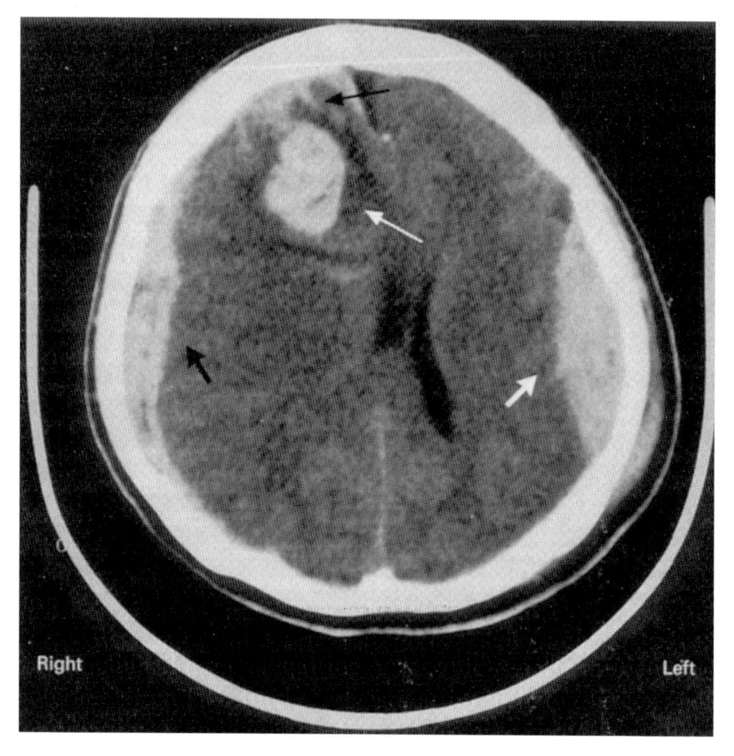

Figure 5.1. The axial section of a computerized tomogram (CT) scan of the head at the level of the lateral ventricles, obtained without the addition of contrast medium, revealed four types of acute post-traumatic intracranial hemorrhage: an epidural hematoma (thick white arrow) and a squamous temporal fracture (which is not shown) on the left side, a laminated subdural hematoma (thick black arrow) on the right side, right-sided periventricular and frontal-lobe contusions containing an intraparenchymal hematoma (thin white arrow), and a subarachnoid hemorrhage (thin black arrow) in the right frontal region. These injuries were sustained in a fall. (Reproduced with permission from Mattiello & Munz, 2001 and the New England Journal of Medicine. Copyright © Massachusetts Medical Society.)

related injury is to rule out a treatable lesion as shown in Figure 5.1 (Mattiello & Munz, 2001). The need for imaging during the more chronic phase, if it develops, is to examine lesions in the context of symptoms and persistence of neurobehavioral deficits. The ultimate goal is to relate neuroimaging findings to treatment and outcome. Various types of functional neuroimaging may be more sensitive in detecting the pathophysiological effects of mild TBI than the routine clinical MR or CT scan. Functional neuroimaging is currently not a widely used imaging procedure, and its clinical potential is just beginning to be understood. For example, recent work by Lewine et al. (1999) has shown the presence of abnormalities on magnetoencephalography (MEG) in mild TBI, where the clinical MR has been assessed to be within normal limits. Also, recent MR spectroscopy (MRS) studies (Friedman et al., 1998; Garnett, Blamire, Corkill et al., 2000a; Garnett, Blamire, Rajagopalan et al., 2000b) and magnetization transfer imaging (Bagley et al., 1999; Sinson et al., 2001) have all shown abnormalities in cases of mild TBI where standard structural neuroimaging demonstrates a "normal" scan. Similar findings have also been demonstrated with positron emission computed tomography (PET), as well as single photon emission computed tomography (SPECT) (Hofman et al., 2001; Kesler et al., 2000). It is likely that as more research develops using these new functional neuroimaging tools, including computerized electroencephalography (EEG) integrated with three-dimensional MR imaging (Ricker & Zafonte, 2000; Thatcher, North, Curtin et al., 2001), that some forms of functional neuroimaging will become more standard assessment tools in the evaluation of sports-related mild TBI.

Basic CT and MR imaging will be reviewed here focusing on cases of mild TBI followed by a more thorough discussion of various functional neuroimaging techniques. This includes functional MR imaging (fMRI), PET, SPECT, quantitative EEG (qEEG), MEG and MRS. Time, post-injury, and the persistence of post-concussional symptoms, as defined by the Diagnostic Statistical Manual of Mental Disorders – Fourth Edition (DSM-IV™) criteria (American Psychiatric Association, 1994) are typically the standard clinical justification for performing these additional functional procedures.[1] There are currently no universally accepted guidelines regarding the utilization of neuroimaging methods in sports injury. However, there have been

[1] Presence of a mild TBI is usually based on the 1993 criteria of the American Congress of Rehabilitation Medicine as follows:
"A traumatically induced physiological disruption of brain function, as manifested by **at least** one of the following: Any period of loss of consciousness; any loss of memory for events immediately before or after the accident; any alteration in mental state at the time of the accident (e.g., feeling dazed, disoriented, or confused); and focal neurological deficit(s) that may or may not be transient; but where the severity of the injury does not exceed the following: loss of consciousness of approximately 30 minutes; after 30 minutes, an initial Glasgow Coma Scale (GCS) of 13-15; and post-traumatic amnesia not greater than 24 hours." American Congress of Rehabilitation Medicine. (1993). Definition of mild traumatic brain injury. *The Journal of Head Trauma Rehabilitation*, *8*, 86-87.

rather dramatic improvements in structural imaging by CT and MR as well as remarkable advances in functional neuroimaging procedures. As these modalities demonstrate greater clinical utility, a variety of the methods discussed in this chapter will likely become customary practice in evaluating the patient with a sports-related head injury, both acutely and in those who develop persistent symptoms.

To best recognize pathological findings in neuroimaging studies related to mild TBI, it is important to understand that the neuropathology of mild TBI (Gennarelli, Thibault, & Graham, 1998; Saatman, Graham, & McIntosh, 1998; Smith, Chen, Nonaka et al., 1999; Smith & Meaney, 2000; Tang, Noda, Hasegawa et al., 1997; Yoon, Fuse, Shah et al., 1998) may be dominated by physiological, synaptic and biochemical abnormalities rather than gross structural changes, although cytoskeletal and brain parenchymal injuries do occur (i.e., shearing; Alexander, 1995). The smaller the lesion, or in the case of transient physiological abnormalities, they become more and more difficult to detect with current neuroimaging technology. In moderate to severe TBI, diffuse axonal injury (DAI) represents a dominant feature of the brain trauma induced by tensile and shearing forces in the brain (Gennarelli et al., 1998), and these pathologies also play a role in mild TBI. This is touched upon in Chapters 3 and 4 in this book and has also been thoroughly discussed elsewhere (see Bigler, 2001a). Briefly, from an imaging perspective, small shear lesions may produce petechial hemorrhages and such hemorrhages may leave hemosiderin deposits or produce a focal disruption in white matter integrity. Hemosiderin is a degraded blood by-product that has residual iron and therefore is readily detected on some MR imaging such as gradient recalled sequences (see Fig. 5.2). Since it is the axon that is most likely to exhibit shear injury, MR signals changes in the white matter (Fig. 5.2) or presence of hemosiderin, are the most common abnormalities following mild injury. Often these lesions are seen close to the gray-white matter junction. Also, cortical contusion, particularly in the inferior-anterior aspect of the frontal lobes or the inferior-mesial aspect of the temporal lobes, can occur in sports-related head injury, and therefore, these regions should be carefully examined in all types of imaging studies performed on the athlete with a history of head injury.

Acute and Sub-Acute Injury Phase: CT and MR Neuroimaging

As already mentioned, the initial neuroimaging studies following head injury usually are either a head CT or MR scan. While MR provides much better resolution of brain parenchyma than CT, CT is faster, can be performed in the presence of life support or other type of equipment (i.e., certain athletic gear), or in the presence of intracranial metal such as when there is any question of penetrating injury. Since CT is based on X-ray it is excellent in delineation of bone and detection of skull fracture and is also sensitive to hemorrhage

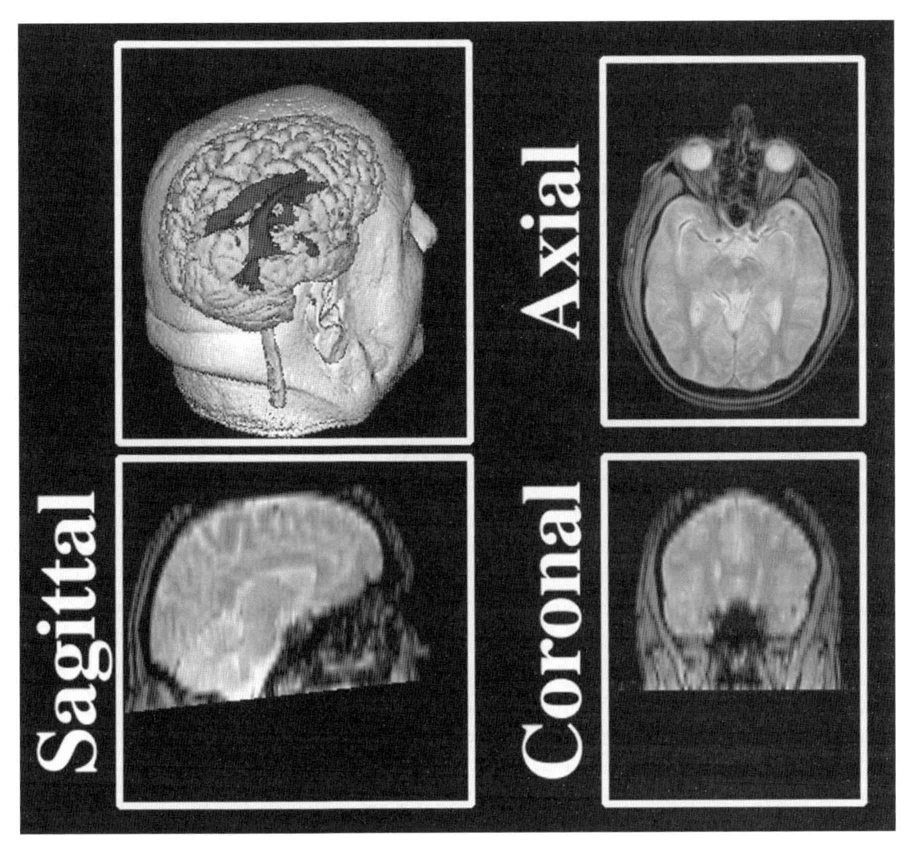

Figure 5.2. The 3-dimensional (3-D) image of the brain shows multiple hemosiderin deposits (black appearing dots), which are thought to be associated with multiple, but small hemorrhagic lesions (i.e., petechial hemorrhages) that occur in response to injury. The individual MR sections that demonstrate some of these lesions are shown in the axial, coronal and sagittal views. This patient sustained a blow to the head when an exploding cylinder struck him imprinting his head into the metallic cylinder. He had an emergency room admission Glasgow Coma Scale (GCS) of 15 and was not admitted to the hospital. Note in the posterior-oblique view of the 3-D MR image how the lesions congregate in the frontal and temporal lobe regions of the brain. Also, often these "shear" injuries occur most dominantly at the white-gray matter junction, which is depicted in the coronal image, in the temporal lobe (from the reader's perspective the black dot in the coronal image).

and edema (Orrison, 2000; Osborn, 1994). Nonetheless, MR provides much better anatomical resolution, which is very important in mild head injury because when lesions are present, they are typically small and, at times, very subtle in their presentation.

For example, the emergently done CT imaging for the patient presented in Figure 5.2 was normal, although he was still definitely symptomatic for sig-

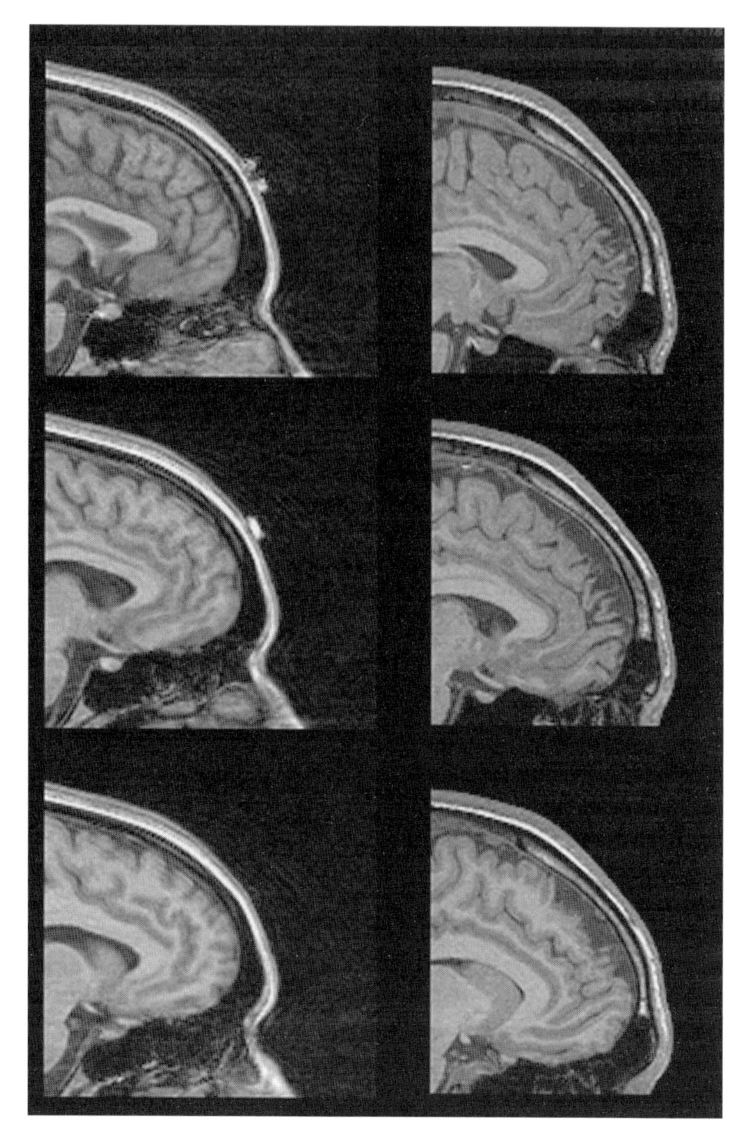

Figure 5.3. The scans on the left are from a patient without specific frontal pathology, age-matched, in comparison to significant frontal atrophy noted in the patient on the right who sustained a mild head injury when thrown from a vehicle that had been involved in a crash. The dark area over the frontal region is excess cerebral-spinal fluid (CSF), that has increased in response to volume loss of the frontal area. The patient had an admission Glasgow Coma Scale (GCS) of 15, but acute computerized tomogram (CT) imaging demonstrated frontal contusion and subarachnoid hemorrhaging. The residuals of that acute frontal injury are the focal frontal pathology observed in the sagittal images portrayed on the right. As might be expected looking at the amount of damage produced by this 'mild' TBI, a significant frontal lobe behavioral syndrome ensued.

nificant concussion from an exploding high-pressure cylindrical filter, which struck his head with such force that his head imprinted the metal casing. The patient was attended to in the emergency room, had a GCS of 15, and was sent home. He had no recall of the injury and had a post-traumatic amnesia of several hours. He had an immediate headache that persisted for days and then gradually diminished but never fully abated by the time the patient was seen for follow-up neuroimaging, approximately a year post-injury. However, he had unrelenting, troublesome problems with concentration, short-term memory and executive function. Subsequent MR imaging demonstrated numerous areas of hemosiderin deposit. Note how they are scattered but tend to be in the frontal and temporal regions of the brain. It can be argued that the focus of pathology in the frontal-temporal areas in TBI is at the basis for the common problems of attention/concentration, impaired short-term memory, changes in temperament and emotion along with deficits in executive functioning (Bigler, 2001a). Accordingly, finding these abnormalities on neuroimaging in this, or any patient with mild TBI, most likely documents the organic basis of the patient's cognitive and neurobehavioral deficits.

Mild cortical contusion can result in underlying atrophy following mild TBI. This is illustrated in Figure 5.3 where a non-seat-belted teenager was thrown from a vehicle on impact. He experienced a brief loss of consciousness but by the time he was evaluated at the emergency room, he was alert and oriented with a GCS of 15. Emergent CT imaging demonstrated subarachnoid blood within the frontal interhemispheric fissure and frontal contusion. The comparative scan on the left demonstrates normal sagittal cuts at similar levels in a non-seat-belted individual. This type of frontal contusion results in atrophic changes of the frontal lobe, which in turn, in this case, were likely at the basis for cognitive (i.e., deficits in attention/concentration and impaired short-term memory), emotional (i.e., labile mood) and behavioral (i.e., amotivational state) changes.

Because of the likelihood of frontal injury in head trauma, combined with the location of the first cranial nerve (olfactory nerve), it is common for some disruption in smell to occur acutely, even in mild TBI. When MR imaging demonstrates inferior frontal damage, these changes in olfaction are likely permanent. This is demonstrated in Figure 5.4, a case in which a young adult male was assaulted by being thrown against a wall (back of head striking first; thus, the frontal contusion is likely a result of a contrecoup injury). There was questionable loss of consciousness, but definite confusion and posttraumatic amnesia (PTA) of several hours. The patient's headache and typical post-concussive symptom's persisted, yet on standard neurological assessment the patient had only impaired smell but no other major abnormality. Normal olfaction never returned and the follow-up MR imaging demonstrated encephalomalacia in the olfactory groove region and anterior-inferior aspect of the frontal lobes bilaterally (see Fig. 5.4). These types of lesions also indicate a likelihood of more generalized inferior frontal damage that often does not disrupt specific cognitive functions but will produce changes in temperament and emotionality. Such changes were observed in this patient.

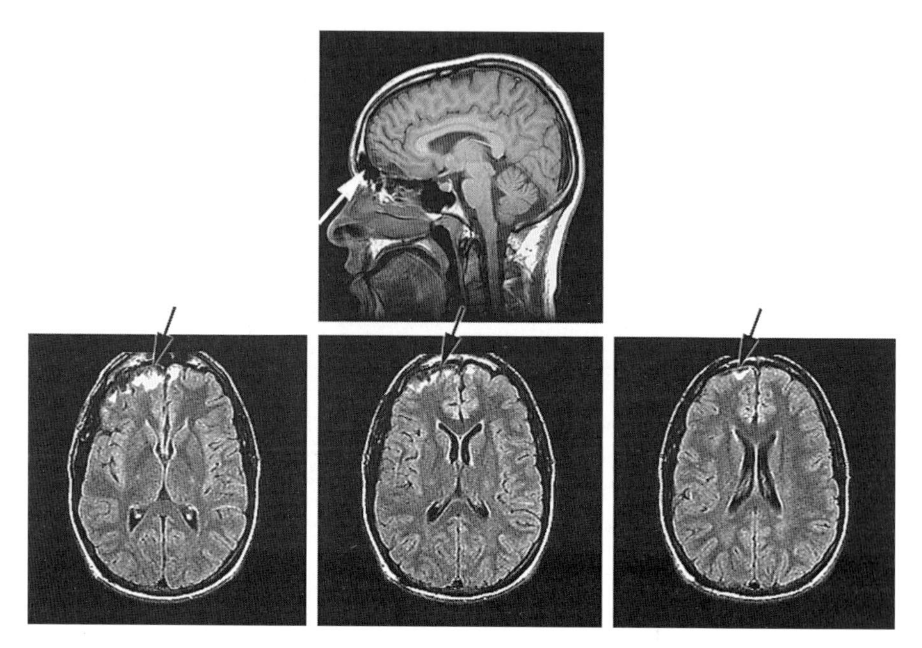

Figure 5.4. Magnetic resonance (MR) imaging more than two years after this patient was assaulted, where he was thrown against a wall. The back of his head struck the wall, but obviously the main injury was a contrecoup frontal injury. The arrows point to encephalomalacic changes that occurred at the site where acute frontal contusions developed. Acutely he had normal neurological exam except for anosmia and no major post-traumatic amnesia. This case demonstrates the common inferior frontal damage that can occur in mild traumatic brain injury. As far as neurobehavioral sequela, this patient developed predominately neuropsychiatric symptoms of poor frustration tolerance, diminished drive and depression, for which he received antidepressant medication. He was able to complete his college education.

As indicated, CT imaging is excellent at detecting skull fracture as demonstrated in Figure 5.5. Often there may be underlying cerebral contusion and edema associated with skull fracture, as was the case with this patient. What is often very important to note is that the acute information may provide critical details that later become clinically useful. For example, in the case present in Figure 5.5, follow-up imaging demonstrated resolution of the hemorrhage and focal edema, with no residual atrophy, but the patient developed behavioral symptoms of change in temperament and personality, consistent with a frontal injury even though follow-up structural imaging did not show lasting "damage" to the frontal area. The presence of frontal involvement in this patient is inferred from the history, presence of a prior frontal skull fracture and prior contusion that undoubtedly left microscopic parenchymal injury and the resulting neuropsychological presentation of the patient. Accordingly, acute neuroimaging findings may be the key to understanding neurobehav-

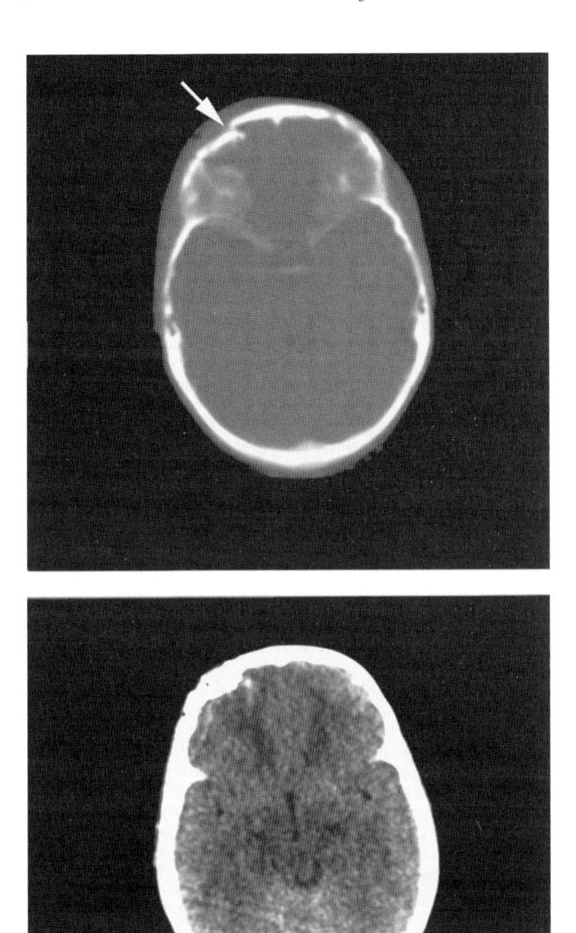

Figure 5.5. (TOP) Bone window computerized tomogram (CT) scan showing fracture (see arrow). (BOTTOM) CT imaging showing some edema and hemorrhage (white areas, just beneath and adjacent to the fracture) over the right frontal area. Although these abnormalities resolved over time such that follow-up imaging was negative, behaviorally the patient demonstrated neurobehavioral changes consistent with frontal lobe damage. A depressed skull fracture, such as this with cortical contusion with hematoma formation, certainly indicates significant focal mechanical deformation to brain parenchyma in this region. Post-mortem studies have shown that when tissues in the regions of such deformation are examined microscopically, neuronal injury is often present (Smith & Meaney, 2000). Accordingly, by understanding where acute imaging findings are abnormal can lead to clinical correlation between brain injury and behavior later on, even when follow-up neuroimaging studies are negative.

ioral sequela of brain injury even when follow-up imaging demonstrates no abnormalities.

Chronic Phase: CT, MR and SPECT Neuroimaging

In terms of structural neuroimaging, at the chronic stage in cases of mild injury, MR imaging is definitely the method of choice (Bigler, 2001a, b; Orrison, 2000). The most common structural deficits are (a) intraparenchymal signal abnormalities, particularly in the white matter and, (b) atrophy, both focal and generalized. However, structural neuroimaging is only part of the clinical

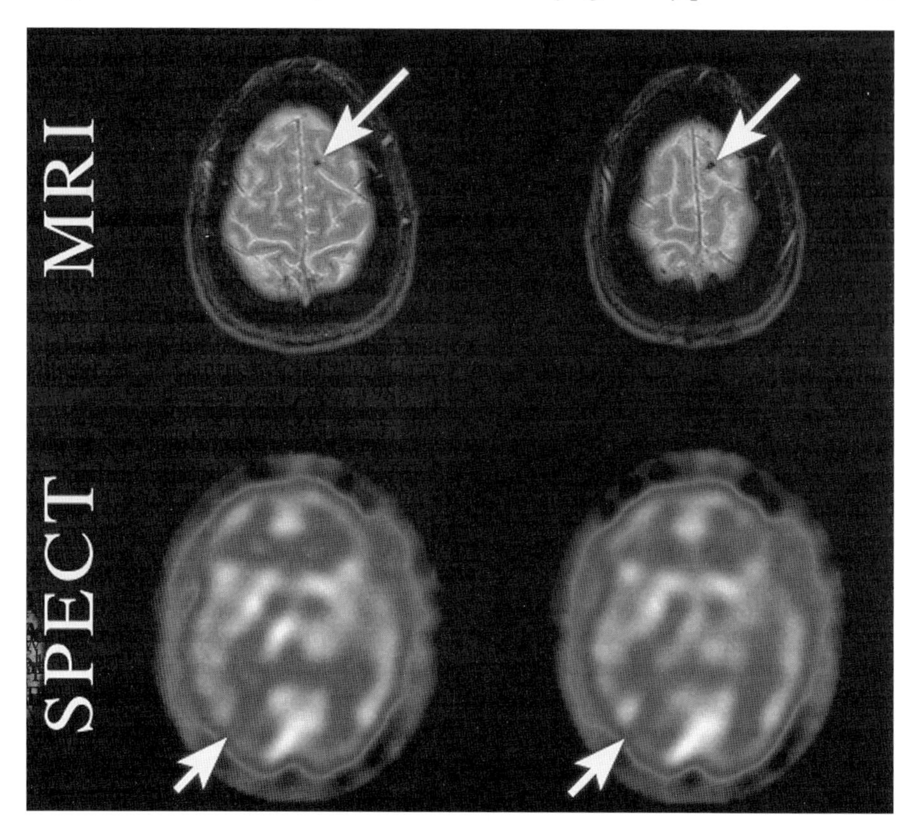

Figure 5.6. This patient sustained a mild head injury and the magnetic resonance (MR) scan shows hemosiderin deposits in the right frontal region but perfusion abnormality on the single photon emission computed tomography (SPECT) in the left posterior area. The relationship between these two findings is probably related to a coup-contrecoup phenomena producing lesions directly opposite one another. Clinically, the patient had the typically post-concussion symptoms of problems with attention/concentration, short-term memory difficulties and depression. Finding such objective abnormalities helps in relating residual symptoms that follow a head injury, to the head injury itself, as opposed to some other etiology.

picture. At this stage, some index of function is also very helpful and this is often done through SPECT scanning, because it is the most commonly used clinical neuroimaging tool in assessing function in the chronic stage (Hofman et al., 2001; Kesler et al., 2000). The importance of using multiple measures in assessing TBI outcome is clearly demonstrated by the findings of both Kesler et al. (2000) and Hofman et al. (2001). In using just structural CT imaging, Hofman et al. found only an 8% abnormality rate in mild TBI. In contrast, by using MR and SPECT, they found 77% of their mild TBI subjects to have an abnormality. Kesler et al. (2000) added a quantitative MR analysis, but also included moderate-to-severe brain injury. It was found by using this multiple approach to the assessment of neuroimaging that approximately 90% of subjects with a head injury had imaging abnormalities; however, when only one imaging modality was used no more than 50% of the subjects had an identifiable injury. One important reason for the hit-rates to increase when multiple neuroimaging measures are used is the different sensitivity in the detection of the residual injury. For example, this is nicely demonstrated in Figure 5.6 where hemosiderin deposition is shown in the superior frontal area on MR imaging. However, SPECT imaging demonstrates disrupted perfusion in the right posterior parietal area, which is the area where a heavy, falling object struck this patient. Together, these structural and functional neuroimaging findings probably represent coup contrecoup injury, but if both had not been done then an incomplete neuroimaging picture would have been present.

Chronic Phase: Functional Neuroimaging

Mild head injury may result in permanent neurobehavioral changes (Alexander, 1995; Hudson, 1996; Ommaya, Salazar, Dannenberg et al., 1996). Functional neuroimaging, as already introduced, provides another method for assessing the long-term consequences of a brain injury. This will be further demonstrated in the sections that follow.

SPECT/PET

SPECT and PET both require the intravascular injection of a radiopharmaceutical. SPECT examinations include methods of evaluating blood-brain-barrier (BBB) breakdown as well as measurements of regional cerebral blood flow or volume. PET imaging relies on the ability to detect positron-emitting radionuclides. Like SPECT, PET imaging involves the intravascular injection of a radiopharmaceutical, however in the case of PET the radionuclides are very short-lived. Through the selection of the appropriate radiolabeled PET compound, it is possible to demonstrate biological and physiological processes involved in human cerebral metabolism. That, in turn, may be related to cognitive deficits.

At resting baseline, generally uniform uptake should be observed and since the outer mantle of the brain is comprised of gray matter, the outer rim should show the highest utilization (typically referred to as perfusion) with less in white matter and no activity in cerebral-spinal fluid (CSF) filled spaces (see Figs. 5.6 and 5.7). Typically there is excellent correspondence between the focal pathology observed on structural imaging and SPECT or PET (Masdeu, Abdel-Dayem & Van Heertum, 1995). In other words, where structural defects are observed there is typically corresponding perfusion defect noted. For example, the case presented in Figure 5.7 is taken about 18 months post-injury where the individual fell during a horse chariot racing activity. As can be seen there is excellent concordance between structural MR imaging and the focal deficit in the parietal area. However, what SPECT or PET does is improve the ability to examine other brain regions that may not have grossly observable structural defect that can be seen on MR or CT, but nonetheless show perfusion abnormality. This improved ability is demonstrated in Figure 5.8 where PET imaging was performed approximately two years after a severe TBI (admission GCS = 5). Follow-up MR imaging demonstrates frontal atrophy, but PET imaging particularly demonstrates a more focal perfusion defect in the frontal area (see arrow).

Fontaine, Azouvi, Remy et al. (1999) using rate of regional cerebral glucose metabolism (rCMRGlu), found a significant relationship between neuropsychological deficit in memory and executive tasks, and decreased rCMRGlu in prefrontal and cingulate cortex. An important implication of these findings is that dysfunctional frontal systems are thought to be, in part, at the basis of sport-related concussion (McCrory & Berkovic, 2002) and post-concussional deficits associated with whiplash (Mosimann, Muri, Felblinger

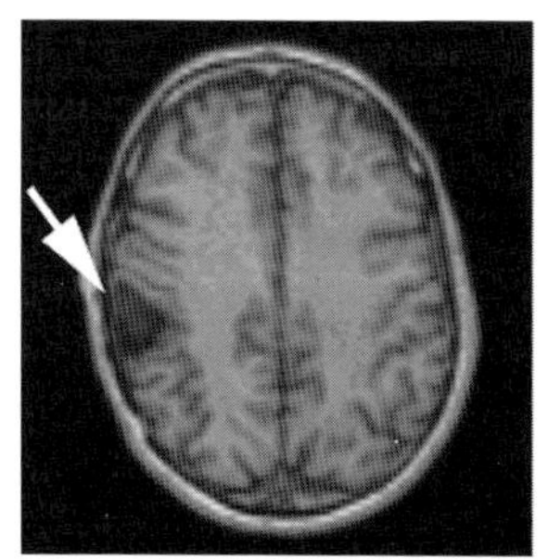

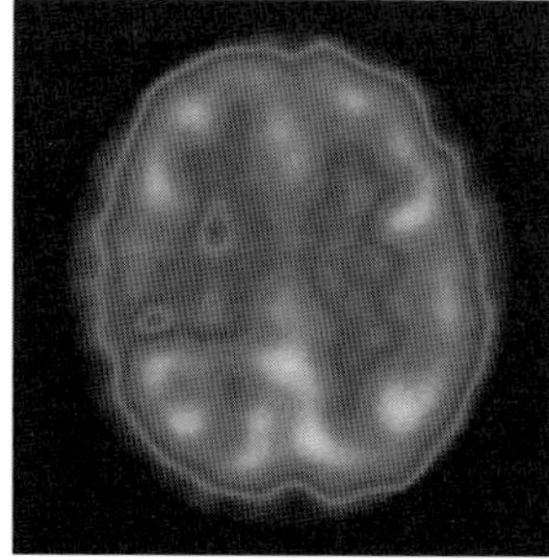

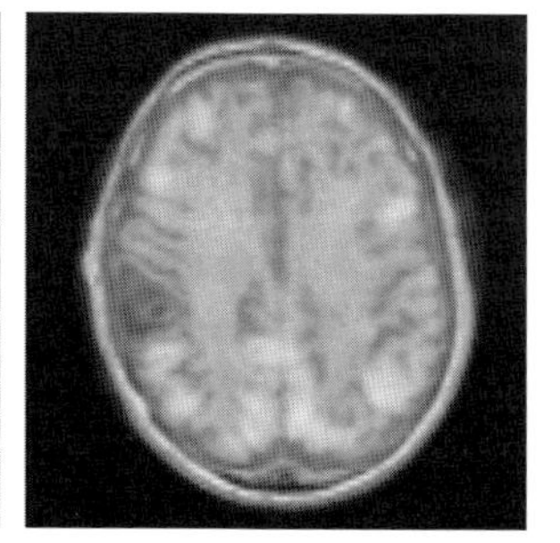

Figure 5.7. The magnetic resonance (MR) image on the left shows a focal area of encephalomalacia as a consequence of focal traumatic brain injury in a sports-related accident (fall in a chariot race). The single photon emission computed tomography (SPECT) scan (MIDDLE VIEW) also demonstrates focal perfusion defect that actually extends somewhat beyond where the focal lesion occurs, which can be best detected by looking at the homologous area in the opposite hemisphere in the fused SPECT image with the MR findings (RIGHT IMAGE). This study demonstrates the utility of SPECT imaging to demonstrate regions of functional impairment in addition to structural imaging findings.

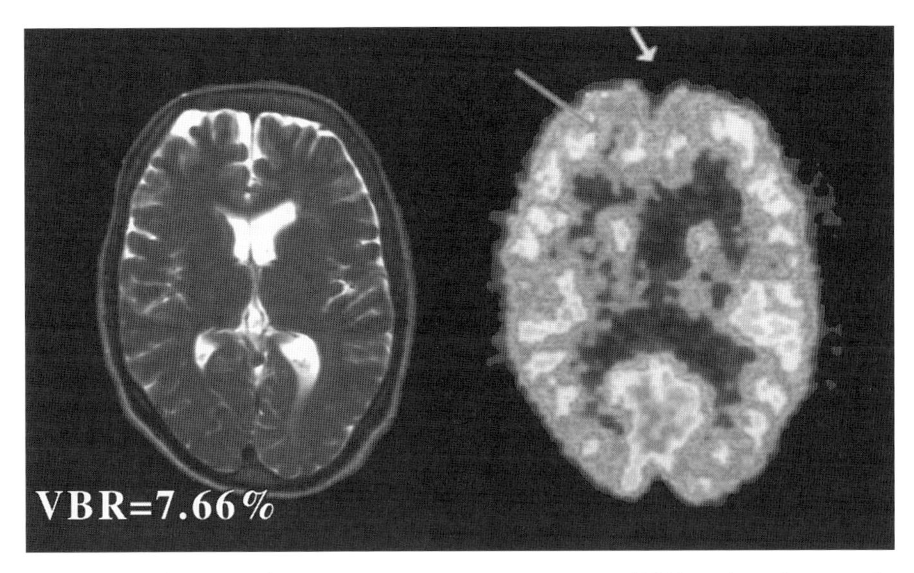

Figure 5.8. This case demonstrates magnetic resonance (MR) and positron emission computed tomography (PET) imaging in the chronic phase. This patient sustained a severe injury (admission Glasgow Coma Scale [GCS] = 5) and the MR imaging performed more that two-years post-injury shows frontal atrophy, but PET imaging actually shows an area of focal perfusion defect (between the two arrows) superimposed upon the more generalized atrophic changes of the frontal lobe. This case demonstrates how functional imaging can be used to more readily pinpoint focal areas of impaired brain function where structural MR imaging show only generalized, non-specific abnormality (i.e., ventricle-to-brain ratio [VBR] of 7.66% indicates generalized atrophic changes).

et al., 2000). Furthermore, Yount, Raschke, Biru et al. (2001) demonstrated atrophic changes in the cingulate gyrus in TBI, adding further documentation of limbic system injury that accompanies TBI (Tate & Bigler, 2000).

MEG

The relatively recent development of large array of biomagnetometer systems has enabled the use of magnetoencephalography (MEG) in the clinical evaluation of a variety of neurological conditions including epilepsy, neoplasms, cerebrovascular disease, psychiatric disorders, learning disorders, developmental disabilities and head trauma. MEG is a method for the detection, localization, and characterization of magnetic fields that emanate from the brain. Current flowing within a wire produces surrounding magnetic fields, and in a similar manner the current flow within neurons produces such a field. Using a sensitive set of magnetic detectors arranged in a helmet design around the head allows for detailed evaluation of the magnetic fields associated with electrical events that occur within the neurons. The recorded neuromagnetic signals appear similar to those identified using electroencephalography (EEG), but can also be mapped as magnetic fields for more precise localization. MEG signals can be recorded spontaneously from the brain, or as a response to a peripheral stimulus.

Obvious abnormalities that reach observable size by MR techniques are straightforward to detect. However, considerable neurological dysfunction can be at a level where structural imaging simply cannot detect an abnormality. This is best exemplified in mild TBI, where the patient may clearly have suffered a brain injury, but no objective abnormal findings are present using standard neuroimaging techniques. MEG has the potential of detecting physiological abnormalities in the absence of any structural defects as demonstrated by Lewine et al. (1999). In this instance MEG studies were performed on TBI subjects who had "normal" MR findings. The MEG, which assesses small magnetic field potentials in brain parenchyma, showed significant abnormalities – sometimes in diffuse patterns – in TBI subjects with no apparent structural abnormality. This is demonstrated in the case presented in Figure 5.9.

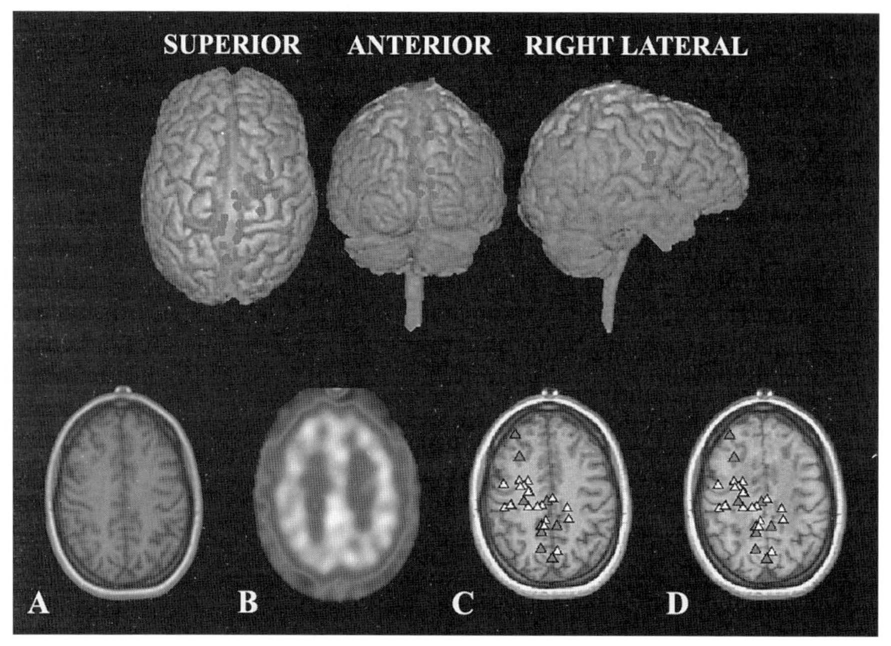

Figure 5.9. Magnetoencephalogram (MEG) findings of abnormality in a patient who sustained a mild-moderate traumatic brain injury (TBI) but who has a normal magnetic resonance (MR) and single photon emission computed tomography (SPECT) scan findings (A, B). Often MEG will show more sensitive detection of abnormalities in mild head injury, even when other imaging findings demonstrate no clinical abnormality. The triangles depict areas of MEG abnormality in axial sections (C, D), which are shown as darker grey shades on the 3-D surface renderings of the brain created by the MR imaging (TOP VIEWS: dorsal left, posterior middle, right lateral).

fMRI

Current clinical fMRI produces images of activated regions of the brain primarily through the detection of the indirect effects of neuronal processes on local blood flow, blood volume, and blood oxygen saturation. fMRI images are typically produced from signal differences between activated and nonactivated image acquisitions. Although this technique originally required the injection of a contrast agent in order to define sufficient differences in signal, methods have now evolved such that contrast injection is not necessary for

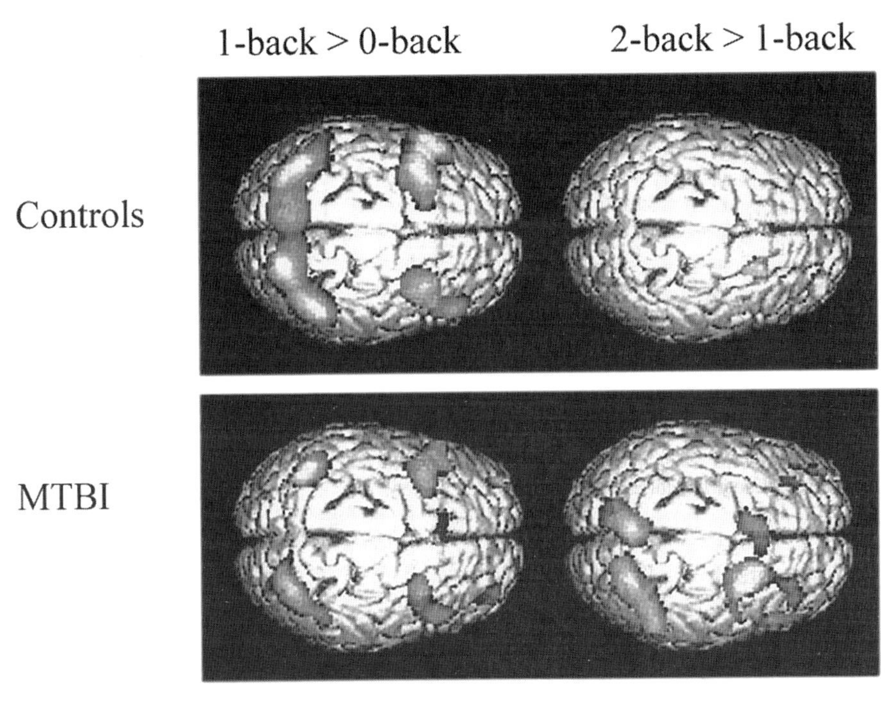

Figure 5.10. Functional magnetic resonance imaging (fMRI) findings in mild TBI from the McAllister et al. (1999) study; this shows that larger areas of recruitment are involved in performing a cognitive task in patients with mild TBI. The location of major cortical activation foci are displayed on a surface-rendered projection showing fMRI patterns of activation performing a task requiring memory and attention. The gyral location of activations (bilateral dorsolateral prefrontal and superior parietal) were similar in both groups from the 0-back to 1-back condition, which is the easier condition. Major differences, however, were observed in the 1-back to 2-back comparison, a more difficult cognitive task, but in controls made easier by the prior experience. Note the more extensive activation of primarily right superior parietal and dorsolateral prefrontal cortex in patients with mild traumatic brain injury (TBI). These findings indicate greater recruitment necessary in the brain that has sustained a mild TBI.

most applications. fMRI is possible on a wide variety of MR systems, and is especially effective at higher field strengths of 1.5 Tesla or above. Clinical MR systems of 3 and 4 Tesla are now becoming more widely available and along with them improved fMRI applications.

The systematic investigations of neurobehavioral correlates of cognitive processes using fMRI technology are in their infancy, even though fMRI techniques have been available for over a decade (see Saykin, Johnson, Flashman et al., 1999). A most interesting study was recently published by McAllister, Saykin, Flashman et al. (1999); they examined fMRI correlates of working memory one month after mild TBI. A synopsis of their findings is portrayed in Figure 5.10. Briefly, they observed that mild TBI subjects required greater activation of brain regions involved in performing working memory than observed in controls. A possible explanation for this finding is that the neuronal network that underlies working memory is disrupted by the injury and greater recruitment is necessary just to maintain function. What is fascinating from this study is that these mild TBI subjects did not differ from controls on most neuropsychological measures, with the exception of several reaction-time tasks on a continuous performance task; however, the TBI subjects significantly endorsed more symptoms of memory problems and likely perceived that their subjective experience was that they had to "work harder" to maintain accurate task performance (see p. 1305, McAllister et al., 1999). In the future, it is likely that fMRI tasks will prove to be exceptional methods for assessing the functional significance of TBI. fMRI techniques may also have application in studying the functional recovery and cerebral reorganization that takes place following brain injury as well (Bilecen, Seifritz, Radu et al., 2000).

As implicated by the above discussion, fMRI has the potential to revolutionize neuropsychological assessment in the evaluation of mild TBI. For example, neurobehavioral probes are being developed that not only reliably show a specific activation pattern of a region in question, but also permit the psychometric assessment of a particular function (i.e., memory; see Gur, Gutierrez, Holdnack et al., 1996). This is shown in Figure 5.11 where a pattern assessing memory shows specific hippocampal activation, in contrast to a self-reflection task that demonstrates frontal activation. Since these areas have a high likelihood of injury in trauma (Bigler, 2001a), it is likely that as neurobehavioral probes are reliably developed they will become standard clinical tools in the assessment of the neurobehavioral effects of mild TBI using the fMRI technology.

qEEG

To date some of the most elegant work accomplished with qEEG and TBI has been that of Thatcher, Camacho, Salazar et al. (1997; 2001). qEEG techniques can also be integrated with MR imaging in the demonstration

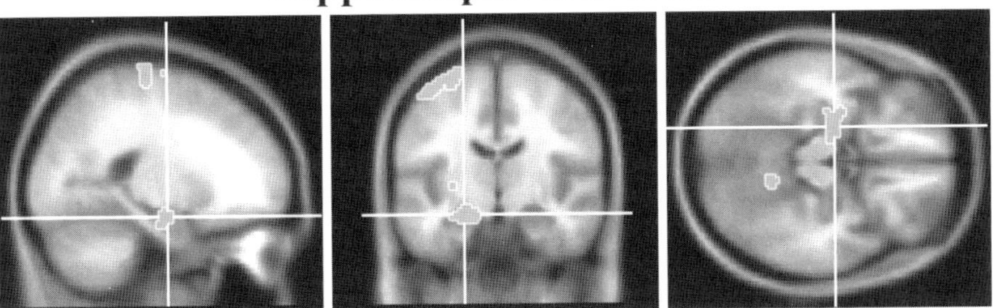

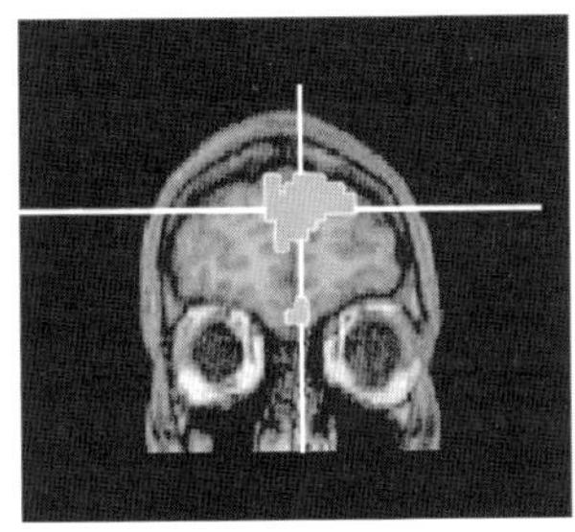

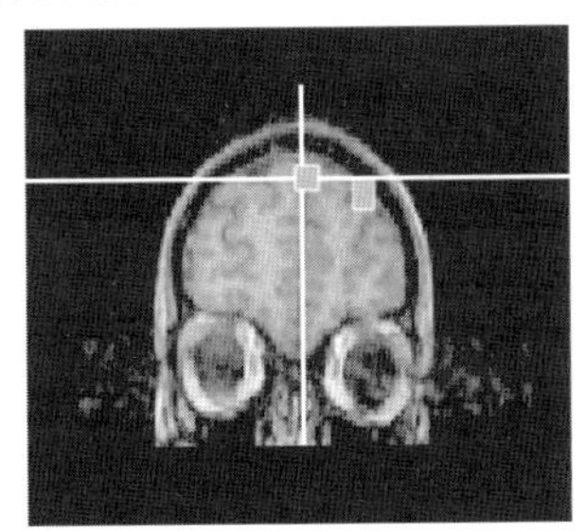

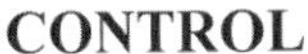

Figure 5.11. Functional magnetic resonance imaging (fMRI) studies are depicted showing specific activation of the hippocampus in a memory task versus frontal activation in a cognitive task of self-reflection. (TOP) The magnetic resonance (MR) images in this panel reflect fused MR images of 5 normal controls in uniform (i.e., Talairach) space in sagittal (LEFT), coronal (MIDDLE), and axial (RIGHT). The task is based on retrieval of new words versus over-learned words. The activation in motor cortex is due to the motor component of responding. (BOTTOM) The fMRI protocol in this task is for the subject to respond to yes/no questions concerning the self (i.e., "I felt happy") versus questions of general knowledge. The individual case presented on the left is from a normal control. The case presented on the right is from a traumatic brain injury (TBI) subject. Note that both are presented in the coronal view. The same activation bar as presented above applies to these cases. As can be seen in the TBI patient, there is less frontal activation from self-reflective thought compared to the non-brain-injured control. If this type of activation can be reproduced in the clinical assessment of TBI patients, it may be the method for simultaneously performing structural and functional assessments of imaging information. (Presented with permission from the lab of Sterling C. Johnson, Ph. D., Barrow Neurological Institute of St. Joseph's Hospital and Medical Center, Phoenix, Arizona.)

of cerebral dysfunction from TBI (Arciniegas, Olincy, Topkoff et al., 2000; Ricker, Muller, Zafonte et al., 2000; Ricker & Zafonte, 2000; Thatcher, Biver, McAlaster et al., 1998; Thatcher et al., 2001). qEEG abnormality can be plotted on the 3-D brain from MR imaging, similar to what was shown in

Figure 5.9 (see also Givens, 1996). These sophisticated technologies provide unique methods for investigating the physiological abnormalities associated with TBI (see Thatcher et al., 2001).

Diffusion-weighted, Tensor Imaging, and Magnetic Resonance Spectroscopy (MRS)

A variety of new neuroimaging techniques or methods of image analysis are becoming available to study the pathological effects of brain injury (Garnett et al., 2000a; Garnett et al., 2000b; Mukherjee, Bahn, McKinstry et al., 2000; Schaefer, Grant & Gonzalez, 2000; Virta, Barnett & Pierpaoli, 1999). Since a major aspect of the pathology responsible for TBI centers on white matter damage (Conti, Raghupathi, Trojanowski et al., 1998), these new methods focus on ways to evaluate the integrity of white matter (Bagley et al., 1999; Thatcher et al., 1997). What is so promising about these methods is that they detect abnormalities that are not seen on conventional clinical MR imaging. As of this writing, no systematic investigation of mild TBI has been conducted using these methods, particularly in sports-related head injury, but they hold tremendous promise because the lesion in sports head injury is likely to be subtle.

Some Clinical Caveats in Neuroimaging of Sports-Related Head Injury

The "functional" defect of a lesion is probably always greater than the structural defect

Figure 5.12 satisfactorily exhibits this point. This patient sustained a moderate to severe injury with multiple hemorrhagic contusions. The focal lesions on MR are very distinct with clear outer boundaries. In contrast, the perfusion abnormalities observed on SPECT imaging are substantially larger. Furthermore, the MEG abnormalities demonstrate even greater regions of abnormal neuronal activity and engaging areas far removed from the focal MR abnormality. Thus, when structural deficits are observed on the CT and MR imaging, even in sports-related mild TBI, there is likely greater physiological disruption that exceeds the boundaries defined by the structural damage per se. Likewise, even in mild TBI the cases that have gone to post-mortem (Blumbergs, Scott, Manavis et al., 1994) show disseminated microscopic lesions. So, even a "small" lesion detected by neuroimaging may merely represent the macroscopic aspect of the lesion and not necessarily the functional connection with behavior, which is likely to be far greater than just the site of the lesion. This is probably why, at least with the current state of neuroimaging-behavioral relationships, that location of an abnormality detected either by CT, MR or SPECT imaging often relates poorly to neuropsychological performance (Bigler 2001a; Hofman et al., 2001).

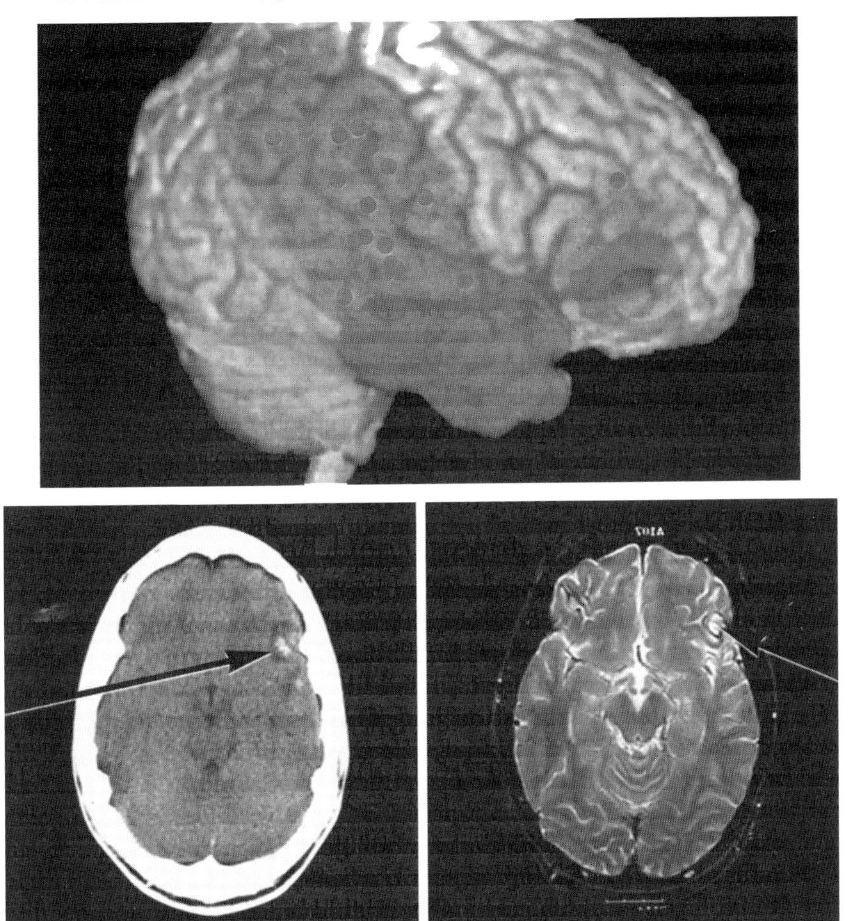

Figure 5.12. (BOTTOM LEFT) The computerized tomography (CT) scan is from the day-of-injury, depicting focal right frontal-temporal injury. (BOTTOM RIGHT) The magnetic resonance image (MRI) scan on the right demonstrates the regions of atrophy, again in the frontal temporal area where the focal injury occurred. (TOP) However, when single photon emission computed tomography (SPECT; darker grey area), magnetoencephalography (MEG) and abnormally low frequency magnetic activity (ALFMA; medium gray with darker grey dots), and magnetic resonance imaging (MRI; darkest grey) are integrated, it is apparent that reliance on just the areas of structural damage result in an underestimation of the area damaged. SPECT imaging demonstrates perfusion abnormalities outside the boundaries of the structural damage, but less that the physiological changes implicated by the MEG findings. This further reinforces the concept that when possible, multiple imaging methods should be undertaken in the full evaluation of the traumatic brain injury (TBI) patient.

The absence of neuroimaging abnormality does not mean the absence of abnormality

In mild head injury, quantitative and functional neuroimaging is often negative. It is always important to understand that pathology may be below the threshold of detection. Quantitative neuroimaging studies (Bigler 2001b) have shown that as a group, patients with mild TBI do not have brain volume loss in response to injury. However, as already reviewed, Lewine et al. (1999) using MEG, and Thatcher et al. (2001) using qEEG, have both shown abnormalities in mild TBI patients who ostensibly have "normal" scan findings. This just means that the pathology is below the gross detection by contemporary structural neuroimaging and that it is likely a physiological disruption of function. In a post-mortem study of mild TBI by Blumbergs et al. (1994) a case is reported where shear injury was histologically confirmed in an individual who had no more than a minute loss of consciousness. Since shear injuries may be very small, such lesions simply may not be detected by neuroimaging, nevertheless can produce significant symptoms. Neuropsychological and neurobehavioral changes maybe the only outward manifestation of the actual underlying neuropathology and even the very best contemporary neuroimaging method may be negative.

Actual lesion size is only modestly related to cognitive and neurobehavioral functioning

A small strategically placed lesion, say in the internal capsule (resulting in paralysis or sensory deficit) or the arcuate fasciculus of the dominant hemisphere (resulting in language deficits), may produce prominent and obvious deficit, whereas large lesions in association cortices may have less obvious effect on behavior. Thus, lesion size often is not much of a predictor of deficit. This may be particularly true in sports injury, because when present, the lesions are typically small, of the petechial hemorrhagic type. Thus, if neuroimaging is negative but sufficient impact injury dynamics are present to injure the brain, or if multiple concussions are present, and valid neurobehavioral deficits consistent with injury are present, clinical judgments need to be made irrespective of the significance, or lack thereof, from neuroimaging studies.

Conclusions

Contemporary neuroimaging provides a range of methods to assess the structural integrity and pathophysiology of mild traumatic brain injury. The type of imaging depends on the patient's clinical history and presentation. New technologies are on the horizon that will likely revolutionize how we image the brain and apply this information to the diagnosis, care, and management of sports-related TBI.

References

Alexander, M.P. (1995). Mild traumatic brain injury: Pathophysiology, natural history, and clinical management. *Neurology*, *45*, 1253–1260.

American Congress of Rehabilitation Medicine. (1993). Definition of mild traumatic brain injury. *The Journal of Head Trauma Rehabilitation*, *8*, 86–87.

American Psychiatric Association. (1994). *Diagnostic and Statistical Manual of Mental Disorders (4th ed.) DSM-IV^{TM}*. Washington, D.C.: American Psychiatric Association.

Arciniegas, D., Olincy, A., Topkoff, J., McRae, K., Cawthra, E., Filley, C.M. et al. (2000). Impaired auditory gating and P50 nonsuppression following traumatic brain injury. *Journal of Neuropsychiatry and Clinical Neurosciences*, *12*, 77–85.

Bagley, L.J., Grossman, R.I., Galetta, S.L., Sinson, G.P., Kotapka, M., & McGowan, J.C. (1999). Characterization of white matter lesions in multiple sclerosis and traumatic brain injury as revealed by magnetization transfer contour plots. *American Journal of Neuroradiology*, *20*, 977–981.

Benson, B.W., Mohtadi, N.G.H., Rose, M.S., & Meeuwisse, W.H. (1999). Head and neck injuries among ice hockey players wearing full face shields vs half face shields. *Journal of the American Medical Association*, *282*, 2328–2332.

Bigler, E.D. (1999a). Neuroimaging in Mild TBI. In N.R. Varney & R.J. Roberts (Eds.), *The Evaluation and Treatment of Mild Traumatic Brain Injury* (pp. 63–80). Mahwah, N.J: Lawrence Erlbaum Associates, Inc.

Bigler, E.D. (1999b). Neuroimaging in pediatric traumatic head injury: Diagnostic considerations and relationships to neurobehavioral outcome. *The Journal of Head Trauma Rehabilitation*, *14*, 70–87.

Bigler, E.D. (1999c). Neuroimaging in traumatic brain injury. In M.J. Raymond, L.C. Bennet, L.C. Hartlage, & C.M. Cullum (Eds.), *Mild Traumatic Brain Injury. A Clinician's Guide* (pp. 11–29). Austin, TX: Pro-ED.

Bigler, E.D. (2001a). The lesion(s) in traumatic brain injury: Implications for clinical neuropsychology. *Archives of Clinical Neuropsychology*, *16*, 95–131.

Bigler, E.D. (2001b). Quantitative magnetic resonance imaging in traumatic brain injury. *The Journal of Head Trauma Rehabilitation*, *16*, 1–21.

Bilecen, D., Seifritz, E., Radu, E.W., Schmid, N., Wetzel, S., Probst, R. et al. (2000). Cortical reorganization after acute unilateral hearing loss traced by fMRI. *Neurology*, *54*, 765–767.

Blumbergs, P.C., Scott, G., Manavis, J., Wainwright, H., Simpson, D.A., & McLean, A.J. (1994). Staining of amyloid precursor protein to study axonal damage in mild head injury. *Lancet*, *344*, 1055–1056.

Colantonio, A., Dawson, D.R., & McLellan, B.A. (1998). Head injury in young adults: Long term outcome. *Archives of Physical Medicine*, *79*, 550–558.

Collins, M.W., Lovell, M.R., & McKeag, D.B. (1999). Current issues in managing sports-related concussion. *Journal of American Medical Association*, *282*, 2283–2285.

Consensus Panel, N.I.H. (1999). Rehabilitation of persons with traumatic brain injury. *Journal of the American Medical Association*, *282*, 974–983.

Conti, A.C., Raghupathi, R., Trojanowski, J.Q., & McIntosh, T.K. (1998). Experimental brain injury induces regionally distinct apoptosis during the acute and delayed post-traumatic period. *Journal of Neuroscience*, *18*, 5663–5672.

Fontaine, A., Azouvi, P., Remy, P., Bussel, B., & Samson, Y. (1999). Functional anatomy of neuropsychological deficits after severe traumatic brain injury. *Neurology*, *53*, 1963–1968.

Friedman, S.D., Brooks, W.M., Jung, R.E., Hart, B.L., & Yeo, R.A. (1998). Proton MR spectroscopic findings correspond to neuropsychological function in traumatic brain injury. *American Journal of Neuroradiology*, *19*, 1879–1885.

Garnett, M.R., Blamire, A.M., Corkill, R.G., Cadoux-Hudson, T.A.D., Rajagopalan, B., & Styles, P. (2000a). Early proton magnetic resonance spectroscopy in normal-appearing brain correlates with outcome in patients following traumatic brain injury. *Brain, 123*, 2046–2054.

Garnett, M.R., Blamire, A.M., Rajagopalan, B., Styles, P., & Cadoux-Hudson, T.A.D. (2000b). Evidence for cellular damage in normal-appearing white matter correlates with injury severity in patients following traumatic brain injury: A magnetic resonance spectroscopy study. *Brain, 123*, 1403–1409.

Gennarelli, T.A., Thibault, L.E., & Graham, D.I. (1998). Diffuse axonal injury: An important form of traumatic brain damage. *Neuroscientist, 4*, 202–215.

Givens, A. (1996). Imaging the neurocognitive networks of the human brain. In E.D. Bigler (Ed.), *Neuroimaging I: Basic Science* (pp. 133–159). New York: Plenum Press.

Gur, R.C., Gutierrez, J.M., Holdnack, J.A., & Mahr, R.N. (1996). Neurobehavioral probes as applied in physiological neuroimaging studies: Methodological considerations. In E.D. Bigler (Ed.), *Neuroimaging I: Basic Science* (pp. 199–214). New York: Plenum Press.

Hofman, P., Stapert, S., van Krooneneburgh, M., Jolles, J., de Kruijk, J., & Wilmink, J. (2001). MR Imaging, single-photon emission CT, and neurocognitive performance after mild traumatic brain injury. *American Journal of Neuroradiology, 22*, 441-449.

Hudson, A.J. (1996). Chronic whiplash. *Neurology, 47*, 615–616.

Kelly, J.P. & Rosenberg, J.H. (1997). Diagnosis and management of concussion in sports. *Neurology, 48*, 575–580.

Kesler, S.R., Adams, H.F., & Bigler, E.D. (2000). SPECT, MR and quantitative MR imaging: Correlates with neuropsychological and psychological outcome in traumatic brain injury. *Brain Injury, 14*, 851–857.

Lewine, J.D., Davis, J.T., Sloan, J.H., Kodituwakku, P.W., & Orrison, W.W. (1999). Neuromagnetic assessment of pathophysiologic brain activity induced by minor head trauma. *American Journal of Neuroradiology, 20*, 857–866.

Masdeu, J.C., Abdel-Dayem, H., & Van Heertum, R.L. (1995). Head trauma: Use of SPECT. *Journal of Neuroimaging, 5*, S53–S57.

Mattiello, J.A., & Munz, M. (2001). Four types of acute post-traumatic intracranial hemorrhage. *New England Journal of Medicine, 344*, 580.

McAllister, T.W., Saykin, A.J., Flashman, L.A., Sparling, M.B., Johnson, S.C., Guerin, S.J. et al. (1999). Brain activation during working memory 1 month after mild traumatic brain injury: A functional MRI study. *Neurology, 53*, 1300–1308.

McCrea, M., Kelly, J.P., Kluge, J., Ackley, B., & Randolph, C. (1997). Standardized assessment of concussion in football players. *Neurology, 48*, 586–588.

McCrory, P.R., & Berkovic, S.F. (2000). Video analysis of acute motor and convulsive manifestations in sport-related concussion. *Neurology, 54*, 1488–1491.

Mosimann, U.P., Muri, R.M., Felblinger, J., & Radanov, B.P. (2000). Saccadic eye movement disturbances in whiplash patients with persistent complaints. *Brain, 123*, 828-835.

Mukherjee, P., Bahn, M.M., McKinstry, R.C., Shimony, J.S., Cull, T.S., Akbudak, E. et al. (2000). Differences between gray matter and white matter water diffusion in stroke: Diffusion-tensor MR imaging in 12 patients. *Radiology, 215*, 211–220.

Ommaya, A.K., Salazar, A.M., Dannenberg, A.L., Ommaya, A.K., Chervinsky, A.B., & Schwab, K. (1996). Outcome after traumatic brain injury in the U.S. military medical system. *The Journal of Trauma: Injury, Infection, and Critical Care, 41*, 972–975.

Orrison, W.W. (2000). *Neuroimaging*. Philadelphia: Saunders.

Osborn, A.G. (1994). *Diagnostic neuroradiology*. St. Louis, MO: Mosby.

Ricker, J.H., Muller, R.-A., Zafonte, R.D., Black, K., Millis, S.R., & Chugani, H. (2001). Verbal recall and recognition following traumatic brain injury: A [^{15}O]-water positron emission tomography study. *Journal of Clinical and Experimental Neuropsychology*, *23*, 196–206.

Ricker, J.H. & Zafonte, R.D. (2000). Functional neuroimaging and quantitative electroencephalography in adult traumatic head injury: Clinical applications and interpretive cautions. *The Journal of Head Trauma Rehabilitation*, *15*, 859–868.

Saatman, K.E., Graham, D.I., & McIntosh, T.K. (1998). The Neuronal Cytoskeleton is at risk after mild and moderate brain injury. *Journal of Neurotrauma*, *15*, 1047–1058.

Saykin, A.J., Johnson, S.C., Flashman, L.A., McAllister, T.W., Sparling, M.B., Darcey, T.M. et al. (1999). Functional differentiation of medial temporal and frontal regions involved in processing novel and familiar words: An fMRI study. *Brain*, *122*, 1963–1971.

Schaefer, P.W., Grant, P.E., & Gonzalez, R.G. (2000). Diffusion-weighted MR imaging of the brain. *Radiology*, *217*, 331–345.

Sinson, G.P., Bagley, L.J., Cecil, K.M., Torchia, M., McGowan, J.C., Lenkinski, R.E. et al. (2001). Magnetization transfer imaging and proton MR spectroscopy in the evaluation of axonal injury: Correlation with clinical outcome after traumatic brain injury. *American Journal of Neuroradiology*, *22*, 143–151.

Smith, D.H., Chen, X.-H., Nonaka, M., Trojanowski, J.Q., Lee, V.-Y., Saatman, K.E. et al. (1999). Accumulation of Amyloid B and Tau and the formation of neurofilament inclusions following diffuse brain injury in the pig. *Journal of Neuropathology and Experimental Neurology*, *58*, 982–992.

Smith, D.H., & Meaney, D.F. (2000). Axonal damage in traumatic brain injury. *Neuroscientist*, *6*, 483–495.

Stuss, D.T. (1995). A sensible approach to mild traumatic brain injury. *Neurology*, *45*, 1251–1252.

Tang, Y., Noda, Y., Hasegawa, T., & Nabeshima, T. (1997). A concussive-like brain injury model in mice (II): Selective neuronal loss in the cortex and hippocampus. *Journal of Neurotrauma*, *14*, 863–873.

Tate, D., & Bigler, E.D. (2000). Fornix and hippocampal atrophy in traumatic brain injury. *Learning & Memory*, *7*, 442–446.

Thatcher, R.W., Biver, C., McAlaster, R., & Salazar, A. (1998). Biophysical linkage between MRI and EEG coherence in closed head injury. *NeuroImage*, *8*, 307–326.

Thatcher, R.W., Camacho, M., Salazar, A., Lindern, C., Biver, C., & Clarke, L. (1997). Quantitative MRI of the gray-white matter distribution in traumatic brain injury. *Journal of Neurotrauma*, *14*, 1–14.

Thatcher, R.W., North, D., Curtin, R., Walker, R.A., Biver, C., Gomez, J.F. et al. (2001). An EEG severity index of traumatic brain injury. *The Journal of Neuropsychiatry and Clinical Neurosciences*, *13*, 77–87.

Virta, A., Barnett, A., & Pierpaoli, C. (1999). Visualizing and characterizing white matter fiber structure and architecture in the human pyramidal tract using Diffusion Tensor MRI. *Magnetic Resonance Imaging*, *17*, 1121–1133.

Weight, D.G. (1998). Minor head trauma: Diagnostic dilemmas. *Psychiatric Clinics of North America*, *21*, 609–624.

Yoon, K.-W., Fuse, T., Shah, P.T., Nguyen, S., & Klein, M.L. (1998). Indirect glutamate neurotoxicity. *Journal of Neurotrauma*, *15*, 141–147.

Yount, R., Raschke, K.A., Biru, M., Tate, D., Miller, M.J., Abildskov, T. et al. (2002). Traumatic brain injury and atrophy of the cingulate gyrus. *The Journal of Neuropsychiatry and Clinical Neurosciences*, *14*, 416–423.

Chapter 6

GENETIC ASPECTS OF TRAUMATIC BRAIN INJURY IN SPORTS

Barry D. Jordan
Burke Rehabilitation Hospital, White Plains, New York;
Weill Medical College of Cornell University New York and New York State Athletic Commission, New York

Traumatic brain injury (TBI) may be encountered in any sport and is considered an important public health concern. Concussion represents the most common type of sports related acute traumatic brain injury (ATBI), however, other types of more severe brain injury such as intracranial hemorrhage and diffuse axonal injury may be encountered. It has been estimated that approximately 300,000 sports related TBIs occur in the United States each year (Centers for Disease Control [CDC], 1997). In addition to ATBI, chronic traumatic brain injury (CTBI) can also be encountered in sports. CTBI represents the cumulative long-term neurological consequences of repetitive concussive and subconcussive blows to the brain (Jordan, 2000). This phenomenon has been principally described in professional boxing, but a clinical variation of the syndrome may be anticipated in tackle football, soccer, ice hockey, and the martial arts (Rabadi & Jordan, 2001).

TBI in sports has the propensity to be associated with significant morbidity and possible mortality. Accordingly, identifying potential risk factors for TBI in sports is of paramount importance. The recognition of potential risk for TBI can lead to more appropriate diagnosis, management and prevention of these injuries. Recent evidence suggests that there may be a genetic predisposition to the effects of TBI. The rationale for this hypothesis extends from our knowledge the genetic and environmental (i.e. head trauma) risk factors for Alzheimer's disease (AD) and the similarities between the neuropathology of cumulative TBI and Alzheimer's disease (AD). The conceptualization of potential genetic contributions to TBI in sports requires an understanding of the pathophysiology of TBI and how it can be influenced by Apolipoprotein E (APOE) genotype.

Amyloid Deposition and Traumatic Brain Injury

Amyloid deposition is a potentially important neuropathological consequence associated with TBI. Several studies have noted increased amyloid deposition following TBI. Smith et al. utilizing a diffuse brain injury model in the pig observed widespread beta amyloid (Aβ) accumulation in damaged neurons (Smith, Chen, & Nonaka, 1999). Transgenic mice, that over-express A , exhibit marked hippocampal atrophy and neuronal death associated with increased Aβ levels in response to TBI (Nakagawa, Nakamura & McIntosh, 1999; Smith, Nakamura & McIntosh, 1998). In humans, severe head injury can trigger amyloid deposition in the brain within days after injury, thus initiating an Alzheimer's disease type process (Roberts, Gentlemen & Lynch, 1991; Roberts, Gentlemen & Lynch, 1994). The presence of diffuse amyloid plaques have been observed in 38% of individuals who sustained a TBI and survived 6 to 18 days (Roberts et al., 1991). After TBI, Aβ is widely distributed throughout the brain and does correlate with the presence of cerebral contusions, intracranial hematoma, axonal injury, ischemic brain damage, brain swelling, or pathology of increased intracranial pressure (Graham, Gentlemen, & Lynch, 1995; Graham, Gentlemen & Nicoll, 1996). Therefore, it has been suggested that the deposition of Aβ is a consequence of the acute phase response of nerve cells to traumatic stress in susceptible individuals (Graham et al., 1995).

Amyloid precursor protein (APP) is a transmembrane glycoprotein and is the source of the Aβ peptide. It has been generally accepted that APP is upregulated during acute traumatic brain injury (Graham et al., 1995) and in fact may be neuroprotective (Mattson, Cheng, Culwell, 1993). The normal cleavage of APP within the Aβ region by α secretase results in the liberation of secreted forms of APP which have been postulated to protect against hypoglycemic injury by reducing calcium and glutamate neurotoxicity. Graham (Graham et al., 1996) noted an increased expression of APP in the pre α cells of the entorhinal cortex and in areas of axonal injury following TBI. It has been suggested that the long-lasting elevation of APP immunoreactivity is secondary to neuronal damage that stimulates astroglial expression (Siman, Card & Nelson, 1989). In contrast to the concept that APP is neuroprotective, it has been hypthesized that the over-expresion and accumulation of APP in neuronal perikarya in response to TBI, may cause degeneration of CA3 neurons in the hippocampus (Murakami, Yamaki, & Iwamoto, 1998).

Abnormal processing of APP will result in Aβ deposition. It has been postulated that APP is synthesized in neurons and delivered to dystrophic nerve endings via fast anterograde axonal transport, where subsequent alterations in the local processing of APP result in deposits of brain amyloid (Koo, Sisodia, & Archer, 1990). The mechanism of altered APP metabolism that produces abnormal amyloid deposition remains to be determined. Several factors may influence the release and processing of APP, which could theoretically result in increased amyloid deposition in TBI. Nitsch (Nitsch, Slack & Wurtman, 1992) noted that stimulation of muscarinic acetylcholine (ACH) m1 and m3 receptor subtypes with carbachol increased the basal release of APP derivatives within minutes of treatment suggesting that pre-existing APP is released in response to receptor activation. Receptor-activated APP release was blocked by staurosporine, thus implying that protein kinases mediate neurotransmitter receptor-controlled APP processing. Another possible mechanism is that increased intracellular calcium secondary to TBI activates calpains which in turn may cleave APP. It has been postulated that the processing of APP is mediated by calpains (Chen, Durr & Fernandez, 2000; Siman, Card & Davis, 1990). Other possible candidates involved in the processing of APP are the cytokines interleukin 1 (IL-1) and interleukin 6 (IL-6). Vandenabeele have suggested that amyloidogenesis in AD results from an IL-1/IL-6 mediated acute phase response in the brain (Vandenabeele & Fiers, 1991). The roles of α,β, or γ secretases in amyloid deposition in TBI remain to be determined. One could speculate that either α secretase activity is decreased and/or the activity of β secretase or γ secretase is increased, resulting in increased amyloidgenesis.

In addition being upregulated in response to injury, APP has been utilized as a marker of axonal injury after TBI (Gentlemen, Nash & Sweeting, 1993; Sheriff, Bridges & Sivaloganathan, 1994). Axonal injury (AI) represents a neuropathological hallmark of TBI secondary to acceleration and deceleration injury to the brain. Traditionally, AI is diagnosed histologically by the presence of axonal retraction balls or clinically by focal hemorrhagic or demyelinating lesions on neuroimaging. However, more recently axonal APP has been utilized as an early marker of axonal injury. It has been postulated that increased axonal APP immunoreactivity occurs as a consequence of the blockage of fast axoplasmic transport of APP (Sheriff et al., 1994).

Evidence of axonal injury has also been documented in milder forms of TBI. Blumbergs (Blumbergs, Scott & Manavis, 1994) observed immunostaining to APP in 5 patients that sustained a concussion but died of unrelated causes 2 to 99 days after brain injury. All of the patients exhibited a Glasgow Coma Scale (GCS) score of 14-15 and experienced loss of consciousness (LOC) 5 minutes or less. Pathologically, axonal injury was noted in the fornix, a major projection of the hippocampus involved in memory function, in all 5 cases. It was suggested that involvement of the fornix may be responsible for the memory disturbances observed in concussed patients. Of interest, lesions of the fimbria-fornix pathway in the rat produce memory impairments and loss of cholinergic activity and are associated with the marked accumulation of APP immunoreactive material in the region of cholinergic fiber degeneration in the hippocampus (Beeson, Shelton & Chen, 1994). This suggests that amyloid deposition may be associated with cholinergic lesions.

Central Cholinergic Neurotransmission and Traumatic Brain Injury

Animal studies suggest that cholinergic neurotransmission may be selectively vulnerable to the effects of TBI and that this disruption is partially responsible for the cognitive impairment associated with TBI. Schmidt and Grady (1995) noted a selective loss of ventrobasal forebrain cholinergic neurons following brief concussive injury in the rat and Gorman (Gorman, Fu & Hovda, 1996) has observed decreases in choline acetyltransferase (CAT) activity in the dorsal hippocampus, frontal and temporal cortices in the rat subjected to brain trauma. Reduced cholinergic neurotransmission has been associated with impaired water-maze learning after parasagittal fluid percussion injury in the rat (Schmidt, Scholten & Maughan, 1999).

Human studies have provided additional evidence of altered cholinergic transmission following TBI. A preliminary human postmortem study noted a decrease in presynaptic cholinergic neurotransmission without affecting muscarinic m1 or m2 receptor binding in the inferior temporal gyrus (Dewar & Graham, 1996). In a follow-up study, Murdoch (Murdoch, Pery & Court, 1998) noted reduced CAT activity in the inferior temporal gyrus, cingulate gyrus, and superior parietal cortex in human postmortem brain from patients that died following head injury compared with age matched controls. It has been suggested that this reduced cholinergic neurotransmission may be responsible for the persistent memory and cognitive impairment following TBI.

Neuropathology of Alzheimer's Disease

The primary neuropatholgical hallmarks of AD are senile plaques and neurofibrillary tangle (NFT) formation. Senile plaques consist of abnormal axonal and dendritic processes (neurites) surrounding extracellular deposits of amyloid. Increased amyloid deposition secondary to either altered amyloidogenesis or abnormal amyloid clearance has been postulated to be the leading pathogenic mechanism in the development of AD (Rosenberg, 2000). Although this amyloid hypothesis suggests that amyloid deposition is necessary but not sufficient to cause AD (Selkoe, 1994), and some investigators have postulated that amyloid deposition is a secondary consequence of the disease process and may not be a direct causation (Roses, 1994). The extent and distribution of NFTs appears to be a more reliable indicator of the severity and duration of AD (Arriagada, Growdon & Hedley-Whyte, 1992). It has been noted that the pattern of amyloid deposits does not correlate with that of NFTs (Braak & Braak, 1996) and cognitive impairment correlates more closely with NFT pathology (Arriagada, 1992) and synaptic loss (Terry, Masliah & Salmon, 1991) which may preceed extracellular amyloid deposition (Masliah, Mallory & Hansen, 1994). Regardless of the primacy of amyloid deposition or NFT formation in the pathogenesis of AD, it is generally agreed that the proximate cause of dementia is neural system destruction, especially in the limbic and association areas, as marked by NFT development and associated synapse and neuron loss (Hyman & Terry, 1994).

Another key issue in the neuropathology of AD, is the reduced cholinergic neurotransmission and its direct association with the memory disturbance in AD (Smith & Swash, 1978). Choline acetyltransferase activity may be reduced by 58 to 90% in selected regions of the AD brain and that this reduced function correlates with dementia severity (Cummings, Vinters & Cole, 1998). Wurtman (1992) suggests that the selective vulnerability of cholinergic neurons in AD may be related choline metabolism. Cholinergic neurons use free choline taken from membrane phosphatidyl choline to synthesize ACH, thus resulting in changes in membrane composition. These changes in membrane composition may make cholinergic neurons more vulnerable by exposing intramembraneous proteins such as APP to proteases (Wurtman, 1992).

Apolipoprotein E and Traumatic Brain Injury: Risk Factors for Alzheimer's Disease

APOE genotype and TBI have been well-established risk factors for the development AD. APOE is a cholesterol transporting molecule in the central nervous system (CNS), that is found in extracellular senile plaques and intraneuronal NFT in AD. APOE exists in three isoforms ε2, ε3, and ε4. APOE ε4 has been well established as a genetic risk factor for both late-onset familial and sporadic AD (Corder, Saunders & Strittmatter, 1993; Saunders, Strittmatter & Schmechel, 1993; Strittmatter, Saunders & Schmechel, 1993). Although APOE ε4 is neither necessary nor sufficient to cause AD (Rosenberg, 2000), a gene dose of ε4 and risk of AD has been noted (Corder et al., 1993; Saunders et al., 1993; Strittmatter et al., 1993). Accumulating epidemiological evidence implicates TBI as a probable risk factor for AD (Lye & Shores, 2000) and individuals who possess the APOE ε4 allele and experience TBI, may be particularly susceptible to developing AD. Mayeaux (Mayeaux, Ottoman & Maestre, 1995) noted a 10-fold synergistic increased risk of AD in individuals with TBI and the presence of APOE e4, whereas an addictive increased risk of AD in patients with head trauma and APOE e4 was observed by Katzman (Katzman, Galosko & Saitoh, 1996). However, in another case control study, although head injury with LOC was associated with increased risk of AD, APOE ε4 was noted to be an independent risk factor the development of AD, that neither modified nor confounded the risk of AD associated with head injury (O'Meara, Kukull & Sheppard, 1997).

Neuropathology of Chronic Traumatic Brain Injury

Histopathological abnormalities in CTBI are similar to those encountered in AD. Intraneuronal NFT composed predominantly of hyperphosphorylated microtubule-associated protein tau represents one of the pathological hallmarks of AD that is also encountered in CTBI. In severe CTBI associated with boxing (i.e. dementia pugilistica) (Jordan, 2000), there is an abundance of NFT and a relative absence of neuritic senile plagues (Corsellis, Bruton & Freeman-Browne, 1973; Corsellis, 1978). Accordingly, one might consider CTBI associated with boxing to be predominantly a "tangle" disease. However, diffuse amyloid plaques have been reported (Roberts, Allsop & Bruton, 1990). The mechanism of NFT formation in CTBI has yet to be elucidated. One could speculate that the predominance of NFTs may be related to AI, however, the relationship between AI and NFT formation has not been established. Using a pig model of diffuse brain injury, accumulation of tau was noted in the cytoplasm of neurons throughout the frontal, parietal, and temporal cortices that correlated with the extent of axonal pathology (Smith et al., 1999). Kanayama (Kanayama, Takeda & Niigawa, 1996) have speculated that the abnormal accumulation microtubule-associated protein 2 (MAP-2) and phosphorylated tau in neuronal perikarya and dendrites in a repetitive head injury model may be related to impaired axonal transport. This hypothesis may explain how AI could be causally related to the formation of NFTs. Roberts (Roberts et al., 1990) utilizing immunocytochemical methods and an antibody raised to the beta-protein present in AD plaques, found that retired boxers with dementia pugilistica and substantial neurofibrillary tangles showed evidence of extensive beta-protein immunoreactive deposits (plaques). These "diffuse" plaques were not visible with Congo red or standard silver stains. Since the degree of beta-protein deposition was comparable to that seen in AD, it was postulated that in dementia pugilistica the pathogenic mechanism of tangle and plaque formation may be similar to that of AD. Support of this hypothesis was provided by Tokuda (Tokuda, Ikeda & Yanugesa, 1991) when these investigators demonstrated tau immunoreactive NFTs and Aβ immunoreactive senile plaques in boxers exhibiting dementia. Another important neuropathologic observation similar to AD has been the presence of ubiquitin in the neurofibrillary tangles in the brains of boxers with dementia and patients with AD (Dale, Leigh & Luthert, 1991). Uhl (Uhl, McKinney & Hedreen, 1982) also presented evidence documenting similarities between CTBI and AD by demonstrating reduced cholinergic activity in a boxer with dementia puglisitica.

Genetic Aspects of Traumatic Brain Injury in Sports

To date, two studies have suggested a genetic predisposition to the neurological consequences of TBI in sports (Jordan, Relkin & Ravdin, 1997;

Kutner, Ehrlanger & Tsai, 2000). In an APOE genotype analysis of 30 active and retired boxers, high exposure boxers (i.e. those with greater than 12 professional bouts) that possessed the ε4 allele exhibited more neurological impairment than those high exposure boxers without the ε4 (Jordan et al., 1997). The ε4 allele had no effect on neurological function in low exposure boxers. In agreement with the boxing study, older active professional football players possessing the APOE ε4 allele scored lower on cognitive tests than did older active players without the allele or younger active players of any genotype (Kutner et al., 2000). In this investigation, age was used as a proxy indicator of exposure. Football players with the ε4 allele performed poorer in the areas of memory, attention, and reaction time. Both studies, although based on relatively small sample sizes, suggest that there may be an interaction exposure to TBI and APOE genotype on neurological outcome in contact/collision sports.

In the clinical literature, several studies support the hypothesis that APOE genotype influences the outcome from TBI, thus suggesting that there is a genetic predisposition to the neurological consequences of TBI. Teasedale (Teasdale, Nicoll & Murray, 1997) in a prospective evaluation of 89 patients sustaining TBI (non-sports related), observed that 17 (57%) of 30 patients with APOE ε4 had an unfavorable outcome at 6 months compared with 16 (27%) of 59 patients without APOE ε4. Unfavorable outcome was defined as dead, vegetative state, or severe disability using the Glasgow outcome scale. Utilizing a different instrument (Functional Independence Measures [FIM]) to assess recovery from TBI, Seliger (Seliger, Lichtman & Polsky, 1997) noted that patients with the APOE ε4 allele experienced a poorer outcome than those without the e4 allele. This differential in recovery was noted in the cognitive domain but not in motor function. Friedman (Friedman, Froom & Sazbon, 1999) also reported a strong association between the APOE ε4 allele and a poor clinical outcome. In this investigation 1 of 27 (3%) of individuals with the APOE ε4 allele had a favorable outcome compared to 13 of 42 (31%) of those without the ε4 allele. A favorable outcome was defined by the absence of dysarthria or dysphasia, lack of behavioral abnormalities, no evidence of severe cognitive impairment, and the ability to live independently. It was also observed that patients with the APOE ε4 allele were 5 times more likely to experience more than 7 days of unconsciousness.

Neurobiology of Apolipoprotein E

In view of the clinical data suggesting a possible genetic influence on neurological outcome after TBI, further understanding of the physiological functions of APOE is necessary. There are several established and putative neurobiological functions of APOE that may effect neurological homeostasis (Table 6.1). The mechanism by which APOE increases the risk of AD and possibly CTBI may directly or indirectly involve several mechanisms. These include

Table 6.1. Postulated and established neurobiological functions of APOE.

Amyloid deposition
Neurofibrillary tangle formation
Cholinergic transmission
Antioxidant activity
Cholesterol transport and metabolism
Regulation of α-1-antichymotrypsin levels
Influence medial temporal lobe atrophy and memory in AD

amyloid deposition, NFT formation, cholinergic transmission, anti-oxidant activity, and the regeneration and repair of CNS injury.

Evidence suggests that APOE acts to promote and/or modulate Aβ fibril formation (Wisniewski, Castano & Golabek, 1994) and the absence of APOE dramatically reduces Aβ deposition (Bales, Verina & Dodel, 1997) and limits neuritic degeneration associated with Aβ deposition (Holzman, Fagan & Mackey, 2000). In postmortem late-onset AD brains, a strong association between the presence of the ε4 allele and increased Aβ deposits compared to patients homozygous for APOE ε3 (Schmechel, Saunders & Strittmatter, 1993). Isoform differences in APOE binding or oxidation of Aβ peptide has also been observed (Strittmatter, Weisgraber & Huang, 1993). It appears that APOE ε3 is much more effective in complexing with Aβ peptide than APOE ε4. The presence of APOE ε4 allele may also promote amyloid deposition in individuals experiencing TBI (Nicoll, Roberts & Graham, 1995). Nicoll (Nicoll et al., 1995) noted that 52% of patients with amyloid deposition following TBI possessed the APOE ε4 allele compared to only 16% of those without amyloid deposition. In addition to APOE, amyloid deposition may also be influenced by other genetic factors. Zunarelli (Zunerelli, Nicoll & Graham, 1996) noted that three out of five individuals with Aβ deposits without the 4 allele, had the 1,1 genotype of presenilin-1(PS-1). It was concluded that if PS-1 genotype influences Aβ deposition but the effect is small and is overwhelmed by that of APOE genotype.

APOE genotype may also influence NFT formation and play a role in neuronal cytoskeletal stability and metabolism. Transgenic mice that overexpress human APOE ε4 exhibited increased hyperphosphorylation of microtubule-associated protein tau in the brain that correlated with the expression of APOE ε4 (Tesseur, Van Dorpe & Spittaels, 2000). In vitro studies indicate that there are isoform-specific interactions of APOE with microtubule-associated protein tau that may regulate intraneuronal tau metabolism and the formation of paired helical filaments and NFT. APOE ε3 binds more avidly to tau forming a biomolecular complex than does APOE ε4 (Strittmatter, Saunders & Goedert, 1994), therefore suggesting that APOE ε4 is more likely to be associated with NFT formation.

APOE may also exert an influence on cholinergic integrity and function. Gordon (Gordon, Grauer & Genis, 1995) noted that APOE deficient mice exhibited markedly lower brain choline acetyltransferase activity in the hippocampus and frontal cortex. It has also been suggested that APOE ε4 allele has a direct impact on cholinergic function in AD (Poirer, 1996). Alzheimer patients that possess the ε4 allele exhibited a more severe cholinergic deficit than AD patients without the ε4 allele (Soininen, Kosunen & Helisalmi, 1995).

Anti-oxidant activity of APOE may play a role in mediating the neuronal maintenance and repair following TBI (Lomnitski, Chapman & Hochman, 1999). APOE ε4 gene increases the susceptibility of CA1 neurons to trauma and oxidative stress through excitotoxic mechanisms (Wallis, Panizzon & Teter, 1999). Postmortem examination of AD brains assessing differing antioxidant activity of APOE isoforms indicate that ε4 has the lowest antioxidant activity and ε2 has the highest antioxidant activity (Tamaoka, Miyatake & Matsuno, 2000). In AD, it has been suggested that mitochondrial/oxidative damage may be more important for cognitive function in patients that carry the ε4 allele (Gibson, Haroutunian & Zhang, 2000).

Chen (Chen, Lomnitski & Michaelson, 1997) reported that APOE deficient mice exhibited an impaired ability to recover from TBI and postulated that APOE may play an important role in neuronal repair. Although the mechanism has not been elucidated, one may speculate that lipid transport may play a role. In the hippocampus of AD patients, APOE mRNA levels are elevated and localize to astroctyes presumed to be involved with lipid uptake where neurons are degenerating or where synaptic modeling is taking place (Zarow & Victoroff, 1998). A differential effect of APOE ε3 and ε4 on neuronal growth has been observed in dorsal root ganglion neuron cultures. APOE ε3 increased neurite outgrowth , whereas APOE ε4 decreased neuronal outgrowth (Nathan, Bellosta & Sanan, 1994). It has been postulated that in response to CNS injury, dysfunctional regulation of phospholipid and cholesterol transport by APOE ε4 during compensatory sprouting and synaptic remodeling may occur (Poirer, 1996).

Genetic Testing in Sports

Confirmation of genetic influences on the outcome from TBI in large, well-defined athletic populations may provide an impetus for genetic testing in sports. Knowledge of an athlete's genetic predisposition to the consequences of TBI, might enable health care providers to better advise athletes about potential risks and implement more appropriate injury prevention and surveillance. However, genetic testing in sports is potentially fraught with ethical and legal issues (Jordan, 1998; Caulfield, 1999). These include confidentiality, possible psychological and emotional burden to the athlete, and the reliability of the genetic testing (Jordan, 1998).

Discussion

Several pathophysiological cascades are initiated at the time of a traumatic event to the brain. Among the vast array of pathological consequences amyloid deposition, NFT formation, and disruption of central cholinergic transmission are essential in understanding the potential genetic contributions to outcome after TBI. Evidence suggests that APOE genotype influences the outcome of TBI via several interrelated mechanisms. It is hypothesized that the following factors are involved in the pathophysiology of CTBI. During impact depolarization following TBI there is an increased release of glutamate and ACH which exerts differential effects on neurobiological function. Increases in glutamate results in increased calcium influx and increased intracellular calcium. This increased intracellular calcium then activates proteases, produces energy failure, and impairs cytoskeletal function. This impaired cytoskeletal impairment results in axonal injury and subsequent interruption of axonal transport in areas rich in cholinergic function. This impairment of axonal transport and increased intracellular calcium increases tau hyperphosphorylation and the formation of NFT. Increased release of ACH secondary to impact depolarization along with cytokines IL-1 and IL-6, and possibly other factors results in the upregulation of APP. This in a setting of impaired axonal transport leads to increased intraneuronal accumulation of APP (a marker of axonal injury). Activated proteases (e.g. ? calpains) and /or other factors yet to be determined result in the abnormal processing of APP, thus initiating amyloid depositon. Thus amyloid deposition and NFT formation are associated with reduced cholinergic function, which is then responsible for the cognitive impairment encountered in CTBI. These above mentioned factors produce an Alzheimer's-like disease process, which is influenced by APOE genotype, therefore providing a genetic predisposition.

Conclusion

In view of the clinical data suggesting a possible genetic influence on neurological outcome after TBI, further investigation utilizing larger well-defined athletic populations is indicated, before genotyping could be utilized to protect the neurological well being of the athlete. Furthermore, the neurobiological functions of APOE and the associations between CTBI and AD need to be further explored.

References

Arriagada, P.V., Growdon, J.H., Hedley-Whyte, T., et al. (1992). Neurofibrillary tangles but not senile plaques parallel duration and severity of Alzheimer's disease. *Neurology*, *42*, 631–639.

Bales, K.R., Verina, T., Dodel, R.C., et al. (1997). Lack of apolipoprotein E dramatically reduces amyloid β-peptide deposition. *Nature Genetics*, *17*, 263–264.

Beeson, J.G., Shelton, E.R., & Chan, H.W. et al. (1994). Age and damage induced changes in amyloid protein precursor immunohistochemistry in the rat brain. *Journal of Comparative Neurology, 342, 69–77.*

Blumbergs, P.C., Scott, G., & Manavis, J. et al. (1994). Staining of amyloid precursor protein to study axonal damage in mild head injury. *Lancet 2, 344,* 1055–1056.

Braak, H. & Braak, E. (1996). Evolution of the neuropathology of Alzheimer's disease. *Acta Neurologica Scandinavica* (Suppl),*165*, 3–12.

Caulfield, T.A. (1999). The law, adolescents, and the APOE ε4 genotype: A view romCanada. *Genetic Testing, 3*, 107–113.

Centers for Disease Control. (1997). Sports-related recurrent brain injuries United States. (MMWR 1997: 46: 224-227). *Journal of the American Medical Association, 277*, 1190–1191.

Chen, M., Durr, J., & Fernandez, H.L. (2000). Possible role of calpain in normal processing of beta-amyloid precursor protein in human platelets. *Biochemical Biophysical Research Communications, 273*(1), 170–175.

Chen, Y., Lomnitski, L., & Michaelson, D.M. et al. (1997). Motor and cognitive deficits in apolipoprotein E deficient mice after closed head injury. *Neuroscience, 80*, 1255–1262.

Corder, E.H., Saunders, A.M., & Strittmatter, W.J. et al. (1993). Gene dose of apolipoprotein E type 4 allele and the risk of Alzheimer's disease in late onset families. *Science, 261*, 921–923.

Corsellis, J.A.N., Bruton, C.J., & Freeman-Browne, C. (1973). The aftermath of boxing. *Psychological Medicine, 3*, 270–303.

Corsellis, J.A.N. (1978). Posttraumatic dementia in Alzheimer's disease. In R. Jatzman, R.D. Terry, & K. Bick (Eds.), *Senile dementia and related disorders* (pp. 125-133). New York: Raven Press.

Cummings, J.L., Vinters, H.V., & Cole, G.M. et al. (1998). Alzheimer's disease. Etiologies, pathophysiology, cognitive reserve, and treatment opportunities. *Neurology, 51*(Suppl), S2–S17.

Dale, G.E., Leigh, P.N., & Luthert, P. et al. (1991). *Journal of Neurology, Neurosurgery and Psychiatry, 54*, 116–118.

Dewar, D. & Graham, D.I. (1996). Depletion of choline acetyltransferase activity but preservation of M1 and M2 muscarinic receptor binding sites in temporal cortex following head injury: a preliminary postmortem study. *Journal of Neurotrauma, 13*, 181–187.

Friedman, G., Froom, P., & Sazbon, L. et al. (1999). Apolipoprotein E e4 genotype predicts a poor outcome in survivors of traumatic brain injury. *Neurology, 52*, 244–248.

Gentlemen, S.M., Nash, M.J., & Sweeting, C.J. et al. (1993). β-amyloid precursor protein (βAPP) as a marker for axonal injury after head injury. *Neuroscience Letters, 160*, 139–144.

Gibson, G.E., Haroutunian, V., & Zhang, H. et al. (2000). Mitochondrial damage in Alzheimer's disease varies with apolipoprotein E genotype. *Annals of Neurology, 48*, 297–303.

Gordon, I., Grauer, E., & Genis, I. et al. (1995). Memory deficits and cholinergic impairments in apolipoprotein E-deficient mice. *Neuroscience Letters, 199*, 1–4.

Gorman, L.K., Fu, K., & Hovda, D.A. et al. (1996). Effects of traumatic brain injury on the cholinergic system in the rat. *Journal of Neurotrauma, 13*, 457–463.

Graham, D.I., Gentlemen, S.M., & Lynch, A. et al. (1995). Distribution of β-amyloid protein in the brain following severe head injury. *Neuropathology and Applied Neurobiology, 21*, 27-34.

Graham, D.I., Gentlemen, S.M., & Nicoll, J.A.R. et al. (1996). Altered β-APP metabolism after head injury and its relationship to the etiology of Alzheimer's disease. *Acta Neurochirurgica,* (Suppl), *66*, 96–102.

Holzman, D.M., Fagan, A.M., & Mackey, B. et al. (2000). Apolipoprotein E facilitates neuritic and cerebrovascular plaque formation in an Alzheimer's disease model. *Annals Neurology, 47*, 739–747.

Hyman, B.T. & Terry, R.D. (1994). Apolipoprotein E, Aβ, and Alzheimer's disease. An editorial comment. *Journal of Neuropathology and Experimental Neurology, 53*, 427–428.

Jordan, B.D., Relkin, N.R., & Ravdin, L.D. et al. (1997). Apolipoprotein Ee4 associated with chronic traumatic brain injury in boxing. *Journal of the American Medical Association, 278*, 136–140.

Jordan, B.D. (1998). Genetic susceptibility to brain injury in sports. A role for genetic testing in athletes. *Physician Sports Medicine, 26*(2), 25–26.

Jordan, B.D. (2000). Chronic traumatic brain injury associated with boxing. *Seminars in Neurology, 20*, 179–185.

Kanayama, G,. Takeda, M., & Niigawa, H. et al. (1996). The effects of repetitive mild brain injury on cytoskeletal protein and behavior. *Methods Find Experimental and Clinical Pharmacology, 18*, 105–115.

Katzman, R., Galosko, D.R., & Saitoh, T. et al. (1996). Apolipoprotein e4 and head trauma: synergistic or additive risks? *Neurology, 46*, 889–892.

Koo, E.H., Sisodia, S.S., & Archer, D.R. et al. (1990). Precursor of amyloid protein in Alzheimer disease undergoes fast anterograde axonal transport. *Proceedings of the National Academy of Sciences, 87*, 1561–1565.

Kutner, K.C., Ehrlanger, D.M., & Tsai, J. et. al. (2000). Lower cognitive performance of older football players possessing apolipoprotein E ε4. *Neurosurgery, 47*, 651–658.

Lomnitski, L., Chapman, S., & Hochman, A. et al. (1999). Antioxidant mechanisms in apolipoprotein E deficient mice prior to and following closed head injury. *Biochimica et Biophysica Acta, 1453*, 359–68.

Lye, T.C. & Shores, E.A. (2000). Traumatic brain injury as arisk factor for Alzheimer's disease: A review. *Neuropsychology Review, 10*(2), 115–129.

Masliah, E., Mallory, M., & Hansen, L. et al. (1994). Synaptic and neuritic alteratons during the progression of Alzheimer's disease. *Neuroscience Letters, 174*, 67–72.

Mattson, M.P., Cheng, B., & Culwell, A.R. et al. (1993). Evidence for excitoprotective and intraneuronal calcium-regulating roles for the secreted forms of the β-amyloid precursor protein. *Neuron, 10*, 243–254.

Mayeaux, R., Ottoman, R., & Maestre, G. et al. (1995). Synergistic effects of traumatic head injury and apoplipoprotein e4 in patients with Alzheimer's disease. *Neurology, 45*, 555–557.

Murakami, N., Yamaki, T., & Iwamoto, Y. et al. (1998). Experimental brain injury induces expression of amyloid precursor protein, which may be related to neuronal loss in the hippocampus. *Journal of Neurotrauma, 15*, 993–1003.

Murdoch, Im., Pery, E.K., & Court, J.A. et al. (1998). Cortical cholinergic dysfunction after human head injury. *Journal of Neurotrauma, 15*, 295–305.

Nakagawa, Y., Nakamura, M., & McIntosh, T.K. (1999). Traumatic brain injury in young,amyloid-beta peptide overexpressing transgenic mice induces marked ipsilateral hippocampal atrophy and diminished Abeta deposition during aging. *Journal of Comparative Neurology, 411*, 390–398.

Nathan, B.P., Bellosta, S., & Sanan, D.A. et al. (1994). Differential effects of apolipoprotein E3 and E4 on neuronal growth in vitro. *Science, 264*, 850–852.

Nicoll, J.A.R., Roberts, G.W., & Graham, D.I. (1995). Apolipoprotein Ee4 allele is associated with deposition of amyloid beta protein following head injury. *Nature Medicine, 1*, 135–137.

Nitsch, R.M., Slack, B.E., & Wurtman, R.J. et al. (1992). Release of Alzheimer amyloid precursor derivatives stimulated by activation of muscarinic acetylcholine receptors. *Science, 258*, 304–307.

O'Meara, E.S., Kukull, W.A., & Sheppard, L. et al. (1997). Head injury and risk of Alzheimer's disease by apolipoprotein E genotype. *American Journal of Epidemiology, 146*, 373–384.

Poirer, J. (1996). Apolipoprotein E in the brain and its role in Alzheimer's disease. *Journal of Psychiatric Neuroscience, 21*, 128–134.

Rabadi, M.H. & Jordan, B.D. (2001). The cumulative effect of repetitive concussion in sports. *Clinical Journal of Sports Medicine, 11*, 194–198.

Roberts, G.W., Allsop, D., & Bruton, C. (1990). The occult aftermath of boxing. *Journal of Neurology Neurosurgery and Psychiatry, 53*, 373–378.

Roberts, G.W., Gentlemen, S.M., & Lynch, A. et al. (1994). β amyloid protein deposition in the brain after severe head injury: implications for the pathogenesis of Alzheimer's disease. *Journal Neurology Neurosurgery Psychiatry, 57*, 419–425.

Roberts, G.W., Gentlemen, S.M., & Lynch, A. et al. (1991). βA4 amyloid protein deposition in brain after head trauma. *Lancet, 338*, 1422–1423.

Rosenberg, R.N. (2000). The molecular and genetic basis of AD: The end of the beginning. The 2000 Wartenberg lecture. *Neurology, 54*, 2045–2054.

Roses, A.D. (1994). Apolipoprotein E affects the rate of Alzheimer disease expression: β-amyloid burden is a secondary consequence dependent on APOE genotype and duration of disease. *Journal of Neuropathology and Experimental Neurology, 53*, 429–437.

Saunders, Am., Strittmatter, W.J., & Schmechel, D. et al. (1993). Association of apolipoprotein E allele ε4 with late-onset famialial and sporadic Alzheimer's disease. *Neurology, 43*, 1467–1472.

Schmechel, D.E., Saunders, A.M., & Strittmatter, W.J. et al. (1993). Increased amyloid β-peptide deposition in cerebral cortex as consequence of apolipoprotein E genotype in late –onset Alzheimer disease. *Proceedings of the National Academy of Sciences, 90*, 9649–9653.

Schmidt, R.H. & Grady, M.S. (1995). Loss of forebrain cholinergic neurons following fluid-percussion injury: implications for cognitive impairment in closed head injury. *Journal of Neurosurgery, 83*, 496–502.

Schmidt, R.H., Scholten, K.J., & Maughan, P.H. (1999). Time course for recovery of water maze performance and central cholinergic innervation after fluid percussion injury. *Journal of Neurotrauma, 16*, 1139–1147.

Seliger, G., Lichtman, S.W., & Polsky, T. et al. (1997). The effect of apolipoprotein E on short-term recovery from head injury. *Neurology, 48*, A213.

Selkoe, D.J. (1994). Alzheimer's disease: A central role for amyloid. *Journal of Neuropathology and Experimental Neurology, 53*, 438–447.

Sheriff, F.E., Bridges, L.R., & Sivaloganathan, S. (1994). Early detection of axonal injury after human head trauma using immunocytochemistry for β-amyloid precursor protein. *Acta Neuropathologica, 87*, 55–62.

Siman, R., Card, J.P., & Davis, L.G. (1990). Proteolytic processing of beta-amyloid precursor by calpain 1. *Journal of Neuroscience, 10*, 2400–2411.

Siman, R., Card, J.P., & Nelson, R.B. et al. (1989). Expression of β-amyloid precursor protein in reactive astrocytes following neuronal damage. *Neuron, 3*, 275–285.

Smith, C.M. & Swash, M. (1978). Possible biochemical basis of memory disorder in Alzheimer's disease. *Neurology, 3*, 471–473.

Smith, D.H., Chen, X.-H., & Nonaka, M. et al. (1999). Accumulation of amyloid β and tau and the formation of neurofilament inclusions following diffuse brain injury in the pig. *Journal of Neuropathology and Experimental Neurology, 58*, 982–992.

Smith, D.H., Nakamura, M., & McIntosh, T.K. et al. (1998). Brain trauma induces massive hippocampal neuron death linked to a surge in β-amyloid levels in mice overexpressing mutant amyloid precursor protein. *American Journal of Pathology, 153*, 1005–1010.

Soininen, H., Kosunen, O., & Helisalmi. et al. (1995). A severe loss of choline acetyltransferase in the frontal cortex of alzheimer patients carrying apolipoprotein ε4 allele. *Neuroscience Letters, 187*, 79–82.
Strittmatter, W.J., Saunders, A.M., & Goedert, M. et al. (1994). Isoform-specific interactions of apolipoprotein E with microtubule-associated proein tau: implications for Alzheimer disease. *Proceedings of the National Academy of Science, 91*, 11183–11186.
Strittmatter, W.J., Saunders, A.M., & Schmechel, D. et al. (1993). Apolipoprotein E: high-avidity binding to β-amyloid and increased frequency of type 4 allele in late-onset familial Alzheimer disease. *Proceedings of the National Academy of Science, 90*, 1977–1981.
Strittmatter, W.J., Weisgraber, K.H., & Huang, D.Y. et al. (1993). Binding of human apolipoprotein E to synthetic amyloid β peptide: isoform-specific effects and implications for late-onset Alzheimer disease. *Proceedings of the National Academy of Science, 90,* 8098–8102.
Tamaoka, A., Miyatake, F., & Matsuno S. et al. (2000). Apolipoprotein E allele_ dependent antioxidant activity in brains with Alzheimer's disease. *Neurology, 54*, 2319–2321.
Teasdale, G.M., Nicoll, J.A.R., & Murray, G. et al. (1997). Association of apolipoprotein E polymorphism with outcome after head injury. *Lancet, 350*, 1069–71.
Terry, R.D., Masliah, E., & Salmon,, D.P. et al. (1991). Physical basis of cognitive alterations in Alzheimer's disease: synapse loss is the major correlate of cognitive impairment. *Annals of Neurology, 30*, 572–580.
Tesseur, I., Van Dorpe, J., & Spittaels, K. et al. (2000). Expression of human apolipoprotein E4 in neurons causes hyperphosphorylation of protein tau in the brains of transgenic mice. *American Journal of Pathology, 156*, 951–964.
Tokuda, T., Ikeda, S., & Yanugesa, N. et al. (1991). Re-examination of ex-boxer's brain using immunohistochemistry with antibodies to amyloid beta protein and tau protein. *Acta Neuropathologica, 82*, 280–285.
Uhl, G.R., McKinney, M., & Hedreen, J.C. et al. (1982). Dementia pugilistic: loss of basal forebrain cholinergic neurons and cortical cholinergic markers. *Annals of Neurology, 12*, 99.
Vandenabeele, P. & Fiers, W. (1991). Amyloidogenesis during Alzheimer's disease due to an IL-1-/IL-6-mediated acute phase response in the brain? *Immunology Today, 12*, 217–219.
Wallis, R.A., Panizzon, K.L., & Teter B. et al. (1999). Protection with MK-801 against susceptibility of mice expressing human apolipoprotein E4 to CA1 neuronal injury from trauma and oxidative stress. *Journal of Neurotrauma, 16*, 986.
Wisniewski, T., Castano, E.M., & Golabek et al. (1994). Acceleration of Alzheimer's fibril formation by apolipoprotein E in vitro. *American Journal of Pathology, 145*, 1030–1035.
Wurtman, R.J. (1992). Choline metabolism as a basis for the selective vulnerability of cholinergic neurons. *Trends in the Neurosciences , 15*, 117–122.
Zarow, C. & Victoroff, J. (1998). Increased apolipoprotein E mRNA in the hippocampus in Alzheimer disease in rats after entorhinal cortex lesioning. *Experimental Neurology, 149*, 79–86.
Zunerelli, E., Nicoll, J.A., & Graham, D.I. (1996). Presenilin-1 polymorphism and amyloid beta-protein deposition in fatal head injury. *Neuroreport, 8*, 45–48

SECTION II

MODELS OF NEURO-PSYCHOLOGICAL ASSESSMENT

EDITED BY

MARK R. LOVELL

Chapter 7

COLLEGIATE AND HIGH SCHOOL SPORTS

Michael W. Collins
University of Pittsburgh Medical Center

Ruben J. Echemendia
Pennsylvania State University

Mark R. Lovell
University of Pittsburgh Medical Center

Introduction and Background

The management of sports-related concussion is currently one of the most hotly debated topics in sport medicine. Much of this debate centers on the determination of when it is safe to return to participation following concussion. This determination is often a difficult one and neuropsychological testing may contribute significantly to the clinical decision making process.

Most experts believe that neurocognitive manifestations of concussion are related to acute metabolic dysfunction (Giza & Hovda, 2001; Hovda et al., 1998). Post-traumatic hyperglycolysis and concomitant decreased cerebral blood flow have been implicated for the cause of this dysfunction. This systematic dysautoregulation, described in detail elsewhere in this text, may not be seen until 2-3 days post-injury and may last for several weeks. Furthermore, it has been postulated that metabolic dysfunction, until fully resolved, may lead to significantly increased neurologic vulnerability if a subsequent trauma (even minor) is sustained. Such metabolic dysfunction is theoretically linked to second impact syndrome and may also form the basis for the less severe, though occasionally incapacitating, presentation of post-concussion syndrome (Cantu, 1986). Although long-term deficits in the form of post-concussion syndrome have been observed from a single concussive event, it is typically assumed that proper management of the concussive injury should lead to good prognosis and minimal deleterious effects with regard to brain function. Conversely, it is our current assumption that returning an athlete to participation prior to complete metabolic recovery may greatly increase the risk of lingering, long-term, or catastrophic neurologic sequelae. As such, acute assessment of injury and determination of existing neurologic difficulties proves critical to the safe management of the concussed athlete.

The focus of this chapter is on the utilization of neuropsychological testing protocols in high school and college athletics. The intent of this chapter is threefold. First, we wish to outline general considerations in the management of the concussed high school and collegiate athlete. To this end, we will emphasize an individualized approach to assessment. Next, we will introduce the reader to two contemporary clinical/research programs that utilize neuropsychological testing protocols for the clinical purpose of managing sports-related concussion. Specifically, the clinical and research protocols of the University of Pittsburgh Sports Medicine Concussion Program and The Pennsylvania State University Concussion Program will be discussed in detail. Although organized differently, these programs both provide sound methodology for the widespread utilization of neuropsychological testing at the college and high school levels of participation. Research using this described methodology has buttressed our theoretical and methodological foundation for advances in our understanding of sports concussion and is likely to be an area of significant growth over the next decade. The third section of the chapter will summarize and review existing peer-reviewed data that outlines the contributions of Sports Neuropsychology at the high school and college levels.

The Need for Neuropsychological Assessment in College and High School Athletics

The determination of lingering difficulties associated with concussion has traditionally proven problematic for a variety of reasons. First, mainstream neurodiagnostic techniques, such as CT scan and MRI, though invaluable in discerning more serious intracranial pathology (e.g. skull fracture, hematoma, parenchymal lesion), are typically insensitive in measuring the subtle effects of concussion. Further, relying on the self-report of the athlete may also prove ineffective because athletes may not be aware of the subtle signs of concussion (e.g. headache, personality changes, memory difficulties, dizziness). In addition, athletes are often taught to "play-through" injury and may minimize symptoms to solidify their playing status and career. Given these issues, ancillary neurodiagnostic strategies have proven critical to the safe management of the concussed athlete. These techniques have also provided a valuable research paradigm from which to gain a better understanding of this complex injury. At the forefront of these approaches is the advent of neuropsychological testing.

Historical Foundation of Sports Neuropsychology

The historical foundation of neuropsychological testing for sports-related concussion began in the college population. Specifically, Jeffrey Barth and colleagues were the first to initiate a prospective research methodology in the mid 1980's with football players in the Ivy League and the University of Pittsburgh (Barth et al., 1989; Macciocchi et al., 1997). For a review of this work, please refer to Chapter 1 of this textbook.

The work of Barth and his colleagues was pioneering in several respects. First, this approach laid the methodological foundation for future neuropsychological studies that built upon their initial findings. Of critical importance was the inclusion of baseline evaluation since individual athletes displayed disparate performance based upon myriad pre-existing factors (e.g. learning disability, cognitive reserve, test anxiety, etc). In addition, this work highlighted the objective nature of neuropsychological evaluation and the ability to uncover even subtle cognitive deficits associated with concussive injury. Notably, however, this initial work also revealed the need for appropriate control groups and the inherent learning or "practice effects" associated with neuropsychological tests. In short, athletes, as a group, revealed ipsitive and relative cognitive deficit, even though they were above baseline levels on each of the individual measures. This finding proved critical to the eventual construction of alternate testing forms and more comprehensive neuropsychological test batteries.

Subsequent to the work conducted by Barth and colleagues, the next systematic utility of neuropsychological testing for sports concussion was implemented with the Pittsburgh Steelers in the early 1990s. This work is discussed elsewhere in this text. This was followed by the development of the NHL League-wide neuropsychological testing program. Such work has resulted in a solid methodological foundation for more widespread utilization of neuropsychological testing protocols for both professional and amateur athletes (Lovell, 2002). In fact, promulgation and utilization of neuropsychological testing protocols for sports concussion management have essentially become the standard for safe management. Evidence of this fact is that neuropsychological testing was recently deemed the "cornerstone" of concussion management by a multi-disciplinary panel of international concussion experts (Aubry et al., 2002). Over the past several years and subsequent to the work by Barth and colleagues, many advances have been made from both a test development and methodological standpoint. We will now review two clinical/research programs that highlight the nature of these advances and illustrate a practical and user-friendly methodology for protocol implementation.

Contemporary Models for the Evaluation of Collegiate and High School Athletes

This section will review two current models of neuropsychological assessment that involve the large-scale participation of collegiate and high school athletes. These models are presented to provide some guidance for researchers and clinicians who desire to implement large scale programs at these levels of participation.

University of Pittsburgh Medical Center (UPMC) Sports Medicine Concussion Program

The UPMC Sports Medicine Concussion program was initiated in September, 2000 and is housed within the Department of Orthopaedic Surgery at UPMC. Dr. Mark Lovell, a neuropsychologist, serves as Director of the newly developed program and Dr. Micky Collins, also a neuropsychologist, serves as Assistant Director. In addition to this core staff, the program also includes Dr. Joseph Maroon, team neurosurgeon of the Pittsburgh Steelers, Dr. Charles Burke, Pittsburgh Penguins physician and Chair of the NHL Concussion Committee, and Dr. Freddie Fu, Departmental Chair of UPMC's Department of Orthopaedic Surgery and head team physician of the Pittsburgh Panthers football team. The daily workings of the program are conducted at the UPMC Center for Sports Medicine, a complex that houses both the Pittsburgh Steelers Football Club and University of Pittsburgh Football Team. The UPMC Sports Concussion Program currently oversees the neuropsychological testing programs for approximately 300 high schools and 100 college programs nationally.

The specific goal of the UPMC Sports Concussion Program is to provide objective clinical data through the use of *ImPACT* (i.e. computerized concussion testing software) to help assist team medical personnel in making safe and appropriate return to play decisions following sports concussion. A second goal is to use this clinical information from a research perspective to investigate a number of pertinent issues regarding management of concussion that have yet to be answered.

The UPMC model emphasizes baseline neuropsychological testing with post-concussion follow-up at 24-48 hours after injury and again five to seven days after injury, and subsequently if needed. In accordance with the recent Concussion in Sports (CIS) group consensus, we also emphasize return to play only after neuropsychological test results have returned to baseline levels and the athlete is symptom free, both at rest and following vigorous physical exertion (Aubry et al., 2002).

There were several driving forces behind the development of the UPMC Sports Concussion Program. Of primary importance was the emergence of neuropsychological testing as a reliable and valid means of assisting in the diagnosis of concussions and in quantifying the severity of the injury. In addition, this program as well as others have grown to fill a growing need for more better concussion assessment technology. As outlined throughout this text, the evolving consensus in the field of sports medicine has been that concussion management "guidelines" (Cantu, 1986; Kelly & Rosenberg, 1997) provide useful information for the initial diagnosis of concussive injury, but are not specific enough to be useful in making individualized return to play decisions regarding return to participation (Collins et al., 1999). In fact the CIS group, which included the developers of the major concussion guidelines, recently agreed that no current guideline system is adequate (Aubry et al., 2002). Through the research efforts described throughout this chapter, as well as through the success of the NFL and NHL neuropsychological testing programs, it is generally understood that individualized evaluation in the form of pre-season/post-injury neuropsychological testing in conjunction with individualized medical management has become the current "cornerstone" in delineating safe return to participation following concussive injury. A second consideration is that many sports medicine physicians (e.g. Primary Care Sports Medicine, Orthopaedic Surgeons) may have only limited knowledge regarding recovery from concussion and may have difficulty detecting the more subtle aspects of injury. Lastly, there is a general paucity of prospective research studies outlining the potential moderating effects of sports concussion and data-driven analysis of acute recovery curves following sports concussion. Thus, there exists a strong need for both research and clinical applications in the area of sports concussion. In short, Sports Neuropsychology should be considered a burgeoning specialty for the application of clinical neuropsychological practice.

The UPMC Sports Medicine Concussion Program rests on the foundation of the National Football League (NFL) and National Hockey League (NHL). However, based on our experience with these more traditional programs, we have recognized the need to institute several important changes that allow us to evaluate large groups of athletes. First, traditional neuropsychological testing is difficult to implement with large groups of athletes due to expense and manpower issues. In fact, it is not uncommon for neuropsychological consultants who work with high school athletes to be asked to perform baseline testing on hundreds of athletes over the course of several days. Second, many of the traditional domains typically assessed with more severe head trauma (e.g. extensive personality, executive, language, malingering assessment) may not be entirely relevant to gain an understanding of the status of the concussed athlete. As outlined above, athletes, in general, are highly motivated to return to sport participation and circumscribed cognitive domains (e.g. speed of processing, verbal/visual/working memory, reaction time) have been shown to be the most sensitive to the effects of mild concussion. In short, sensitive and time-efficient neuropsychological test batteries are critical to the success of Sports Neuropsychology, at the college and high school level. Third, another issue of concern in working with college or high school athletes is the need for serial evaluations. This requires the re-administration of the test or test battery multiple times and raises issues regarding improvement in performance based on exposure rather than on clinical recovery. These "practice effects" may complicate the interpretation of test results and need to be carefully evaluated (Echemendia & Petukian, 2001). In fact, given the need for baseline assessment and serial post-injury evaluation, it is not uncommon that an athlete may be evaluated up to five times over the course of one months time. Thus, reliable and reproducible test forms for each measured domain becomes essential to the successful assessment of sports related concussion. A final concern, which is particularly relevant at the college and high school level, is the clear communication of test results and interpretive hypotheses to those generally unfamiliar with the nomenclature of neuropsychology.

While neuropsychological testing provides important diagnostic information, it should be emphasized that neuropsychological testing provides only on piece of the diagnostic puzzle (Guskiewicz, 2001). Symptom data, prior history of concussion, moderating variables (e.g. learning disability, general neurological history), the athletes general response to injury, and personality factors may all prove critical to delineating a safe return to competition (see Echemendia & Cantu, Chapter 26 in this volume). Thus, specific clinical interview skills and the accumulation of relevant demographic/history data also prove critical to the management of the concussed athlete.

With the forgoing issues in mind, a decision was made in 1995 to begin the construction of the ImPACT computerized neuropsychological test battery. To date, over 7,500 baseline evaluations have been completed and post-concussion evaluations on over 600 high school and college athletes have been completed.

UPMC Sports Concussion Program Protocol

Pre-season baseline evaluation

High school and collegiate at-risk athletes (e.g. football, soccer, wrestling, lacrosse) are typically administered ImPACT to establish a "baseline" level of neurocognitive functioning. The baseline session typically takes place prior to the beginning of the athletic season, before any physical contact is sustained. With appropriate facilities (software can be networked into laboratory), computerized testing can be conducted in a group format of up to 20-25 athletes per session (depending upon number of computers available). An athletic trainer or other familiar with ImPACT should closely proctor each session. Though ImPACT is a user-friendly program, the eventual success of the program rests on an athletes' optimal performance at the baseline session.

Follow-up evaluations

Following suspected concussion, athletes typically undergo a second evaluation using ImPACT. Such testing is usually conducted within 72 hours of suspected injury. Baseline data from the first evaluation may serve as a direct comparison to determine the athlete's recovery from injury. This evaluation can be conducted by the team athletic trainer or physician and also takes approximately 20 minutes to complete. The tests used in the follow-up phase of the evaluation are identical (though stimuli will be randomized) to those utilized in the baseline phase to allow for the direct comparison of results. Re-testing is typically conducted at regular intervals (e.g. days 5, 10 post injury) to determine "recovery curves" for both neurocognitive and self-report symptomatology. An extensive clinical report is generated after the post-concussion evaluation outlining demographic information, concussion/medical history, raw data of ImPACT test modules, neurocognitive composite scores, symptom profile, and graphs displaying the athletes pre-post injury performance.

Post-injury consultation

The most critical phase of the post-concussion evaluative process is the interpretation of the data generated from ImPACT. ImPACT is a neuropsychological test instrument and should be reviewed by a neuropsychologist or other professional formally trained in interpreting the data. ImPACT should also be viewed as a clinical "tool" that provides objective data for which to make post-injury management recommendations and return to play decisions. We wish to stress that post-concussion neurocognitive data *and* self-report symptomatology should be given equal consideration when determining recovery from injury. Given the complexity of concussive injury, it is not uncommon that self-report symptomatology will resolve earlier than neurocognitive deficits or vica/versa.

Although having baseline data is optimal (given the individual variability in cognitive ability/symptom presentation), any athlete who sustains a concussion may be evaluated effectively with ImPACT. Our current database at UPMC consists of approximately 7,500 high school, college, and professional athletes. Thus, extensive normative data is available for post-injury comparison and facilitation of appropriate post-injury management directives.

We have found that data derived from ImPACT may be utilized to help with a number of management directives. For example, following the first post-concussion evaluation, the data allows the clinician to ascertain the general severity of the concussion, which can be communicated to the athlete him/herself, the team medical staff, and potentially the coaching staff. This may serve as a prognostic barometer for return-to-competition. Moreover, the cognitive abilities affected by concussion are also the requisite skills required in the classroom. Thus, data derived from ImPACT may help the athlete receive appropriate academic support during the period of recovery. Lastly, it is well-known that athletes recovering from concussion will have an exacerbation of symptomatology during exertional activity (whether it be cognitive or physical exertion). Thus, ImPACT may serve as a barometer for when an athlete can begin to be exerted and pushed from both mental and physical standpoint. We have found that reduced activity during the acute stages of recovery helps to facilitate recovery from concussive injury. Thus, athletes with minimal impairment on ImPACT might be pushed earlier from a physical standpoint, whereas those with discernable impairment may be managed more conservatively.

A final point of emphasis is the importance of a multi-disciplinary approach to concussion management. As a Sport Neuropsychologist, one needs to effectively work within a system that involves multiple disciplines and frames of reference. Work in this area will inevitably involve consultation or collaboration with athletic training, physical therapy, primary-care sports medicine, orthopaedic surgery, neurology, and neurological surgery. The success of the UPMC Sports Concussion Program has been predicated upon effective communication with such professionals, practical application of the aforementioned methodology, and solid relationships that have formed with consultant organizations. An overriding goal of the UPMC Sports Concussion Program is to assist sports medicine practitioners in making more informed, objective, and scientifically-based decisions regards post-concussion management and return-to-play directives.

ImPACT was developed specifically for assessing sports-related concussion. The computer program measures multiple aspects of cognitive function in athletes, including attention span, working memory, sustained and selective attention, response variability, and several dimensions of verbal/visual memory. Reaction time is also measured to one-hundredth of a second across individual test modules (10 modules total) and allows for an assessment of processing speed as the player fatigues. Importantly, the program also consists of a 21-item self-report symptom scale and demographic/history form that precedes the neuropsychological measures. The program, in its entirety, is a user-friendly, Windows-based program that can be administered by an athletic trainer or physician with minimal training. Further, athletes can be tested in a group format since the software can be networked into school, university, or team computer laboratories. The test battery consists of a near infinite number of alternate forms by randomly varying the stimulus array with each module. This feature was built into the program to minimize the practice effects that have limited the usefulness of more traditional neuropsychological tests. The program, as a whole, takes approximately 20 minutes to complete.

The Penn State University Concussion Program

The Penn State program began as a result of frustration that arose when using neuropsychological tests within a more traditional context that did not allow baseline testing. The frustration was the result of not knowing the athletes' "pre-morbid" status on neurocognitive tests. Although we were convinced of the utility of using neuropsychological tests in sport-related concussion, we were very uncomfortable using group normative data to ascertain whether a player had returned to "normal functioning." In 1995, a pilot program named the Penn State Cerebral Concussion program was initiated to systematically examine the effects of mTBI on college athletes using a neuropsychological screening battery. The program was based on the pioneering work of Dr. Barth and his colleagues as well as Dr. Lovell's work in professional football. Since there was relatively little information on what tests or batteries would be most effective with this population, many colleagues in neuropsychology were contacted and asked to provide their input. We were particularly interested in identifying tests that had demonstrated reliability and validity with concussion and TBI populations, were short, easily administered and had multiple forms (if possible).

Prior to 1995, much of the work that had been conducted with sports neuropsychology in the United States was with football. We were interested in developing a comprehensive program that included a variety of men's and women's sports. Initially, athletes from the football, ice hockey, soccer (men and women), and basketball (men and women) teams were selected as "at risk" for concussion. Athletes from tennis, swimming, and baseball were selected as the "low risk" group. Since that time we have added the wrestling team, men's and women's lacrosse, and men's and women's rugby. In addition, we have worked with the men's ice hockey team from Princeton University for three years and more recently have added Princeton's football, women's ice hockey, men's and women's soccer, and men's and women's lacrosse.

An important consideration in developing any college neuropsychological concussion program is that it requires a tremendous amount of work and cooperation among a wide group of individuals. This is particularly true of a multi-sport program that involves hundreds of athletes, as well as scores of athletic trainers, physicians and coaches. We have been very fortunate to work with many enlightened coaches at Penn State and Princeton. We have also had the good fortune of developing excellent collegial relationships with team physicians and athletic trainers at both institutions.

The Penn State Concussion program assesses athletes at baseline, ideally prior to contact participation in sport. A unique aspect of this program is the assessment of injury very early in the recovery process. Athletes sustaining a concussion were routinely tested at 2 hours post injury and again at 48 hours, one week, and one month post injury. Throughout the six seasons that the program has been in existence, the neuropsychological measures have been subjected to multiple analyses. These data have resulted in the addition and deletion of measures. The initial battery consisted of the PASAT, a 5 word list learning task, Boston Naming Test, COWAT, SDMT, Stroop, Trail Making Test, Visual Search and Attention Test, VIGIL, and Digit Span. The five-word list learning task was deleted after one season due to marked ceiling effects and was replaced with the HVLT. Subsequently, the PASAT was deleted because of the significant frustration that it caused with many of the athletes and the lack of unique variance that it captured. Digits forward was also deleted due to lack of sensitivity. The VSAT was replaced with the Penn State Cancellation Test and the BVMT-R was added to more fully assess visuospatial learning and memory. During 2001, the ImPACT neuropsychological test battery was also included for the purposes of research.

The program was initially funded by the university's Graduate Research Office and the Department of Psychology. Since 1999 the program has been funded in part by the National Operating Committee on Standards for Athletic Equipment (NOCSAE). To date, baseline data have been collected on approximately 800 athletes and a total of 70 concussive events have been recorded. Retrospective data from this project revealed relatively high rates of concussion in our athletes prior to their collegiate career: 29.8% of football players, 41.2% of men's soccer players, 42.2% of women's soccer players, 55.8% of ice hockey players, 36.8% of men's basketball players, and 31.3% of women's basketball players (Echemendia, 1999).

Sports Neuropsychology for the High School and College Athlete: An Overview of Existing Data

The UPMC and Penn State Concussion Testing Programs provide a meaningful clinical protocol to help quantify an athletes level of functioning to help delineate management directives and return to play data. Taken together, these programs have evaluated hundreds of athletes in this regard. Potentially more important, however, is the solid research methodology inherent in this clinical protocol. Of obvious importance is the fact that baseline/post-concussion neuropsychological testing provides an opportunity to sensitively quantify the injury and research germane areas of inquiry that have yet to be explored in the literature. The intent of this section of the chapter is to review existing neuropsychological studies that have been performed with high school or college athlete populations.

Research Pertaining to College Athletics

Based upon the Ivy League work conducted by Barth and colleagues (described earlier), Collins and colleagues initiated a second multi-site college study of football players during the 1997–1998 seasons. This program involved the baseline testing of 393 college football players from Michigan State University, the University of Florida, the University of Pittsburgh, and the University of Utah (Collins, Lovell, & McKeag, 1999). A variant of the Pittsburgh Steelers Neuropsychological Test Battery was utilized and several retrospective analyses were conducted examining the effects of prior concussions on baseline cognitive performance. Preliminary findings revealed that those athletes with a history of two or more prior concussions performed significantly more poorly at baseline on tests measuring speed of information processing and executive function. Further, presence of a diagnosed learning disability, in combination with a history of multiple concussions, was found to especially attenuate baseline neuropsychological function. Lastly, prospective, baseline-post injury data was collected on 19 athletes diagnosed with concussion during the course of the study. Relative to matched, non-injured football player controls, these injured athletes displayed significantly impaired (and below baseline) performance on the Hopkins Verbal Learning Test (verbal memory). Overall, relative to controls, deficits were noted out to day 7 post-injury, especially in terms of memory and overall speed of information processing. Importantly, injured athletes' self report of symptoms resolved 3-5 days after injury. This latter finding highlighted the importance of objective neuropsychological testing since athletes may attempt to minimize or be generally unaware of overall difficulties. It should be noted that Lovell and Collins (1998), based upon the same database, also published a much more abbreviated study examining neuropsychological function in Michigan State University football players. This study presented test-retest (baseline-post season) data from the neuropsychological test battery, showing the relative stability of the battery over time. Further, prospective pre-post injury data was presented on four cases of concussion revealing discernable impairment with processing speed and word fluency out to 5 days from injury.

Another prospective neuropsychological study of sport-related concussion in college athletes was conducted by Echemendia and his colleagues (Echemendia & Petukian, 2001) using the previously described methodology of the Penn State Program. Using the baseline – posttest paradigm, these researchers evaluated 29 injured male and female athletes from football, men's ice hockey, and men's and women's soccer and basketball. Twenty non-injured athletes were also serially evaluated and served as controls. Athletes were evaluated using a comprehensive neuropsychological screening battery at baseline and within 2 hours of injury, 48 hours, 1 week, and 1 month post-injury. Using MANOVA, statistical and clinically meaningful differences were found between injured athletes and controls at 2 hours after concussion with injured athletes experiencing deficits in verbal learning, verbal memory, and attention/concentration. At 48 hours post-injury significant differences were found between concussed athletes and controls. Controls performed better than their injured counterparts on 20 of 23 measures of NP functioning comprising working memory, verbal learning, verbal memory, divided attention, and speed of information processing. Injured athletes performed worse at the 48-hour assessment than they did at the 2 hour assessment, whereas the control group *improved* during that period. At one week post-injury the controls continued to outperform the concussion group on 20 of the 23 NP indices but the overall MANOVA was not significant. Since the study was exploratory, univariate ANOVA's were examined and 4 indices were found to statistically differentiate the two groups: visual-motor speed, working memory, sustained attention and concentration, and reaction time. However, since the MANOVA was not significant these results can only be considered suggestive although they do raise the possibility that some athletes with concussion may have neurocognitive deficits as much as 7 days following injury. At one month post injury, an unusual finding emerged in that the injured group outperformed the control group on one measure. The finding was interpreted in light on increased motivation among the concussed athletes and decreased motivation on the part of controls.

This study was important since it is the first prospective college neuropsychological analysis of concussed female athletes as well as non-football male athletes. It was also the first study to use a neuropsychological test battery to assess athletes within 2 hours of concussive injury. The use of the two-hour assessment interval allowed for an evaluation of the progression of cognitive and neurobehavioral symptoms from a point in closer proximity to the injury than had been done previously. The test intervals led to a finding that in many instances neuropsychological functioning actually decreased from the 2 hour test period to the 48 hour test period, a finding that is highly consistent with the neurochemical cascade documented in the animal literature. Clearly, more studies with these populations are needed to better determine potential gender and sports-specific moderating effects of injury.

Preliminary data from this project (Echemendia, 1999) that have subsequently been replicated with a much larger sample size reflected no differences in neuropsychological test performance between those athletes reporting no history of concussion and those reporting a history of one or more concussions. This finding is in contrast to the Collins et al. (1999) study that found baseline differences as a function of number of concussions prior to baseline testing. These data also revealed significant differences in neuropsychological test scores among different sports, underscoring the need for individualized baseline testing.

The Penn State program has more recently focused on the potential danger of "heading" the ball in soccer. Some studies have suggested that the practice of heading the ball in soccer may lead to significant declines in neurocognitive functioning. Unfortunately, many of these studies failed to tease out the effects of heading from the consequences of concussion. Petukian, Echemendia, and Macklin (2000) conducted a prospective pilot study with the Penn State men's and women's soccer team. The study employed a prospective cross-over design where each team received neuropsychological testing prior to and following a planned heading practice. One half of the participants engaged in the heading practice on day one and the other half engaged in a non-heading practice designed to elicit the same level of physical activity. In the following practice two days later the groups were switched allowing for each player to serve as his or her own control. The results yielded no significant differences on posttest scores between the heading and non-heading groups suggesting that in this small pilot study of college athletes there were no acute effects of heading.

McCrea and colleagues in (2002) have now published several interesting studies of acute recovery in college athletes utilizing a cognitive screening approach called the Standardized Assessment of Concussion (SAC). The SAC is a brief (approximately 5 minute), on-field mental status exam intended to measure immediate memory (5 word serial learning task), concentration, and delayed recall (recall of 5 words after 5 minutes). In addition, the SAC assesses orientation and includes a brief neurologic screening. Approximately 500 football players were baseline tested with this abbreviated battery of tests and 33 athletes were retested within 24 hours and again within 48 hours following concussive injury. All post-injury evaluations were conducted on the sideline by Athletic Trainers. No controls were utilized for this study and the baseline scores of those not concussed were used as group normative data. Following concussion, the total SAC score was significantly lower than that of the baseline total SAC score of those not concussed. Furthermore, individual subtest scores in the area of memory and concentration were also significantly lower compared with the normal baseline scores. All scores returned to normal within 48 hours of injury. It was concluded that the SAC is a sensitive test measuring the acute (i.e. on-field) effects of concussion and may serve as an important sideline tool to immediately diagnose the injury. However, it is important to recognize the obvious disparity between recovery patterns using the SAC (athletes recover within 48 hours) versus more formal neuropsychological evaluation (athletes reveal deficits out to at least day 7 post-injury). In our opinion, this highlights the importance of a more comprehensive approach to assessment. As outlined by McCrea, the SAC should serve only as an initial, on-field diagnostic measure and *should not* replace more formal neuropsychological evaluation to determine safe return to participation following concussion. Using the SAC in isolation may actually prove harmful since the measure clearly produces false negatives and lingering deficits in athletes' function are likely to be present.

Lastly, a recent study conducted by Collins, Iverson, Lovell et al. (2003) has examined on-field predictors of neuropsychological and symptom deficit in a relatively large sample (N = 78) of concussed high school and college athletes. This data was collected from the previously described UPMC Sports Concussion Program. In this analysis, "good" and "poor" outcome groups were formed based upon results derived from ImPACT at approximately 3-days post-injury. Specifically, good outcome (N = 44 athletes) was defined as the athletes exhibiting no measurable impairment (relative to baseline) in terms of both neurocognitive (i.e. memory) and symptom functioning (i.e. symptom inventory) as measured by ImPACT. Conversely, "poor" outcome (N = 34 athletes) was defined as a 10-point increase in symptom reporting and 10-point decrease in memory functioning (exceeding the 80% confidence interval on ImPACT). Subsequent analyses were conducted examining the presence of on-field markers of injury in these outcome groups. Odds ratios revealed that athletes demonstrating "poor" outcome were over 10-times more likely to have exhibited any presence of on-field retrograde amnesia when compared to those demonstrating "good" outcome. Similarly, athletes in the poor outcome group were approximately 4-times more likely to have exhibited any degree of on-field post-traumatic amnesia. There were no differences between groups in terms of on-field presence of loss of consciousness or brief (< 5 minutes) disorientation. Such findings are potentially quite germane since traditional concussion management "guidelines" (which are not data-driven or empirically-based) base severity of injury on the loss of consciousness construct. These findings question the validity of this approach and emphasize the relative importance of amnesia in predicting outcome.

Research Pertaining to High School Athletics

Although the focus of this chapter has thus far been on the evaluation of the collegiate athlete, the model of conducting large-scale neuropsychological testing has recently been extended to the high school level. This represents an important step as the younger athlete represents the largest at-risk population and has historically been overlooked.

To date, there have been only a few neuropsychological studies of high school athletes and most of these studies have been conducted through the University of Pittsburgh Sports Medicine Concussion Program. Although much more research data is urgently needed with this age group and numerous studies are currently underway, the results of initial studies suggest lingering post-concussive neuropsychological deficits lasting seven days or more in high school athletes. For example, Lovell, Collins, and Iverson (2003) and Lovell, Collins, and Iverson (in press) have recently documented memory deficits lasting at least seven days in a group of mildly injured or "dinged" high school athletes who would fall within the Grade 1 classification system within existing concussion guideline systems. All athletes in this sample demonstrated on-field symptoms that had completely resolved within 15 minutes of trauma. No high school athlete in the sample returned to play. Memory deficits were measured by computerized neuropsychological testing (ImPACT) and a control-group was utilized. Interestingly, though athletes demonstrated demonstrable memory deficits out to day 7 post-injury, self-reporting of symptoms resolved by day 4 post-trauma. Such data is in accordance with previous studies described above utilizing paper-and-pencil neurocognitive testing. Such findings bring into question the common practice of returning mildly concussed athletes to the playing field during the same contest in which they are injured. These data directly contradict widely used grading systems, such as the American Academy of Neurology. Such data also highlight the sensitivity of a computerized neuropsychological testing protocol in delineating the subtle aspects of concussive injury.

A recent study conducted by Collins, Field, and Lovell (2003) was also published examining the issue of post-concussion headache in a large sample of concussed athletes (N =110 athletes). In this study, athletes with no degree of headache at day 7 post-concussion were compared to those athletes experiencing any degree of headache. Findings from this analysis revealed that athletes reporting headache performed significantly worse on ImPACT composite scores in the areas of reaction time and memory, as well as these athletes reporting a greater number of other post-concussion symptoms. Such data highlight the need for conservative management in high school athletes demonstrating any degree of post-concussion headache. This symptom appears predictive of incomplete recovery following injury. Recent published data collected on a large sample of concussed high school athletes has also suggested cumulative effects of concussion (Collins, Iverson, Lovell et al., 2003). More specifically, athletes with a history of three or more concussions were found to be much more likely to experience a loss of consciousness, amnesia or other mental status changes at the time of their next injury, compared to a group with no concussion history. Lastly, a recent study published by Field, Collins, Lovell and colleagues (In press, 2003) compared recovery rates from concussion in a large sample of high school and college athletes (N = 92). Interesting, concussed high school athletes demonstrated prolonged memory dysfunction compared to concussed college athletes. Specifically, high school athletes performed significantly worse than age-matched controls at 7 days post-injury. College athletes, despite apparently suffering more severe in-season concussions, displayed commensurate performance with matched-control subjects by day 3 after concussion. Once again, self-report of post-concussion symptoms by athletes was not predictive of poor performance on neurocognitive testing. Such data are interesting since they seem to indicate a lengthened recovery process from concussion in high school athletes. Such data also call into question the usage of concussion "guidelines" that assume a standard implementation for all age groups and playing levels.

In summary, recent data derived from this body of research appears to indicate a need for careful post-injury evaluation for *any* high school athlete diagnosed with concussion. Such data call into question the common practice of returning high school athletes to play following a "bell-ringer" or concussive incident where symptoms clear expeditiously. Findings from this research indicate that a prudent approach may be to remove any high school athlete from sport participation until proper post-injury evaluation by a qualified physician or clinician with appropriate training. Data derived from multiple researchers also appears to indicate a potential delayed-onset of symptoms (neurocognitive deficits, self-report symptoms) following injury and that recovery may not be a linear process. As such, serial on-field and comprehensive post-injury evaluation (in the form of neuropsychological testing) appears indicated. This is especially germane since the reviewed studies indicate quicker recovery from perceived symptoms as compared to more formal neurocognitive test data. A potential hypothesis in lieu of these findings is athletes may minimize symptomatology in hopes of a quicker return to the playing field. Lastly, the reviewed study indicated more prolonged recovery following concussion in high school athletes is an important preliminary finding which further underscores the need for conservative management in the high school concussed athlete.

Summary

This chapter has provided an overview of neuropsychological assessment within the college and high school environments. We are pleased to report that work with college and high school athletes is currently an area of considerable activity and numerous clinical and research program have been established at both levels. Within the next five years, we expect continued growth in interest in concussion in these athletes and are confident that this research will lead to substantial innovations regarding diagnosis, management, and treatment of concussion.

References

Aubry, M., Cantu, R., Dvorak, J., Graf-Baummann,, T., Johnston, K., Kelly, J. et al. (2002). Summary and agreement statement of the 1st International Conference on Concussion in Sport, Vienna 2001. *Clinical Journal of Sport Medicine, 12,* 6–11.

Barth, J., Alves, W., Ryan, T.V., Macciocchi, S.N., Rimel, R.W., Jane, J.A., & Nelson, W.E. (1989). Mild head injury in sports: Neuropsychological sequelae and recovery of function. In H. Levin, H. Eisenberg, & A. Benton (Eds.), *Mild Head Injury* (pp. 257–275). New York, NY, Oxford University Press.

Cantu, R.C. (1986). Guidelines for return to contact sports after a cerebral concussion. *Physician and Sports Medicine, 14*(10), 75–83.

Collins, M.W., Grindel, S.H., Lovell, M.R., Dede, D.E., Moser, D.J., Phalin B.R. et al. (1999). Relationship between concussion and neuropsychological performance in college football players. *Journal of the American Medical Assocation, 282*(10), 964–970.

Collins, M.W., Lovell, M.R. & McKeag, D.B. (1999). Concussion Management Guidelines. *Journal of the American Medical Association, 282,* 2283–2284.

Collins, M.W., Lovell, M.R., Iverson, G.L., Cantu, R.C., & Maroon, J.C. (2002). Cumulative effects of concussion in high school athletes. *Neurosurgery, 51,* 1175–1181.

Collins, M.W., Field, M., Lovell, M.R., Iverson, G.L., Johnston, K.M., Maroon, J., & Fu, F.H. (2003). Relationship between postconcussion headache and neuropsychological test performance in high school athletes. *American Journal of Sports Medicine, 31,* 168–173.

Collins, M.W., Iverson G., Lovell, M.R., McKeag, D.B., Norwig, J., & Maroon, J. (2003). On-field predictors of neuropsychological and symptom deficit following sports-related concussion. *Clinical Journal of Sport Medicine, 13,* 222–229.

Echemendia, R.E. (1999). Penn State Cancellation Test, Personal Communication Test.

Echemendia, R.E. & Petukian, M. (2001). Neuropsychological test performance prior to and following sports-related mild traumatic brain injury. *Clinical Journal of Sports Medicine, 11,* 23–31.

Field, M., Collins M.W., Lovell M.R., & Maroon, J. (in press). Does Age play a role in recovery from sports-related concussion? A comparison of high school and college athletes. *Journal of Pediatrics.*

Giza, C.C. & Hovda, D.A. (2001). The neurometabolic cascade of concussion. *Journal of Athletic Training, 36,* 228–235.

Guskiewicz, K.M. (2001). The Concussion puzzle: 5 compelling questions. *Journal of Athletic Training, 36*, 225–226.

Hovda, D.A., Prins, M., Becker, D.P., Lee, S., Bergsneider, M., & Martin, N. (1998). Neurobiology of concussion. In J. Bailes, M.R. Lovell, & J.C. Maroon (Eds.), *Sports-Related Concussion.* St. Louis, Quality Medical Publishers.

Kelly, J.P. & Rosenberg, J.H. (1997). Diagnosis and management of concussion in sports. *Neurology*, 48, 575–580.

Lovell, M.R., Collins, M.W., Iverson, G.L., Johnston, K., & Bradley, J. (in press). Grade 1 or "ding" concussions in high school athletes. *American Journal of Sports Medicine.*

Lovell, M.R. & Collins, M.W. (1998). Neuropsychological assessment of the college football players. *Journal of Head Trauma Rehabilitation, 13*(2), 9–26.

Lovell, M.R. The relevance of neuropsychological testing for sports-related head injuries. (2002). *Current Sports Medicine Reports, 1*(1), 7–12.

Lovell, M.R., Collins, M.W., Iverson, G.L., Maroon, J.C., Field, M., Cantu, R.C. et al. (2003). Recovery from mild concussion in high school athletes. *Journal of Neurosurgery, 98*, 296–301.

Macciocchi, S., Barth, J., Alves, W., Rimel, R.W., & Jane, J.A. (1997). Neuropsychological functioning and recovery after mild head injury in collegiate athletes. *Neurosurgery, 39*(3), 510–514.

McCrea, M., Kelly, J.P., Randolf, C., Cisler, R. & Berger, L. (2002). Immediate neurocognitive effects of concussion. *Neurosurgery, 50*(5), 1032–1040.

Petukian, M., Echemendia, R.E. & Macklin, S. (2000). The acute neuropsychological effects of heading in soccer: a pilot study. *Clinical Journal of Sports Medicine, 10*(2), 971–973.

Chapter 8

YOUTH HOCKEY

Rudolph Hatfield, Linas Bieliauskas, Paula Begloff, Brett Steinberg, and Mary Kauszler
University of Michigan Health System
V.A. Medical Center, Ann Arbor, Michigan

High school athletic programs offer a wide variety of competitive sports in which students can participate. Students may choose to concentrate on a single sport, or participate in several different athletic activities. Competitive high school sports programs are designed to allow the contestants to develop themselves physically and socially, as well as offering potential college scholarships to accomplished players. While participation in high school athletics offers numerous benefits to the participants, the students participating in high school athletic programs are also at an increased risk for injury even though high school athletic programs devote numerous resources to injury prevention (Thurman, Branche, & Scniezek, 1998).

The type of injury that may result from participation in high school athletics will depend on the specific activity itself. Contact or collision sports like ice hockey and tackle football would be expected to have significantly more acute injuries than baseball or golf (Powell & Barber-Foss, 1999). Collision sports might also be expected to result in significantly more concussions than non-contact sports. For example, Powell and Barber-Foss (1999) collected information from high school athletic programs regarding injury type and frequency occurring over a three-year period. Data was collected from 246 NATA-certified athletic trainers nationwide. Ten major high school sports were surveyed and all of the sports reported at least some incidence of concussion. Tackle football reported the highest rate (about 63% of all reported concussions) and this sport was followed by high school wrestling (about 11% of all reported concussions). Ice hockey, which might also be expected to result in injuries, was not included in the study.

We know of no formal comparisons for injury rates between adolescent ice hockey players and participants in other high school sports. However, given that the manner in which the game of ice hockey is played, we would expect that the potential for injuries resulting from play may be as prevalent as in football. First, the rules instituted in ice hockey allow for player substitutions to be made without stoppage of the game itself. Thus, players typically spend 60-120 seconds on the ice and are allowed to rest until they return to their optimal level of play. This ensures that active contestants are not fatigued and are able to perform at their best possible level throughout the contest. Short playing shifts also allow players to withstand the physical rigors of the game and deliver punishing checks and blocks throughout the game. Second, the speed at which hockey players are able to travel is quite fast, allowing for some significant impacts when players collide with one another. Third, the playing field itself is more likely to be harder and much more unyielding in ice hockey than in football. Falls on the ice may be more likely to result in an injury than falls on a grass playing field, even with the heavy padding that the players wear. Fourth, unlike a football field, the ice hockey rink is surrounded with a wooden barrier into which players frequently collide or are driven into, providing another source of potential for injury. Thus when players collide, the initial contact may be with another player followed by contact with the boards and/or the ice. Such a sequence could actually increase the potential for injury during collisions. Finally, flying pucks or intermittent fights may also result in a player receiving concussion, although data gathered from professional hockey indicates that fighting accounts for a relatively small percentage of concussions (Lovell & Burke, 2000). Nonetheless, collisions with another player or with a barrier may result in both rotational and deceleration injuries that can lead to the tearing and sheering of neurons that result in the syndrome know as diffuse axonal injury (DAI).

The effects of concussions (often referred to as Post Concussion Syndrome) were once thought to be transient. Deficits on neuropsychological testing following a concussion most often consist of deficits of attention, information processing, memory, visuospatial skills, and executive functions. Once an individual no longer exhibited any overt symptoms or confusion, they were considered to have recovered. More recently however, neuropsychological assessments of individuals receiving concussions after automobile accidents have suggested that there may be residual effects following some concussions such as difficulties with concentration and memory, dizziness, and headache (Wrightson & Gronwell, 1981). Moreover, the effects of repeated concussions have received considerable attention in professional sports (research indicates that players who sustain one concussion are 4 to 6 times more likely to receive subsequent concussion). This is particularly true of the National Football League and National Hockey League, where several high-profile players have been forced to retire after experiencing cognitive declines, especially memory loss, related to multiple concussions. The effects of concussion in high school and collegiate football players have also been investigated to some extent (e.g., Lovell & Collins, 1998); however, less attention has been given to hockey players at lower levels of play. Given the nature of their sport, even junior level hockey players could experience high incidences of low-grade concussions. A single concussion, and especially repeated concussions, occurring in adolescence, might also potentially result in some cognitive repercussions for a competitor in adulthood.

Perhaps the most through and efficient method of documenting changes in the neurobehavioral functioning in an individual is by means of neuropsychological assessment. Given the serious potential for concussion in high school hockey, it is worth investigating the effects on neuropsychological functioning that can occur in a player who receives a concussion. To our knowledge, there are no published studies on the effects of concussion in adolescent hockey players. There may be differences in rates of recovery, residual effects, etc. with this group not observed with adult players. Furthermore, in order to ascertain the potential for injury in junior level hockey it would be helpful to track the incidence and severity of concussion in a high school or junior level ice hockey program. A standard program of neuropsychological assessment and continued monitoring of the players could benefit the health and well being of the young players by identifying any changes in a player's cognitive abilities following a concussion. Individuals receiving concussions could also be followed with repeated assessments comparing their performances to some baseline measure in order to determine if and when they should be allowed to return to play.

Neuropsychological assessment and follow-up of junior hockey players could be structured similarly to neuropsychological assessment programs in professional sports (i.e., Bleiberg, Halpern, Reeves, & Daniel, 1998). Ideally as described by Bleiberg et al. (1998), players would receive a baseline neuropsychological evaluation at the beginning of the playing year. Players would then be monitored during practice and actual competition by their coaching staff and trainers. In the event a player receives a CONCUSSION, the coach or trainer would use a standard sideline assessment evaluation to assess the player's level of functioning and the severity of the concussion (McCrea et al., 1998). Moreover, players experiencing concussions would be withheld from further play and practice until a repeat neuropsychological evaluation could be performed. Such a repeat neuropsychological evaluation would be best if it were scheduled within 24–48 hours of the player's concussion. If the repeat neuropsychological test results indicated that the player was unable to perform to his baseline level in any of the neurobehavioral domains assessed, he would be withheld from further play and practice. Subsequent neuropsychological evaluations would be administered. The player would continue to be retested until he returned to his baseline level of cognitive functioning over all of the areas assessed. Once he returned to baseline he could then be allowed to participate in practice and actual competition, providing he was not experiencing any other neurological symptoms (i.e., headache, blurred vision, etc) or residual effects (i.e., nausea, psychiatric distress). In an effort to ensure that the player would not be at risk for further injury, a multidisciplinary approach incorporating other guidelines for allowing and athlete to return to play following concussion could be entertained as well (see Cantu et al., 2000 for a list of alternative guidelines). A program structured in this manner could better help identify the potential for concussion in adolescent hockey players, chart their recovery time, and determine any lasting residual effects. Furthermore, a program with such information could be used in conjunction with coaches and athletic trainers to help minimize the risk of second impact syndrome (Cantu, 1995) or other potentially hazardous complications associated with a player receiving a concussion. The effects of second impact syndrome can lead to a rapid cognitive deterioration and even death.

We were fortunate enough to be able to implement a program of neuropsychological assessment in a team of junior league hockey players. The players that participated in the current study were 44 high school junior league hockey players. Consent was obtained from players and their guardians before they participated in the study. The players were part of a developmental program that was designed to give top U.S.16 to 17 year-old hockey players a chance to compete against high-caliber competition from around the nation and around the world. The comprehensive training program provided for these high school athletes included a full hockey facility, weight room, and a boxing facility complete with a boxing ring. The players were encouraged to learn to box and actually engaged in regular sparring sessions and heavy bag work as part of their training regimen. The inclusion of boxing was believed to be an excellent way to condition the players as well as to provide them with training in self-defense in the event that they became involved in a scuffle on the ice. It is possible that participants could experience low grade concussions occurring during boxing training and did not report this to either their coaches or trainers. Another factor that could possibly increase the potential for injury in this particular group of players was the level of their competition. In order to develop these players to their maximum potential the team competed against teams composed of players that were several years older. Thus, these junior players were continually pitted against older, potentially stronger players, which could increase the probability of being injured due to collisions or being checked by an opposing player.

Neuropsychological assessment of Junior Hockey Players

The ages of the players at the time of their baseline testing ranged from 15 to 18 years old (with a mean age of 16.57 years). Players were interviewed and asked if they had ever experienced a previous concussion prior to the baseline testing. Fifteen of the 44 players (34 percent of the team) reported experiencing a concussion prior to their baseline evaluation. Of those 15 players reporting a previous concussion, 5 players (11 percent of the team) reported experiencing 2 or more concussions prior to their baseline evaluation. Table 8.1 displays the number of players reporting having experienced a previous concussion in each age group.

The players were then assessed for their neuropsychological functioning. Each player received a baseline neuropsychological evaluation prior to the

Table 8.1. Ages of players reporting a CONCUSSION prior to baseline neuropsychological testing.

Age	Total Number of Players	1 Prior Concussion	> 2 Prior Concussions
15	1	1	0
16	21	5	1
17	18	3	4
18	4	1	0

start of the hockey season. The choice of the particular neuropsychological tests used in the assessment of these players was made on the basis of several criteria: First, the entire test battery had to be brief and yet provide adequate measurement across all general domains of neuropsychological functioning; testing had to be completed in one hour or less. Second, the potential for multiple assessments of a player in a relatively brief time period also necessitated the need to select neuropsychological tests that had parallel forms or were not susceptible to learning effects. Third, the tests also had to be appropriate for use with 15-18 year-olds. On the basis of these criteria, 14 relatively well researched and established neuropsychological tests were selected to be used in the assessment of the junior hockey players. These tests were judged to acceptably meet the aforementioned criteria. (The reaction time test, motor tests, and the Trail Making tests have no parallel forms. Nonetheless they were included in our battery as both are considered to be sensitive measures to even mild cognitive dysfunction). Baseline evaluations and subsequent follow-up evaluations were approximately one hour in length, all tests were believed to be appropriate for the age group being tested, and tests that were especially susceptible to practice effects had at least one alternate form that was readily available. Our brief test battery covered several domains including intellect, attention, memory, visual spatial functioning, motor functioning, executive functioning, and emotional functioning. [1]

[1] For an estimate of general intellect we used the Peabody Picture Vocabulary Test-III (Dunn & Dunn, 1997). We utilized 2 measures of attention, the Digit Span subtest from the WAIS-III (Wechsler, 1997) for short term attention and the Symbol Digit Modalities Test (Smith, 1982) for complex attention. Aspects of complex attention and executive functioning were also measured by the Stroop Test (Stroop, 1935) and the Trail Making Test (Army Individual Test Battery, 1944). Verbal memory was measured by the Selective Reminding Test (SRT: Hannay & Levin, 1985) and nonverbal memory by the Visual Spatial Learning Test (VSLT: Malec, Ivnik, & Hinkeldey, 1991). The Controlled Oral Word Association and Animal Naming Tests (Benton & Hamsher, 1989) measured the expressive language domain of verbal fluency. Manual dexterity was measured by the Grooved Pegboard Test (Klove, 1963), motor speed by the Finger Tapping Test (Halstead, 1947), and strength by the Grip Strength Test (Reitan & Wolfson, 1993). Reaction time was measured using the Lafayette Multi-Choice Reaction Timer (Model #: 63014). Emotional functioning was measured with the Symptom Check List-90-Revised (SCL-90-R: Derogatis, 1977).

A modified form of the Standardized Assessment for Concussion (SAC: McCrea et al., 1998) was used as a sideline measure to ascertain if a player had received a concussion during play. When a player was suspected to have experienced a concussion he was removed from play and assessed with the sideline evaluation by a coach or a trainer. The player was able to return to the game if he was able to satisfactorily pass the sideline assessment. If not, then the player was withheld from play and a repeat neuropsychological evaluation was performed. Players receiving concussions were typically followed and reevaluated with the neuropsychological tests 24-72 hours after experiencing their concussion. However, in one case a player did not report his symptoms to his coaches or trainers until several days following his concussion and his first follow-up evaluation did not take place until nine days after his concussion (see the case of Player F later in this chapter). Once a player was evaluated his results were compared to the baseline results. If the player's repeat neuropsychological test results were not equivalent to his test results at his baseline performance he was withheld from play and subsequent follow-up neuropsychological evaluations were performed. Domains of functioning that were deemed to have returned to the player's baseline level on successive repeat neuropsychological evaluations were not retested in the follow up assessments. This helped lessen the time burden associated with testing for each player and also most likely helped to let the player know that he was recovering. We did not follow a specific time schedule for the reevaluations, but instead follow-up evaluations were rescheduled on an individual basis. Successive follow up evaluations were performed at the request of the player or coaching staff, when either the player or coaching staff felt that the player's mental facilities had improved enough so that he was functioning at or near his pre-concussion level. Therefore, the time that elapsed between repeat evaluations varied from player to player.

Baseline Comparisons of Previously Concussed VS. Previously Non-concussed Players

We were interested if the players who had reported experiencing a concussion before the start of their current season would demonstrate any significant cognitive differences from their teammates who had not had a previous concussion. Statistical analysis using the MANOVA procedure failed to reveal any significant differences on any of the neuropsychological measures between the players that did not report experiencing prior concussion and those players that did report experiencing a prior concussion (Wilks' Lambda, $F_{(10, 23)} = 1.15$, $p = .37$). The only measure that approached significance was the Digits Backward portion of the Digit Span subtest of the WAIS-III ($p = .06$). Digits Backward theoretically involves holding the set of numbers in working memory and manipulating the number set while the subject recites them in reverse sequence. Such a difference between previously concussed and nonconcussed individuals would be consistent with the effects of Post Concussion Syndrome; however, the relatively small sample sizes may have at least in part resulted in a lack of statistical power that prohibited traditional parametric tests to detect significant differences between the groups. We also computed estimates of effect size for each comparison, all of which were relatively small with Eta Squared values ranging from 0.0 to .10 (see Cohen, 1992). Given the small effect sizes obtained from the analyses, the groups were judged to be functioning equivalently on all neuropsychological domains at baseline.

Recovery of Function following Concussion

Six of the players sustained a concussion over the course of the season and were subjected to repeat neuropsychological evaluations until they were able to produce test scores that approximated their baseline performance. These players ranged from 16-18 years of age. Sideline evaluations of the players performed by coachers or trainers indicated that all 6 players had received a Grade 1 concussion. A Grade 1 concussion is generally defined as a period of confusion with little or no amnesia and no loss of consciousness (See Cantu, 2000 for a review of the various grading systems). None of the 6 players had more than one concussion over the season; however, of the 6 players, 3 had reported experiencing a concussion prior to their baseline neuropsychological evaluation (one of the players had experienced 2 concussions prior to his baseline testing). As previously mentioned, return to baseline level of functioning was determined by comparing the player's most recent test results to his baseline results. A licensed Ph.D. neuropsychologist reviewed all test results. We did not use a statistical algorithm to determine whether a player's performance during his repeat assessment was equivalent to his baseline performance, but instead this determination was based on a qualitative comparison of the test data by the clinician.

Recovery time was variable over the group as the number of repeat neuropsychological assessments performed on these players ranged from 1-4. The time period from the date of player's concussion to the player having been judged to have returned sufficiently close enough to their baseline performance to allow a return to play ranged from 5-175 days. However, a retrospective analysis based on a statistical comparison of each player's last neuropsychological performance to his baseline performance indicated that two of the players did not return to their baseline performance on several of the neuropsychological indices (e.g., see case study of Player F in this chapter). By the clinician's interpretation, one player was judged to have returned to his baseline following one repeat evaluation, one player returned to baseline following 2 evaluations, three players needed to complete 3 evaluations before being allowed to return to play, and one player still had not totally reached his baseline performances following 4 repeat assessments.

A post hoc analysis of the data was undertaken to determine the specific neuropsychological variables that demonstrated a decline following a concussion. As all 6 of the players were judged to have experienced a Grade 1 concussion, the severity of the concussion was not considered to be a significant confounding factor in a comparative analysis of the 6 players. Moreover, since there were no statistically significant differences between previously concussed and non-concussed players on any of the neuropsychological measures at the baseline evaluation, having a prior history of concussion also was not considered to interact with any of the current comparisons.

Due to the small number of players who actually reported a concussion over the season, traditional statistical comparisons lacked sufficient statistical power to reveal significant group differences between non-concussed and recently concussed players. In order to perform a meaningful comparison and offset this lack of statistical power, the players' scores on each neuropsychological test were standardized. First, means and standard deviations were calculated using the baseline test data for the entire team for each individual test indicator. The baseline performance was then standardized using a Z score distribution. We operationally defined a decrease of one-half of a standard deviation below the player's baseline performance to represent a substantial difference from the player's previous performance (Cohen, 1992). Likewise, given this standard, performances within one half of a standard deviation of the players' performance would not be considered to represent a substantial change from their previous score.

The results indicated that the specific tests demonstrating declines from previous levels varied substantially from individual to individual, but tests that place a high load on complex attention and memory were most affected in all six individuals. Table 8.2 displays the number of standard deviations above or below the player's baseline performance that a particular test result was on subsequent testing sessions.

Attention

As can be seen from Table 8.2, one player (Player A) demonstrated difficulties with immediate attention (Digit Span and Symbol Digit Modalities tests) and with his ability to generate lists of words beginning with a pre-specified letter or from a pre-specified category (fluency tests) 2 days following his concussion. His difficulties with attention had not resolved 2 weeks later (results at Test 2) but were completely resolved one month later (results at Test 3). None of the other players experienced substantial decrements to their performance on tests of attention following their concussion. Three players of the 6 concussed players exhibited initial decrements in their performance on the Trail Making Test, a test of psychomotor speed, sequencing, and the ability to simultaneously alternate between 2 conceptual sets. These difficulties resolved in a week or less for all 3 players as all of the players returned to near baseline rather quickly on this measure.

Table 8.2. Test performances demonstrating a decrease from baseline following an neuropsychological effects of MTBI in six junior hockey players.

Player Test number following MTBI	Fluency (letter)	Fluency (category)	Digits Backward	Trails A	Trails B	SDM	SRT Total Recall	SRT LTS	SRT CLTR	VSLT Dsum	VSLT Psum
A.											
Test 1	1.30	.860	2.50	–	–	1.70	.680	1.76	–	2.29	–
Test 2	1.00	1.52	1.66	–	–	1.70	.880	1.24	–	2.94	–
Test 3	–	–	–	–	–	–	–	–	–	–	–
B.											
Test 1	–	–	–	–	.67	–	1.85	–	–	.77	–
Test 2	–	–	–	–	–	–	–	–	–	–	–
C.											
Test 1	–	–	–	–	–	–	–	.96	.85	–	–
Test 2	–	–	–	–	–	–	–	–	–	–	–
D.											
Test 1	–	–	–	1.72	.78	–	1.07	1.32	1.35	–	–
Test 2	–	–	–	1.07	2.12	–	2.72	4.39	2.10	–	–
Test 3	–	–	–	–	–	–	–	–	–	–	–
E.											
Test 1	–	–	–	.67	–	–	.96	.79	1.11	–	.62
Test 2	–	–	–	–	–	–	3.10	2.29	2.73	1.53	1.54
Test 3	–	–	–	–	–	–	.68	.77	–	1.15	1.23
F.											
Test 1	–	–	–	–	–	–	4.27	4.49	3.45	2.29	5.35
Test 2	–	–	–	–	–	–	2.52	2.12	3.22	1.52	.62
Test 3	–	–	–	–	–	–	1.07	2.03	1.35	–	–
Test 4	–	–	–	–	–	–	1.07	1.59	.94	–	–

Note: Numerical values in the cells represent the number of standard deviations the test falls ***below*** *the player's baseline performance on the same test. SMD = Symbol Digit Modalities Test; SRT = Selective reminding Test; LTS = Long Term Storage; CLTR = Continuos Long Term Retrieval; Dsum = Visual Spatial Learning Test correct designs placed following a delay; Psum = Visual Spatial Learning Test correct positions.*

Memory Recovery in Players that Experienced a Concussion

As can be seen from Table 8.2 all of the players exhibited some decrease in their memory performance following their concussion. The Selective Reminding Test (SRT: Hannay & Levin, 1985) and the Visual Spatial Learning Test (Malec, Ivink, and Hinkeldey, 1991) were used to assess verbal and nonverbal memory functions respectively in the players. The neuropsychological distinction between verbal and nonverbal memory is an old one in neuropsychology and has been empirically validated. It is assumed that memory for verbal material is a relatively localized function of the left cerebral hemisphere in the vast majority of right-handed individuals, whereas memory for nonverbal material is relatively a function of the right cerebral hemisphere. Verbal memory could be affected from either a direct impact to the left side of the head or a collision that results in a rotational type injury affecting the entire brain. Nonverbal memory could likewise be affected in a similar fashion involving an impact to the right side of the head or a rotational type injury. Our findings concerning verbal memory deficits following a CONCUSSION and recovery are discussed first.

Verbal memory recovery

The SRT consists of a list of 12 unrelated words that are read to the subject. The subject's task is to recall as many words as possible from the list. After the first recall attempt, any words that were missed are repeated to the subject and he is immediately asked to recall the entire list again. The procedure is subsequently repeated either 12 times in this manner or until the subject is able to recall all the words from the list on 3 consecutive trials. We also included a delayed recall condition and a multiple choice recognition paradigm following the delayed recall trial. Delayed recall occurred 30 minutes following the player's last learning trial. Several indices are calculated from the subject's SRT performance, which reflect verbal learning and memory. Total recall represents the total number of words recalled over the learning trials. Long-term storage (LTS) represents the number of words recalled on 2 or more consecutive trials, whereas consistent long-term retrieval (CLTR) corresponds to the total number of words recalled without the need for reminding. As can be seen in Table 8.2, five of the six players initially displayed a decrease in their LTS and total recall of the SRT items. The initial magnitude of the decrease in these indices varied substantially across the group, ranging from about two-thirds of a standard deviation to over four standard deviations for total recall, and from eight tenths of a standard deviation to nearly four and a half standard deviation decrease for LTS. CLTR was decreased substantially in four of the six players and revealed a loss of about eight tenths of a standard deviation to a loss of nearly three and a half standard deviations. Verbal memory recovery rate was also variable for the group ranging from 5-164 days, although 2 of the players (Player E and Player F) did not completely return to within one-half of a standard deviation of their baseline performance on some of the verbal memory indices.

Recovery for nonverbal memory

Nonverbal memory was assessed using the Visual Spatial Learning Test (VSLT), a test that requires a subject to memorize the location of seven cardboard visual designs on a 6 × 4 grid. The designs are difficult to describe in verbal terms; therefore this task may place more emphasis on memory processes that occur in the right cerebral hemisphere. Like the SRT the subject can complete several learning trials to learn the correct location and position of the designs (in this case only 5 trials as opposed to 12 trials in the SRT). After each learning trial the subject is shown the correct arrangement of the designs, and asked to try again. The correct designs are mixed in with a number of incorrect distracter designs to make the task more difficult. There is also a 30-minute delay following the fifth learning trial, after which the subject must place the designs on the grid solely from memory. Several indices can also be computed for the VSLT, among which are the number of correct designs placed following the delay (Dsum) and the number correctly positioned (Psum).

As can be seen from Table 8.2, four of the players demonstrated a decrease in at least once index of the VSLT following their concussion. *Dsum* (the number of correctly placed designs) decrements ranged from about eight-tenths of a standard deviation to nearly three standard deviations from baseline, whereas *Psum* (number of correctly positioned designs) decrements ranged from about six-tenths of a standard deviation to over five standard deviations from baseline. Visual memory appeared to have a more rapid recovery time in the group than did verbal memory, ranging from 2-68 days; however, Player E's VSLT indices were not within one half of a standard deviation from baseline on his final assessment ten days after his CONCUSSION; therefore, it is unclear how much longer he would have taken to return to his baseline performance.

Summary of Findings for Memory Tests

From a practical aspect, the psychometric test results suggest that decreased memory for verbal material may be the cognitive ability that demonstrates the greatest initial decline following a concussion in younger athletes, even when the player experiences a low grade concussion. Moreover, recovery rates for verbal memory loss in younger individuals may vary substantially. Recovery was not felt to be affected by the severity of the concussion in this small sample as all players were judged to have experienced a Grade 1 concussion based on the sideline assessment performed by a qualified coach or trainer. Verbal memory is a complicated process that is composed of several different processes that includes but certainly is not limited to attention, consolidation, and retrieval. This finding, while based on a very small sample, suggests that perhaps more focus should be placed on assessing verbal information processing, verbal recall, effects of interference on learning and recall for verbal material, and recovery rates for junior league players experiencing a concussion. Larger sample sizes (perhaps by utilizing many different teams in large scale collaborative studies) and using other sophisticated measures such as the Wechsler Memory Scale-III or the California Verbal Learning Test-II might help provide further information concerning recovery rates and potential residual effects following a concussion. However, many of these tests do not have multiple parallel forms and therefore may be particularly suspect to practice effects.

Nonverbal memory also demonstrated variable recovery rates in the players. While the effects of a concussion did not appear as salient on nonverbal memory tests as verbal memory tests, the relative loss of memory for nonverbal information following a concussion is still quite striking. Moreover, memory for visual information is also a complicated process that consists of multiple functions. More complex measures of nonverbal memory recovery following a concussion would also shed light on what specific processes are compromised as well as their recuperation.

In summary, while there was some variability in the specific neuropsychological domains that demonstrated a decline from their baseline level following a concussion. Results indicate that memory, especially verbal memory, was the area that was most affected. Nearly all of the players made a fairly rapid recovery, which would be expected when young players are involved. One would expect greater neuroplasticity and quicker recuperative powers in younger individuals. In support of this notion, there is a body of empirical literature that has demonstrated that younger individuals recover more rapidly from head injury than older individuals with the same level of impairment (e.g., Russell, 1971). Moreover, Wrightson and Gromwell (1981) found that individuals injured in sports competitions had significantly fewer prolonged complaints than did subjects with equivalently severe automobile-related head injuries. We would expect that ambitious players trying to impress coaches and potential scouts would be motivated to make a quick recovery and most of these players were anxious to return to play. However, as can be seen in Table 8.2, there were 2 of the players who had fully returned to their baseline level of functioning on memory indices at their last neuropsychological evaluation. We now turn to the case of Player F and discuss his results in more detail.

The Case of Player F

Player F was a 16 year-old competitor who was checked into the boards by a player from the opposing team. Player F did not experience a loss of consciousness, but did feel some lightheadedness and dizziness immediately following the collision; he did not report experiencing a concussion prior to this incident during his playing career. He had no amnesia, but he began experiencing a headache within a few minutes of the collision. He continued play and then later he sat out his next two shifts. He did not immediately inform anyone of his condition. He then finished playing in the game and also finished playing in the tournament in which the team was involved. Nine days following his concussion, he was still experiencing severe headaches in the

Table 8.3. Neuropsychological test results for player F (raw data).

TEST	Baseline	9 days post MTBI	54 days post MTBI	74 days post MTBI	164 days post MTBI
Peabody Picture Vocabulary Test-III	102	99	–	–	–
Digit Span (Percentile)	37	37	–	–	–
Symbol Digit Modalities Test (correct)	66	60	76	–	–
Selective Reminding Test					
Long Term Storage (Percentile)	79	14	49	50	57
Continuous Long Term Retrieval (Percentile)	95	4	7	62	71
Visual Spatial Learning Test					
Correct Designs (Raw Total)	35	29	31	32	34
Correct Position (Raw Score)	34	17	30	32	33
Controlled Oral Word Association (Raw Total)	29	37	36	–	–
Animal Naming (Raw Total)	23	22	26	–	–
Trail Making Test (Part A, seconds)	15	17	14	–	–
Trail Making Test (Part B, seconds)	51	59	47	–	–
Reaction Time Test-Simple (m seconds)	365	323	240	–	–
Reaction Time Test-Choice (m seconds)	366	450	298	–	–
Grooved Pegboard Test-Right (seconds)	52	58	62	55	–
Grooved Pegboard Test-Left (seconds)	59	63	66	62	–

frontal portion of head. Player F was an good student, but now he became very nauseated when reading. At one point he reported vomiting 11 times while trying to read his schoolwork. He was examined by a neurologist who decided that he had received a Grade One concussion and recommended an urgent head scan. Player F was also withheld from all physical exertion and physical contact until his headaches could be controlled. CT scan of the brain revealed scattered hypodensities in the cortex and subcortex in both hemispheres thought to represent possible diffuse axonal injury; however, this was not confirmed by a follow up MRI scan of the brain. He was also reevaluated with neuropsychological testing. Table 8.3 displays Player F's baseline neuropsychological evaluation and subsequent follow-up evaluations.

As depicted in Table 8.3, nine days following his concussion, Player F displayed markedly decreased memory for verbal information and decreased memory for nonverbal information. Choice reaction time (reaction time requiring the subject to discriminate between stimuli and respond to specific stimuli) was also affected and there were subtle changes in Player F's manual dexterity. Language functions appeared relatively uncompromised. Fifty-four days following Player F's concussion he continued to display decreased verbal memory, but memory for visual material was improved and reaction time performance was better than his baseline level (possibly due to a practice effect). He still complained of headaches, but not nausea. Seventy-four days following his concussion, Player F's memory for verbal information had improved substantially, but was not at baseline. One hundred and sixty four days post concussion, verbal memory performance was still substantially lower than baseline (see Table 8.2 and Table 8.3). While no further neuropsychological tests were performed, it is clear from the tables that Player F's neuropsychological data indicated that he abstinence from physical contact might be entertained. Given that 164 days had elapsed between his concussion and his final evaluation, and that he continued to demonstrate memory difficulties, it may have been prudent that he refrain from contact sports for several months to a year.

Also of interest are Player F's scores on a self-report measure of psychological stress following his concussion. Figure 8.1 depicts his score on three general measures of psychological distress measured by the SCL-90-R.

The SCL-90-R lists the symptoms and complaints common to medical and psychiatric patients. The three overall indices of concern here are: the Global Severity Index (GSI), which measures an overall level of distress; the Positive Symptom Index (PSDI), which represents the average distress level across the items; the Positive Symptom Total (PSD), the total of symptoms for which any level of distress is reported. Each scale has an average score of 50 with a standard deviation of 10 and scores over 60 indicate areas of concern. As can be seen in Figure 8.1, Player F reported little psychological distress at base-

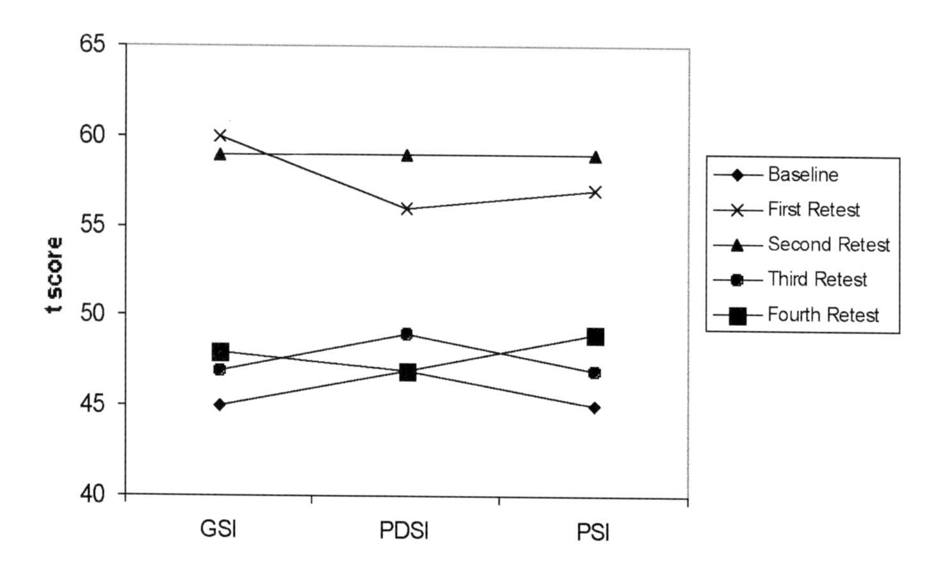

Note: GSI = Global Severity Index; PDSI = Positive Symptom Distres Index; PSI = Positive Symptom Index.

Figure 8.1. Player F's psychological distress following his MTBI.

line, but reported a significant increase in his psychological distress following his concussion. This increase in emotional distress was driven by an increase in his obsessive-compulsive, anxious, and depressive symptoms. Player F also endorsed a significantly higher number of health concerns from his baseline evaluation such as a nearly constant headache, difficulty sleeping, difficulty with motivation to perform schoolwork, and markedly decreased energy. As can be seen in Figure 8.1 Player F continued to display significant levels of psychological distress 54 days following his concussion. Seventy-four days following Player F's concussion, much of his overall psychological distress had abated; however inspection of the individual subscales indicated that he was still expressing a significantly high number of ruminations and obsessive behaviors compared to baseline. At 164 days following his concussion his SCL-90-R major indices were essentially at baseline.

Thus, parallel to Player F's significant cognitive decline following his concussion was a drastic increase in his psychological distress. While this increase in psychological distress observed in individuals with moderate to severe brain injury is hypothesized to reflect organic etiologies, the source of the distress observed in individuals with a concussion is less clear. Given that Player F's psychological distress abated as his cognitive status improved we suspect that this distress was reactive in nature. However, the case of Player F does raise some interesting concerns regarding compliance with the assessment process. We discuss this and other issues briefly in our summary.

Summary

We were able to make a number of statistical comparisons and to investigate the effects of concussion based on data gathered from a team of promising high school age hockey players. Our finding that 34% of the players had a prior concussion and about 13% experienced a concussion during a single season is consistent with the overall estimates for football (see Barth et al., 1989). Furthermore, no psychometric test differences between the previously concussed and nonconcussed players were observed at the initial baseline evaluation. We would expect younger individuals to recover more quickly from the effects of concussion due to greater neuro-plasticity and better recuperative powers. This idea is supported by research with young rats subjected to varying levels of fluid percussion brain injury (e.g. Prins et al., 1996). However, there is also evidence that children and adolescents are more susceptible to second impact syndrome than are adults (Cantu, 1995). Prins et al. (1996) also found that young rats compared to adult rats demonstrated significant hypoperfusion in response to their injuries. Thus, high school athletes that may be back in competition before being fully recovered may find themselves at increased risk for potentially more serious damage. Moreover, there are no recorded cases of second impact syndrome in which the individual was older than 21 years of age (Erlanger, 1999) suggesting that the potential for such an injury is limited to younger individuals. In this context, another serious dilemma to the athlete involved in contact sports is the potential for permanent damage from multiple concussions. Cantu suggests that susceptibility to a second brain injury has two components, an acute phase and a more chronic phase, each composed of different physiological sequale.

Neurocognitive deficits following concussion in our group of players occurred in areas of attention, information processing, and memory. These effects are consistent with the empirical investigations on the neurobehavioral effects of Post Concussion Syndrome (Katz & Deluca, 1992). Regarding the observed memory dysfunction in our group, we also found that verbal memory deficits were observed to some extent in all six of the injured players but not nonverbal memory deficits. Levin et al. (1982) found that the severity of verbal memory deficits in adolescents but not in young children was related to the severity level of closed head injury. The severity of visual memory deficits was related to the severity of injury in both young children and adolescents. The researchers accounted for their findings by noting that visual memory functions are established relatively early in development, whereas verbal memory is rapidly developing in adolescents but not well developed in younger children. Thus, verbal memory deficits may be expected to be more salient than visual memory in junior level players receiving a concussion. These deficits resolved rather quickly in four of our six players experiencing a concussion which is also consistent with prior research (i.e., Ruff et al., 1989). However, two players did not exhibit a complete return to baseline functioning as memory indices were still more than a standard deviation below the baseline level at their last neuropsychological evaluation. There is evidence that a small number of individuals either demonstrate either prolonged recovery from concussion or do not completely resolve at all (Dikmen, McClean, & Terrkin, 1986). Moreover, the severity of the concussion (loss of conscious versus no loss of consciousness) does not appear to impact the magnitude of the cognitive deficits observed in these individuals (Leininger et al., 1990). It is unclear if this group of individuals is more vulnerable to potential second impact syndrome effects, but our findings taken in context with prior research argue for close monitoring of any player suspected of having a concussion. Nevertheless, it is noted that the player showing the most significant cognitive change, Player F, appeared to be experiencing the effects of an initial impact only.

The case of Player F raises some interesting issues regarding the use of neuropsychological testing in junior level sports. Player F received a grade one concussion during a game, yet he continued to play for several games. Player F did not report his symptoms to us and subsequently experienced quite a bit of physical, psychological, and neurocognitive distress. We have no way of knowing if he was involved in any other significant collisions as he continued to play that may have exacerbated his concussion. His distress and return to baseline may have not been so complicated had he reported his difficulties immediately to his coaches. While the coaching staff initially received our program quite enthusiastically, the players appeared to regard it as a nuisance as the season wore on. In this regard, it is certainly quite likely that not all concussions were reported during the season. We believe that coaches and players would benefit from through information about the potential effects of multiple concussions. Players and coaches alike view playing with an injury as "good for the team." Working through an injury and the ability to "play with pain" are old principles that are instilled in athletes at an early age. However, playing a contact sport with a concussion is certainly more hazardous than playing with a sprained ankle. Both athletes and coaches could benefit from education regarding the residual effects of concussion and the risks associated with additional trauma following a concussion. Perhaps a short seminar and discussion concerning the effects of concussion during the preseason and subsequent short follow-up discussions as players are injured during the season could better educate players and coaches. In this manner, athletes and coaches alike could better appreciate the benefits of a sound neuropsychological assessment program.

Based on our findings we offer several directions for clinical applications of neuropsychological assessment in junior level hockey as well as potential directions for future research:

1. Baseline neuropsychological testing of junior level hockey players should be implemented in order to follow the resolution of symptoms in players experiencing an concussion. Education and strong communication between the neuropsychologist and the team could promote better compliance with the assessment program.
2. Our results indicate that verbal memory is the cognitive domain most significantly affected following a concussion. Sideline assessment following a suspected concussion as well as any follow up assessments should thoroughly assess for verbal memory loss.
3. Standardized sideline assessment of players in junior hockey is crucial to quantify the immediate neurocognitive effects of an concussion and make an informed decision of whether to allow a player to return to play or withhold the player for more extensive testing.
4. Neuropsychological tests are quite sensitive for monitoring concussion-related cognitive symptoms and their resolution. Neuropsychological evaluations of concussed players should be utilized along with other information (e.g. neurological evaluation) in determining a player's fitness to return to play following a concussion.
5. Neuropsychological assessment of the immediate and prolonged cognitive effects of concussion may be useful for determining the symptom patterns and resolution of cognitive deficits in junior level hockey players.

References

Army Individual Test Battery. (1994). Manual of Directions and Scoring. Washington, DC: War Department, Adjutant General's Office.

Barth, J.T., Alves, W.M., Ryan, T.V, Macciocchi, S.N., Rimel, R. W., Jane, J.J. et al. (1989). Mild head injury in sports: Neuropsychological sequelae and recovery of function. In H.S. Levin, H.M. Eisenberg, A.L. Benton (Eds.), *Mild Head injury* (pp. 257–277). New York, NY: Oxford University Press.

Benton, A. & Hamsher, KdeS. (1989). *Multilingual Aphasia Examination.* Iowa City, Iowa: AJA Associates.

Cantu, R.C. (2000). Overview of concussion. In R.C. Cantu (Ed.), *Neurologic Athletic Head and Spine Injuries* (pp. 76-79). Philadelphia, Pennsylvania: W.B. Sanders.

Cantu, R.C., Bailes, J.E., & Wilberger, J.E. (2000). Guidelines for return to contact or collision sport after a cervical spine injury. In R.C. Cantu (Ed.), *Neurologic Athletic Head and Spine Injuries* (pp. 153–160). Philadelphia, Pennsylvania: W.B. Sanders.

Cohen, J. (1992). A power primer. *Psychological Bulletin, 112*, 155-159.

Derogatis, L.R. (1977). *SCL-R Administration, Scoring, and Procedures Manual.* Baltimore: Clinical Psychometrics Research Unit, John Hopkins School of Medicine.

Dikmen, D., McClean, A., & Terrkin, N. (1986). Neuropsychological and psychological consequences of mild head injury. *Journal of Neurology, Neurosurgery, and Psychiatry, 49*, 1227–1232.

Dunn, L.M., & Dunn, L.M., (1997). *Norms Booklet for the PPVT-III: Peabody Picture Vocabulary Test Third Edition.* Circle Pines: Minnesota: American Guidance Service.

Erlanger, D.M., Kutner, K.C., Barth, J.T., & Barnes, R. (1999). Neuropsychology of sports-related head injury: Dementia Pugilistica to Post Concussion Syndrome. *Clinical Neuropsychologist, 13*(2), 193–209.

Halstead, W.C. (1947). *Brain and Intelligence.* Chicago: University of Chicago Press.

Hannay, J.H. & Levin, H.S. (1985). Selective reminding test: An examination of the equivalence of four forms. *Journal of Clinical and Experimental Neuropsychology, 7*, 251-263.

Katz, R. & DeLuca, J. (1992). Sequelae of minor traumatic brain injury. *American Family Physician, 5*, 1491-1498.

Klove, H. (1963). Clinical Neuropsychology. In F.M. Forster (Ed.), *The Medical Clinics of North America.* New York: Saunders.

Levin, H.S., Eisenberg, H.M., Wigg, N.R., & Kobayashi, K. (1982). Memory and intellectual ability after head injury in children and adolescents. *Neurosurgery, 11*(5), 668-673.

Lovell, M. R. (1999). Evaluation of the professional athlete. In: J.E. Bailes, M.R. Lovell, & J.C. Maroon, (Eds.), *Sports Related Concussion.* St Louis, Missouri: Quality Medical Publishing.

Lovell, M.R., & Burke, C.J. (2000). Concussions in ice hockey: The national hockey league program. In R.C. Cantu (Ed.), *Neurologic Athletic Head and Spine Injuries.* Philadelphia, Pennsylvania: W.B. Sanders.

Lovell, M.R. & Collins, M.W. (1998). Neuropsychological assessment of the college football player. *Journal of Head Trauma and Rehabilitation, 13*(2), 9-36.

Malec, J.F., Ivnik, R.J., & Hinkeldey, N.S. (1991). Visual spatial learning test. *Psychological Assessment, 3*, 82-88.

McCrea, M.M., Kelly, J.P., Randolph, C.R., Kluge, J., Bartolic, E., Finn, G. et al. (1998). Standardized assessment of concussion (SAC): On site mental status

evaluation of the athlete. *Journal of Head Trauma and Rehabilitation, 13*(2), 27–35.
Powell, J.W. & Barber-Foss, K.D. (1999). Traumatic brain injury in high school athletes. *Journal of the American Medical Association, 282*(10), 958–963.
Prins, M.L., Lee, S.M., Cheng, C.L., Becker, D.P., & Hovda, D.A. (1996). Fluid percussion brain injury in the developing and adult rat: A comparative study of mortality, morphology, intracranial pressure and mean arterial blood pressure. *Brain Research. Developmental Brain Research, 95*(2), 272–82.
Reitan, R.M. & Wolfson, D. (1993). *The Halstead-Reitan Neuropsychological Test Battery: Theory and Clinical Interpretation.* Tucson, AZ: Neuropsychology Press.
Ruff, R.M., Levin, H.S., Mattis, S., High, Jr, W.M., Marshall, L.F., Eisenberg, H.M., & Tabaddor, K. (1989). Recover of memory after mild head injury: A three-center study. In H. Levin, H. Eisenberg, & A. Benton (Eds.), *Mild head injury* (pp. 176–188). New York: Oxford Press.
Smith, A. (1982). *Symbol Digit Modalities Test (SDMT). Manual (Revised).* Los Angeles: Western Psychological Services.
Stroop, J.R. (1935). Studies of interference in serial verbal reactions. *Journal of Experimental Psychology, 18*, 643–662.
Thurman, D.J., Branche, C.M., & Sniezek, J.E. (1998). The epidemiology of sports-related traumatic brain injuries in the Untied States: Recent developments. *Journal of Head Trauma Rehabilitation, 13*, 1–8.
Wechsler, D. (1997). *WAIS-III Administration and Scoring Manual.* San Antonio, TX: Psychological Cooperation.
Wrightson, P., & Gronwell, P. (1981). Time off work and symptoms of a minor head injury. *Injury,* 12, 445–451.

Chapter 9

SOUTH AFRICAN RUGBY UNION

A. Shuttleworth-Edwards, M. Border, I. Reid, and S. Radloff

An earlier version of this paper was presented at the 24th mid-year annual meeting of the International neuropsychological Society, Brasilia, Brazil SARAH Network of Hospitals, July 2001. The research was supported by grants from Rhodes University; the Chris Burger/Petro Jackson Players Fund; the South African Rugby Football Union (SARFU). Acknowledgements are due to the following former Clinical Masters students for research assistance: Tessa Ackermann, Ruth Ancer, Taryn Beilinsohn, Lisa Bold, Arlene Dickenson, Melissa Finkelstein. Correspondence should be sent to Professor Ann Edwards, National Sports Concussion Initiative (NSCI), Psychology Clinic, Rhodes University, Grahamstown, South Africa. E-mail: a.edwards@ru.ac.za

Introduction

In South Africa neuropsychological research on concussion has focussed on Rugby Union,[1] with an emphasis on persistent rather than acute and subacute

[1] Rugby Union is one of a cluster of rugby football games which originated from soccer, the oldest and most widely played of all the football games (Micheli & Riseborough, 1974). In 1823 a schoolboy at Rugby school in England, whilst playing soccer, picked up the ball and ran with it to put it across the goal line. Over a period of thirty years this approach took on and developed into the completely separate game of rugby football, which later splintered and developed into several modes: Rugby Union; Rugby League; American football; and Australian Rules football. Rugby Union is now an extremely popular and fast-growing spectator sport worldwide, which is played at school, University and professional levels in countries such as England, Wales, Scotland, America, Canada, Argentina, France, Japan, Australia, New Zealand, Zimbabwe and South Africa.

effects. The term 'concussion' is used here to denote 'mild traumatic brain injury', being broadly defined as a traumatically induced alteration in mental status which may, or importantly, may not involve loss of consciousness (Maroon et al., 2000). Persistent consequences are taken to be those which last beyond three months, which is when studies on sports-related concussion indicate that recovery on cognitive test function following a concussion has generally levelled off (Barth et al., 1989; Hinton-Bayre, Geffen, Geffen, McFarland & Friis, 1999; Maddocks & Saling, 1996; Shuttleworth-Jordan, Puchert & Balarin, 1993; Wilberger, 1993).

The South African research on players of Rugby Union has developed abreast of similar research on American football (Collins et al., 1999; Wilberger, 1988), Australian Rules football (Cremona-Meteyard & Geffen, 1994), and soccer in the USA, the Netherlands and Scandinavia (Abreau, Templer, Schuyler, & Hutchison, 1990; Matser, Kessels, Jordan, Lezak & Troost,1998; Matser, Kessels, Lezak, Jordan & Troost, 1999; Tysvaer & Løchen, 1991; Tysvaer,1992; conference paper of Witol & Webbe, 1993, in Baroff, 1998). All of these studies demonstrate the presence of unremitting neuropsychological deficit amongst the various contact sports' playing groups. Repeatedly, the functional modalities most affected appear to be speed of information processing, and/or verbal and non-verbal memory both immediate and delayed. Further there is evidence from some studies of persistent postconcussive symptoms amongst these groups (e.g. Abreau et al., 1990; Tysvaer, 1992). To the authors' knowledge, the only neuropsychological research thus far on Rugby Union has been conducted in South Africa. This is with the exception of a study by Pettersen and Skelton (2000) who used Canadian rugby players as a laboratory population on which to study the effects of glucose on memory performance. Results from their study confirm the presence of subtle residual deficits in cognition for Rugby Union players with a history of recurrent concussions. Again the deficits identified were specifically in the areas of delayed verbal and non-verbal memory and verbal attention.

In 1996, a large on-going study on players of Rugby Union was initiated by the present authors in collaboration with the South African Rugby Football Union (SARFU) and the MRC/UCT Exercise Research Unit in Cape Town. The aim of this chapter is to present a preliminary overview of results derived from the first three phases of this ongoing study which were conducted on two adult national teams and a schoolboy cohort. The analysis is located within the framework of Brain Reserve Capacity theory as formulated by Satz (1993).

Dangerousness of Rugby Union

Rugby Union is classified as one of the world's dangerous sports due to body collisions (Hillis, McIntyre, Maclean, Goodwin & McKenna, 1994; Wekesa,

Asembo & Njororai, 1996), and is considered to be one of the sports with the highest dynamic and static demands (Hillis et al., 1994). Jakoet and Noakes (1998) conducted a study on injury frequency sustained by the 416 rugby players from 16 countries participating in the 1995 Rugby world Cup. They confirm a very high injury risk in Rugby Union especially amongst the best players in the game, thereby challenging any view that superior fitness, skill and experience will lower risk of rugby injury. It is of concern that injury rates in Rugby Union appear to be increasing (Garraway, Lee, Hutton, Russell & Macleod, 2000; Jakoet & Noakes, 1998). Most Rugby Union injuries occur during the tackling phase of play followed by rucks and mauls, and dangerousness increases in association with greater speed of the game, larger size of the players, and higher levels of competitiveness (Jakoet & Noakes, 1998).

A comparison of the incidence of overall injury for three types of football played at Eton revealed Rugby Union to be the most dangerous (Briscoe, 1985). Garraway et al. (2000) report an injury rate for professional Rugby Union players which is 50% higher than the highest rate reported for Rugby League. Similarly Walker (1985) reports an incidence of injuries for Rugby League players which is lower when compared with figures of serious injury from Rugby Union series. Typically across a spectrum of adult and schoolboy studies on Rugby Union head, face and neck injuries make up a large proportion of all injuries (McKenna, Borman, Findlay & de Boer, 1986; Macleod, 1993; Myers, 1980; Nathan, Goedeke & Noakes, 1983; Roux, Goedeke, Visser, van Zyl, & Noakes, 1987; Roy, 1974; Ryan & McQuillan, 1992; van Heerden, 1976). This figure is commonly between 25-30% of injuries, with three studies citing proportions as high as from 37-52% of all injuries (McKenna et al., 1986; Myers, 1980; Seward, Orchard, Hazard & Collinson, 1993). Specifically, Seward et al. (1993) report the incidence of head and neck injuries as 37.3% for Rugby Union compared with 28.5% for Rugby League and only 14.4% for Australian Rules football. Finally, in terms of positional influences on exposure to concussion, it is confirmed that for rugby, as with football at adult level, forwards sustain a significantly higher frequency of injuries per se, and more injuries to the head and neck than backs (Davies & Gibson, 1978; Gissane, Jennings, Cumine, Stephenson & White, 1997; Lingard, Sharrock & Salmond, 1976; Jakoet & Noakes, 1998; Seward et al., 1993).

With reference to rugby head injury with definitive CNS involvement, Nathan et al. (1983) identified the percentage of concussion during a *single* rugby season at a South African high school to be 21.5%. On the basis of self-reports, Shuttleworth-Edwards, Ackermann, Beilinsohn, Border and Radloff (2001a) established an average historical incidence of 2.3 (range 0 -7) concussions per rugby playing schoolboy in a survey of three South African schools' top teams, compared with an average incidence of only 0.4 (range 0-1) for an equivalent group of field hockey players. Self-report incidence data on concussion in Rugby Union obtained by Shuttleworth-Edwards and colleagues for two adult professional teams (open and Under-21) were considered to be without value due to gross under-reporting as is known to occur amongst contact sports players at professional levels (Sturmi, Smith, & Lombardo, 1998). In this instance there was probably fear of being withdrawn from future participation in the game by their employment agency (the South African Rugby Football Union) under whose auspices the testing was conducted. The figures yielded were lower than self-reports for the equivalent noncontact sport cricket and field hockey controls, and lower than for schoolboy level rugby which renders them highly implausible. However, the extent of concussion risk in Rugby Union can be extrapolated further from a number of other sources.

For instance, Wills and Leathem (2001) report that Rugby Union accounts for the highest rate of sport-related brain injury in New Zealand, and identified that in one season of New Zealand club rugby 30% of players reported at least one CNS related head injury. A high concussion incidence of 42% has been reported for university American football players over a series of seasons (Barth et al., 1989), which is comparable to a concussion incidence of 47.2% reported for high school players of American football (Langburt, Cohen, Akhthar, O'Neill, & Lee, 2001). In relation to this, Pettersen and Skelton (2000) note Barth's figures and report the incidence of concussion in adult Rugby Union to be even higher than that of American football at 50%. Green and Jordan (1998) claim that concussion is a fairly common event in major league soccer, reporting a rate of 0.31 per 1000 hours of athlete exposures, and 21% of the players in their cohort had sustained at least one concussion. However, Garraway and Macleod (1995) report a concussion incidence of double this for amateur Rugby Union players of 0.62 per 1000 playing hours.

Thus, from the comparative studies reported above, a highly consistent picture emerges, which is that compared with soccer, American football, Rugby League and Australian Rules football, Rugby Union appears to be the most dangerous per se, and is also the most susceptible to incidences of concussion. Accordingly, players of Rugby Union are an important target for sports concussion research. This was the impetus for the current South African project referred to above, from which a series of preliminary indications have been presented in national and international forums (Reid et al., 1999; Shuttleworth-Edwards et al., 2001a; Shuttleworth-Edwards, Border & Radloff, 2001b). From the outset it was deemed of heuristic value to locate this South African research in a theoretical context, which will be elaborated on below.

A Theoretical Perspective for Research in Sports Mild Head Injury

Specifically in the field of mild head injury, literature searches reveal that the overall tenor of publications resides firmly on the a-theoretical side, with the focus on data-gathering, data collations, and related discussions along descriptive dimensions. A prime example is the well-known text Levin, Eisenberg and Benton (1989), which provides the substance of a conference on mild head injury in which theoretical expositions and experimental models are restricted to the area of neuroscience. As is pointed out in the review of this collation by Adams and Putnam (1991), the section on neuropsychology per se is `most disappointing', showing a lack of sophistication in the attribution of meaning to isolated study effects, and providing only one report (that of Ruff and co-researchers) which moves in the direction of generalizability via the pooling of collaborative data from a three-centre study.

In addition to Levin et al.'s (1989) text, a number of seminal articles appeared in the 1980s (Barth et al., 1983; Binder, 1986; Boll, 1985), all of which served to ignite a new appreciation that mild head injury was probably an overlooked problem that might be the cause of significant neuropsychological dysfunction. Again, however, these contributions are empirically oriented, and restricted on an explanatory level to discussions of neuropathological contributions in relation to behavioural outcome. However, albeit not at a high level of theoretical operation, there is a conceptual thrust in these reports which goes beyond the mere presentation of empirical data, and which serves to alert readers to the potential hazards of mild head injury. All of them emphasize the *variability* in mild head injury outcome, depending on the interactive factors of injury in relation to differential individual demographic characteristics and premorbid factors. Boll (1985) and Binder (1986) both highlight enhanced possibilities for positive effects following mild head injury due to factors which reduce brain reserve such as older age, a prior head injury, and marginal pre-existing coping strategies. Barth et al. (1983) point out that they found a trimodal distribution of minimal, mild and moderate to severe neuropsychological impairment related to reduced cognitive efficiency, and factors such as older age and less education.

In contrast to the crop of consciousness raising literature of the 1980s with respect to the potential hazards of mild head injury, a number of major reviews have subsequently appeared which present a somewhat opposite thrust (Binder, 1997; Binder, Rohling, & Larrabee, 1997; Satz et al., 1997; Satz, 2001), all indicating that the maximum prevalence of persistent neuropsychological deficit is likely to be small. However, these more recent reviews focus heavily on the weight of a vast array of empirical findings, and discussion mainly revolves around the empiric presence or absence of relatively short-term *group* mild head injury effects rather than broader and more intricate theoretical issues. Compared with earlier reviews there appears to be less reticence expressed, and even less theoretical reflection ventured, around the meaning of the overall apparently null outcome. The overriding tone of these reviews is to dampen health concerns around mild head injury, and leaves an impression that null outcome (as long as it has been reliably established from a methodological point of view) means that recovery has indeed occurred and that this is the end point of the story.

However, the indication from Brain Reserve Capacity (BRC) theory as formulated by Satz (1993) himself, suggests that this should not be assumed to be the case.

In terms of Satz's formulation, the BRC concept is linked to the notion of a *threshold factor* that exists prior to the presentation of symptoms due to dysfunction in the central nervous system. The idea is that in the pre-clinical stages of neurological damage or disease, individual differences exist in terms of brain reserve capacity that account for *variable* instances of protection from or vulnerability to symptom onset. In essence the following suppositions from BRC apply: (i) there will be individual differences in risk of clinically detectable dysfunction in association with neural damage due to differences in brain reserve capacity which serve to protect against, or cause vulnerability to functional impairment; (ii) the presence of a premorbid vulnerability factor implies lowered brain reserve capacity, and hence greater likelihood of functional impairment; (iii) there will be an aggregation effect of reduced brain reserve capacity which will serve to increase vulnerability to functional impairment, due to the combined presence of premorbid vulnerability factors and/or the overlay of single or multiple instances of neurological damage or disorder and/or enhanced task challenge. The theory poses a number of vulnerability factors which imply reduced brain reserve capacity and therefore predispose individuals to earlier symptom onset including, low education and IQ, older age, the presence of a psychiatric or neurological disorder, a prior head injury, and a specific area of cognitive deficiency including a learning disability. A vast body of research can be called upon to support the BRC suppositions (see Satz, 1993).

The important point that arises out of BRC theory for research purposes in Rugby Union, is that due to different levels of pre-existing cerebral reserve in association with the onset of neural attrition, it must be expected that the presentation of symptomatology will occur differentially between individuals. Subtle individual differences such as level of IQ and education may cause threshold variance, as well as intensity of exposure to concussion in association with positional differences in play. This has methodological implications for the analysis of results, in that it implies the rugby playing group will not be homogenous, and it is essential that studies should take account of *individual* outcome in the isolation of effects. This is possible via the examination of standard deviations and distribution of scores between groups (see earlier examples of the present authors' work: Reid et al., 1999; Shuttleworth-Edwards et al., 2001a).

However, a further mode of analysis is to calculate the percentage of deficit across measures for sports playing groups which can then be compared with the percentage of deficit for an equivalent control group. This is a method that arguably has more immediate clinical relevance than the statistical comparison of group effects. For example, Zakzanis (1998), expresses concern about drawing fallacious conclusions with respect to brain-behaviour relations via sole reliance on quasi-experimental group comparisons.

Thus, some of the most influential boxing and soccer studies have adopted the research mode which calculates the percentage of players revealing cognitive deficit (for example, Casson et al., 1984; Kaste et al., 1982; Matser et al., 1999; Tysvaer & Løchen, 1991). Illustrative data from these studies appear in Table 9.1. In addition to such findings in respect of *objective* cognitive test data, are studies which reflect on the extent of postconcussive symptoms amongst players of contact sport. Tysvaer (1992), reports that 30% of former Norwegian soccer players complained of permanent postconcussive problems, including headaches, irritability, dizziness, neck pain, drowsiness, concentration and memory problems. A number of other studies report more generally on the persistent presence of postconcussive symptoms in players of contact sport which are not as prevalent for controls, including research in respect of adult soccer (Abreau et al., 1990), junior ice hockey (Gaetz, Goodman, & Weinberg, 2000), and American high school football (Gerberich, Priest, Boen, Straub, & Maxwell, 1983). In these studies specificity of outcome in terms of percentages of players with symptoms is not made available. However, the studies typically allude to the unremitting presence of headaches, blurred vision, dizziness, memory and thinking amongst players of these sports.

Accordingly, in order to investigate the additive effect of repetitive sports mild head injury, it was decided to conduct a comparative analysis of percentages of players with objective test deficit and reported postconcussive symptoms from the present authors' study on South African Rugby Union. Based on empirical reports on the incidence and outcome of concussive head injury in rugby football sports as reviewed above, and in terms of BRC theory it was hypothesized that due to the aggregation effect of repeated concussion

Table 9.1. Percentage of individuals with cognitive deficit in boxing and soccer.

Kaste et al. (1982) Trail Making Test	86% Boxers	No control group
Casson et al. (1984) Any Test *	100% Boxers	No control group
Tysvaer and Løchen (1991) Trail Making Test Any Test *	 32% Soccer 81% Soccer	 0% Control group 49% Control group
Matser et al. (1999) Complex Figure Test-Recall	27% Soccer	7% Control group
Wisconsin Card Sorting Test	39% Soccer	13% Control group

* Players who show deficit on any test in the neuropsychological battery used (See text)

via participation in Rugby Union, in association with longer or more exposed positional play, and/or in association with a prior cognitive vulnerability, the following would occur in respect of impairment (operationalized as objective signs of cognitive deficit on testing, and/or self-reported post-concussive symptoms): (i) rugby players would show more impairment than noncontact sport controls; (ii) forward players would show more impairment than backline players; (iii) older and higher level players would show more impairment than younger players; (iv) players who had a recorded history of a learning problem would show more impairment than noncontact sport controls with a recorded history of a learning problem.

Methodology

A three-phase neuropsychological investigation into persistent effects following concussion (comprising objective tests of cognitive function and a questionnaire tapping a wide range of subjective postconcussive sequelae) was conducted on players of Rugby Union in South Africa.

Participants

Rugby groups were made up of participants from three levels of play as follows: national open players (mean age 27.5), national under-21 players (mean age 19.7) and school players (mean age 17.3). These groups were compared with an appropriate noncontact sport control group from the national open cricket players (mean age 27.1) and/or national open field hockey players (mean age 23.2), and school field hockey players (mean age 17.0). Cricket and field hockey are sports which are not characterized by multiple concussions due to collisions between players or players to ground, such as occur as an inevitable part of the game in Rugby Union. Whereas ice hockey has a high incidence of concussion (Gaetz et al., 2000), field hockey has one of the lowest rates of concussion amongst field sports, being significantly lower than both football and Rugby Union (Powell & Barber-Foss, 1999; Shuttleworth-Edwards et al., 2001a) which renders it by contrast a highly suitable control group.

Participants for the main study were excluded with a history of substance abuse; a neurological or psychiatric condition; a prior moderate or severe head injury for any reason (i.e. loss of consciousness in excess of 30 minutes or hospitalization with Glasgow-Coma Scale <13); any prior grade failure, and/or a recorded leaning problem. The main sample consisted of 26 national open rugby players (15 forwards and 11 backs), 19 national under-21 rugby players (11 forwards and 8 backs), 47 school rugby players (28 forwards and 19 backs), and, as control groups, 21 national open cricketers, 21 national open field hockey players and 34 schoolboy field hockey players. All comparative groups, including subgroups of forwards and backs, were equivalent for age, education, and IQ with the exception of the national under-21 rugby players who were significantly lower than field hockey controls with respect to all these variables. Six school boys with a prior history of a learning problem were excluded from the main study. They formed two subgroups for further comparative purposes, consisting of 3 rugby players with a learning problem (Mean IQ 113.5), and 3 field hockey players with a learning problem (Mean IQ 101.0).

Assessment procedure

Participants were tested individually by psychology graduates who were trained and experienced in the administration of psychometric tests. Rugby players were assessed pre-season in order to exclude the acute and subacute effects of concussion. The assessment procedure consisted of the administration of a demographic questionnaire, a self-reported postconcussive symptom questionnaire, followed by a neuropsychological test battery. The postconcussive symptom questionnaire consisted of 31 items clustered within the four symptom categories of 'Behavioural', 'Emotional', 'Physiological/ Neurological', and 'Cognitive'. The assessment battery was replicated for each phase of the study, barring a few refinements that were incorporated into the school phase to enhance test sensitivity and/or validity, including some additional tests and updated versions of Wechsler subtests. The tests used included: (i) *a measure of general intellectual functioning* (to provide an estimate of premorbid IQ), and (ii) *neuropsychological measures within five modalities* known to be sensitive to the non-specific effects of diffuse brain injury in association with closed head injury, as follows:

General intellectual functioning (for an estimate of premorbid IQ). *National open rugby, national open cricket, national under-21 rugby, national open field hockey:* South African Wechsler Adult Intelligence Scale (SAWAIS) – Picture Completion and Comprehension subtests. *School rugby and school field hockey:* Wechsler Adult Intelligence Scale III (WAIS III) – Picture Completion and Vocabulary subtests; National Adult Reading Test (NART). **Specific modalities: (i) Attention and Concentration.** *All groups:* SAWAIS Digit Span subtest – Forwards and Backwards. *School rugby and field hockey:* WAIS III Letter-number Sequencing subtest (LNS); STROOP Neuropsychological Screening Test. (ii) **Visuoperceptual scanning speed.** *All groups:* SAWAIS Digit-Symbol Substitution subtest; Trail Making Tests A and B. (iii) **Memory:** *All groups:* Wechsler Memory Scale (WMS) Associate Learning subtest; Digit-Symbol Incidental recall: Immediate; Digit-Symbol Incidental recall: Delayed; Wechsler Memory Scale (WMS) Visual Reproduction subtest; (iv) **Verbal fluency.** *All groups:* Words-in-One-Minute Unstructured Verbal Fluency Test; Structured Verbal Fluency Test – 'S' Words. (v) **Fine hand motor dexterity.** *All groups:* Sequential Finger Tapping Test.

Descriptive Data Analysis. **Cognitive tests.** For each comparative group the number of players who showed neuropsychological test deficit was calculated. Deficit on individual tests was determined according to the degree to which a test score deviated significantly from the norm in the direction of poor performance, as follows: (i) None – the test score is within 1 standard deviation from the norm; (ii) Mild – the test score is equal to or greater than 1 standard deviation from the norm but less than 2 standard deviations; (iii) Moderate/Severe – the test score is equal to or greater than 2 standard deviations from the norm. The most appropriate available normative data for each of the tests were used, the same standard being applied for rugby and equivalent control group participants. **Postconcussive Symptom Questionnaire.** The number of players within each comparative group who answered 'never', 'sometimes' or 'often' for each one of the 31 items were calculated.

Statistical Analyses. Group comparisons of percentages of test deficit ('none', 'mild', or 'moderate/severe') or postconcussive symptoms ('never', 'sometimes', or 'often') were conducted using Pearson's chi-square test. In order to highlight the most indicative findings, results were extracted for descriptive comment if they met the following criteria: (i) *$p<0.05$; (ii) ~$0.05<p<0.15$; and/or (iii) # difference between comparative groups of 30%+. For ease of presentation, the percentages of players with the presence of any objective test deficit (mild and moderate/severe) or any postconcussive symptomatology (sometimes and often) were combined and appear in Tables 9.2, 9.3, 9.5 and 9.6. On occasion the significance was clearly attributable to symptoms which occurred 'often' amongst a rugby group compared with controls, rather than a combination of 'sometimes' and 'often', in which case this is specified on the table. Statistical analyses were not conducted on the small subgroups of schoolboys with a history of a learning problem. The comparative percentages of individuals with deficit for these two subgroups (Rugby Union and field hockey) appear in Table 9.4.

Discussion

The objective cognitive test results for the adult national open and under-21 rugby players (Table 9.2), demonstrate remarkably consistent support for greater deficit amongst rugby playing groups in relation to controls, and forwards in relation to backs, in each of the functional areas of speed of information processing, memory, verbal fluency and hand motor dexterity. Amongst the two adult teams (Table 9.3) there was only one result that went in the opposite direction to the hypotheses (10% of field hockey players had deficit compared with 0% of open rugby players on one trial of the Sequential Finger Tapping test). On its own this result could be attributed to chance variation, especially in that this particular task is conducted manually and measured in seconds with a stopwatch, and is probably the least reliable test in the battery.

In contrast to outcome for the two adult teams, at the school level (Table 9.2) there was only one result in support of more deficit for rugby versus controls, which was on one trial of hand motor function. In isolation this result may be attributed to chance as much as due to neurological dysfunction. However of interest (Table 9.3) are results that suggest marginally less deficit for school rugby forwards compared with backs consistently across visual memory tests and for unstructured verbal fluency. This is not in keeping with the hypothesis that rugby forwards will show more problems than backs due to their known greater exposure to head injury. However, it appears that positional stances may be less entrenched at school level than at older levels of play, such that in this cohort deleterious effects of concussion are showing up amongst backs on visual memory and verbal fluency

Table 9.2. Percentages of individuals with cognitive deficit (1 SD+). Results in support of hypothesis: Rugby > Controls; Forwards > Backs.

Speed of Information Processing		
Digit Symbol Substitution (DSS)	23% Open Rugby	5% Cricket *
	40% Open Forwards	0% Open Backs *
	23% Open Rugby	5% Field Hockey ~
	42% Under 21 Rugby	5% Field Hockey *
	55% Under 21 Forwards	25% Under 21 Backs #
Trail Making Test B	19% Open Rugby	0% Cricket ~
	33% Open Forwards	0% Open Backs ~
	32% Under 21 Rugby	5% Field Hockey ~
Memory		
DSS: Incidental Recall – Immediate	47% Open Forwards	9% Open Backs ~
	31% Open Rugby	5% Field Hockey ~
WMS Visual Reproduction – Delayed	23% Open Rugby	5% Field Hockey ~
WMS Associate Pairs Hard – Immediate	19% Open Rugby	0% Field Hockey ~
	11% Under 21 Rugby	0% Field Hockey ~
Verbal Fluency		
Unstructured	79% Under 21 Rugby	33% Field Hockey *
	53% Open Forwards	18% Open Backs #
Hand-Motor Function		
Sequential Finger Tapping Preferred Hand	26% Under 21 Rugby	5% Field Hockey ~
	46% Under 21 Forwards	0% Under 21 Backs ~
	26% School Rugby	12% School Field Hockey ~
Sequential Finger Tapping Non-Preferred Hand	37% Under 21 Rugby	0% Field Hockey *
	55% Under 21 Forwards	13% Under 21 Backs ~

Note: Results selected for presentation were delineated from the Chi-Squared analyses according to the following criteria: * p<0,05; ~ 0,05< p< 0,15; # difference of 30%+

Table 9.3. Percentages of individuals with cognitive deficit (1 SD+). Results not in support of hypothesis: Controls > Rugby; Backs > Forwards.

Memory		
DSS Incidental Memory:		
– Immediate	11% School Forwards	37% School Backs ~
– Delayed	4% School Forwards	21% School Backs ~
WMS Visual Reproduction		
– Immediate	4% School Forwards	26% School Backs ~
– Delayed	4% School Forwards	21% School Backs ~
Verbal Fluency		
Structured	4% School Forwards	21% School Backs ~
Hand-Motor Function		
Sequential Finger Tapping Non-Preferred Hand	0% Open Rugby	10% Cricket ~

Note: Results selected for presentation were delineated from the Chi-Squared analyses according to the following criteria: * p<0,05; ~ 0,05< p< 0,15; # difference of 30%$^{+}$

tasks. Such a notion is supported by the concussion incidence derived on this school cohort, in which there was a marginally lower number of concussions reported for forwards compared with backs, and one of the backs reported a history of seven concussions compared with a maximum of five amongst forwards. A comparative analysis of means and standard deviations for this same school sample (Shuttleworth-Edwards et al., 2001a), also indicated problems for rugby players on the WMS Associate Pairs delayed recall task. (This was a task that could not be incorporated into the present analysis due to the absence of an independent normative standard by which to calculate the extent of individual deficit).

Overall, therefore, taking the two school rugby analyses into consideration, even at this early stage of play, there appear to be a number of subtle indicators of incipient neurocognitive dysfunction, particularly in the area of memory function. More alarming indications, however, arise from the small subset of analyses of schoolboys with a history of a learning problem (see Table 9.4). There is substantially increased fall-out amongst rugby players with the prior vulnerability factor of a learning problem in the areas of attention and concentration, information processing speed, and visual memory. The rugby subgroup with a learning problem had a higher estimated IQ than the field hockey subgroup with a learning problem (113.5, 101.0, respectively), yet the percentage of cognitive deficit for these rugby players clusters around 67%, compared with close on zero indication of deficit across tests

Table 9.4. School Rugby and School Field Hockey players with a prior learning disability. Percentages of individuals with cognitive deficit (1 SD+).

Attention and Concentration		
Digits Backwards	100% School Rugby	0% School Field Hockey
Letter Number Sequencing	67% School Rugby	0% School Field Hockey
STROOP	67% School Rugby	33% School Field Hockey
Speed of Information Processing		
Trail Making Test A	33% School Rugby	0% School Field Hockey
Trail Making Test B	67% School Rugby	0% School Field Hockey
Memory		
DSS Incidental Memory:		
– Immediate	67% School Rugby	0% School Field Hockey
– Delayed	33% School Rugby	0% School Field Hockey

for the field hockey players. Albeit the subgroup sample numbers are small, the findings are commensurate with the research of Collins et al. (1999), who demonstrate significantly increased cognitive deficit in football players with repeated concussions and a learning disability compared with concussed football players without a learning disability.

With respect to outcome for self-reported postconcussive symptoms (see Table 9.5), as with the objective test data, these were substantially prevalent for the national adult level rugby players compared with controls, and forwards in relation to backs. For both of the adult teams, similar problems cluster together in each of the emotional, behavioural, physical/neurological and cognitive areas. Also, although not quite as prevalent, there are higher percentages of school rugby players compared with equivalent controls who report postconcussive symptoms in each one of these areas.

It is of note, however, (see Table 9.6), that there is a marked reversal of findings on a few key physical and cognitive areas (i.e. headaches, eyesight and attention and concentration), where the open rugby group report substantially fewer symptoms than the controls. This is explicable in terms of underreporting by these top professional rugby players of symptoms that might obviously be considered a threat to their participation in the game. As noted earlier, the concussion rate reported by this same cohort was absurdly low, and headaches in particular would be associated with evidence for concussion and therefore guardedly reported. Similarly, problems with vigilance (attention) and eyesight would have obvious implications for high level

Table 9.5. Percentages of individuals with reported postconcussive symptoms In support of hypothesis: Rugby > Controls; Forwards > Backs.

Emotional		
Depression	53% Open Forwards	18% Open Backs ~
	82% Under 21 Forwards	50% Under 21 Backs #
Appetite Problems	27% Open Forwards	0% Open Backs ~
Sleep Difficulties	36% School Rugby	18% School Field Hockey ~
Restlessness	53% Open Forwards	18% Open Backs ~
Worry	67% Open Forwards	36% Open Backs #
	82% Under 21 Forwards	50% Under 21 Backs ~
Anxiety	80% Open Forwards	27% Open Backs *
Irritability	100% Under 21 Forwards	63% Under 21 Backs ~
Sensitive to Noise	27% Open Rugby	10% Field Hockey ~
	42% Under 21 Rugby	10% Field Hockey ~
Behavioural		
Argumentativeness	62% Open Rugby	33% Cricket ~
	80% Open Forwards	36% Open Backs *
Short-tempered (Often)	16% Under 21 Rugby	0% Field Hockey ~
	64% Under 21 Forwards	25% Under 21 Backs #
Aggressive	42% Under 21 Rugby	14% Field Hockey *
Easily Angered	91% Under 21 Forwards	38% Under 21 Backs *
Easily Angered (Often)	13% School Rugby	0% School Field Hockey ~
Physical/Neurological		
Headaches	73% Under 21 Forwards	25% Under 21 Backs *
Clumsiness	42% Under 21 Rugby	10% Field Hockey *
	25% School Forwards	6% School Backs ~
Fatigue	63% Under 21 Rugby	33% Field Hockey ~
Clumsy Speech	50% Open Rugby	29% Cricket ~
	58% Under 21 Rugby	33% Field Hockey ~
	53% School Rugby	32% School Field Hockey ~
Slurred Speech	27% Under 21 Forwards	0% Under 21 Backs ~
Hearing	11% School Forwards	0% School Backs ~
Cognitive		
Memory	47% Open Forwards	0% Open Backs *
	55% Under 21 Forwards	25% Under 21 Backs ~
Sustained Attention	73% Open Rugby	48% Cricket *
	82% Under 21 Forwards	50% Under 21 Backs ~

Note: Results selected for presentation were delineated from the Chi-Squared analyses according to the following criteria: * p<0,05; ~ 0,05< p< 0,15; # difference of 30%+

Table 9.6. Percentages of individuals with reported postconcussive symptoms not in support of hypothesis: Controls > Rugby.

Emotional		
Worry	34% School Rugby	53% School Field Hockey ~
Physical/Neurological		
Headaches	35% Open Rugby	81% Cricket *
	35% Open Rugby	61% Field Hockey *
Eyesight	4% Open Rugby	19% Cricket *
Weakness in Limbs	11% School Rugby	27% School Field Hockey ~
	8% Open Rugby	24% Field Hockey ~
Cognitive		
Attention & Concentration	31% Open Rugby	57% Field Hockey ~

Note: Results selected for presentation were delineated from the Chi-Squared analyses according to the following criteria: * $p<0,05$; ~ $0,05< p< 0,15$; # difference of 30%+.

sports performance and might be underreported. The perception of greater limb weakness by both the adult level and school level field hockey players compared with rugby players suggests a hockey cohort effect, and could be associated with participation in a game which is much more dependent on fleet-footedness than body power as required in rugby. Increased 'worry' for school field hockey players is an isolated finding in this younger group, which goes against the hypotheses. It is difficult to explain, and may be attributed to pre-selected differences or to chance.

Summary and Conclusions

In summary, the overwhelming weight of evidence appears to be in the direction of support for the primary hypotheses derived from BRC theory which is that rugby players will show more impairment than noncontact sport controls, and problems will be enhanced amongst older, positionally more exposed and more cognitively vulnerable rugby players. The most robust cluster of deleterious effects for the objective test data appears in the area of speed of information processing followed by memory, which accords with prior sports studies as reviewed earlier. The percentages of deficit amongst these adult rugby players (for most part around 30 to 40% for speed of information processing, and up to 47% for memory) appears similar to those reported on comparable tasks for soccer, and about half that reported for boxers (see Table 9.1). For rugby schoolboys with a learning problem, percentages of deficit on a number of tests of speed of information processing and attention and concentration rise exponentially to figures comparable to those from boxing, ranging from 67%-100%. Evidence for this degree of risk of cognitive fall-off has caused medical outrage in respect of professional boxers, and implies that equivalent concern may be applicable to schoolboy rugby players with such prior cognitive vulnerability.

For postconcussive symptoms, the percentage of problems over a wide spectrum of reported neurobehavioural areas appears to be around 20-30% more than controls, which accords with the figure of 30% cited earlier from Tysvaer (1992) for the percentage of soccer players who report persistent postconcussive symptoms. What is of particular concern are deleterious neurobehavioural signs across *all three rugby groups* for speech-related functions, and aggressive/argumentative type behaviours, which imply frontal lobe involvement typically associated with closed head injury. Further of concern, is a high percentage of self-reported problems in the areas of memory and sustained attention across both adult rugby teams, especially for forwards, which provides cross-validation in respect of this outcome for rugby players, as well as cross-validation for problems with memory and sustained attention on the objective test data established in respect of adult rugby players. (The tests in the category of speed of information processing could equally be classified as tests of sustained attention). It is of note that for a number of key self-report neurobehavioural and cognitive dimensions that are so indicative of brain-related dysfunction (i.e. aggressive type behaviours, speech and memory problems), there were no results that implied problems for controls. Generally, for both the cognitive test data and the postconcussive symptoms, the results which seem to run in the opposite direction, are either explicable in terms of the particular cohort, or of such an isolated nature as to have little substance. Across three different levels of participation in Rugby Union, together with similar findings for American football and soccer, the chance that these are pre-selected differences rather than the consequences of repeated exposure to concussion, is rendered extremely unlikely.

The high injury rate per se, as well as the high incidence of concussion in Rugby Union, appear to be greater than that reported in any of the other field contact sports. The problems delineated here for Rugby Union players can be seen to have *clinical* significance in that the mode of investigation in the present study is based on an analysis of the *proportion (i.e. number)* of Rugby Union players who show neuropsychological signs selectively in the areas known to be most susceptible to damage in association with closed head injury. Importantly, an alternative set of analyses on these same cognitive test data, comprising direct comparisons of group mean and variability effects, pointed to the same areas of deficit for rugby players in speed of information processing and memory, all significant at probability levels of less than 0.01 ($p<0.01$). Further, the findings of the research across these three levels of play gain potency contextualized within the postulates of BRC theory. In particular, the theory alerts to the potential for subclinical effects which may become apparent with longer exposure to the game or prior cognitive vulnerability (as demonstrated across these studies), as well as under conditions of increased task challenge with potentially devastating consequences, such as in the context of school and university examinations. Finally, increased risk of dementia in association with repetitive sports-related head injury is a potentially dire consequence that needs to be factored in.

Thus, ethical issues around the participation of minors in a sport such as Rugby Union needs to be seriously addressed. This is particularly so for those whose cerebral reserve is already compromised due to prior learning disability or neurological disorder. As a start it would appear imperative to discourage any compulsory or routine participation in the sport, especially in the case of children and adolescents. Rather, participation should occur only following properly informed consent in which the potential for insidious brain-related consequences in association with the game are fully acknowledged. Further, screening procedures should be in place in order (i) to identify vulnerable players such as those with prior compromised cognitive function, (ii) to monitor those playing in the more hazardous forward positions, and (iii) to guide return-to-play decision for those who are concussed. Generally, as indicated in relation to the wider spectrum of contact sports (Maroon et al., 2000; Shuttleworth-Edwards & Border, 2002; Woijtys et al., 1999), it would appear essential to involve neuropsychologists in the management of concussion in Rugby Union, for both educative and screening purposes.

References

Abreau, F., Templer, D.I., Schuyler, B.A., & Hutchison, H.T. (1990). Neuropsychological assessment of soccer players. *Neuropsychology, 4*, 175–181.

Adams, K.M. & Putnam, S.H. (1991). What's minor about mild head injury? *Journal of Clinical and Experimental Neuropsychology, 13*, 388–394.

Baroff, G.S. (1998). Is heading a soccer ball injurious to brain function? *Journal of Head Trauma Rehabilitation, 13*, 45–52.

Barth, J.T., Macciocchi, S.N., Giordani, B., Rimel, R., Jane, J.A., & Boll, T.J. (1983). Neuropsychological sequelae of minor head injury. *Neurosurgery, 13*(5), 529-532.

Barth, J.T., Alves, W.M., Ryan, T.V., Macciocchi, S.N., Rimel, R.W., Jane, J.A. et al. (1989). Mild head injury in sports: neuropsychological sequelae and recovery of function. In H.S. Levin, H.M. Eisenberg, & A.L. Benton (Eds.), *Mild Head Injury* (pp. 257–575). Oxford: Oxford University Press.

Binder, L.M. (1986). Persisting symptoms after mild head injury: A review of the postconcussive syndrome. *Journal of Clinical and Experimental Neuropsychology, 8*, 323–346.

Binder, L.M. (1997). A review of mild head trauma. Part II: Clinical implications. *Journal of Clinical and Experimental Neuropsychology, 19*, 432–457.

Binder, L.M., Rohling, L.M., & Larrabee, G.J. (1997). A review of mild head trauma. Part I: Meta-analytic review of neuropsychological studies. *Journal of Clinical and Experimental Neuropsychology, 19*, 421–431.

Boll, T.J. (1985). Developing issues in clinical neuropsychology. Journal of Clinical and Experimental Neuropsychology, 7, 473-485.

Briscoe, J.H. (1985). Sports injuries in adolescent boarding school boys. *British Journal of Sports Medicine, 19*, 67–70.

Casson, I.R., Siegel, O., Sham, R., Campbell, E.A., Tarlau, M., & DiDomenico, A. (1984). Brain damage in modern boxers. *Journal of the American Medical Association, 251*, 2663–2667.

Collins, M.W., Grindel, S. H., Lovell, M.R., Dede, D.E., Moser, D.J., Phalin, B.R. et al. (1999). Relationship between concussion and neuropsychological performance in college football players. *Journal of the American Medical Association, 282*, 964–70.

Cremona-Meteyard, S.L. & Geffen, G.M. (1994). Persistent visuospatial attention deficits following mild head injury in Australian Rules football players. *Neuropsychologist, 32*, 649–662.

Davies, J.E. & Gibson, T. (1978). Injuries in Rugby Union football. *British Medical Journal, 2*, 1759–1761.

Gaetz, M., Goodman, D., & Weinberg, H. (2000). Electrophysiological evidence for the cumulative effects of concussion. *Brain Injury, 14*, 1077–1088.

Garraway, W.M., Lee, A.J., Hutton, S.J., Russell, E.B.A.W., & Macleod, D.A.D. (2000). Impact of professionalism on injuries in rugby union. *British Journal of Sports Medicine, 34*, 348–351

Garraway, M. & Macleod, D. (1995). Epidemiology of rugby football injuries. *The Lancet, 345*, 1485–1487.

Gerberich, S.G., Priest, J.D., Boen, J.R., Straub, C., & Maxwell, R.E. (1983). Concussion incidences and severity in secondary school varsity football players. *American Journal of Public Health, 73*, 1370–1375.

Gissane, C., Jennings, G.C., Cumine, A.J., Stephenson, S.E., & White, J.A. (1997). The Australian *Journal of Science and Medicine in Sport, 29*, 91–94.

Green, G.A. & Jordan, S.E. (1998). Are brain injuries a significant problem in soccer? *Clinics in Sports Medicine, 17*, 795–809.

Hillis, W.S., McIntyre, P.D., Maclean, J., Goodwin, J.F., & McKenna, W.J. (1994). ABC of sports medicine: sudden death in sport. *British Medical Journal, 309*, 657–660.

Hinton-Bayre, A.D., Geffen, G.M., Geffen, L.B., McFarland, K.A., & Friis, P. (1999). Concussion in contact sports: reliable change indices of impairment and recovery. *Journal of Clinical and Experimental Neuropsychology, 21*, 70–86.

Jakoet, I. & Noakes, T.D. (1998). A high rate of injury during the 1995 Rugby World cup. *South African Medical Journal, 1*, 45–47.

Kaste, M., Kuurne, T., Vilkki, J., Katevuo, K., Sainio, K., & Meurala, H. (1982). Is chronic brain damage in boxing a hazard of the past? *The Lancet, 27*, 1186–1188.

Langburt, W., Cohen, B., Akhthar, N., O'Neill, K., & Lee, J.C. (2001). Incidence of concussion in high school football players of Ohio Pennsylvania. *Journal of Child Neurology, 16*, 83–85.

Levin, H.S., Eisenberg, H.M., & Benton, A.L. (Eds.). (1989). *Mild Head Injury*. New York: Oxford University Press.

Lingard, D.A., Sharrock, N.E., & Salmond, C.E. (1976). Risk factors of sports injuries in winter. *The New Zealand Medical Journal, 83*, 69–73.

Macleod, D.A.D. (1993). Risks and injuries in rugby football. In G.R. McLatchie & C.M.E. Lennox (Eds.), *The soft tissues. Trauma and sports injuries* (pp. 371–381). London: Butterworth-Heinemann Ltd.

Maddocks, D. & Saling, M. (1996). Neuropsychological deficits following concussion. *Brain Injury, 10*, 99–103.

Maroon, J.C., Lovell, M.R., Norwig, A.T.C., Podell, K., Powell, J.W., & Hartl, R. (2000). Cerebral concussion in athletes: evaluation and neuropsychological testing. *Neurosurgery, 47*, 659–669.

Matser, J.T., Kessels, A.G.H., Jordan, B.D., Lezak, M.D., & Troost, J. (1998). Chronic traumatic brain injury in professional soccer players. *Neurology, 51*, 791–796.

Matser, J.T., Kessels, A.G.H., Lezak, M.D., Jordan, B.D., & Troost, J. (1999). Neuropsychological impairment in amateur soccer players. *Journal of the American Medical Association, 282*, 971–973.

McKenna, S., Borman, B., Findlay, J., & de Boer, M. (1986). Sports injuries in New Zealand. *New Zealand Medical Journal, 99*, 899–901.

Micheli, L.J. & Riseborough, E.M. (1974). The incidence of injuries in rugby football. *Journal of Sports Medicine, 2*, 93–97.

Myers, P.T. (1980). Injuries presenting from rugby union football. *The Medical Journal of Australia, 2*, 17–20.

Nathan, M., Goedeke, R., & Noakes, T.D. (1983). The incidence and nature of rugby injuries experienced at one school during the 1982 rugby season. *South African Medical Journal, 64*, 132–137.

Pettersen, J.A. & Skelton, R.W. (2000). Glucose enhances long-term declarative memory in mildly head-injured varsity rugby players. *Psychobiology, 28*, 81–89.

Powell, J.W. & Barber-Foss, K.D. (1999). Traumatic brain injury in high school athletes. *Journal of the American Medical Association, 282*, 958–963.

Reid, I., Shuttleworth-Jordan, A.B., Ancer, R., Dickinson, A., Radloff, S., & Jakoet, I. (1999). To scrum or not to scrum: First report from the RU-SARFU rugby head injury study [Abstract]. *Journal of the International Neuropsychology Society, 5*, 283.

Roux, C.E., Goedeke, R., Visser, G.R., Van Zyl, W.A., & Noakes, T.D. (1987). The epidemiology of schoolboy rugby injuries. *South African Medical Journal, 71*, 307–313.

Roy, S.P. (1974). The nature and frequency of rugby injuries. A pilot study of 300 injuries at Stellenbosch. *South African Medical Journal, 48*, 2321–2327.

Ryan, J.M. & McQuillan, R. (1992). A survey of rugby injuries attending an accident and emergency department. *Irish Medical Journal, 85*, 72–73.

Satz, P. (1993). Brain reserve capacity on symptom onset after brain injury: A formulation and review of evidence for threshold theory. *Neuropsychology, 7*, 273–295.

Satz, P. (2001). Mild head injury in children and adolescents. *Current Directions in Psychological Science, 10*, 106–109.

Satz, P., Zaucha, K., McCleary, C., Light, R., Asarnow, R., & Becker, D. (1997). Mild head injury in children and adolescents: a review of studies (1970-1995). *Psychological Bulletin, 122*, 107–131.

Seward, H., Orchard, J., Hazard, H., & Collinson, D. (1993). Football injuries in Australia at the élite level. *The Medical Journal of Australia, 159*, 298–301.

Shuttleworth-Edwards, A.B., Ackermann, T., Beilinsohn, T., Border, M., & Radloff, S. (September, 2001a). *A study on the effects of cumulative mild head injury in high school rugby*. Paper presented in Shuttleworth-Edwards, A.B. (Chair), Sports related head injury. Symposium convened at the 8th National Conference of the SA Clinical Neuropsychological Association (SACNA), University of Cape Town.

Shuttleworth-Edwards, A.B., & Border, M.A. (2002). Computer based screening in concussion management: use versus abuse. *British Journal of Sports Medicine, 36*, 473.

Shuttleworth-Edwards, A., Border, M., & Radloff, S. (2001b). Participation in contact sport: A case of mild head battering with long-term additive effects [Abstract]. *Journal of the International Neuropsychology Society, 7*, 405-406.

Shuttleworth-Jordan, A.B., Puchert, J., & Balarin, E. (1993). Negative consequences of mild head injury in rugby: a matter worthy of concern. In R. Plunkett & S. Anderson (Eds.). *Proceedings of the 5th National Neuropsychology Conference*. Durban: South African Clinical Neuropsychological Association (SACNA).

Sturmi, J.E., Smith, C., & Lombardo, J.A. (1998). Mild brain trauma in sports. Diagnosis and treatment guidelines. *Sports Medicine, 25*, 351-358.

Tysvaer, A.T. (1992). Head and neck injuries in soccer. Impact of minor trauma. *Sports Medicine, 14*, 200-213.

Tysvaer, A.T. & Lochen, E.A. (1991). Soccer injuries to the brain. A neuropsychologic study of former soccer players. *The American Journal of Sports Medicine, 19*, 56-60.

Van Heerden, J.J. (1976). 'n Ontleding van rugbybeserings. *South African Medical Journal, 50*, 1374-1379.

Walker, R.D. (1985). Sports injuries: rugby league may be less dangerous than union. *The Practitioner, 229*, 205-206.

Wekesa, M., Asembo, J.M., & Njororai, W.W.S. (1996). Injury surveillance in a rugby tournament. *British Journal of Sports Medicine, 30*, 61-63.

Wilberger, J.E. (1988). Minor head injury in athletes. *Neurotrauma Medical Report, 2*, 3-4.

Wilberger, J.E. (1993). Minor head injuries in American football. Prevention of long term sequelae. *Sports Medicine, 15*, 338-343.

Wills, S.M. & Leathem, J.M. (2001). An investigation of brain injury incurred in New Zealand club-grade rugby [Abstract]. *Journal of the International Neuropsychology Society, 7*, 405.

Wojtys, E.M., Hovda, D., Landry, G., Boland, A., Lovell, M., McCrea, M. et al. (1999). Concussion in sports. *The American Journal of Sports Medicine, 27*, 676-686.

Zakzanis, K.K. (1998). Methodological commentary: Brain is related to behavior (p< .05). *Journal of Clinical and Experimental Neuropsychology, 3*, 419-427.

Chapter 10

AUSTRALIAN RULES FOOTBALL AND RUGBY LEAGUE

Anton D. Hinton-Bayre and Gina Geffen
Cognitive Psychophysiology Laboratory, University of Queensland, Australia

Introduction

Research on traumatic brain injury (TBI) sustained in contact sport is important for many reasons. Many people who regularly participate in contact sports are at a significant risk of sustaining concussion. Sport and recreation activities frequently rate as one of the top five causes of mild TBI (Bazarian et al., 1999; Sosin, Sniezek, & Thurman, 1996). Although it is believed that the majority of cases of single uncomplicated mild TBI and sports concussion lead to short-term neurobehavioural dysfunction, followed by full recovery, a sufficiently clear understanding of the sequelae is not currently available. Moreover, the high incidence of repeat concussion in contact sport has lead to concerns over protracted sequelae, traumatic encephalopathy, and even death due to second impact syndrome (Cantu, 1998). Perhaps the most problematic aspect of the diagnosis and management of concussion is the difficulty in reliably identifying a pathological change in the brain following trauma (McCrory, Johnston, Mohtadi, & Meeuwisse, 2001; Hovda et al., 1999). Contemporary imaging techniques regularly fail to reveal abnormality in cases of concussion, with diagnostic criteria relying almost solely on neurological indicators (Johnston, McCrory, Mohtadi, & Meeuwisse, 2001). The difficulty in identifying the underlying pathology of concussion is reflected in popular definitions of the injury, which rely almost exclusively on behavioural observation and assessment (see Johnston et al., 2001). Consequently, early attempts to standardise the diagnosis and management of concussion in sport have been based on clinical judgement with little empirical substance. The standardization of appropriate assessment techniques would provide an empirical basis for management of concussion in contact sport. A growing body of evidence suggests that of the various techniques available, neuropsychological assessment of brain function may be the most sensitive to dysfunction in concussion. The validation of such assessment in the context of contact sport has risen rapidly since 1995. Trauma sustained within the context of contact sport is likely to be of the mildest form seen in human activity (Alexander, 1995) and provides a model for examining the sequelae of TBI. The study of TBI in contact sport allows a unique opportunity to assess function before trauma occurs, permitting a more sensitive analysis of the effects of concussion on subsequent recovery. Thus, we see at least two reasons for neuropsychology to focus more attention on TBI in the sporting arena: (1) to gain a better understanding of minimal brain trauma, (2) to investigate the potential role of neuropsychological assessment in the management of sports-related TBI.

The present chapter examines the research of neuropsychological assessment in the contact sports of Rugby League (RL) and Australian Rules Football (commonly referred to as AFL – Australian Football League). Following a brief historical review of the development of neuropsychological assessment of concussion in contact sport in Australia, the empirical work that has been conducted over the past 15 years in AFL is examined. Research relevant to the assessment of immediate mental disruption following concussion will be considered first. This will be followed by a discussion of the research on the post-acute stage (days-weeks following concussion), and finally the problem of the limited amount of research on persistent and cumulative effects is discussed. The major part of this chapter will focus on our more recent work with Rugby League players. This research has sought to validate neuropsychological assessment in contact sport, with particular attention directed to how these results may be applied to the management of concussion.

Historical review

The antecedents of neuropsychological assessment in AFL can be traced back to the use of standard neurological screening techniques in the 1980s. In particular, measures of mental status, including orientation, recent memory, and short-term recall were becoming common place in the on-site diagnosis of concussion (Dicker, 1989; McCrory, 1989). Nonetheless, the decision of whether a concussed athlete was recovered remained one based on clinical intuition, player honesty in reporting any difficulties, and the reliance of knowledge acquired through studies of boxing trauma and mild traumatic brain injury in the general population. The first reports on the potential use of neuropsychological assessment in AFL were made in the late 1980s. Dicker and Maddocks (1988) provided a preliminary report of the utility of the Digit Symbol Substitution test in objectively monitoring the recovery of brain function following concussion. At a similar time, Cremona-Meteyard and Geffen (1994) sought to quantify the presence of acute and chronic cognitive function deficits following concussion.

In the early 1990s Shuttleworth-Jordan and colleagues investigated the effects of concussion in South African Rugby Union (RU) players. However, this research appeared to be an isolated investigation. Despite the international popularity of RU, particularly in the Oceanic region and some European countries, there had been little published on the neuropsychological effects of concussion in this sport. By the mid-1990s, AFL research was ongoing and for the first time concussion in RL was addressed. Earlier research into AFL concussions was particularly focussed on the clinical features of the injury (Maddocks, Dicker, & Saling, 1995; McCrory, Bladin, & Berkovic, 1997). At the same time, Hinton-Bayre, Geffen and colleagues (1997, 1999, 1999) sought to further examine the utility of neuropsychological assessment in the post-acute management of concussion in rugby league players. A more comprehensive research program based in Victoria (a state in Australia) has been underway since 2000 examining many aspects of the science and clinical management of concussion in Australian Rules and Rugby players. Preliminary outcomes from this research will be briefly discussed in this chapter and is further considered in the computerized testing chapter of this book.

Australian Rules Football

AFL is unique to Australia with the first recorded match contested in 1877. The game was originally developed by Irish settlers, hence it shares many characteristics of Gaelic football.[1] While the game was once located almost exclusively in Victoria, it has become the most popular contact sport in the

[1] An AFL match is contested between two teams with 21 players a side, with 18 on the field for each team at any one time. There are set field positions with players located at various positions around the field (usually positioned in opposing pairs), and as there is no off-side rule, all players move freely around the field. The game is played on an oval field with four scoring posts located at either end of the ground. 'Goals' (6 points) are obtained by kicking an oval ball directly through the middle two posts. 'Behinds' (1 point) are obtained when the ball passes between a middle post and an outer post, or whenever the ball passes between the two outer posts and is not directly kicked. The ball is moved around the field either by kicking, hand-balling (where the ball is struck with a closed fist), or running with the ball. Throwing is not permitted. In general play, there is continual contesting for possession of the ball, in which players can be bumped out of the way or tackled. When a player catches the ball directly from a kick from any player (known as a 'mark'), the catching player is permitted to take an unimpeded kick. A match is played in quarters over a two-hour period.

country with over 385,000 regular participants recorded in 1993 (approximately 2% of the 1993 national population) (National Health and Medical Research Council of Australia, 1994). Hard protective equipment is not permitted, and soft head-gear is worn by a minority of players at the senior level. The nature of the game is such that players regularly leap into the air to catch the ball. Players are permitted to use another player as a step to gain extra height in order to mark the ball, and thus falls from heights of 3 to 4 metres are not uncommon. Only in the case of a more severe injury is the game stopped. Concussions regularly result from direct player contact whilst contesting the ball, from a player striking their head on the ground, and more rarely from striking a scoring post. It is not surprising that the focus of neuropsychological research in Australia was initially on AFL. While the incidence of more severe head trauma in contact sport is extremely rare, the incidence of concussion is far more prevalent (Orchard, Wood, Seward, & Broad, 1998). A retrospective study by Maddocks, Saling, and Dicker (1995) indicated that 60% of active professional AFL players had a history of concussion.

Similar to studies conducted in American football, research on AFL players has also examined the sensitivity and utility of neuropsychological assessment in the management of concussion, while attempting to gain a better understanding of the functional deficits resulting from the injury. Neuropsychological assessment research of concussion in AFL has focused on three basic areas that will be addressed in turn: (a) on-site evaluation, (b) recovery of function, and (c) cumulative and chronic effects.

On-site evaluation

In many instances of concussion a demonstrable loss of consciousness is not present. However, a concussed athlete may demonstrate confusion and amnesia yet retain motor function and even continue to play (Yarnell & Lynch, 1973). Team physicians were encouraged to implement systematic sideline evaluation of orientation, recent memory and short-term recall (Dicker, 1989). These practices were conducted to ascertain the presence of confusion and amnesia and thus assist in the recognition and diagnosis of concussion. Subsequent reports of systematic evaluation revealed that orientation was not reliably impaired following concussion in AFL (Maddocks, Dicker, & Saling, 1995). However, evidence for impaired recent memory was found. Questions such as "Who did you play last week?", "How did you get to the game today?", and "Which side scored first?" successfully identified concussed players. The routine use of such questions has become prevalent in the sideline assessment of concussion. Collateral research has suggested that the presence and duration of retrograde amnesia varies non-linearly with time following trauma (McCrory & Maddocks, 1994). Immediately following trauma, players were able to clearly recall events almost up to impact (less than a minute). However, when reassessed 10 mins later the amnesic period had 'ballooned' to 21 minutes on average, before returning to a 3½ minute period when assessed finally at 24 hours post trauma. Thus the use of retrograde amnesia in the management of concussion was considered questionable unless the time of assessment was specified. The majority of concussion management guidelines rely on the presence and duration of various post-trauma signs and symptoms. AFL concussion research has indicated that systematic assessment of anterograde and retrograde amnesia will assist in the diagnosis of concussion.

Recovery of function

It has long been known that difficulties persist beyond the resolution of immediate signs and symptoms of mild traumatic brain injury. While exaggeration of symptoms following mild TBI is often suspected in contexts other than professional contact sport, the concern with sportspeople is that they are likely to minimise subjective complaints of physical or somatic symptoms in order to return to participation. Therefore, objective performance based measures of brain function were sought to assist in the clinical decision process of determining recovery. A preliminary examination of the potential use of neuropsychological tests reported pre-post performance of 13 concussed AFL players on the Digit Symbol test. When compared to preseason performance, players completed significantly fewer items on the Digit Symbol when retested within 24 hours of trauma (Dicker & Maddocks, 1988). Concussed players' performance was reported to be equivalent to preseason performance by 5 days post trauma. Furthermore, players with a period of post-traumatic amnesia (PTA) in excess of 30 minutes were reported to demonstrate slower return to baseline levels. However, only two players had PTA exceeding 30 minutes. Unfortunately, performance measures such as the Digit Symbol are highly susceptible to practice effects (Hinton-Bayre, Geffen, Geffen et al., 1999). Without a comparably assessed control group to ascertain what performance levels should result from repeated measurement, it could not be clearly determined whether improved performance was due to recovery of function or simple re-exposure to test materials.

In a follow-up to their 1989 study, Maddocks and Saling (1996) employed an age-matched control group of AFL referees (n = 10), and a more comprehensive battery, which included the Digit Symbol, a four-choice reaction time test, and the Paced Auditory Serial Addition Task (PASAT). Significant differences were found between concussed AFL players (n = 10) and controls on the Digit Symbol and reaction time test when reassessed at 5 days post-trauma. Concussed players were comparable to their preseason performance at 5 days, whereas controls demonstrated significant improvement. This work confirmed that a simple return to preseason performance may actually under-estimate deficits, as concussed players had not demonstrated the relative improvement that would have been expected had they not been injured. Recent work with AFL players has suggested that indices from the computerized protocol 'Cogsport' were more sensitive to concussion induced cognitive deficits (Collie, Darby, & Maruff, 2001). After screening 240 AFL players preseason on Cogsport, the Trail Making Test and Digit Symbol, 15 players sustained concussion and were retested at two and 14 days post trauma. It was found that reaction time variability and information processing speed indices were impaired on Cogsport, yet performance on the traditional tests was found not to change following concussion. However, it would appear that computerized tests are not immune to methodological concerns like practice effects as control players tended to demonstrate reduced performance variability on retesting (Makdissi et al., 2001). While computerised assessment provides many benefits, the psychometric properties of such measures requires greater investigation to ensure acceptable validity.

The data clearly indicate that performance on neuropsychological measures of speed of information processing appears to significantly decline following trauma. Based on the methodology employed, concussion in AFL appears to be a brief and transient phenomenon. The actual demonstration of recovery on such measures must take into account the influence of practice to clearly determine when recovery of function has occurred. The AFL research suggests that clear declines in performance from preseason on sensitive tests, such as the Digit Symbol, may only be apparent when post-trauma assessment occurs within minutes of injury. Testing for a significant decline in the days following concussion appears to be complicated by practice effects, as concussed players show no change in performance when compared to preseason data, whereas controls demonstrate practice effects. It is this 'absence of practice' that has been used to infer impaired brain function following concussion. This is similar to earlier interpretations by Barth and colleagues (1989).

Persistent and cumulative effects

There is limited support for persistent difficulties following concussion in AFL. Within days of concussion it has been reported that players did not show evidence of MRI or EEG abnormalities, symptom complaints, impairment on a neuropsychological test, or subsequently impaired playing performance (McCrory et al., 1997). Earlier AFL studies relied almost exclusively on standardised neuropsychological tests, usually the Digit Symbol. Using an experimental task of covert orientation of attention, it was demonstrated that a sample of 9 concussed AFL players were found to show no benefit in speed of response after valid cuing at two weeks post trauma (Cremona-Meteyard & Geffen, 1994). This relative impairment for concussed players was still present one year post trauma. It is noteworthy that six of the nine players used in the study reported a history of previous concussions. Thus the deficit observed at one year may be suggestive of cumulative effects of repeated trauma. The persistent deficit could also have resulted from injuries that occurred between the 2 week and 1 year follow-up, but were never reported, even though players were questioned about this.

The possibility for cumulative effects should not be underestimated. A retrospective study of 198 professional AFL players revealed that 55 had sustained two or more concussions (Maddocks, Saling, & Dicker, 1995). Performance on the Digit Symbol was recorded for each of these groups, yet no significant difference was found. No player had sustained a concussion in the 6 months prior to the study, again suggesting no clear evidence of cumulative effects resulting from concussion in AFL. These data are retrospective and based on subjective report, which is not methodologically ideal. Yet, similar methodology applied to soccer players was reported to reveal impaired performance (Matser et al., 1998, 1999). A comparative study controlling for level and history of participation would be instructive.

Rugby League

Rugby football is believed to have originated in the 1820s at 'Rugby School' in England.[2] The separation of Rugby League from Rugby Union did not occur until many decades later in 1895. Rugby League was first played in Australia at the turn of last century. The international popularity of Rugby League has continued to develop with 21 countries competing at the recent 2000 Rugby League World Cup. Like AFL, protective gear is not mandatory. Many players wear some form of shoulder protection, yet few professionals wear soft head-gear. Again, hard helmets are not permitted. Most head injuries in RL result from tackling, affecting both offensive and defensive players. The most common mechanisms of concussion appear to be from the offensive player being hit in the head during an attempted tackle (tackling above the shoulder is an illegal play), or a player's head striking another part of a player or the ground (Hinton-Bayre, 2000). It is not uncommon for a

[2] In a game of RL there are 17 players on each side, with 13 on the field at any one time. There are set field positions in RL and an off-side rule is present. A regulation RL field is rectangular with a set of 'uprights' shaped like the letter 'H' positioned in the centre of a 'try-line' at either end. The main objective of the game is to place an oval-shaped ball over the try-line by hand, this is known as a 'try' and is worth 4 points. After a try is scored a player will attempt to score a 'conversion' by kicking the ball, which is placed on the ground, between the two vertical poles of the uprights above the transverse pole. A conversion is worth 2 points, and may also be attempted after some penalties. A 'field-goal' worth 1 point may be attempted from a drop-kick at any time during regular play. In general play, the ball is passed by hand backwards, whilst territory is gained by running forward. Advancing or offensive players in possession of the ball are 'tackled' by an opposing player or players. Possession of the ball is exchanged after 6 tackles, notwithstanding a penalty. As such, a tackle is effected more than twice a minute on average. RL is played in two 40 minute halves.

player to receive dual trauma during a tackle, first contacting with another player before striking the ground.

Over recent years our major research interest has been in concussion in rugby league players. There were several reasons for focussing on this population. Rugby League is the fourth most popular contact sport in Australia, behind AFL, soccer, and Rugby Union (NHMRC, 1994). When examining elite football injury rates, the highest relative frequency of concussion has been found in Rugby League (8.5%), over twice the incidence of AFL (3.6%) (Seward, Orchard, Hazard, & Collinson, 1993). Rugby League has been reported to be the leading cause of mild head trauma presenting to hospital emergency departments in the Australian state of Queensland (Epidemiological and Health Information Branch, Queensland Health, 1993). Furthermore, recent epidemiological data have confirmed that rugby codes produce the highest incidence of injury, head injury, and loss of consciousness (Queensland Injury Surveillance Unit, 2000).

From a neuropsychological perspective there were three main areas of interest: (a) to investigate which measures were most sensitive to concussion in contact sport, (b) to determine the expected time-course of recovery following concussion, and (c) to gain a better understanding of the long-term and potentially cumulative effects of concussion. The research summarised below addressed each of these areas.

Sensitivity of neuropsychological assessment

Over the last 25 years several standard neuropsychological measures have been found to be sensitive to mild TBI in the general population. Research in AFL has tended to be reliant for the most part on the Digit Symbol test (Dicker & Maddocks, 1988; Maddocks et al., 1995; Maddocks & Saling, 1996; McCrory et al., 1997). Hinton-Bayre, Geffen and McFarland (1999) compiled a screening battery similar to that proposed by Lezak (1995) covering attention, psychomotor speed, cognitive flexibility, information processing ability, learning and memory for rapid assessment and detection of subtle change (Binder, Rohling, & Larrabee, 1997). The tests we selected were chosen on several criteria, including: (a) demonstrated sensitivity in general or contact sport mild TBI, (b) availability of alternate forms – or facility of production of such forms, (c) brevity of administration, and (d) breadth of functions possibly impaired following mild trauma. The selected tests and the functions they assess are presented in Table 10.1. We also employed tests to assess pre-morbid intellectual functioning (NART-R, Spot-the-Word) to examine their purported resistance to head injury (Crawford, Parker, & McKinlay, 1992).

A total of 86 professional rugby league players underwent baseline assessment on the protocol outlined in Table 10.1. During the course of a single competitive season 13 players were independently diagnosed as hav-

Table 10.1 Psychometric tests and cognitive constructs assessed.

Test		Constructs[a]
Auditory Verbal Learning Test		Immediate memory span, verbal learning, interference tendencies, short- and long-term retention, retrieval efficieny
Controlled Oral Word Association Test		Verbal fluency
Dodrill-Stroop Colour-Word Test		Executive function, selective attention, cognitive flexibility, response inhibition
Symbol Digit Modalities Test		Visual scanning and tracking, psychomotor speed, associative learning
Digit Symbol Substitution Test		Complex attention, psychomotor speed, visuo-motor coordination
Speed of Comprehension Test		Language comprehension, syntactic and semantic processing, rate of information processing
Digit Span	Forwards	Efficiency of attention
	Backwards	Mental tracking, working memory
Spot-the-Word		Lexical decision, verbal intelligence estimate
National Adult Reading Test		Verbal intelligence estimate

[a] Adapted from Lezak (1995) and Spreen and Strauss (1998).

ing sustained a concussion. An uninjured control group equivalent for age, education, estimated IQ and number of previous concussions was formed. Concussed players were retested within 24-48 hours of injury, with control players being retested at a similar time following a game. Table 10.2 presents test scores for concussed players on the regular indices interpreted for each test, taken at preseason and 2 days post trauma. Comparative scores for control players are presented in the lower section of Table 10.2. Several measures including the AVLT, COWAT, Stroop, Digit Span, and NART-R were administered individually preseason. However, because access to players' time was limited, several tests were adapted for group administration, including Speed of Comprehension, Spot-the-word, Digit Symbol and Symbol Digit. All measures were administered individually following concussion in follow-up testing. This procedure was kept constant across concussed and control players.

No evidence of relatively impaired performance was found of the AVLT, COWAT, Digit Span, Spot-the-Word, and NART-R following concussion. Concussed players recorded reduced performance on Digit Symbol, Symbol Digit, and Speed Comprehension upon retesting 24-48 hours after trauma. Control players showed no change in performance on retesting. Relative impairment was also seen on the Dodrill-Stroop test. When required to read colour words printed in incongruent coloured ink in Part A, concussed

Table 10.2. Psychometric test performance pre- and post-concussion.

Concussed (n = 13)	Preseason M (SD)		Post Injury – 2 days M (SD)		t
AVLT Trial 1	6.8	(1.3)	5.7	(1.4)	2.55*
Trial 5	11.5	(1.8)	11.8	(2.0)	0.58
Trial 7	9.9	(2.7)	9.7	(2.8)	0.46
Total (1-5)	47.6	(8.5)	45.9	(7.0)	1.15
COWAT	40.4	(7.9)	43.1	(9.0)	1.84
Stroop A	80.0	(11.9)	86.2	(13.7)	3.17*
Stroop B	152.2	(15.9)	154.2	(19.7)	0.56
Digit Span Forward	7.2	(1.2)	7.6	(1.0)	1.16
Digit Span Backward	5.6	(1.6)	5.5	(1.3)	0.14
Silly Sentences[a]	73.3	(10.9)	57.8	(15.0)	3.98**
Symbol Digit[a]	61.7	(11.4)	55.7	(10.8)	2.85*
Digit Symbol[a]	73.7	(7.7)	68.2	(6.2)	2.65*
Controls (n = 13)					
AVLT Trial 1	5.8	(1.6)	6.5	(1.3)	1.23
Trial 5	12.4	(2.1)	11.6	(2.1)	0.15
Trial 7	10.2	(3.0)	10.3	(2.6)	0.46
Total (1-5)	48.5	(8.0)	49.3	(7.4)	0.36
COWAT	33.6	(7.8)	36.8	(7.7)	1.47
Stroop A	92.3	(19.5)	94.7	(19.6)	1.07
Stroop B	204.4	(63.9)	185.8	(55.6)	2.50*
Digit Span Forward	6.5	(1.1)	6.8	(1.4)	1.00
Digit Span Backward	5.5	(1.0)	5.4	(1.7)	0.20
Silly Sentences[a]	69.6	(11.0)	68.2	(9.7)	1.29
Symbol Digit[a]	62.0	(8.0)	63.0	(8.4)	0.90
Digit Symbol[a]	68.3	(11.8)	70.8	(7.0)	1.36

Note. AVLT = Auditory Verbal Learning Test, COWAT = Controlled Oral Word Association Test. [a] n = 10; ** $p < .01$; * $p < .05$.

players were significantly slower on retesting, whereas control player performance was stable across the two testing sessions. Conversely, on Part B where the colour-word must be ignored and the colour of the ink must be named concussed players showed no change in performance on retesting, yet control players completed the task significantly faster on the second occasion.

These results suggest that concussion resulted in a selective impairment on tests requiring some element of visual processing. However, this interpretation should not be overstated. The verbal measures employed did not tax speed of information processing to the same extent as the visual measures. Reductions in information processing speed, usually secured in a timed attention task, have been referred to as the hallmark cognitive effect of concussion (Binder et al., 1997). The somewhat anomalous result on Stroop

A may reflect a selective attention deficit, with concussed players having difficulty ignoring anticipated requirements of Stroop B when retested following trauma (Brooks, Fos, Greve, & Hammond, 1999; Stablum, Mogontale, & Umilta, 1996). As the impetus for test selection was clinically-driven, an analytical examination of underlying processes is only made tentatively.

Recovery From Concussion

Several studies have demonstrated that concussion leads to impaired performance on standard clinical neuropsychological tests. Consequently, the use of sensitive psychometric measures as objective indices of recovery after concussion in sport has been recommended by several authors (see Grindell, Lovell, & Collins, 2001). However, effective and valid utilisation of such tests in the context of managing sports-related concussion requires further standardisation. The applied use of psychometric tests in the assessment of concussion in sport presents unique challenges to the neuropsychologist.

One of the benefits of assessing the effects of concussion in contact sport is the ability to collect pre-injury data on cognitive function. Concussed players can be reassessed and compared to their own pre-injury performance. Analyses of within-subject variations in performance are far more powerful than between subject differences or comparisons to non-specific normative data (Brooks, 1987). However, preseason screening of contact sport players must be undertaken within a limited window of opportunity. To assess a large group of people within a brief period, session length must be considered. All prospective studies to date have limited assessment schedules to 30-45 minutes, far more brief than the regular neuropsychological assessment. Finally, given pre-season data, recovery of function may be considered on an individual basis. None of the group-analysed studies of concussion in sport have provided adequate criteria for making individual decisions.

Recovery from the acute effects of concussion has been measured as a return to pre-season performance (e.g. McCrory et al., 1997) and the convergence of change scores in serial retesting so that concussed and uninjured controls show similar variations in performance (e.g. Macciocchi et al., 1996). The 'pre-injury' method of determining recovery fails to adequately control for practice effects and thus may underestimate impairment. A return to pre-injury levels may again appear to be face-valid recovery but is only defensible when uninjured players show no deviation from baseline. The 'convergence' method controls for practice effects and the expectation that above pre-injury levels may be a better indication of normal performance, but is severely limited without suitable retest normative data.

Practice Effects

Repeated assessment necessitates consideration of practice effects, as initial deficit and monitoring of improvement may be confounded. Three strategies were employed to control practice effects in the context of neuropsychological assessment in Rugby League (Hinton-Bayre, Geffen, Geffen et al., 1999). First, alternate forms of all tests were employed. Second, given that many studies seem to indicate that improved performance is greatest from first to second assessment, measures were given twice preseason. In this way, the individual player acts as their own control facilitating a clear deficit post-trauma, and allowing a return to baseline to more accurately reflect recovery of function. Third, uninjured control players provided retest normative data to facilitate the generation of cut-scores for determining the presence of ongoing deficits. The derivation of cut-scores was based on the Reliable Change Index (RCI). This was adjusted for practice effects, as indexed in control players (Chelune et al., 1993). An individual's expected score upon retesting would be their original score plus the mean practice effect, seen in a control sample. If the obtained retest score was close enough to the expected retest score (within the 90% confidence interval), then a judgment of no impairment was made.

Preliminary preseason data on 71 professional rugby league players retested within 1-2 weeks showed that 80% and 73% of players demonstrated improved performance on retesting for the Digit Symbol and Speed of Comprehension tests respectively. These results have several implications. First, whether or not preseason data are available to compare with performance following trauma, retest norms will be required in order to control for the effects of practice. Second, practice effects may depend on type of measure employed. Tests involving some component of timed performance appear to be differentially affected by repeated administration. Third, improved performance was noted even when alternate forms were utilised. Thus alternate forms are a necessary, but not sufficient method of controlling practice effects. Fourth, the retest interval appears to be of great importance. Retest intervals of around one year tend not to result in improved performance (Lovell & Collins, 1998; Temkin, Heaton, Grant, & Dikmen, 1999). Retest interval and magnitude of practice effect appear to be inversely related. As many psychometric texts remind us, the reliability and validity of a test are features of its use, rather than characteristics of the test itself. Establishing retest normative data that mirror the testing schedule desired in pre/post concussion assessment would be of great assistance to the clinician in terms of ascertaining the presence of deficit and rate of recovery.

Neuropsychological Test Performance Following Concussion

Data were collected on a sample of 21 rugby league players before and after concussion. Four players experienced a loss of consciousness (LOC), all less than 1 minute. In total 14 players experienced a period of post-traumatic amnesia (PTA) without LOC. Of the 14 players presenting with PTA but no LOC, PTA was less than 10 minutes in six players, and from 10 minutes to 3 hours in the remaining eight players. A brief period (< 5 minutes) of confusion was reported in the remaining three players. Concussed players were assessed twice preseason and up to three times following trauma; 1-3 days, 1-2 weeks, and 3 to 5 weeks. Seven of the 21 players had received only one preseason exposure to tests, due to sustaining concussion prior to completion of baseline assessment.

In a series of mixed factorial analyses of variance, it was shown that profiles of performance on each of the three tests (Digit Symbol, Symbol Digit, & Speed of Comprehension) differentiated concussed from control players (see Fig. 10.1). Across the measures the concussed players consistently demonstrated a significant decline in performance from preseason to 2 days (median) following trauma. At a median of 10 days following trauma, on average concussed players recorded performances comparable to their preseason performance across the three sensitive tests. On the Symbol Digit and Speed of Comprehension tests no further improvement was seen upon retesting. This result would suggest that a return to preseason levels of performance on these measures would be sufficient to demonstrate recovery, providing two preseason exposures were administered. However, even with dual preseason assessment, control players demonstrated improved performance upon later serial retesting on the Digit Symbol. A return to preseason levels on the Digit Symbol may be insufficient to reliably qualify as recovery.

The group data analyses indicated that recovery from concussion sustained in RL is measurably longer, with evidence of relative impairment at 10 days on the Digit Symbol, than seen in prospective studies of other contact sports, namely AFL (Maddocks & Saling, 1996; McCrory et al., 1997) and American football (e.g. Macciocchi et al., 1996). It is difficult to state whether this is due to differences in methodology (ie, testing schedule, tests used) or differences in the actual injuries sustained. Severity of injury appears to be comparable across various codes of football on average. It is possible that the mechanism of injury differs according to style of play. For example, in our study of RL players the common cause of concussion was the 'high' tackle, which accounted for one-third of the injuries recorded. While it would seem likely that a similar situation is likely in both AFL and American Football, the authors are not aware of any detailed published research on nature of contact leading to concussion. A great deal may be learnt from investigating the mechanics of concussion in the human model of contact sports (McIntosh, McCrory, & Comerford, 1999).

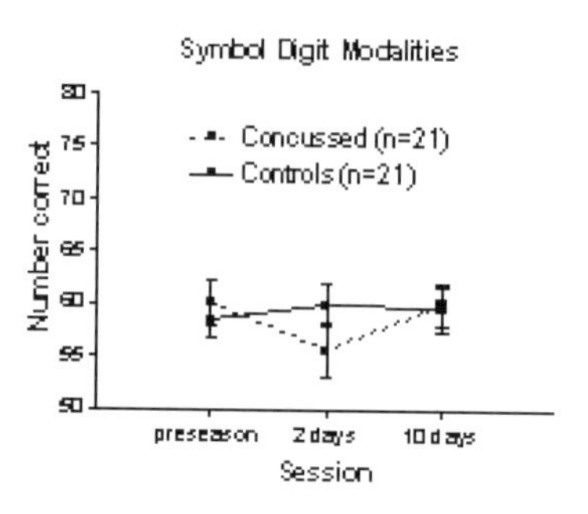

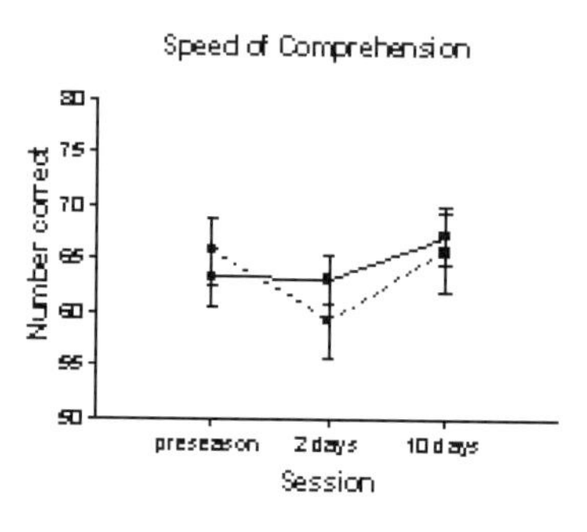

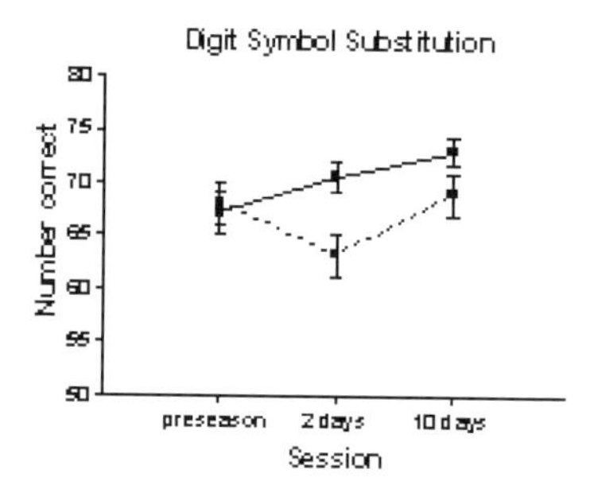

Figure 10.1. Serial retesting of concussed and control players on sensitive neuropsychological tests.

Measuring Significant Variations in Individual Cases

In a growing number of applied psychology settings where pre versus post comparison of measurement is required, normative data for change scores is gaining popularity. The first documented application of the Reliable Change Index (RCI) in neuropsychology was in a study of cognitive performance pre versus post epilepsy surgery (Chelune et al., 1993). The RCI takes into account measurement error in determining the probability and thus significance of a given change score (Jacobson & Truax, 1991). Chelune and colleagues (1993) adjusted the RCI for practice (RCI-P) by calculating the difference between Time 1 and Time 2 performance, adding the mean change observed in controls, and dividing by the standard error of the difference between scores. In this way confidence intervals may be constructed to determine probability of a change score centred on the participant's score adjusted for practice. Scores that exceed ± 1.645 represent a significant improvement or deterioration in performance, based on 90% confidence intervals. It is noteworthy that this is not the only means of determining reliable change. There is still conjecture over the most appropriate formulae to employ (see Erlanger, Feldman, & Barth, 2001; Temkin et al., 1999), though the difference between results yielded by most approaches appear to have trivial clinical significance.

Our preliminary results of the 21 concussed players analysed above (Hinton-Bayre, Geffen, Geffen et al., 1999) indicated that 18 players (85%) demonstrated 'significantly' impaired performance on at least one of the three tests (Digit Symbol, Symbol Digit, & Speed of Comprehension) when first reassessed 2 days following trauma. At 10 days following trauma 10 concussed players (48%) were still significantly impaired on at least one test. Group based data had suggested return to preseason performance on average by 10 days, when almost half of the players were still markedly below the desired level. It must be noted however, that the RCI-P was able to correct for ongoing practice effects, for example from Time 2 to Time 3, Time 3 to Time 4 an so on, as was donc in this work. The hit-rate for any individual measure was less impressive (see Table 10.3), with no test identifying more than 57% of players as impaired 2 days post-trauma. Table 10.3 presents the number of concussed and control players demonstrating significant change based on RCI-P scores from both preseason to 2 days post trauma, and preseason to 10 days post-trauma. It was also noted that reliability coefficients were greater between Time 2 and 3 (r = .91-.94), than Time 1 and 2 (r = .62-.82). This result was interpreted as suggesting that repeated testing reduces measurement error, making a dual baseline approach a more powerful one when wanting to potentially identify small changes in performance following trauma. Players impaired at 10 days were followed up again at 1 month post trauma. At this time all concussed players demonstrated return to a practice-corrected pre-injury level, except one who subsequently relocated before further investigation could be conducted. This style of individual analysis highlights the potential loss of information when focus is given solely to group based data.

Symptom Reporting as a Measure of Impairment and Recovery

Thus far the present section has focussed on the effects of concussion on cognitive performance. Concussion is also known to precipitate a multitude of other signs and symptoms. This information is often used in the recogni-

Table 10.3. Number of players demonstrating significant change on tests from preseason to 2 days, and preseason to 10 days.

Test	Performance	Concussed n=21	Concussed (n=14)	Uninjured Controls n=21	Uninjured Controls (n=14)
Preseason – 2days					
Speed of Comprehension	Deteriorated	9	(7)	1	(1)
	Improved	2	(1)	0	(0)
Symbol Digit	Deteriorated	11	(8)	1	(0)
	Improved	1	(0)	1	(0)
Digit Symbol	Deteriorated	12	(9)	2	(2)
	Improved	0	(0)	1	(1)
Preseason – 10 days					
Speed of Comprehension	Deteriorated	8	(6)	1	(1)
	Improved	1	(0)	1	(0)
Symbol Digit	Deteriorated	1	(1)	1	(1)
	Improved	2	(1)	2	(1)
Digit Symbol	Deteriorated	3	(2)	1	(1)
	Improved	0	(0)	1	(1)

Note. Values presented in parentheses represent those players receiving two baseline preseason assessment sessions.

tion, diagnosis, and management of the injury both in and out of the sporting arena. In many instances concussion may immediately be presumed as players are slow to get up after the trauma or display some evidence of impaired coordination. However, in 23% of concussions recorded the traumatic incident was not witnessed by experienced qualified sports-trainers, and injuries went unnoticed until the players volunteered themselves from the field with symptomatic complaints (Hinton-Bayre, 2000). This reinforces the need for objective measures of mental function for on the field and on the sideline, including protocols for the management of suspected concussion.

Immediately following trauma the most common signs/symptoms were headache, amnesia, disequilibrium, visual disturbance, dizziness, nausea, feeling in a daze, and to a lesser extent, loss of consciousness. In most cases the concussed players experienced several of these symptoms. Furthermore, few players complained of ongoing symptoms (Hinton-Bayre, Geffen, Geffen et al., 1999). Often symptoms were reported to have resolved within the same day or early the next. This is despite findings that cognitive performance was impaired in several players for 10 days or more (Hinton-Bayre, Geffen, Geffen et al., 1999). Conversely, in the general mild TBI literature it is frequently suggested that concussion symptoms persist longer than impaired psychometric performance.

One possible interpretation is that somatic symptoms and disturbances to cognition following concussion may be dissociable. However, it is more likely that players are seeking to minimise symptoms in order to return to play sooner. In line with this interpretation, concussed players showed a sharp decline in overall reporting of symptom frequency and severity upon serial retesting. Control players reported a stable pattern of symptom reporting across time. Furthermore, at 10 days post trauma control players complained more frequently of symptoms such as fatigue, weakness, dizziness, and irritability. It is possible that concussed players only reported symptoms they believed were a result of concussion. Also it is possible that symptoms did indeed decline in concussed players as they had more restricted training and match exposure following trauma. The inclusion of an orthopaedic control group would help to resolve this issue, whilst helping to refine the specificity of changes in performance tests to concussion. Nonetheless there is a real potential for players, particularly professionals, to minimise symptoms in the days following trauma in order to return to play quickly. The role of the more objective performance measures cannot be overstated in the sporting context. The quality of the clinician-player relationship may also be important. A commitment to educating staff and players, as well as establishing rapport is essential to eliciting honest responses and best performance from players.

Validity of Concussion Severity Gradings

There are over 17 different guidelines published for the management of concussion in sport. The dilemma for the sports health professional is deciding which one to choose, particularly as many argue such guidelines are wholly reliant on opinion rather than scientific data (Johnston et al., 2001). We attempted to evaluate the three most popular of these guidelines, at least in terms of reported use (American Academy of Neurology, AAN, 1997; Cantu, 1986; Colorado Medical Society, 1991). All of these guidelines rely on establishing the severity of the presenting trauma in order to prescribe a period of abstinence from contact sport. Severity is regularly based on duration of immediate symptoms and the presence and duration of LOC or PTA.

When contrasting the proportions of concussed players demonstrating significant declines in performance, there was no apparent relationship between concussion severity grading for any of the management guidelines and recovery of cognitive performance (see Table 10.4) (Hinton-Bayre & Geffen, 2002). Moreover, players presenting with a mild concussion that may have been permitted to return to play went on to record significantly reduced performance. Conversely, in the few cases where a brief LOC occurred, psychometric deficits were not even present at 2 days post-trauma. While it is

Table 10.4. Number of concussed players demonstrating deteriorated performance according to concussion severity[a].

Grading System	Severity Grade	No. players $n = 21$	Time post trauma 2 days		10 days	
American Academy of Neurology (1997)						
	1	4	3	(75)	3	(75)
	2	13	12	(92)	7	(54)
	3	4	3	(75)	0	(0)
Robert C. Cantu (1986)						
	1	10	9	(90)	7	(70)
	2	11	9	(82)	3	(27)
	3	0	0	(0)	0	(0)
Colorado Medical Society (1991)						
	1	3	3	(100)	1	(33)
	2	14	12	(86)	9	(64)
	3	4	3	(75)	0	(0)

[a] Figures in parentheses represent the percentage of players impaired.

premature to make any strong statements about the implications of these results, the data suggest that regularly used indices of severity (viz. LOC & PTA) as referred to in current guidelines do not predict subsequent cognitive impairment and recovery. Arbitrary gradings of severity do not appear justified and empirically-derived classifications of severity are worthy of investigation.

Chronic and Cumulative Effects

It is a widely held belief that the effects of repeated brain trauma are cumulative. There is evidence suggesting that repeat trauma, concussive and sub-concussive, leads to persistent impairment in sports such as boxing (see Heilbronner in this book) and soccer (see Matser in this book). A recent retrospective study in American footballers also suggested a history of repeated concussion leads to poorer psychometric test performance, but only in those with a history of learning disorder (Collins et al., 1999).

We gathered a retrospective concussion history from 119 RL players. Where possible, reports were checked against available medical records. It was found that 88% of active RL players had a history of concussion during their career, with 60% reporting multiple concussions. When players were separated according to a history of zero, one or two+ concussions, no significant differences were seen between these three groups on the three tests found to be sensitive at the post-acute stage following trauma. Furthermore, no evidence of relatively impaired ability to benefit from practice was found when contrasting the same frequency of head injury categories in a sub-group of 71 players who completed two assessments 1-2 weeks apart. Further analysis was conducted, as simply accounting for number of concussions may not sufficiently account for performance variations. We considered that severity and recency of trauma may also contribute to deficits. Yet, hierarchical multiple regression analyses incorporating data on the severity, recency and number of concussions failed to predict psychometric test performance, after demographic variables were entered.

It was also considered that a history of concussion, at least in active players, may serve to prolong recovery following a repeat concussion. Evidence of delayed, but seemingly complete recovery, from repeat concussion was reported by Gronwall and Wrightson (1975). Interestingly, no attempt has been made to replicate this finding. The 21 concussed players assessed prospectively were reanalysed to determine whether a more classically 'significant' history of trauma led to relatively delayed recovery. Given the small number of players involved, data were analysed separately according to a history of more severe (LOC versus no LOC), more recent (last season versus over two seasons ago), and more frequent (1 previous versus 2+). There was no evidence of differential recovery in any of the comparisons. The results obtained suggested that concussion, at least in active RL players, does not result in long - term impairment even in the case of a history of repeated trauma.

Unfortunately, given the numbers involved in the study we were not able to investigate the interactive effects of severity, recency and number of previous concussions. Furthermore, to effectively undertake a prospective assessment of repeated concussion requires an extremely large sample to even attempt meaningful analyses. In the 43 concussions recorded from following around 100 players per season over three years only six repeat incidents were recorded. This will no doubt be an underestimate as many players change clubs over competitive seasons. This factor alone markedly affects the efficiency of running a longitudinal prospective study of concussion at the professional level. Clearly, more research on the potential of cumulative effects is required. In particular, the potential association between concussion and other co-morbid factors would be of interest, as was observed with learning disorder in American footballers (Collins et al., 1999).

Conclusions

There is little doubt that sports neuropsychology has grown rapidly over the past 15 years. Neuropsychological assessment has demonstrated a role in the diagnosis and management of concussion in sport, particularly high-risk contact sports. The present chapter sought to summarize the extent of neuropsychological practice and research in the sports of AFL and RL in Australia. In re-iterating the major findings generated by the studies reviewed, relevant contrasts will be made with the existent work in other high-risk sports, many of which are covered in this book.

Prospective and retrospective data have shown that concussions occur frequently in AFL and RL. These two sports have been the focus of Sports Neuropsychology in Australia as they represent the sports with the highest absolute and relative incidence rates of concussion respectively. The majority of 'active' professional players have a history of concussion and many of these players report multiple incidents. While there are several studies reporting the incidence rates of concussion, there are comparatively little data on the immediate and ongoing effects of such injuries. Furthermore, an evidence-based approach to the management of concussion has barely begun. The research for AFL and RL was presented separately to provide the reader with a perspective of the different foci of various research groups involved in the study of contact sport concussion. However, data from both codes are considered together in summarising evidence. There is insufficient evidence to consider that concussions sustained in one football code should be qualitatively different from those in another, particularly as the mechanisms of injury are likely to be similar. As such, the main findings from the chapter are discussed in terms of neuropsychological assessment in sport and implications for management.

One of the most concerning aspects of the RL study conducted is that a considerable number of concussions were not recognized by training staff. These players only manifested cognitive disturbances or other non-observable symptoms (eg. headache). Given that players may minimize symptoms, the use of more objective performance measures seems pertinent. Studies with concussed AFL players indicated that measures of recent memory were most sensitive to cognitive disturbance immediately (within minutes) following concussion. Measures of orientation did not distinguish concussed players from controls. Furthermore, performance on the Digit Symbol test appears to be impaired in concussed players relative to their preseason performance within minutes of injury. Thus, it appears that there is a number of measures available to assist in the identification of concussion, including the Standardized Assessment of Concussion (SAC) developed with American footballers (McCrea, 2001). Ongoing work is underway to standardize the use of such measures in an applied setting.

Similar to prospective studies in American football, both AFL and RL concussion research has suggested that the majority of such injuries present with brief periods of amnesia or confusion, with incidents involving a loss of consciousness occurring infrequently. Furthermore, performance on standard psychometric measures suggest that recovery on average will occur within 5-10 days of concussion, consistent also with American football findings. Our research has indicated that measures of speed of information processing appear to be the most sensitive to the effects of concussion. The interpretation that a deficit in speed of information processing is a hallmark of closed head injury involving acceleration/deceleration forces is consistent with several studies of mild TBI in the general population (Binder et al., 1997). However, we would recommend the use of such tests as a screen, and only in cases where more detailed assessment is not possible. An attempt was made to validate popular concussion management guidelines without success. The presence and duration of amnesia/unconsciousness did not appear to be related to recovery from concussion as measured by sensitive psychometric tests (Hinton-Bayre & Geffen, 2002). It may be that in the case of mild TBI, brief periods of mental status aberration are not related to later cognitive function. More work is required in this area to assist in the development of scientifically supported management strategies and to better understand the nature of mild brain trauma in general.

Most prospective studies of concussion take one preseason index of test performance, as opposed to two preseason sessions in the RL work. Our data suggest that not only will a dual preseason exposure to tests increase the hit-rate for deficit, but players will also demonstrate longer recovery periods. Many studies suffer from inadequate attempts to control for practice effects, which are of particular importance when using repeat sessions with brief retest intervals. Furthermore, the use of clinical change scores, such as the RCI-P, permit estimates of individual variations in performance. Use of such a technique in the RL study indicated that while recovery for players on average returned to a practiced preseason level at 10 days post trauma, almost half of the players demonstrated continued impairment up until 1 month post trauma. The sensitivity of measures appears to be somewhat dependent on the methodology employed, not just the type of measure.

Perhaps the most controversial area surrounding concussion is the potential effect of repeated trauma leading to longer-term difficulties as seen in some boxing and soccer studies. No AFL or RL study to date has found strong evidence for chronic or cumulative effects from concussion resulting in those sports, though prospective data are lacking. Despite taking into account not only the number of previous injuries, but also the severity and recency of such injuries, no long-term effects were reported or demonstrated on performance measures. However, the synergistic relationship between repeated trauma and other factors such as learning disorder, genetic vulnerability, or even advancing age were not accounted for. Obviously, more detailed prospective studies are required.

To summarize, sports neuropsychology continues to develop in Australia. Much of the work completed complements studies performed on American footballers in the US. However, there is still considerable work to be done to ensure that the most sensitive measures are being used in a reliable and valid manner. Furthermore, the effects of concussion in contact sport from the immediate symptoms to the potential chronic difficulties, requires more detailed collaborative research. There are several sports with a high-risk of concussion inherent and there are also several models of assessment present in the literature. A more coordinated approach to research would be of enormous benefit to the development of knowledge concerning the injury and the effective implementation of neuropsychological assessment in the management of concussion.

References

Alexander, M.P. (1995). Mild traumatic brain injury: Pathophysiology, natural history, and clinical management. *Neurology, 45*, 1253–1260.

American Academy of Neurology (AAN), Quality Standards Subcommittee. (1997). Practice parameter: The management of concussion in sports (summary statement). *Neurology, 48*, 581–585.

Barth, J.T., Alves, W.M., Ryan, T.V., Macciocchi, S.N., Rimel, R.W., Jane, J.A., & Nelson, W.E. (1989). Mild head injury in sports: Neuropsychological sequelae and recovery of function. In H.S. Levin, H.M. Eisenberg & A.L. Benton (Eds.), *Mild Head Injury* (pp. 257–275). New York: Oxford University Press.

Bazarian, J.J., Wong, T., Harris, M., Leahy, N., Mookerjee, S., & Dombovy, M. (1999). Epidemiology and predictors of post-concussive syndrome after minor head injury in an emergrency population. *Brain Injury, 13*, 173–189.

Binder, L.M., Rohling, M.L., & Larrabee, G.J. (1997). A review of mild head trauma. Part I: Meta-analytic review of neuropsychological studies. *Journal of Clinical and Experimental Neuropsychology, 19*, 421–431.

Brooks, D.N. (1987). Measuring neuropsychological and functional recovery. In H.S. Levin, J. Grafman, & H. M. Eisenberg (Eds.), *Neurobehavioral recovery from head injury* (pp. 57–72). Oxford, Oxford University Press.

Brooks, J., Fos, L.A., Greve, K.W., & Hammond, J.S. (1999). Assessment of executive function in patients with mild traumatic brain injury. *The Journal of Trauma: Injury, Infection, and Critical Care, 46*, 159–163.

Cantu, R.C. (1986). Guidelines for return to contact sports after a cerebral concussion. *Physician and Sportsmedicine, 14*, 10.

Cantu, R.C. (1998). Second impact syndrome. *Clinics in Sports Medicine, 17*, 37–44.

Chelune, G.J., Naugle, R.I., Luders, H., Sedlak, J., & Awad, I.A. (1993). Individual change after epilepsy surgery: Practice effects and base-rate information. *Neuropsychology, 7*, 41–52.

Collie, A., Darby, D., & Maruff, P. (2001). Computerised assessment of athletes with sports related head injury. *British Journal of Sports Medicine, 35*, 297-302.

Collins, M.W., Grindel, S.H., Lovell, M.R., Dede, D.E., Moser, D.J., Phalin, B.R. et al. (1999). Relationship between concussion and neuropsychological performance in college football players. *Journal of the American Medical Association, 282*, 964–970.

Colorado Medical Society. (1991). *Report of the Sports Medicine Committee: Guidelines for the Management of Concussion in Sports.* (Vol. Revised). Denver: Colorado Medical Society.

Crawford, J.R., Parker, D.M., & McKinlay, W.W. (1992). *A handbook of neuropsychological assessment.* Hove, U.K.: Lawrence Erlbaum.

Cremona-Meteyard, S.L., & Geffen, G.M. (1994). Persistent visuospatial attention deficits following mild head injury in Australian Rules Football players. *Neuropsychologia, 32*, 649–662.

Dicker, G. (1989). Concussion management. Paper presented at the *Grand Final Symposium*, Melbourne, Australia.

Dicker, G., & Maddocks, D. (1988). An objective measure of recovery from concussion in Australian Rules footballers. *The Australian Journal of Science and Medicine in Sport, December*, 17.

Epidemiology and Health Information Branch. (1993). *Injuries (with particular reference to head injuries)* (Information Circular No. 19E). Brisbane: Queensland Health.

Erlanger, D., Feldman, D.J., & Barth, J.T. (2001). Statistical techniques for interpreting post-concussion neuropsychological tests. *British Journal of Sports Medicine, 35*, 370–371.

Grindell, S.H., Lovell, M.R., & Collins, M.W. (2001). The assessment of sport-related concussion: the evidence behind neuropsychological testing and management. *Clinical Journal of Sport Medicine, 11*, 134–143.

Gronwall, D., & Wrightson, P. (1975). Cumulative effect of concussion. *Lancet, 2*, 995–997.

Hinton-Bayre, A.D. (2000). Psychometric assessment and the management of concussion in contact sport. *Unpublished doctoral thesis*. University of Queensland, Australia.

Hinton-Bayre, A.D., Geffen, G.M., & McFarland, K.A. (1997). Mild head injury and speed of information processing: A prospective study of professional rugby league players. *Journal of Clinical and Experimental Neuropsychology, 19*, 275–289.

Hinton-Bayre, A.D., Geffen, G.M., Geffen, L.B., McFarland, K., & Friis, P. (1999). Concussion in contact sports: Reliable change indices of impairment and recovery. *Journal of Clinical and Experimental Neuropsychology, 21*, 70–86.

Hinton-Bayre, A.D., Geffen, G.M., & McFarland, K.A. (1999). Sensitivity of neuropsychological tests to the acute effects of concussion in contact sport. In B. Murdoch, D. Theodoros, & E. Ward (Eds.), *Brain Impairment and Rehabilitation: A National Perspective* (pp. 75–81). Brisbane: Academic Press.

Hinton-Bayre, A. D. & Geffen, G. (2002). Severity of sports-related concussion and neuropsychological test performance. *Neurology, 59*, 1068-1070.

Hovda, D.A., Prins, M., Becker, D.P., Lee, S., Bergsneider, M., & Martin, N. (1999). Neurobiology of concussion. In J.E. Bailes, M.R. Lovell, & J.C. Maroon (Eds.), *Sports-related concussion* (pp. 12–51). St Louis, MO: Quality Medical Publishing.

Jacobson, N.S., & Truax, P. (1991). Clinical significance: A statistical approach to defining meaningful change in psychotherapy research. *Journal of Consulting and Clinical Psychology, 59*, 12–19.

Johnston, K.M., McCrory, P.R., Mohtadi, N.G., & Meeuwisse, W. (2001). Evidence-based review of sport-related concussion: clinical science. *Clinical Journal of Sports Medicine, 11*, 150–159.

Lezak, M.D. (1995). *Neuropsychological Assessment* (3rd ed.). Oxford: Oxford University Press.

Lovell, M.R., & Collins, M.W. (1998). Neuropsychological assessment of the college football player. *Journal of Head Trauma Rehabilitation, 13*, 9–26.

Macciocchi, S.N., Barth, J.T., Alves, W., Rimel, R.W., & Jane, J.A. (1996). Neuropsychological functioning and recovery after mild head injury in collegiate athletes. *Neurosurgery, 39*, 510–514.

Maddocks, D., Dicker, G., & Saling, M. (1995). The assessment of orientation following concussion in athletes. *Clinical Journal of Sports Medicine, 5*, 32–35.

Maddocks, D., Saling, M., & Dicker, G. (1995). A note on normative data for a test sensitive to concussion in Australian Rules footballers. *Australian Psychologist, 30*, 125–127.

Maddocks, D., & Saling, M. (1996). Neuropsychological deficits following concussion. *Brain Injury, 10*, 99–103.

Makdissi, M., Collie, A., Maruff, P., Darby, D.G., Bush, A., McCrory, P. et al. (2001). Computerised cognitive assessment of concussed Australian Rules footballers. *British Journal of Sports Medicine, 35*, 354–60.

Matser, E.J.T., Kessels, A.G., Jordan, B.D., Lezak, M.D., & Troost, J. (1998). Chronic traumatic brain injury in professional soccer players. *Neurology, 51*, 791–796.

Matser, E.J.T., Kessels, A.G., Lezak, M.D., Jordan, B.D., & Troost, J. (1999). Neuropsychological impairment in amateur soccer players. *Journal of the American Medical Association, 282*, 971–973.

McCrea, M. (2001). Standardized mental status assessment of sports concussion. *Clinical Journal of Sport Medicine, 11*, 176–181.

McCrory, P. (1989). Concussion background/Acute management. Paper presented at the *Grand Final Symposium*, Melbourne, Australia.

McCrory, P.R., Bladin, P.F., & Berkovic, S.F. (1997). Retrospective study of concussive convulsions in elite Australian rules and rugby league footballers: phenomenology, aetiology, and outcome. *British Medical Journal, 314*, 171–174.

McCrory, P.R., Johnston, K.M., Mohtadi, N.G., & Meeuwisse, W. (2001). Evidence-based review of sport-related concussion: basic science. *Clinical Journal of Sports Medicine, 11*, 160–165.

McCrory, P., & Maddocks, D. (1994). Memory disturbance after concussive brain injury. Paper presented at the *International Conference of Science and Medicine in Sport*, Brisbane, Australia.

McIntosh, A.S., McCrory, P., & Comerford, J. (1999). Biomechanics of head injures in Australian Rules football. *Journal of Science and Medicine in Sport, 2 (Suppl.)*, 56 [Abstract].

National Health and Medical Research Council. (1994). *Football injuries of the head and neck*. Canberra: Australian Government Publishing Service.

Orchard, J., Wood, T., Seward, H., & Broad, A. (1998). Comparison of injuries in elite senior and junior Australian Football. *Journal of Science and Medicine in Sport, 1*, 82–88.

Queensland Injury Surveillance Unit. (2000). Sports injuries. *Injury Bulletin, 59*, 1–6.

Seward, H., Orchard, J., Hazard, H., & Collinson, D. (1993). Football injuries in Australia at the elite level. *The Medical Journal of Australia, 159*, 298–301.

Shuttleworth-Jordan, A.B., Balarin, E., & Puchert, J. (1993). Mild head injury effects in rugby: Is playing the game really worth the cost? *Journal of Clinical and Experimental Neuropsychology, 15*, 403.

Sosin, D.M., Sniezek, J.E., & Thurman, D.J. (1996). Incidence of mild and moderate brain injury in the United States, 1991. *Brain Injury, 10*, 47–54.

Spreen, O., & Strauss, E. (1998). *A Compendium of Neuropsychological Tests* (2nd ed.). New York: Oxford University Press.

Stablum, F., Mogentale, C., & Umilta, C. (1996). Executive functioning following mild closed head injury. *Cortex, 32*, 261–278.

Temkin, N.R., Heaton, R.K., Grant, I., & Dikmen, S. S. (1999). Detecting significant change in neuropscyhological test performance: A comparison of four models. *Journal of the International Neuropsychological Society, 5*, 357–369.

Yarnell, P., & Lynch, S. (1973). The 'ding' amnestic state in football trauma. *Neurology, 23*, 196–197.

Chapter 11

SOCCER

Erik J.T. Matser
Neuroscience Centre, Erasmus University Rotterdam, The Netherlands

Fons A.G.H. Kessels
Research Unit Patient Care, University Hospital of Maastricht, The Netherlands

Mark R. Lovell
Sports Medicine Concussion Program, The University of Pittsburgh Medical Center

Introduction

Mild traumatic brain injury (concussion) is common in soccer and can occur for a variety of reasons. In recent years, the potential for brain injury in soccer players has captured news headlines and has created much controversy internationally. Recently, an apparent case of second impact syndrome (SIS) in a junior soccer player shocked the Dutch soccer community. In the United States, there has also been a growing interest in the potential for brain injury in soccer players that has resulted in increased scientific study and public inquiry. In fact, a recent national scientific committee have been established to more formally study the potential for concussive brain injury (IOM, 2001). Within the public sector, the issue of concussions in soccer has also been a prominent one and has resulted in some communities banning heading of the ball in recreational youth soccer athletes (NY Times, 2001).

The study of concussions in soccer in an important one. Soccer is easily the most popular sport in the world and is played by over 250 million people, including large numbers of children of both sexes. Given the immense popularity of the sport internationally, it is somewhat surprising that of scientific knowledge regarding the potential risks of brain injury is based on only a handful of published studies. However, interest in this area is rapidly expanding and it is likely that research conducted over the next five years will likely have a determining influence on the direction of medical management of concussion for decades to come.

This chapter will review existing research regarding the prevalence and potential for both short-term and long-term neurocognitive consequences of concussions in soccer. In addition, this chapter will also suggest new methods of scientific inquiry that may change the course of research in the near future. Finally, the new concussion management recommended by the Federation Internationale de Football Association (FIFA) will be reviewed and possible injury prevention strategies will be discussed.

Epidemiology of Concussions in Soccer

The exact incidence of traumatic brain injury related to sports in general can only be estimated at the current time. World-wide estimates of the incidence of concussion of all causes range from 152 to 430 cases per 100.000 population per year (Jennett & Macmillan, 1981). The percentage of brain injuries related to sports ranges from 3% to 25%. Based on these figures, the rates of sports-related brain injuries could theoretically range from 5 to 68 cases with a median value of 42 per 100.000 person years (Kraus, 1991). Other studies show that, of all traumatic brain injuries, 10% to 22% are treated in hospitals and it is estimated that 11% of all hospital treated TBI in children and adolescents are sports related (Lehman, 1987; Frenquelli, Ruscito, Sicciolo, Rizzo, & Massarelli, 1991; Hansen, Pless and Blavvers, 1991). Studies designed to identify all individuals who seek medical attention after TBI report that only 16% to 20% are admitted suggesting significantly higher incidence rates than those cited above (Fife, 1987). Unlike sports such as American football, both male and female participants enjoy soccer and studies have suggested comparable rates of concussion in both sexes at the high school level (Powell & Barber-Foss, 1999). Furthermore, National Collegiate Athletic Association (NCAA) statistics reported an incidence for concussion of .14 per 1,000 athletic exposures for males and .15 per 1,000 for females.

Although soccer is considered to be safe by the general public compared to sports such as American football and Ice Hockey, the American Academy of Pediatrics has recently classified soccer as a contact/collision sport (American Academy of Pediatrics, 1998). Although rare, fatal neurologic injuries in soccer have also been reported. During the period 1931 to 1976, 26 fatal traumatic brain injuries were attributed to English soccer players, including 8 that were attributed to heading the ball (Hughes, 1974). In the United States, from 1979 to 1993, 18 fatal accidents were reported from players running into goalposts (Demarco & Reeves, 1994). Another four fatal accidents in high school soccer have also been documented between 1980 and 1988 (Mueller & Cantu, 1990). Furthermore, widespread media attention has lead to increasing public awareness of the potential risks of soccer.

Potential Causes of Brain Injury in Soccer

Concussions in soccer may have several potential causes. One of the most common causes of injury is the contact of the head with other body parts. More specifically, head to head, head to other body part (e.g. elbow or knee) and head to ground contact occur relatively frequently in soccer and have acknowledged by most researchers as being contributing factors with regard to concussion.

The formal study of concussion in soccer athletes has a relatively recent history. Initial studies of concussion in soccer athletes were conducted in Scandinavia. In Norway, Tysvaer provided much of the early documentation of the consequences of concussion in soccer athletes. He documented that 33% of retired amateur soccer players showed brain ventricular dilation and a high percentage (81%) of these players demonstrated memory impairment compared to age matched controls. In additional research, Tysvaer further demonstrated that 36 out of 128 former amateur soccer players complained of permanent neurologic symptoms such as headaches, neck pain and dizziness (Tysvaer & Lochen, 1991; Sortland & Tysvaer, 1989; Tysvaer, Storli & Bachen, 1989; Tysvaer & Storli, 1981). Although these early studies served to heighten awareness within the medical community at the time, there relevance to the current concussion literature has been questioned for several reasons. First, these documented neurological decline in athletes who played with a heavier leather ball whose weight significantly increased when matches were played in wet conditions. Second, these were retrospective studies and the exact mechanism of injury in these athletes was unclear.

More recently, Matser and his colleagues have published findings that suggesting neuropsychological deficits in Dutch soccer athletes (Matser, Kessels, Lezak & Troost, 1998). In studying 53 elite professional soccer players, 54% experienced one or more grade 3 concussions during their professional careers. In addition, 79% percent of the players reported head to head collisions, which could be classified as grade 1 and grade 2 concussions (mental alterations with no LOC). The median number of soccer matches played annually was 50 (range 25–70) and the median of the number of practices per week was six (range 4–9). Compared to control objects (elite middle distance runners and swimmers) the professionals performed poorer on verbal and visual memory, planning and visuoperceptual tasks. The differences remained significant after adjustments for confounding variables (the number of concussions not related to soccer, alcohol consumption, level of education and the number of general anaesthesias). These psychometric test scores also remained significant after a Bonferroni correction. An increasing number of headers and grade 3 concussions incurred during soccer participation were associated negatively with memory, visuoperceptual, and planning capacity. Field position also influenced performance on neuropsychological testing. Forward and defensive players performed significantly poorer on visuoperceptual and verbal- and visual memory tasks.

In a later study, 33 amateur soccer players were studied (Matser, Kessels, Lezak & Troost, 1999). Twenty-seven percent incurred one grade 3 concussions and 33% reported 2 to 5 grade 3 concussions in their soccer careers. The median number of balls headed in a match was 8.5 (range 0–20). Compared to control objects (middle distance runners and swimmers) amateur soccer players exhibited impairments in planning and memory. These scores remained statistically after Bonferroni correction and after adjustments for confounding variables (concussions unrelated to soccer, alcohol intake, level of education, and number of general anaesthesias). Concussions incurred in soccer were inversely correlated with performances on planning, attention and visual and verbal memory tasks.

The findings of the studies reviewed above suggest that the blows to the head incurred in soccer play may result in cognitive impairment, and that the kind of impairment players sustain can vary according to their position on the field. In the Dutch studies, concussions tended to compromise abilities for visual analysis and planning, and aspects of attention, but also appeared to affect both verbal and visual memory, possibly reflecting the diffuse nature of concussions. Although these patterns tend to characterize specific playing roles, the overall findings indicate that serious soccer players who engage in many hours of practice and play each year are likely to sustain cognitive deficits associable to the nature and frequency of the blows to the head.

Heading of the Soccer Ball: Neuropsychological Consequences?

Although few researchers would dispute the role of direct blows to the head as a causative agent in concussion, the specific role of heading the ball is a more controversial one. It has been suggested that the use of the head to direct the soccer ball may be analogous to the repetitive blows to the head in boxing (Rabadi & Jordan, 2001), producing a pattern of chronic traumatic brain injury or CTBI. The potential mechanism of injury is rapid shifting of brain tissue within the skull cavity, presumably resulting in changes in brain physiology that render the brain more vulnerable for a period of time after the first "injury" (see Chapter 4 by Giza and Hovda, in this volume). However, research in this area has only recently started to evolve. One particularly intriguing study has recently been published by Slemmer and his colleagues (Slemmer, Matser, De Zeeuw & Weber, 2002). This study, investigated the effects of single and repeated mild stretch forces in vitro, in cultured mouse hippocampal cells. After repeated injury, neurtites appeared beaded and damaged, a finding that was not observed following a single insult. In addition, nerone-specific enolase (NSE) levels were elevated after repeated insults. These results were consistent with an earlier study in human subjects that found that elevated NSE levels correlated with poor outcome (Hermann et al., 1999).

In addition to an emerging body of evidence form the animal literature, proponents of the role of heading in chronic traumatic brain injury (CTBI) have also cited the second impact literature as evidence that two of more mild blows to the head during this presumed period of increased vulnerability can result in dramatically increased intracranial pressure, infrequently resulting in death (Cantu, 1998). For instance, a junior player in the Netherlands died recently after being hit on the head (header) after being symptomatic from a previous blow to the head (player to player collision). Another cited source of support for the role of heading in the development of CTBI is the report that migraine headaches that are associated with heading of the ball (Matthews, 1972). However, as migraine headaches most often occur independently of brain injury, this line of evidence is currently unclear and deserves further study.

Biomechanical Aspects of Heading the Soccer Ball

It has been estimated that professional soccer players play approximately 300 division games and head the ball more than 2000 times during their career (Jordan, Green, Galanty, Mandelbaum, & Jabour, 1996, 1996; Tysvaer & Storli, 1981). Forward players and defenders typically headed the ball more often than midfield players. A recent Dutch study showed an average of 800 headers per team in 50 matches in a single professional soccer season (range 500–1300) (Matser et al., 1998). Current soccer balls weigh 396 to 453 g, and the speed of the ball can reach 60 to 120 km/h. It has been calculated that a ball kicked with half power from a distance of 10 m travels 83.2 km/h and hits the head with an impact of 116 kPa. Kicked with full power the ball hits the head with 200 kPa (Von Schneider et al., 1975). Moreover, traditional leather balls can increase in weight up to 20% when wet. However, this is not an issue with modern synthetic balls.

Neuropsychological Sequelae of heading the Ball. What is the current evidence?

The question of whether or not heading the soccer ball results in either acute or chronic changes in brain function has become one of the most hotly debated issues within sports medicine circles. At least part of the reason for this controversy has been the lack of conclusive research regarding that clearly establishes a link between heading and brain injury. In particular, there has been a shortage of prospective research designed to separate the effects of heading from concussive effects due to other types of insult that occur within the context of a soccer match (e.g. collision of heads, etc.). The following represents a review of the few studies that attempted to address this issue.

Evidence supporting the role of headers

In an article that sparked significant international debate, Matser et al. (1998) studied eighty-four active elite professional soccer players from several professional premier league soccer club in the Netherlands. Although baseline testing was not undertaken, each athlete underwent extensive neuropsychological evaluation. The number of headers in one professional season and the number of soccer related concussions was investigated concerning cognitive functioning. Cognitive tests were administered post-injury that measured abstract reasoning, planning, memory, attention, mental speed, fluency and visuo-perception. The studied cohort consisted of forward players (26%), midfield players (40%), defense players (32%) and 2% of the players were goalkeepers. The players headed the ball 500 times an average in one single season (range 70–1260), an average of 10 headers in a single match. Forward and defense players headed the ball more often than midfield players. The neuropsychological test scores were adjusted for age, level of education, alcohol intake, the number of general anaesthesias and the number of concussions not sustained in soccer. In addition, 85% of the professionals interviewed complained of (sub)concussive symptoms such as headaches, dizziness, visual disturbances and/or feeling lightheaded after heading drills and headers of soccer balls who were kicked with full force (goalkeeper kicks, or corner/free kicks). On the contrary, a study in USA high school soccer players showed no relation between the number of headers and cognitive impairments (Kirkendall, Jordan & Garrett, 2001). One possible explanation is the level of play of the studied participants in the Dutch and American cohorts, with professional level players experiencing difficulties as a result of the increased velocity of the ball at impact and the more frequent heading of the ball. In addition, another Dutch study showed that the cognitive impairments found in amateur soccer players were mainly caused by the number of soccer related concussions and not the number of headers (Matser et al., 1999). Because the amount of headers is presumably much higher in the professionals than in the amateur players, the neurologic problems caused by headers could be a problem that becomes evident more in professional rather than amateur soccer players.

More recently, Downs and Abwender (2002) compared neuropsychological test performance between a group of 32 soccer athletes and 29 swimmers. They hypothesized that the soccer group would perform more poorly on testing than the swimmers due to an increased risk of head injury in this group. Soccer athletes were reported to have performed more poorly on 6 of 11 neuropsychological measures after controlling for the effects of age. However, this study did not specifically examine the role of headers and therefore contributes little to our understanding of the role of heading the ball. Furthermore, since no baseline testing data is reported, it is uncertain whether other factors may have accounted for differences between the two groups.

Evidence that does not support the role of headers

In one of the early studies designed to evaluate the potential role of heading the soccer ball in mild traumatic brain injury, Jordan et al. (1996) compared 20 members of the United States Men's National Team were compared to the 20 elite male track atheltes. Symptoms of concussion were related to concussions received while playing soccer but not to number of years of participation in the sport or to number of times that the athlete headed the ball.

In a later prospective study designed to help separate the effect of heading from other potential causes of concussion, Petukian, Echemendia and Macklin (2000) conducted a a pilot study with the Penn State men's and women's soccer team. The study employed a cross-over design where each team received neuropsychological testing prior to and following a planned heading drills. One half of the participants engaged in the heading practice on day one and the other half engaged in a non heading practice designed to elicit the same level of physical activity. In the following practice two days later the groups were switched allowing for each player to serve as his or her own control. The preliminary data following a single season did not indicate any decline in neuropsychological test scores between those athletes who headed the ball frequently and those who did not. In fact, subjects actually performed better on some of the tests following the heading drills, suggesting "practice effects for repeated exposure to the tests. This may have obscured small changes in test performance.

In another study that failed to support the role of heading in brain injury, Guskiewicz (2002) and his collageues did not demonstrate any difference on neuropsycological testing of 91 soccer atheltes, compared to 96 non-soccer atheltes (women's field hockey, women's lacrosse, male baseball players and 53 non-athlete control subjects. In addition, there was no significant relationship between history of soccer-related concussion and either scholastic aptitude or neuropsychological functioning. Soccer athletes had an average of 15.3 season of participation as well as a higher incidence of prior concussions and exposure to heading the ball but falied to demonstrate any difference on a modified Pittsburgh Steelers Test Battery, completed at the beginning of their Freshman or Sophomore year of college.

As highlighted by our review of the literature, the issue of whether or not heading of the soccer ball results in acute or chronic brain injury has yet to conclusively been put to rest. To date, most of the evidence to support the role of heading the ball as a contributor to brain injury is based on retrospective analysis of athletes who have neurocognitive sequelae following participation in the sport. Prospective studies are currently in progress and will hopefully provide more definitive information regarding this important issue.

New Management Guidelines for Minimizing the Effects of Concussion in Soccer Athletes

Concussions in soccer, which soccer players may refer to as 'dings', 'having your bell rung' and 'seeing stars' have received increasing attention due to concerns about longer-term effects. Most concussions cause a temporary disruption in mental functioning and most concussion symptoms seen in amateur and professional soccer players fade within a week or two (see Table 11.1).

Kelly and Rosenberg (27) define concussion as a trauma induced alteration in mental status that may or may not involve loss of consciousness. Some frequently observed features of concussion are vacant stare, inability to focus attention, disorientation, incoordination, emotional lability, memory deficits, slowed reaction time, slowed mental- and motor speed, problems with planning and judgement, and difficulties in processing novel or complex visual spatial stimuli. According to AAN norms (1997) (28) concussions are graded in three categories:

Grade 1 concussion: Transient confusion, no LOC (loss of consciousness) and a duration of mental status abnormalities of < 15 minutes.

Grade 2 concussion: Transient confusion, no LOC and a duration of mental status abnormalities of > 15 minutes

Grade 3 concussion: LOC, either brief (seconds) or prolonged (till 15 minutes)

Contusion: LOC > 15 minutes.

However, in Europe the AAN notation for concussion is not in use, for example in the Netherlands only a concussion grade three is classified by neurologists and general practicioners as a 'concussion' or 'commotio cerebri'. The use of different classification systems for MTBI causes confusion and it is preferable that the AAN 1997 grading system for concussion will be in use on a mondial level. In addition, when presenting our studies in the USA we've had to explain that the concussions documented in our studies were all concussions grade 3.

Our interest in soccer related concussions started after we've studied amateur boxers before and after a boxing match (29). The median number of head punches sustained during an amateur match was 8 (range 0–31). Sixty-five percent of the boxers received 10 or fewer head punches and 35% of the boxers incurred more than 10 head punches in a match. Thirteen percent of the fights ended in a knock out or referee stops contest. In this inception cohort study there was an inverse correlation between weight and the number of head punches regarding cognitive performance. The cognitive impairments involved planning, memory and attention problems. Moreover, Knock Outs (grade 3 concussions) were significant predictors for planning and memory impairments in the amateur boxers. The findings in this study made us curious about the association between head/brain injuries in soccer, the most popular sport in the world.

In studying 7 professional premier league soccer teams in the Netherlands 2 out of 11 players incurred grade 3 concussions during one single season (season 1999–2000). Most of the concussed players were forward and defense players and head to head collisions were the main cause of inflicting concussion, another common cause of concussion was head to body contact (players running into each other, players kicked to the head) and some players were concussed by balls to the head delivered from free kicks. Although most players seem to recover quickly from concussion, 33% of the amateur soccer players who sustained a soccer related concussion still encounter chronic cognitive problems (26).

In studying 53 elite professional soccer players (22), 54% experienced one or more grade 3 concussions during their professional careers. In addition, 79% percent of the players reported head to head collisions which could be classified as grade 1 and grade 2 concussions (mental alterations with no LOC). The players reported a median of 800 headers (range 50 to 2100) during competitive matches in one soccer season (an average of 16 headers in a single match). Moreover, the median of the number of soccer matches played annually was 50 (range 25 to 70) and the median of the number of practices per week was six (range 4–9). Compared to control objects (elite middle distance runners and swimmers) the professionals performed poorer on verbal and visual memory, planning and visuoperceptual tasks. The differences remained significant after adjustments for confounding variables (the number of concussions not related to soccer, alcohol consumption, level of education and the number of general anaesthesias). These psychometric test scores also remained significant after a Bonferroni correction. An increasing number of headers and grade 3 concussions incurred during soccer participation were associated negatively with memory, visuoperceptual, and planning capacity. Field position also influenced performance on neuropsychological testing. Forward and defensive players performed significantly poorer on visuoperceptual and verbal- and visual memory tasks. Forward and defensive players headed the ball more often and experienced a higher frequency of soccer related concussion.

In studying 33 amateur soccer players (26), 27% incurred one grade 3 concussion and 33% reported 2 to 5 grade 3 concussions in their soccer careers. The median number of balls headed in a match was 8.5 (range 0–20). Compared to control objects (middle distance runners and swimmers) amateur soccer players exhibited impairments in planning and memory. These scores remained statistically after Bonferroni correction and after adjustments for confounding variables (concussions unrelated to soccer, alcohol intake, level of education, and number of general anaesthesias). Concussions incurred in soccer were inversely correlated with performances on planning, attention and visual and verbal memory tasks.

Study Synthesis

The findings of the studies presented above indicate that the blows to the head incurred in soccer play may result in cognitive impairment, and that the kind of impairment players sustain can vary according to their position on the field. The patterns peculiar to each type injury appeared with a fair degree of consistency in each study. Thus, players who do the most headers display more problems with both visual and verbal memory, and may suffer deficits in visual analysis and planning, and slowing on tasks requiring focussed attention and visual scanning. Concussions tend to compromise abilities for visual analysis and planning, and aspects of attention, but may also involve both verbal and visual memory reflecting the diffuse nature of concussions. Although these patterns tend to characterize specific playing roles, the overall findings indicate that serious soccer players who engage in many hours of practice and play each year are likely to sustain cognitive deficits associable to the nature and frequency of the blows to their heads receive.

Soccer related concussions and aging:
Although it can be difficult for young athletes to imagine growing old, one of the most significant demographic factors all over the world over the past centuries has been the steady growth in life expectancy at birth. When premature death is prevented and longevity is increased, the question of the quality of life during the remaining life years is an important one.

In one aspect, aging had become almost synonymous with cognitive impairment. However, as the collision sport studies show, cognitive impairment is not exclusively a disease of the elderly. It can occur at any age especially when one considers MCI due to (cumulations of) traumatic brain injurie at young age. Mild Cognitive Impairment (MCI) has been defined as a clinical entity. Persons with MCI have memory impairments beyond what would be expected for age. These persons have relatively normal general cognitive function and activities of daily living. When compared to age and education-matched normal persons, measures of learning are significantly impaired. There are several definitions for MCI with small differences in symptomatology. According to Zaudig, 1992 two types of MCI are described (30):

Type 1: (A) memory impairment alone (STM and LTM memory)

Type 2: (A) memory impairment + (B) deficit in at least one other higher cortical function, but not interfering significantly with daily living (ADL).

According to the MCI classification of Zaudig 1992, the professional soccer players with intense careers, who sustained multiple concussions and who headed the ball often suffer from type 2 MCI. This may be of importance in later life because it is known from aging studies that subjects over 60 years with MCI develop dementia at a rate of 10-15% per year, in contrast with age-matched controls subjects, who develop dementia at a rate of 1-2% per year (30). In addition, persons who sustained TBI were found to express Alzheimer's disease a median of eight years younger than persons with no history of traumatic brain injury (31). However, the authors of the MCI studies underline that MCI is not necessarily developing in AD: some persons have MCI relatively static.

Future Directions

Concussions in soccer, have received increasing attention due to concerns about long-term neurocognitive consequences. As is the case with other sports detailed throughout this text, most concussions cause a temporary disruption in mental functioning and most concussion symptoms seen in amateur and professional soccer players fade within a week or two. However, exact management directives for safe return to play have been lacking and more general return to play guidelines have frequently been employed in the absence of more specific guidelines.

Recently, the Federation Internationale de Football Association (FIFA) in conjunction with the International Olympic Committee (IOC) and the International Ice Hockey Federation (IHF) assembled a group of physicians, neuropsychologists and sports administrators in Vienna Austria to continue to explore methods of reducing morbidity secondary to sports related concussion. The deliberations that took place during this meeting lead to the publication of a document outlining recommendations for both the diagnosis and management of concussion in sports (Aubry et al., 2001).

One of the most important conclusions of this meeting was that none of the previously published concussion management guidelines were adequate to assure proper management of every concussion. Although a complete discussion of these recommendations are beyond the scope of this chapter, the group emphasized the implementation of neuropsychological testing, whenever possible. The recognition of neuropsychological testing as a key element of the post-concussions evaluation process represented a particularly important development in the diagnosis and rehabilitation of the concussed athlete. The use of baseline neuropsychological testing was specifically recommended whenever possible. In addition, a graduated return to play protocol was emphasized. This protocol emphasizes the following elements:

1. Removal from contest following and signs/symptoms of concussion.
2. No return to play in current game
3. Medical evaluation following injury
4. Stepwise return to play
   a. No activity and rest until asymptomatic
   b. Light aerobic exercise
   c. Sport-specific training
   d. Non-contact drills
   e. Full-contact drills
   f. Game play

It was specifically recommended that each step would, in most circumstances, be separated by 24 hours. Furthermore, any recurrence of concussive symptoms should lead to the athlete dropping back to the previous level. In other words, if an athlete is asymptomatic at rest and develops a headache following light aerobic exercise, the athlete should return to complete rest. The Vienna group further recognized that conventional structural neuroimaging studies are usually normal following concussive injury and should be employed only when a structural lesion is suspected. The group further suggested that functional imaging are in the early stages of development but may provide valuable information in the future.

Prevention of Concussion in Soccer Athletes

Thus far, this chapter has focused primarily on the neuropsychological aspects of soccer related brain injury, and on appropriate management of the injury. However, the issue of prevention of injury has become an increasingly popular topic of discussion and is an extremely important issue. Obviously, the goal of medical personnel, parents and fans alike should be to promote safety and minimize injury whenever possible.

Protective headgear in soccer

As concussions in soccer have received increasing attention, the potential use of protective headgear has been discussed in both medical and lay circles. The focus on the development of protective headgear is understandable given the participations of millions of youth soccer athletes and the active involvement and concern of their parents as coaches and fans. However, scientific evidence to suggest that protective headgear will prevent concussion is currently lacking. Furthermore, it in unlikely that helmets or other types of protective headgear will result in elimination of the risk of concussion in the sport. In fact, helmets in other sports have not specifically been developed to prevent concussion but rather to prevent injuries such as skull fracture (Crisco, 2001).

As emphasized throughout this text, concussive injury represents a complex neurometabolic event that occurs due to the shifting of brain tissue within the skull and may not even require direct trauma to the head. Clearly, concussions occur frequently in sports that require the use of helmets such as American football and Ice Hockey. Furthermore, it is also important to emphasize that the use of helmets in contact sports is likely to have the effect of decreasing the exercise of player caution in protection of the head and could actually result in an increase in the velocity at which head collisions occur, if athletes feel less vulnerable to injury. The "spearing" type of injury that is currently commonplace in American Football represents an example of this phenomenon and is thought to result in the most severe concussive injuries within this sport. Although we applaud the intent of protecting the health of soccer athletes and the exploration of all potential safeguards, it appears to be premature to promote the adoption of protective headgear at this point in time.

Heading technique

In attempt to increase safety within the sport of soccer, some authors have suggested the teaching of proper heading techniques at the youth level. This represents an important issue that, if implemented in younger players, could result in an overall reduction of concussion related to poor technique.

Correct heading of the soccer ball should involve the use of the frontal bone to contact the ball. Furthermore, the neck muscles should be properly flexed to prevent acceleration of the head. In addition, it has been recommended that the lower body should be in-line with the head and neck to increase the resistant mass (Asken & Schwartz, 1998). Since concussions are known to occur as a result of rapid movement of the skull inside the skull cavity, minimization of whipping of the head may reduce injury. Green and Jordan (1998) have further suggested 10 actions to promote safer play, some of which relate to proper heading technique. Ultimately, biomechanical studies are necessary to better quantify the forces involved in heading of the soccer ball under specific conditions. Studies of this nature are currently underway and promise to yield important information. For instance, The impact forces involved in heading of the soccer ball is currently under study though the electromyographic analysis of three different header types (shooting, clearing and passing) in US Division I intercollegiate female soccer players. (Bauer, Thomas, Cauraugh, Kaminski, & Hass, 2001). Increased muscle activity was observed in the neck during the jumping approach, which appeared to stabilize the connection between the head and body. This was felt to stabilize the head-neck complex. In addition, studies that rely on the use of non-human head forms is now underway to provide information regarding the biomechanical forces that are involved in heading.

Player behavior and enforcement of the rules

Although generally regarded as a "clean" sport, injury can and does occur as a result of overly aggressive play. In particular, the concussions may occur as a result of elbowing, rough tackling or other types of body contact. Certainly, some amount of body contact is inevitable and some injuries may be of an accidental nature. However, overly aggressive play may result in needless injury. Limiting this type of behaviour through enforcement of rules represents an important aspect of minimization of concussions on the playing field. Enforcement of the rules is important at all levels but is particularly important at the professional or elite amateur level as younger players often emulate the behaviour of these athletes.

Directions for Research

The forgoing review has focused on existing research in the area of soccer related concussion. As emphasized throughout this chapter, current research has been limited to a relatively small number of scientific studies and most published studies have been of a retrospective rather than a prospective nature. This has resulted in questions regarding the attribution of neurocognitive decline to a particular causative agent (e.g. heading the ball, number of prior concussions, etc.).

Within the past two years, there has been a trend towards the adoption of research designs that will hopefully provide more conclusive information. In particular, attempts to study the acute effects of heading via analysis of neuropsychological test results before and after participation in controlled heading drills has yielded important initial results. However, if this line of research is to be successful in the future, it will be important to develop more sensitive assessment tools that are relatively free of practice effects that obscure change in neuropsychological test performance. Computer-based neuropsychological testing may provide one such improvement in testing methods in the future.

In addition to improving our neuropsychological testing technology, the implementation of functional brain imaging techniques holds great promise of the future. Early results from the University of Pittsburgh Functional Brain Imaging program have suggested that subtle changes in brain function that last days after injury can be detected in mild (Grade 1) concussions. It is hoped that this technology can be applied to the measurement of changes in brain function following the participation of non-concussed athletes in heading drills. Although somewhat logistically difficult to implement, studies of this nature could provide very valuable data. In addition, it will be important to continue to study the long-term consequences of heading the ball through the longitudinal study of non-concussed athletes over years of participation. Studies of this nature could help to separate the effects of neurocognitive deficits due to sub-concussive blows from those that are the result of concussive injuries. Similarly, new developments in basic neuroscience research should continue to yield important information regarding possible cellular changes following mild neurological insult.

Finally, much more research is needed regarding specific populations of soccer athletes. At the current time, little is know about the relative risk of injury in different age groups or between males and females. Given documented differences between younger and older athletes with regard to response to more severe brain injury, more research regarding high school athletes and below is urgently needed. In addition, although preliminary information data has not suggested significant differences between male and female athletes (Lovell & Hagen, 2001), this is an area that requires additional study.

Summary

Close observation and reliable neuropsychological assessment of the brain injured soccer player is critical to the prevention of a more serious injury and potential cumulative neuropsychological impairment. As highlighted by this chapter, the sport of soccer is currently undergoing significant research scrutiny regarding the issue of concussion and it is likely that this area of research will continue to expand over the next decade. Ultimately, it is hope that current research that is underway with college and professional athletes will have an impact on the care of the younger athlete and will result in practical strategies for in creasing the safety of younger athletes throughout the world.

References

American Academy of Pediatrics Policy Statement (AAPPS). (1998). Recommendations for participation in competitive sports. *The Physician and Sportsmedicine, 16*, 165–167.

Asken M.J. & Schwartz R.C. (1998). Heading the ball in soccer: What's the risk of brain injury? *The Physician and Sportsmedicine, 26*, 211–220.

Aubry, M., Cantu, R., Dvorak, J., Graf-Baumann, T., Johnston, K.M., Kelly, J. (2001). Summary and agreement statement of the 1st international symposium on concussion in sport, Vienna, 2001. *Clinical Journal of Sports Medicine, 12*, 6–11.

Bauer, J.A., Thomas T.S., Cauraugh J.H., Kaminski T.W., & Hass C.J. (2001), *Journal of Sports Science, 19*(3), 171–179.

Cantu, R.C. (1998). Second-impact syndrome. *Clinics in Sports Medicine, 17*, 37–44.

Crisco, T. (2001). *Studies of soccer and football players. In Is Soccer Bad for Children's Heads? Summary of the IOM workshop on neuropsychological Consequences of Head Impact in Youth Soccer*. Institute of Medicine, 9–12.

DeMarco, J. & Reeves, C. (1993). Injuries associated with soccer goalposts, United States, 1979-1993. *Journal of the American Medical Association, 271*,1233.

Downs, D.S. & Abwender, D. (2002). Neuropsychological impairment in soccer athletes. *Journal of Sports Medicine and Physical Fitness, 42*(1), 103–107.

Fife, D. (1987). Head injury with and without hospital admission: Comparison of incidence and short time disability. *American Journal of Public Health, 77*, 810–812.

Frenquelli, A., Ruscito, P., Sicciolo, G., Rizzo, S., & Massarelli, N. (1991). Head and neck trauma in sporting activities: review of 208 cases. *Journal of Craniomax Surgery, 19*, 178–181.

Green, G.A. & Jordan, S.E. (1998). Are brain injuries a significant problem in soccer? *Clinical Sports Medicine, 17*(4), 795–809.

Guskiewicz K., Marshall, S.W., Broglio, S.P., Cantu, R.C., & Kirkendall D.T. (2002). No evidence of impaired neurocognitive performance in collegiate soccer players. *American Journal of Sports Medicine, 2*, 157–162.

Hansen T.B., Pless, S., & Bravvers, M. (1991). Cranial injuries among children in the county of Ringkobing. *Ugeskr Laeger, 15*, 2447–2479.

Hermann, M., Curio, N., Jost, S., Wunderlich, M.T., Synowitz, H., & Wallesch, C.W. (1999). *Retor Neurol Neurosci, 14*, 109–114.

Hughes, R. (1974). Head damage. A warning to all players. *The Sunday Times,* Nov 10.

Institute of Medicine (IOM) (2001). Is soccer bad for children's heads? Summary of the *IOM Workshop on Neuropsychological Consequences of Head Impact in Youth Soccer.* Washington, D.C. National Academy Press.

Jennett, B. & MacMillan, R. (1981). Epidemiology of head injury. *British Medical Journal, 282,* 101–104.

Jordan, S.E., Green, G., Galanty, H.L., Mandelbaum, B.R. & Jabour, B.A. (1996). Acute and chronic brain injury in United States National Team soccer players. *American Journal of Sports Medicine, 24,* 205–210.

Kirkendall, D.T., Jordan, S.E., & Garrett, W.E. (2001). Heading and head injuries in soccer. *Sports Medicine, 31*(5),369–386.

Kraus, J.F. (1991). Epidemiologic features of injuries to the central nervous system. In D.W. Andersen (Ed.). *Neuroepidemiology, a tribute to Bruce Schoenberg* (pp. 333–357). Boca Raton, FL: CRC Press.

Lehman, L.B. (1987). Nervous system sports-related injuries. *American Journal of Sports Medicine, 15,* 494–499.

Lovell, M.R. & Hagen, T. (2001). Gender issues in sports-related concussion. A presentation at the *AOSSM International Soccer Symposium,* Beverly Hills.

Matthews, W.B. (1972). Footballer's migraine. *British Medical Journal, 2*(809), 326–327.

Matser, J.T., Kessels, A.G.H., Lezak, M.D., & Troost, J. (1998). Chronic traumatic brain injury in professional soccer players. *Neurology, 51,* 791–796.

Matser, J.T., Kessels, A.G.H., Lezak, M.D., & Troost, J. (1999). Neuropsychological impairment in amateur soccer players. *Journal of the American Medical Association, 282,* 971–973.

Mueller, F.O., Cantu, R.C. (1990). Catastrophic injuries and fatalities in high school and college sports, 1982–1988. *Medicine and Science in Sports and Exercise, 22,* 737–741.

New York Times (2001). Concerns about heading by youth soccer players sets off debate. November, s6.

Powell, J.W. & Barber-Foss, K.D. (1999). Traumatic brain injury in high school athletes. *Journal of the American Medical Association, 282,* 958–963.

Petukian, M., Echemendia, R.J., & Macklin, S. (2000). *Clinical Journal of Sports Medicine, 10*(2), 104-109.

Rabadi, M.H. & Jordan, B.D. (2001). The cumulative effect of repetitive concussion in sports. *Clinical Journal of Sports Medicine, 11,* 194–198.

Slemmer, J.E., Matser, E.J., De Zeeuw, C.I., & Weber, J.T. (2002). Repeated mild injury causes cumulative damage to hippocampal cells. *Brain, 125,* 2699–2709.

Sortland, O. & Tysvaer, A.T. (1989). Brain damage in former association football players. An evaluation by cerebral computed tomography. *Neuroradiology, 31,* 44–48.

Tysvaer, A.T. & Lochen, E.A. (1991). Soccer injuries to the brain. A neuropsychological study of former soccer players. *The American Journal of Sports Medicine, 19,* 56–60.

Tysvaer, A.T., Storli, O., Bachen, N.I. Soccer injuries to the brain. (1989). A neurologic and electroencephalographic study of former players. *Acta Neurologica Scandinavia, 80,* 151–156.

Tysvaer, A.T., Storli, O. (1981). Association Football Injuries to the Brain. A Preliminary Report. *British Journal of Sports Medicine, 15,* 163–166.

Von Schneider, P.G. & Lichte, H. (1975). Untersuchungen zur Grosse der Krafteinwirkung beim Kopfballspiel des Fussballers. *Sportartzt und Sportmedizin, 26,* 222–223.

Chapter 12

AMERICAN PROFESSIONAL FOOTBALL

Mark R. Lovell
Director, UPMC Sports Medicine Concussion Program, Director, NFL Neuropsychology Program
Pittsburgh, Pennsylvania

William Barr
NYU Comprehensive Epilepsy Center, New York

Introduction

Over the past decade, the study of mild traumatic brain injuries (mTBI) in American professional football athletes has become an intense area of focus and has influenced the development of similar projects in other sports. During this period, the neuropsychologist has increasingly played an important role in shaping MTBI management strategies with the NFL and at all level of sports (Lovell, 1998). In fact, the neuropsychological model developed for use within the NFL has also played an influential role in development of the Neuropsychology program within the National Hockey League (Lovell & Burke, 2000) and within the college and high school ranks (Lovell, Collins, Iverson & Maroon, 2003). This chapter will describe the current Neuropsychology program within the National Football League and will focus specifically on the role of the neuropsychologist within the context of professional football.

The Use of Neuropsychological Testing in American Professional Football-Historical Roots

The use of neuropsychological assessment procedures within professional football has been a recent phenomenon. The first large scale study of concussion in athletes (football players) was carried out at the college level and involved the cooperative efforts of the University of Virginia, the Ivy League schools, and the University of Pittsburgh (Barth et al., 1989). This project is discussed elsewhere within this text and will not be discussed in detail in this chapter. Although the University of Virginia study was conceptualized a research project and data gleaned through this study were not used directly to make clinical, return to play decisions, this study helped to establish a model of neuropsychological assessment that could be adapted for more clinical use. As a result of frustration with existing return-to-play guidelines, which were based almost totally on player signs and symptoms, a neuropsychological evaluation program was instituted with the Pittsburgh Steelers in 1993 by Drs. Mark Lovell and Joseph Maroon (Lovell, 1996, Lovell, 1998; Maroon et al., 2000) and with the active participation of John Norwig, A.T.C. and Dr. Julian Bailes and Anthony Yates. This represented the first clinically oriented project within professional sports structured to assist team medical personnel in making return to play decisions, following a suspected MTBI. This approach involved the baseline evaluation of each athlete prior to the beginning of the season to provide the basis for comparison, in the event of an injury during the season. Testing was then repeated within 24 to 48 hours after a suspected MTBI, and again prior to the return of the athlete to contact.

During the 1993 season, the neuropsychological testing program was limited to the Pittsburgh Steelers and involved the baseline evaluation of 23 NFL athletes. Athletes within the project volunteered to be evaluated. During these seasons, neuropsychological testing was successfully utilized to assist in determining player readiness to return to the playing field. The project continued to expand to other athletes on the Steelers roster throughout the 1994 season and testing was effectively employed to evaluate a number of injured athletes during that season. During the 1994 season, there were injuries to several "high profile" athletes both within the Steelers organization and throughout the league that served to heighten the awareness of the potential danger of MTBI's. This, in turn, highlighted the need for a more comprehensive and systematic approach to the study of MTBI and lead to the formation of the NFL Subcommittee of Mild Traumatic Brain Injury. This committee has been chaired by Dr. Elliot Pellman of the New York Jets and is composed of NFL team physicians, athletic trainers and equipment managers, as well as neurosurgical, biomechanical and neuropsychological consultants (Dr. Mark Lovell). Over the past six seasons, this committee has overseen multiple projects within the NFL designed to better understand MTBI. In addition to supporting the Neuropsychology program discussed within this chapter, this committee has spearheaded research on the epidemiology of MTBI, the investigation of protective equipment (e.g. mouth guards and helmets) and has more recently overseen an innovative approach for testing helmet characteristics in the laboratory.

Neuropsychological Evaluation of the Professional Athlete

Before implementing a neuropsychological testing program with professional athletes, we realized that some changes would have to be made from routine clinical practice. Neuropsychological assessment of MTBI typically involves an interview combined with a test battery that may take 4-6 hours or more to complete. Before extending this methodology for use in the NFL, we understood that the assessment process would have to be very brief to accommodate to the athletes' busy schedules and to address the need to evaluate a large volume of athletes in a limited time period. As a result of these factors, a 30-minute test battery was developed, with the goal of evaluating injured athletes at multiple time points. Details of this methodology are reviewed below:

The NFL Test Battery

Table 12.1 provides a listing of the neuropsychological tests that have now been formally adopted by the NFL Subcommittee on Mild Traumatic Brain Injury. All NFL teams as now are participating in the program are currently utilizing this approach. This test battery has recently been revised with the addition of the several tests from *the Wechsler Adult Intelligence Scale-III* (Wechsler, 1997).

The *Hopkins Verbal Learning Test* (HVLT, Brandt, 1991) consists of a 12-word list that is presented to the athlete on three consecutive trials. In its revised version, the athlete is assessed for recall after each presentation and again following a 20-minute delay period. The *Brief Visuospatial Memory Test-Revised* (BVMT-R, Benedict, 1997) evaluates visual memory and involves the presentation of six abstract spatial designs on three consecutive trials. Similar to the *HVLT*, the athletes recall following each trial and his delayed recall is evaluated. Both the *HVLT* and the *BVMT-R* have six equivalent forms, which minimize practice effects and makes them ideal for use with athletes who are likely to undergo evaluation on multiple occasions throughout the course of their careers. The *Trail Making Test* (Reitan, 1958) consists of two parts and requires the athlete to utilize spatial scanning and mental flexibility skills. The *Controlled Oral Word Association Test* (Benton & Hamsher, 1978) the athlete to recall as many words as possible that begin with a given letter of the alphabet, within a 60 second time period. This is completed for three separate letters and provides a measure of verbal fluency. In addition to the neuropsychological tests mentioned above, it is important

Table 12.1. NFL Neuropsychological test battery.

Test	Ability evaluated
Orientation Questions (Lovell, 1996)	Retrograde and anterograde amnesia, orientation to place and time
Hopkins Verbal Learning Test (HVLT) (Brandt, 1991)	Memory for words (verbal memory)
Brief Visuospatial Memory Test-Revised (BVMT-R) (Benedict, 1997)	Visual memory
Trail Making Test (Reitan, 1958)	Visual Scanning, mental flexibility
Controlled Oral Word Fluency (Benton and Hamsher, 1978)	Word fluency, word retrieval
WAIS-III Symbol Search (Wechsler, 1997)	Visual scanning, visual search
WAIS-III Digit Symbol (Wechsler, 1997)	Visual scanning, information processing
WAIS-III Digit Span (Wechsler, 1997)	Attention span
Post-Concussion Symptom Inventory (Lovell, 1996)	MTBI symptoms
Delayed recall from HVLT Delayed recall from BVMT-R	Delayed memory for words Delayed memory for designs

to monitor the athlete's symptoms. The *Post-Concussion Symptom Inventory* has recently been developed and is currently being utilized by both the NFL and NHL (Lovell, 1996; Lovell & Collins, 1998).

As can be seen in Table 12.1, the NFL test battery was constructed to evaluate multiple aspects of cognitive functioning, while being relatively brief. It is heavily oriented towards the evaluation of attentional processes, visual scanning and information processing, although the test battery also evaluates verbal memory, coordination and speech fluency. Past research in neuropsychology has identified these as the cognitive functions most likely to be affected by concussion. The tests that made up the battery were administered using standardized instructions to avoid variation in test results across testing sessions and across teams. The most recent version of the NFL test battery has recently undergone factor analysis and four principal factors have emerged: 1) visual attention; 2) verbal attention; 3) visual memory, and; 4) verbal memory. The tests that make up this test battery have also been found to be sensitive to concussion, in preliminary studies that have evaluated the ability of component tests to discriminate concussed from non-concussed athletes (Collins et al., 1999).

Timeline of the Evaluation

Baseline testing

Pre-season baseline evaluation of the athlete is important for several reasons. Individual players vary significantly with regard to their level of performance on tests of memory, attention/concentration, mental processing speed and motor speed. Athletes may perform poorly on the more demanding tests because of pre-injury learning disabilities, attention deficit disorder or other factors such as test taking anxiety. One also needs to consider the possibility that the effects of previous concussions might affect the athlete's test performance.

Brief sideline assessment

The neuropsychologist is usually not the first professional to evaluate the concussed athlete. The team athletic trainer or physician usually completes the on-field evaluation of the athlete. The athlete should be evaluated both for signs (observed by staff) symptoms (reported by athlete) of concussion. Although these brief assessment tools are helpful in quantifying cognitive emerging cognitive deficits immediately after injury, they are not sufficiently sensitive to be utilized in making return to play decisions. Under no circumstances should sideline testing be utilized as a substitute for formal neuropsychological testing.

The sideline evaluation should involve an assessment of the player's orientation to place, game, and details of the contest. The athlete's recall of events preceding the collision (retrograde amnesia) should also be evaluated. The athlete's ability to learn and retain new information (anterograde amnesia) should also be tested via a brief sideline memory test. The player should be asked to repeat three to five words until they can so consistently. They should be checked for recall of this list within five minutes. Brief tests of attention span such as backward recitation of digits or months of the year are also useful. Finally, the player should be observed for emerging post-concussive symptoms such as headache, nausea, imbalance or on-field confusion (Kelly & Rosenberg, 1997).

Testing following concussion

Whenever possible, the initial neuropsychological evaluation of the athlete should take place within 24 to 48 hours of the suspected concussion. We have found that athletes at all levels are prone to under-report symptoms in hopes of a speedy return to competition (Lovell, 2001). Therefore, even when athletes appear to be symptom free, a neuropsychological evaluation is recommended to evaluate more subtle aspects of cognitive functioning such as information processing speed and memory. If the athlete displays any cognitive deficits on testing or continues to exhibit post-concussive symptoms, a follow-up neuropsychological evaluation is recommended within 5 to 7 days after injury, prior to return to play. This time interval represents a useful and practical time span and also appears to be consistent with animal brain metabolism studies which have demonstrated metabolic changes in the brain which persist for several days following injury (Hovda et al., 1998). The pre-season baseline evaluation of the athlete is important for several reasons. Individual players vary significantly with regard to their level of performance on tests of memory, attention/concentration, mental processing speed and motor speed (Lovell, 1998. Athletes may perform poorly on the more demanding tests because of pre-injury learning disabilities, attention deficit disorder or other factors such as test taking anxiety.

Practical and Methodological Challenges In Working With Professional Football Athletes

The neuropsychologist may be faced with initial resistance when attempting to implement a concussion assessment program with a professional sports franchise. First, the neuropsychologist is likely to be met with initial skepticism for introducing something new to the team. For success, one must have the full cooperation of the coaching staff as well as the team medical and athletic training staff. Developing a good working relationship with the athletic trainers is a must for scheduling evaluations and for communication with the athletes. The players must have the understanding that the testing is occurring for their benefit and is an endeavor that is valued by the entire organization. The players are likely to respond in a positive manner if the baseline testing is voluntary, but strongly recommended by the team as part of their routine preseason physical examination.

After receiving the "green light" to implement the neuropsychological testing program, the team neuropsychologist must then often with misconceptions regarding the nature and purpose of the testing. Players often react to the neuropsychologist as a "shrink" that is trying to "get inside of the their "head." Alternatively, if not explained thoroughly, neuropsychological testing may inappropriately viewed as "IQ testing" that could be used against him by scouts or by management to make decisions about his intellectual capacity. The neuropsychologist should thoroughly explain the nature and the purpose of the testing prior to each session to clear up any misconceptions. It should be explained that the test results should be used to provide objective information regarding the presence or absence of cognitive dysfunction secondary to concussion. The players should realize that their injury status will not rest solely on the results of the testing and represents one piece of the diagnostic puzzle. This information will be used by team officials as one of many factors that will aid in their decision regarding return to play.

In working with professional athletes, it is imperative that the team neuropsychologist has at least a basic understanding of the game of football, including the rules and the role of players at various team positions. It is best to develop a professional yet friendly and confident relationship with the players. It is important not to portray oneself as a fan, but as a skilled professional who is there for a purpose. Caring and professionalism will ultimately lead to trust.

While the neuropsychologist may initially be viewed inaccurately based on pre-existing stereotypes, he/she should be aware of his/her own prejudice regarding athletes. In particular the image of the "dumb jock" is an inaccurate characterization and the neuropsychologist will soon learn that professional athletes are a group of college-educated individuals that have risen to the top of their ranks, through the combination of intelligence and athleticism. The athletes, for the most part, perform well on neuropsychological tests and approach the testing with a similar level of competitiveness that they exhibit on the playing field. Many may even desire immediate feedback on their performance and how their scores compare to those from other players. This can be handled by providing some assurance of their adequacy without divulging test scores of team members.

Symptom Minimization in Professional Athletes

While some MTBI victims in neuropsychological practice may exaggerate symptoms or malinger for litigation purposes, professional athletes are more likely to minimize their symptoms or attempt to "fake good" in order to return to play as quickly as possible. The neuropsychologist should be able to recognize such attempts. In addition, the group testing of athletes creates the potential for athletes to share information regarding the testing process, thus diminishing the value of the test results. For example, when evaluating a large number of players at baseline, it is important to use 3 or more alternate forms of the tests, as players are known to share test information with their team mates (e.g. words from a list learning test). In one such case, players in the training room were observed playing a game composed of reciting lists of words beginning with various letters (similar to verbal fluency testing).

Within the context of professional sports, questions may naturally arise regarding who is chosen for baseline evaluations and where and when the testing will occur. While testing of the entire team is recommended, many teams give priority to high-profile quarterbacks, running backs, and receivers that are perceived to be "at risk" for concussion. However, one must also consider whether a player is a member of the special teams, including punt and kickoff coverage, where all players involved in open-field blocking and tackling may be placed at risk for developing concussion.

There is no perfect answer regarding ~~for~~ the question of when to perform baseline neuropsychological testing. When working with professional teams, one will quickly learn that the players have very busy schedules including practice and classroom meetings. During the off-season, they may have other professional or social commitments that make it difficult to complete testing during this time. In addition, testing during preseason training camp is nearly impossible as a result of the tight schedule of practices and other team activities. There is typically no time in the weeks immediately prior to the season. As a result, many teams have opted to have their players undergo neuropsychological testing in April, May or June during "mini-camps" or during off-season conditioning programs. At that point, the neuropsychologist may be in a position to test rookies coming into the system and newly acquired veterans who have not undergone testing with other teams. Additional testing on a smaller scale can be accomplished subsequently to account for any roster changes made prior to the first kickoff of the season.

Baseline testing is best accomplished through use of a team of examiners. We have found it particularly useful to employ graduate students and clinical staff that have obtained training and experience in test administration and scoring. Testing is typically performed in a two- to four-hour time-block with players scheduled every half-hour. Space is often an issue. Examiners are placed in separate rooms on site at the team training facility in offices typically housing team trainers and medical staff.

The Role of the Neuropsychologist within the Team Medical Staff

The inclusion of the neuropsychologist in professional football is a relatively recent development. In fact, at the current time, the role of the neuropsychologist in professional sports is rapidly evolving and expanding. This is understandable since most sports medicine physicians had only limited experience with the field of Neuropsychology and most neuropsychologists had not previously worked within the sports medicine environment. Initially, neuropsychologists were viewed with some suspicion and apprehension. Questions naturally arose regarding how neuropsychological test information could potentially change decision-making protocol and how the inclusion of yet another professional (in addition to team physicians, athletic trainers and dentists) might affect medical staff dynamics. However, these issues have rapidly dissipated as neuropsychologists have gained experience within the professional sports environment (please see Chapter 21 this volume for a more thorough discussion of consultation issues).

Future Directions

Neuropsychological consultation is now provided to nearly all NFL teams. Many teams have traditionally used the league-endorsed battery of tests, thus yielding a potentially large amount of data for research. While efforts to combine data from multiple teams are underway, a number of obstacles do exist. Many feel that presenting aggregate statistics on neuropsychological test scores might propagate stereotyped views of the NFL athlete. One strategy to circumvent this issue would be to simply analyze change scores from baseline in those athletes who have concussions. Another approach would be to analyze the proportion of players whose post-concussion scores exceed an empirically derived cutoff. With the social and economic issues and concerns now inherent in professional sports, alternative methods of data analysis need to be considered to proceed with any form of organized research program.

Most will agree that the data obtained from neuropsychological testing of NFL players can provide useful information for improving management of concussions in athletes, as well as teaching us something about recovery from mild traumatic brain injury in the non-sports population. Based on the establishment of a large sample of athletes who have undergone baseline testing *prior* to injury, it is possible to better determine the time course for acute recovery as well as establishing the relationship between non-cognitive symptoms such as headaches and dizziness and cognitive deficits in the area of attention and memory. In addition to studying the acute recovery process, more long-range longitudinal questions could also be used to address such as the impact of multiple concussions on long-term functions (Collins et al., 2002). This topic is currently being debated actively in sports-medicine circles, Serial testing might help identify who these players are at an earlier point in time, thus preventing more serious injury.

In addition to yielding important information regarding the recovery process, the NFL program may grow to include neuropsychologists in roles other than as concussion specialists. For example, some teams have inquired about the use of neuropsychological data for predicting performance on the field. For instance, performance on a specific neuropsychological test might be used to predict which players might be most susceptible to making certain types of penalties. Other questions may eventually arise with regard to whether neuropsychological test scores can be used in any way to predict overall success as an NFL player.

Neuropsychological test data might also be used to determine individual strengths and weaknesses in cognition that would be informative for coaches in their interactions with players. For example, one team requested their neuropsychologist to perform additional testing on a player who was having great difficulty learning the program of team plays and signals. After additional testing, extending well beyond the baseline concussion battery, it was determined that the player had a significant learning disability that interfered with his ability to learn and remember through reading or any form of verbal input. Alternatively, the player was found to have good perceptual skills and a very strong visual memory. Further success was enhanced by encouraging coaches to communicate the plays to him through demonstration or film and to give him hand signals during the game. While this type of neuropsychological assessment can be useful, this places the neuropsychologist outside of the traditional role as part of the medical team and creates a potential conflict of interest if the test data is utilized to select (or cut) certain players.

While the program described above represents the standard for neuropsychological testing in 2002, professional football will no doubt follow the trend towards the utilization of computerized neuropsychological testing in sports. Currently, approximately one-half of NFL teams are using computer-based testing (e.g. ImPACT) and this trend is likely to continue in the future. Various approaches to computer-based neuropsychological assessment are described elsewhere in this text and therefore will not be reviewed here (see Chapter 20).

Summary

This chapter has reviewed the potential uses of neuropsychological testing with professional athletes and has reviewed current research in the area. The current large-scale program being conducted with the NFL has been reviewed. The use of neuropsychological testing has evolved rapidly from being virtually unheard of in the early 1990s to widespread current acceptance. In fact, neuropsychologist's have gradually become accepted valued team members in many NFL franchises and this trend promises to continue as team medical staff continue to seek better methods of making return to play decisions. As the NFL program began in response to pressing clinical issues, the research potential of this project has yet to develop fully. We anticipate that research in this area will increase rapidly over the next five years-leading to exciting new discoveries regarding recovery from mTBI.

References

Barth, J., Alves, W., Ryan, T.V., Macciocchi, S.N., Rimerl, R.W., Jane, J.A. et al. (1989). Mild head injury in sports: Neuropsychological sequelae and recovery of function. In H. Levin, H. Eisenberg & A. Benton, (Eds.), *Mild Head Injury.* New York, NY: Oxford University Press.

Benedict, R.H.B. (1997). *Brief Visuospatial Memory Test-Revised.* Odessa, FL: Psychological Assessment Resources, Inc.

Benton, A. & Hamsher, K. (1978). *Multilingual Aphasia Examination.* Iowa City: University of Iowa Press.

Brandt, J. (1991). The Hopkins Verbal Learning Test: Development of a new memory test with six equivalent forms. *Clinical Neuropsychologist, 5,* 125–142.

Collins, M.W., Grindel, S., Lovell, M.R., Dede, D.E., Moser, D.J., & Phalin, B.R. et al. (1999). Relationship between concussion and neuropsychological performance in college football players. *Journal of the American Medical Association, 282*, 964–970.

Collins, M.W., Lovell, M.R., Iverson, G.L., Cantu, R., Maroon, J.C., & Field, M. (2002). *Neurosurgery 51,* 1175–1181.

Hovda, D.A., Prins, M., Becker, D.P., Lee, S., Bergsneider, M., & Martin, N. (1998). Neurobiology of concussion. In J. Bailes, M.R. Lovell & J.C. Maroon (Eds.), *Sports-Related Concussion* (pp. 12-51). St. Louis: Quality Medical Publishers.

Kelly, J.P. & Rosenberg, J.H. (1997). Diagnosis and management of MTBI in sports. *Neurology, 48,* 575–580.

Lovell, M.R. (1996, February). Evaluation of the professional athlete. Paper presented at the *First Annual Sports Related Concussion Conference*, Pittsburgh, PA.

Lovell, M.R. (1998). Evaluation of the professional Athlete. In J.E. Bailes, M.R.Lovell, & J.C. Maroon (Eds.), *Sports-Related Concussion*. St. Louis: Quality Medical Publishers, 200-214.
Lovell, M.R. & Collins, M.W. (1998). Neuropsychological assessment of the college football player. *Journal of Head Trauma Rehabilitation, 13*(2), 9–26.
Maroon, J.C., Lovell, M.R., Norwig, J., Podell, K., Powell, J.W., & Hartl, R. (2000). Cerebral concussion in athletes: evaluation and neuropsychological testing, *Neurosurgery, 47*, 659–672.
Reitan, R. (1958). Validity of the Trail Making Test as an indicator of organic brain damage. *Perceptual and Motor Skills, 8*, 271–276.
Smith, A. (1982). *Symbol Digit Modalities Test Manual*. Los Angeles, CA: Western Psychological Services.
Wechsler, D. (1997). *Wechsler Adult Intelligence Scale-III*. San Antonio. *The Psychological Corporation*.

Chapter 13

PROFESSIONAL ICE HOCKEY

Mark R. Lovell
Co-Director, NHL Neuropsychology Program

Ruben J. Echemendia
Pennsylvania State University
Co-Director, NHL Neuropsychology Program

Charles J. Burke, III
University of Pittsburgh Medical Center
Director, NHL Concussion Project

Introduction

The evaluation of concussion in professional hockey players has recently become an area of intense interest over the past five years. The most recent outgrowth of this interest has been motivated by a desire to protect the health of hockey athletes and has resulted in the development of comprehensive concussion evaluation program within the National Hockey League (NHL) (Anderson & Lovell, 1999; Lovell & Burke, 2000). This program has been structured to identify athlete's immediately after injury and to avoid exposure to further injury by premature return to the ice. The NHL program has also been developed to answer a number of important research questions. This chapter will provide an overview of the concussion program that has been developed for the NHL and the current league-wide evaluation and management protocol will be reviewed with special reference to return-to-play issues.

The importance of the neuropsychologist within the sport of ice hockey has recently been signified by several developments. First, a recent summary document published under the auspices of the International Ice Hockey Federation, FIFA and the International Olympic Committee (Aubry et al., 2001) has identified neuropsychological assessment as the "cornerstone" of the concussion evaluation process. This development has lead to the request for an increasing number of neuropsychologists within both amateur and professional sports. Second, within the context of the NHL, neuropsychologists now play an important role not only in the baseline assessment of the athletes but are also now highly involved in return to play decision making.

Biomechanics of concussion in the hockey athlete

The pathophysiology of concussion has been detailed elsewhere in this text (see Chapter 4, this volume) and will not be reviewed further in this chapter. However, there are several aspects of ice hockey that deserve specific mention. Today's professional hockey players are typically larger, faster and better conditioned than in the past generations, resulting in a fast-paced and sophisticated game. In fact, all NHL rosters contain athletes who weigh over two hundred pounds. Furthermore, a modern NHL player may reach speeds of almost 30 miles per hour during a game situation. In addition, the continuous substitution of rested players into the game maintains this level of competitiveness throughout the game.

Most of the concussions sustained by professional hockey athletes are the result of high-speed collisions. This can result in both deceleration and rotational injuries during which brain axons are stretched or torn (Povlishock & Coburn, 1989) and also results in significant metabolic dysfunction within the brain (Hovda et al., 1998). As detailed elsewhere in this text, concussive injury does not require direct trauma to the head and therefore is not necessarily prevented through the use of protective headgear. In addition, direct contact of the head with the glass, boards, stick, elbow or ice may result in direct trauma to the skull as well as contusion of the brain in more severe cases. The hockey helmet may be important in protecting the athlete against this type of injury. Finally, periodic fights on the ice may also result in a concussion, although in our experience, these incidents account for a relatively small number of injuries.

The National Hockey League (NHL) Concussion Program

The NHL concussion program was initiated in 1997 to minimize concussive injuries in NHL players and involves the cooperative efforts of the NHL Players Association, the NHL team physicians, athletic trainers and consulting neuropsychologists. Initially, one of the primary goals of the project was to gather systematic league-wide statistics regarding the incidence of concussion and to better understand the recovery process. At the time of the institution of this program, a concussion tracking evaluation form was developed that is completed by the team physician following a suspected concussion. This form has now been changed to include the physician's initial assessment of signs and symptoms of concussion as observed by the team physician and athletic trainer. This information is then transferred to a central league-wide database at the University of Pittsburgh for later study.

In addition to the concussion surveillance database, which involves input both from NHL team physicians and athletic trainers, a league-wide neuropsychological testing program was mandated by the NHL to assist in the assessment of player's neurocognitive status following a suspected concussion. This program will be detailed briefly below.

Rink-side Evaluation

The initial evaluation of the concussed college or professional hockey player begins on the ice or at rink-side and the athletic trainer or team physician usually completes the first assessment of the athlete's status. In evaluating the athlete following a suspected concussion, it is important to evaluate both the player's cognitive status (via formal mental status testing) as well as reported symptoms. To facilitate the identification of concussion immediately after suspected injury, a standard protocol has been adopted that involves the evaluation of initial symptoms as well as a brief mental status evaluation based on the McGill ACE examination (Johnston, Lassonde, & Pito, 2001). Portions of the ACE are utilized by the NHL initial evaluation. While the initial assessment of concussion is very important in diagnosing the injury, we need to stress that this type of brief evaluation *is not* meant to provide a comprehensive evaluation of signs/symptoms of concussion and is not a substitute for further in-depth evaluation.

This examination provides an initial assessment of the player's orientation to place, game, and details of the contest. Retrograde amnesia refers to the athlete's recall of information preceding the injury and is an important marker of injury severity. The ability to learn and retain new information (anterograde amnesia) should also be tested via a brief sideline memory test. We suggest requiring the athlete to learn and retain a five-word list, which is contained within the ACE. The sequential pointing to body parts represents another potential method of evaluating memory in the athlete for whom English represents a second language. Regardless of whether sequence learning or word list learning procedures are used, the athlete should be checked for recall of this list within approximately five minutes. Brief tests of attentional capacity such as recitation of digits in backward order or backward recitation of months of the year are also useful but are not sufficient to evaluate concussion. Finally, the player should be observed for emerging non-cognitive post-concussive symptoms such as headache, nausea, dizziness, imbalance or on-ice confusion. The athlete should also be observed for the development of motor incoordination or any change in behavior.

Neuropsychological Assessment

The formal neuropsychological evaluation of the athlete is structured to take place within 24 to 48 hours of the suspected concussion, whenever possible. Although many athletes may appear to be symptom free, a neuropsychological evaluation is recommended to evaluate more subtle aspects of cognitive functioning such as information processing speed and memory. Follow-up neuropsychological evaluation is recommended within 5 to 7 days after injury if any abnormalities are presents at the time of initial follow-up. This time interval represents a useful and practical time span and also appears to be consistent with animal brain metabolism studies which have demonstrated metabolic changes in the brain which persist for days following injury (Hovda et al., 1998).

In designing a league-wide neuropsychological evaluation program, there were a number of factors that were considered. Time is always a factor in professional athletes and is a particularly significant issue in ice hockey. First, multiple languages are spoken within the NHL and some athletes may have a limited grasp of the English language. Therefore, a number of neuropsychological tests have been selected that require relatively little familiarity with the English language and can be easily explained. In addition, English-based tests such as word lists and verbal fluency tasks are omitted with non-native English speakers.

In addition to the language issue, the logistics of a typical professional hockey travel schedule (which often includes two to three week road trips) has required the development of a "network approach" through which injured players can be evaluated at nay point in time during a road trip. If a player is injured while in their non-home city, the athletic trainer under the supervision of the opponent's team physician completes the initial rink-side evaluation. If neuropsychological testing is indicated, the neuropsychological consultant for the opponent's team completes the evaluation and passes these results on to the neuropsychologist from the player's team. The neuropsychologist then provides consultation to the athlete's team physician who makes the return to play decision.

Importance of Baseline Testing in Professional Hockey

As is noted elsewhere throughout this text, the importance of the baseline evaluation of the athlete cannot be overemphasized. Pre-injury differences in performance between athletes in the areas of attention, memory and processing speed are common in athletes. For instance, some players perform poorly on the more demanding tests because of pre-injury learning disabilities, attention deficit disorder or other factors such as test taking anxiety. In addition, differences in language competency mentioned above can also result in differences in performance on testing. The use of baseline testing also allows for the evaluation of the player over time and will assist the NHL in tracking athletes throughout their careers.

The National Hockey League Neuropsychological Test Battery

As noted earlier, the application of neuropsychological testing within the sport of ice hockey strategies to ice hockey provides specific challenges. As with all organized sports, time pressures and the need for efficiency must be balanced with the need for sampling of multiple domains of neuropsychological functioning. Specifically, the test battery should be constructed to evaluate the athletes functioning in the areas of attention, information processing speed, fluency and memory. In addition, procedures should be selected that have multiple equivalent multiple forms or that have been thoroughly researched with regards to the expected "practice effects." The test battery of tests adopted for the NHL study was constructed with these factors in mind. The NHL test battery was developed by the Neuropsychological Advisory Board who serves as supervisors of the neuropsychological testing component of the program. This group was initially comprised of Drs. Mark Lovell and Ruben Echemendia (co-Directors) and by Drs. William Barr and Elizabeth Parker. Current board members are Drs. Lovell, Echemendia, Barr, and Drs. Liza Kozora and Don Gerber. The test NHL battery can be administered in approximately 30 minutes. The specific tests that make up the battery are listed in Table 13.1.

As the majority of these tests have been described in other chapters in this text, they will not be reviewed further on this chapter.

Table 13.1. NHL neuropsychological test battery.

Test	Ability Evaluated
Orientation Questions	Retrograde and anterograde amnesia, orientation to place and time
Concussion Symptom Inventory	Post-concussive symptoms
Hopkins Verbal Learning Test (HVLT) * (Brandt, 1991)	Word learning
Brief Visuospatial Memory Test-Revised (Benedict and Groninger, 1995)	Visual (shape) memory
Color Trail Making (D'Elia et al., 1989)	Visual scanning, mental flexibility
Controlled Oral Word Association Test * (Benton and Hamsher, 1978)	Word Fluency, word retrieval
Penn State Cancellation Test (Echemendia, 1999)	Visual scanning, attention
Symbol Digit Modalities (Smith, 1982)	Visual scanning, immediate memory
Delayed recall from HVLT	Delayed recall for words

*Suggested for English speaking athletes only.

In addition to the neuropsychological tests utilized in the NHL test battery, the neuropsychologist should be careful to evaluate non-cognitive symptoms of concussion. To this end, the NHL program utilizes a *Symptom Self-Rating* Inventory, which is administered at the time of the initial evaluation and at every subsequent follow-up evaluation.

The Role of Neuropsychological Assessment in Return to Play Decisions

The decision to return a hockey player to the ice following a concussion should be made only after carefully consideration of a number of factors and the evaluation of the player's medical history, concussion symptoms and performance on neuropsychological testing. Although there is no simple formula for making return-to-play decisions and these decisions should be made on an individual basis, we will provide a general framework for making these difficult decisions. The neuropsychologist plays an important role as members of the team of professional who make return to play decisions.

Player concussion history

The team neuropsychologist, physician or athletic trainer should gather a complete concussion history of all athletes under his or her care. Although this issue is still actively debated, it has been suggested that multiple concussions may result in permanent brain injury and resulting disability (Gronwall & Wrightson, 1975; Collins et al., 1999; Collins et al., 2002). Although there is currently no absolute cutoff point at which a player should no longer compete, our experience with professional athletes has suggested that athletes who sustain multiple concussions within the same season may be at increased risk for permanent disability. Therefore, the player's concussion history should be taken into consideration when return to-play decisions are being made and athletes who have suffered multiple concussions should be evaluated particularly carefully.

Performance on initial rink side cognitive screening

The athlete should be evaluated utilizing mental status evaluation or cognitive screening such as the rink-side cognitive screening evaluation described earlier. This type of brief testing should ideally be incorporated into the player's pre-season baseline assessment to assure that the athlete can pass the screening items prior to injury. Specifically, the player should be evaluated for amnesia for events occurring before the injury (*retrograde amnesia*) and after the injury (*post-traumatic amnesia*). Additionally, the athlete should be evaluated for disruption of orientation and attentional processes. In general, the items that comprise the rink-side screening evaluation are sufficiently simple that athletes should be expected to complete all items successfully. If the player fails this evaluation, he should be observed and formal neuropsychological testing should be recommended.

Evaluation of post-concussion symptoms

At the NHL level, the player's post-injury symptoms as measured initially at rink side via the mental status card and by the concussion symptom inventory at the time of the neuropsychological evaluation. The athlete's report of symptoms should be evaluated both at rest and following exertional activities such as riding a stationary bicycle. If the player remains asymptomatic during this type of activity, we recommend re-evaluation of the player's symptoms during and following non-contact skating, prior to returning the athlete to play.

Neuropsychological test results

Neuropsychological testing has proven to be sensitive to even variations in neurocognitive function in athletes and represents the one of the most sensitive methods of documenting changes in cognitive processes following concussion (Hinton-Bayre, Geffen, McFarland, & Friis, 1999; Lovell & Collins, 1998; Lovell et al., 2003). However, at the current time exact standards for determining readiness to play have yet to be derived and each athlete's performance should be evaluated individually. Our experience with professional athletes has indicated that test performance following a concussion is variable depending on the nature of the injury (i.e. blow to the head vs. deceleration injury), severity of injury, and the players concussion history). We suggest that *any decline* in test performance following a concussion should be viewed as potentially significant. Although this strategy may eventually prove to be somewhat conservative, the adverse consequences of returning an athlete to the ice prematurely following a concussion argue for caution in medical decision-making.

Important Research Questions

In addition to providing important clinical data to the team physician, the NHL program has been structured to help to answer a number of important questions regarding sports-related concussion. This project should eventually allow the NHL to track the rate of concussion for season-to-season, team-to-team and conference-to-conference and will promote science-based decision-making. In addition, one of the primary goals of this project is to help answer basic return-to-play questions such as: 1). How long should an athlete wait to return to maximize safety or prevent further injury? 2) How many concussions during any given season that should result in termination of play for that season; 3) what specific criteria should be utilized in making return-to-play decisions? For instance, is loss of consciousness an important factor in determining recovery or other factors such as duration of amnesia or concussion symptoms relatively more important?

Although not a stated goal of the NHL program, this project may eventually help to clarify issues regarding the myriad of existing concussion management guidelines. More specifically, large-scale projects such as the NHL concussion program hopefully will eventually yield evidence-based concussion strategies, which are based on a number of factors including the results of neuropsychological testing.

Additionally, the NHL concussion project will promote a better understanding of the role of neuropsychological testing in the assessment of athletes. The project will specifically answer questions such as: 1) which neuropsychological tests are sufficiently reliable and valid to allow their continued and more widespread use throughout organized athletics? What neuropsychological cutoff scores should be utilized in making return to play decisions and what confidence intervals will be utilized? and; 3) to what extent do players' self-report symptoms correlate with objective neuropsychological test results. As is detailed in Chapter 18 of this volume, the correlation between neuropsychological test results and athlete symptoms self-report is an imperfect one. This dissociation between symptoms and neuropsychological performance may be a function of a variety of factors, which include the involvement of both neurological and non-neurological processes (e.g. brain vs. vestibular systems), limitations of current testing or other processes. Hopefully, the NHL project will help to answer some of these questions in the future.

Summary

This chapter has provided a summary of the NHL concussion program and has focused on important issues regarding the evaluation and management of the concussed hockey player. Given the preliminary nature of this project, a clinical rather than a research perspective has been presented and issues important to clinical decision-making have been discussed. It is hoped that the NHL concussion program will result in a decrease in sport-related concussions and to a better understanding of sports-related concussion. It is also hoped that this project and other like it will promote better evaluation and management strategies for amateur athletes. As noted throughout this chapter, the neuropsychologist has come to play an increasingly important role in clinical decision-making within professional hockey. It is anticipated that this role will continue to evolve over the next decade and beyond.

References

Anderson, P.E. & Lovell, M.R. Testing in Ice Hockey: the expanding role of the neuropsychologists. In J.E. Bailes, M.R. Lovell & J.C. Maroon (Eds.), *Sports-Related Concussion* (pp. 215-225). St. Louis: Quality Medical Publishers.

Aubry, M., Cantu, R., Dvorak, J., Johnston, K., Kelly, J., Lovell, M.R. et al. (the concussion in Sport Group) (CIS). (2002). Summary and agreement statement of the first International Conference on Concussion in Sport. *British Journal of Sports Medicine, 36*, 6-10.

Collins, M.W., Grindel, S.H., Lovell, M.R., Dede, D.E., Moser, D.J., Phalin, B.R. et al. (1999). Relationship between concussion and neuropsychological performance in college football players. *Journal of the American Medical Association, 282*(10), 964–970.
Collins, M.W., Lovell, M.R., Iverson, G.L, Cantu, R., Maroon, J.C., & Field, M. (2002). Cumulative effects of concussion in high school athletes. *Neurosurgery, 51,* 1175–1181.
Gronwall, D. & Wrightson, P. (1975). Cumulative effects of concussion. *Lancet, 2,* 995–997.
Hinton-Bayre, A., Geffen, G.M., McFarland, K., & Friis, P. (1999). Concussion in contact sports: Reliable change indices of improvement and recovery. *Journal of Clinical and Experimental Neuropsychology, 21,* 70–86.
Hovda, D.A., Prins, M., Becker, D.P., Lee, S., Bergsneider, M. & Martin, N. Neurobiology of concussion. (1998). In J.Bailes, M.R. Lovell & J.C. Maroon (Eds.), *Sports-Related Concussion.* St. Louis: Quality Medical Publishers.
Johnston, K.M., Lassonde, M., Pito, A. (2001). A contemporary neurosurgical approach to sport-related head injury: The McGill concussion protocol. *Journal of the American College of Surgeons, 192,* 515–524.
Lovell, M.R. (1999). Evaluation of the professional athlete. In J.E. Bailes, M.R. Lovell, & J.C. Maroon (Eds.), *Sports-Related Concussion* (pp. 200–214). St. Louis: Quality Medical Publishers.
Lovell, M.R. & Collins, M.W. (1998). Neuropsychological assessment of the college football players. *Journal of Head Trauma Rehabilitation, 13*(2), 9–26.
Lovell, M.R. & Burke, C.J. (2000). Concussion in the professional athlete: the NHL Program. In R.E. Cantu (Ed.), *Neurologic Athletic Head and Spine Injuries*(pp. 109–116). Philadelphia, W.B. Saunders.
Povlishock, J.T. & Coburn, T.H. (1989). Morphopathological change associated with mild head injury. In H.S. Levin, H.M. Eisenberg & A.L. Benton (Eds.), *Mild Head Injury.* New York: Oxford.

Chapter 14

BOXING

Robert L. Heilbronner
Northwestern University Medical School and
University of Chicago Hospitals

Lisa D. Ravdin
Weill Medical College of Cornell University and
New York Presbyterian Hospital

Introduction

In recent years, an extensive literature has accumulated regarding the health hazards associated with boxing. Research and anecdotal reports have demonstrated that boxers are subject to both acute (e.g. contusions, concussion, intracranial hemmorhages, etc.) and chronic neurologic injuries (e.g. "punch drunk syndrome" or dementia pugilistica). This chapter is not intended to serve as a forum on the moral and ethical issues related to boxing; for that, the reader is referred to a series of articles and editorials published by the Journal of the American Medical Association (Enzenauer, 1994; Haines, 1994; Ludwig, 1986; Lundberg, 1986, 1994; Patterson, 1986; Sammons, 1989). Neither is it meant to be an exhaustive review on the neurologic and psychiatric syndromes associated with boxing, which can be found elsewhere (Jordan, 1987; Mendez, 1995). The intent of this chapter is to provide the practicing clinical neuropsychologist with information about some of the common changes in neuropsychological performance, which are likely to occur as a result of engaging in amateur and professional boxing.

The following areas will be presented: a) epidemiology of boxing deaths and acute neurologic injuries; b) the biomechanics and pathology of a punch; c) the effects of multiple subconcussive head blows; d) neuropsychological syndromes in boxing (e.g., acute neurologic injuries; groggy states; and chronic traumatic brain injury); e) risk factors associated with chronic traumatic brain injury (cTBI) in boxers; and f) a review of neuropsychological studies on professional and amateur boxers.

Epidemiology

In 1980, there were estimated to be about 5,000 professional boxers licensed in the United States and 25,000 worldwide (Morrison, 1986) although the precise number is unknown. As a sport, boxing is regulated by state or local boxing commissions established under law in 46 states, five territories, and the District of Columbia. In 1983, Georgia, Oklahoma, South Carolina, and Wyoming were the only states not to have boxing statutes (Council on Scientific Affairs, 1983). Licensed boxers are known to move between states for scheduled bouts and there are reports that some of them may fight under assumed names in different states. There is often an incomplete and disorganized exchange of information between many state boxing commissions regarding the identification and medical conditions of these licensed boxers.

There are at least 25,000 amateur boxers in the United States (Council on Scientific Affairs, 1983), many of them teenagers who fight an average of about 20 fights per year and whose careers last approximately five years (Morrison, 1986). About 15,000 of these amateur boxers are registered with the Amateur Boxing Federation (ABF), formerly the National Amateur Athletic Union (AAU) Junior Olympic Boxing Program. An additional 12,500 amateur boxers participate in the Golden Gloves Association boxing program (Council on Scientific Affairs, 1983). In recent years, "tough man" and "tough woman" boxing contests have been staged in various states throughout the country. These contests are poorly organized, are not sanctioned by appropriate state boxing commissions, and they usually involve poorly conditioned, unlicensed amateurs.

Boxing deaths

Deaths from boxing are widely publicized events. Surprisingly, however, the number is actually quite low. Sources of data for fatality rates for boxing are rare, since the exact number of amateurs and professional boxers in the world is unknown. One recent estimate indicates a fatality rate of 0.13 deaths per 1,000 participants per year (Council on Scientific Affairs, 1983). This is lower than or close to the rates of other high risk sports such as college football (0.3); motorcycle racing (0.7); scuba diving (1.1); mountaineering (5.1); hang gliding (5.6); sky diving (12.3); and horse racing (12.8). Gonzales (1951) reviewed deaths resulting from various sports in New York City between 1918 and 1950 and found more deaths occurred in baseball and football than in boxing. McCown (1959) reported only two boxing deaths among 20,505 professional boxers in New York from 1953 to 1977.

Fatalities occur less often among amateurs than professionals. Among 645 fatalities from 1918 to 1983, only one third of them were amateurs. This averages to about 3 deaths per year compared with nine to 10 deaths per year from all boxing. According to one source, the usual cause of boxing deaths was subdural hemorrhage (Payne, 1968). The mechanism of injury is related to the rotational acceleration of the head from a blow sufficient enough to cause a rupture of the bridging or connecting veins. This can result either from the direct effects of the head blow or from sudden impact deceleration of the head against the floor or ringpost (Lampert & Hardman, 1984).

Acute neurologic injuries

There have been a number of epidemiologic studies which have analyzed the frequency of acute neurologic injuries in amateur and professional boxing (Jordan, 1987). The majority of amateur studies indicate that permanent and irreversible neurologic dysfunction rarely occurs. During the years 1981 and 1982, 48 out of a total of 547 bouts (8.7%) in the USA Amatuer Boxing Federation National Championships had to be discontinued because of head trauma (Estwanick, Boitano, & Ari, 1984). A comparable degree of head injuries was reported at the US Military Academy during the period of 1983-1985, where 22 out of the 294 boxing related injuries were head trauma (Welch, Stiler, & Kroeten, 1986). The majority of these occurred during the actual fights more than in practice. In general, it appears that head injuries are not a frequent occurrence in well-supervised boxing programs. Perhaps, this reflects greater safeguards and an increased sensitivity to the potential harm that can result from a direct blow to the head.

Two studies have investigated the frequency of acute neurologic injuries in professional boxers. Mc Cown (1959) observed 325 knockouts (KO's) and 789 technical knockouts (TKO's) among 11,173 participants. Of those KO'd, only ten boxers required hospitalization. Jordan and Campbell (1986) reviewed all acute boxing injuries among professional boxers in New York State from August 1982 through July 1984. There were 376 injuries in 3110 rounds fought, 262 of which were head injuries. This yielded a frequency of 0.8 head injuries per ten rounds and 2.9 head injuries per ten boxers. According to these authors, rarely did the head injury result in neurologic dysfunction, as measured by standard neurologic exam: neuropsychological measures were not included.

From these epidemiologic studies we can conclude that deaths and acute neurologic injuries do occur in boxing, with a greater frequency in the professional ranks. Compared to other competitive sports, however, the number of deaths due to boxing is actually quite low, although the data are imprecise because the exact number of amateurs and professional boxers in the world is unknown. In recent years, there have been fewer deaths and less severe neurologic injuries, at both the amateur and professional level. This may reflect improved safeguards, increased medical supervision, better equipment, and more forced layoffs and retirements. It may also reflect increased awareness on the part of ringside physicians, athletic trainers, and the boxers themselves. Correspondingly, increasingly sensitive methods of assessment, including neu-

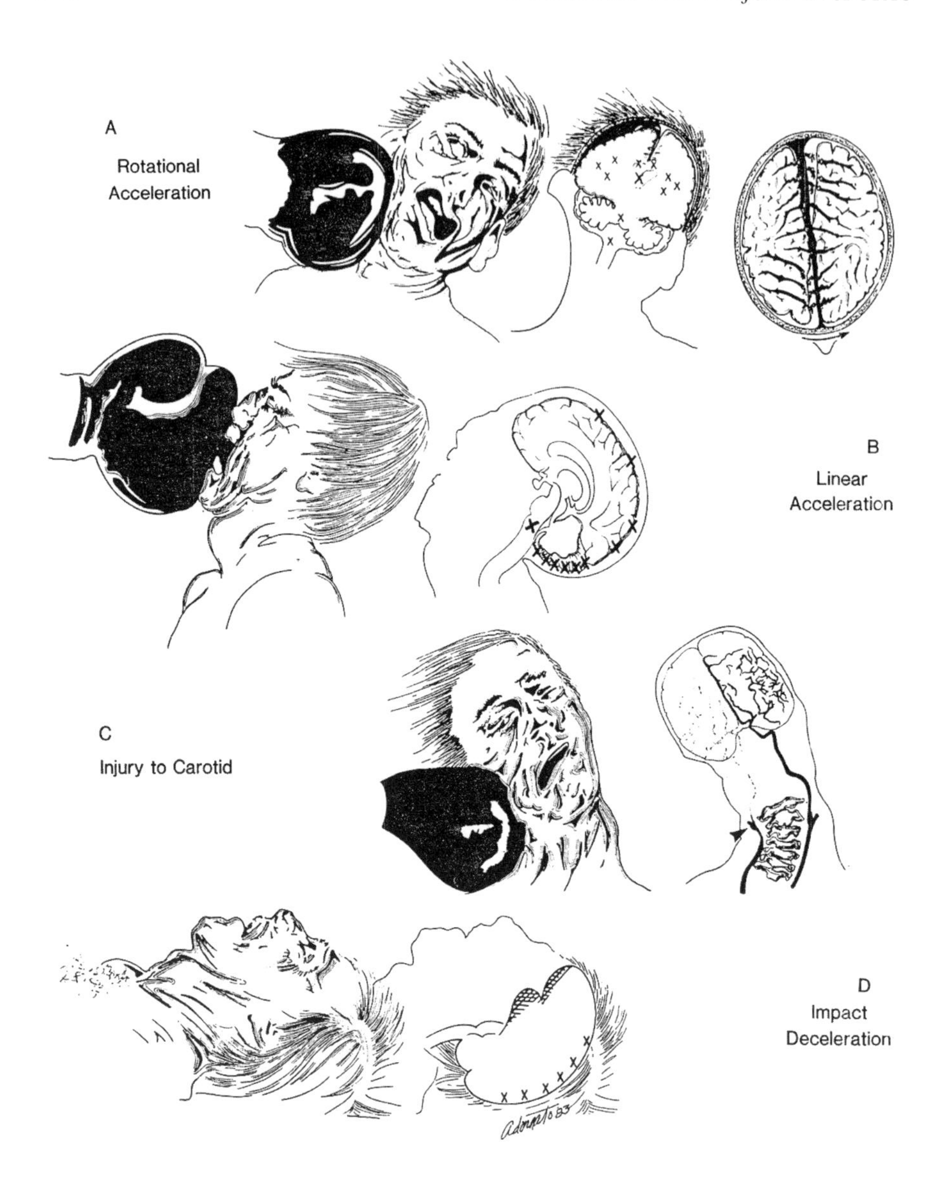

Figure 14.1. Acute brain damage induced by the following. A, Rotational (angular) acceleration causing rotational movement of brain resulting in subdural hematoma by tears of stretched veins and diffuse axonal injury by damage to long fiber tracts in white matter, corpus callosum, and brain stem. B, Linear acceleration of head causing gliding contusions in parasagittal regions of cerebral cortex, ischemic lesions in cerebellum, and axonal damage in brain stem. C, Injury to carotid and compression of carotid sinus cause generalized ischemia of brain. D, impact deceleration of head by falls against ropes or mat causes contrecoup lesions of orbital surface of frontal lobes and tips of temporal lobes as well as gliding contusions.

ropsychological tests, are being used to demonstrate evidence of less obvious indications of brain injury from boxing, especially in professional boxers.

The Biomechanics and Pathology of a Punch

The concussive properties of a punch are related to the manner in which the blow is delivered and how the mechanical forces are transferred and absorbed through the cranium (Jordan, 1987). A punch thrown from the shoulder, such as a roundhouse or hook, tends to deliver more force than a straight forward jab. The force transmitted by a punch is directly proportional to the mass of the glove (which weighs anywhere from 10 to 12oz.) and the velocity of the swing; it is inversely proportional to the total mass opposing the punch (Parkinson, 1982). The essential feature of a punch is that the force must be sufficient enough to accelerate the skull.

Lampert and Hardman (1984) described acute and chronic morphological changes in the brains of boxers and ascribed these changes to different varieties of accelerational forces (Fig. 14.1). *Rotational or angular acceleration* occurs when a punch causes a rotational movement of the skull and the brain lags behind causing the blood vessels to shear and stretch. A groggy fighter who has lost control of his neck muscles presents a head that is most susceptible to this type of acceleration. *Linear acceleration* occurs from blows directly to the face in an anterior to posterior direction. This has been shown to cause gliding contusions and focal ischemic lesions, particularly in the cerebellum (Unterharnscheidt & Sellier, 1971). Sudden acceleration may also produce hyperextension of the neck, known to cause axonal damage in the medullopontine angle and reticular formation, resulting in a KO. *Blows to the neck* can cause injury to the carotid artery. Dissecting aneurysms or occlusions by thrombus may result as well as increased reflex mechanisms causing hypotension and bradycardia associated with decreased blood flow to the brain (Unterharnscheidt & Sellier, 1971). *Impact deceleration* is produced when boxers hit the ropes or mat after a KO. The fall on the back of the head may result in contre-coup contusions of the orbital surface of the frontal lobes and anterior aspects of the temporal lobes. All of these types of acceleration injuries are followed by cerebral edema, increased intracranial pressure, and ischemia (Lampert & Hardman, 1984). With increased pressure, tonsilar herniation may occur and hemorrhagic necrosis at the points of herniation will develop. Death results from ischemia and hemorrhages in the midbrain and upper pons after such herniation. Although head gear used by amateur boxers may minimize the impact of a head blow and reduce the likelihood of facial laceration and contusions, it may actually increase the inertial force of acceleration, especially angular acceleration, through an increase in the surface size around the head. This could conceivably result in more severe concussion.

Results of animal studies indicate that different types of acceleration forces differ in their ability to produce cerebral concussion (Gennarelli et al., 1982).

Rotational acceleration more commonly induces a concussion and diffuse axonal injury whereas linear forces are less likely to promote a KO, but can produce focal damage. Moreover, the centripital forces of rotational injuries do not cause damage to the mesencephalic centers of consciousness as much as the temporal and limbic areas (Ommaya & Gennarelli, 1974). Direct impact to the head is not a requirement of concussion; whiplash injuries have been shown to produce loss of consciousness in animals (Ommaya & Gennarelli, 1974). In a boxing match, the distinction between these different types of acceleration forces becomes blurred because the impact of a punch usually results from a combination of forces and the effects of a whiplash.

Contact phenomena, which can be described as the local mechanical damage to the brain secondary to the impact of a blow, is also an important determinant of brain injury and/or skull fracture (Gennarelli et al., 1982). In boxing, rarely is the impact of a blow sufficient to produce a skull fracture; however, focal brain contusions remain a real possibility. Theoretically, the head gear used by amateur boxers may be important in reducing the impact of a blow and it can reduce the risk of contact phenomenon, although this remains to be demonstrated. Once a boxer is knocked down, and strikes his head on the floor mat, a rapid deceleration (impact deceleration) occurs that can result in contrecoup damage to orbital frontal and anterior temporal cortices.

Infrequently, the acute effect of multiple head blows in a single bout can result in permanent and irreversible brain damage. Subdural hematomas (SDH), which are the most common acute pathologic brain injury in boxing, account for 75% of all acute brain injuries and they are the leading cause of boxing fatalities (Unterharnscheidt & Sellier, 1971). Subdural hematomas usually result from the tearing of bridging veins secondary to acceleration of the skull from a blow (Lampert & Hardman, 1984). Less frequently, acute brain lesions due to boxing include epidural hematomas, subarachnoid hemorrhages, intracranial hemorrhages, and diffuse brain contusions without associated hemorrhages. Intracerebral hemorrhages occur primarily in the parasagittal regions of the cortex and subcortical white matter, deep white matter, the corpus callosum, and cerebellar peduncles (Lampert & Hardman, 1984). Microscopically, acute closed head trauma can result in diffuse degeneration of the cerebral white matter secondary to axonal damage (Stritch, 1956). This diffuse axonal injury (DAI) occurs at the time of the head trauma and is not the result of complicating factors such as hypoxia, brain edema, or increased intracranial pressure (Adams, Graham, Murray, & Scott, 1982). At autopsy, unless DAI is associated with hemorrhages, it can be easily missed (Lampert & Hardman, 1984).

Effects of Multiple Subconcussive Head Blows

Although the knockout punch is usually a goal of the boxer, there is evidence to support the notion that subconcussive head blows may be the real cause of brain injury in boxers, especially the chronic brain damage seen in a subset of boxers with extensive fight histories. In animal studies, using mechanically-produced blows to the head to simulate punches received by a boxer, Unterharnscheidt (1975) demonstrated that the administration of one subconcussive blow produced no behavioral or histopathological lesions. However, multiple subconcussive blows repeated at 5 to twenty second intervals (like in a bout), produced severe permanent brain damage due primarily to circulatory changes. The primary loci of injury included partial or total loss of Purkinje cells and glial proliferation in the cerebellum, and moderate glial proliferation in the white matter of the cerebrum. More severe deficits were produced by increasing the number of head blows; after only 15 head blows, the animals evidenced irreversible weakening of their forelegs. Compared to more severe impacts delivered less often, multiple subconcussive head blows in rapid succession produced more severe brain damage.

Several studies have found a positive relationship between the number of bouts a boxer has fought, and the likelihood of developing neurological, psychiatric, or histopathological symptoms of boxers encephalopathy (Corsellis, Bruton, & Freeman-Browne, 1973; Critchley, 1957; Isherwood, Mawdsley, & Ferguson, 1966; Ross, Cole, Thompson, & Kim, 1983). In a study conducted by Casson et al. (1982), CT abnormalities (mostly cortical atrophy) of five of ten active professional boxers correlated with the number of bouts fought. None of the boxers were knocked out more than twice in their career, leading the authors to conclude that the number of bouts-brain damage relationship was likely due to the cumulative effects of subconcussive head blows. Evidence suggests that the cumulative effects of multiple subconcussive blows is the likely mechanism by which chronic brain damage in boxers is produced (Jordan, Jahre, Hauser et al., 1992a,b). The neuropathological damage in the brains of boxers (e.g., cavum septum pellucidum; cerebellar abnormalities; cerebral scarring and atrophy; degeneration of specific nuclear groups like the substantia nigra, locus ceruleus, and nucleus basalis of Meynert; and neurofibrillary tangles (Corsellis et al., 1973; Stiller & Weinberger, 1985) is never reported in any other sports, and no other sport involves such a large number of repeated and intentional blows to the head.

Any discussion about repeated head trauma in sports must include the concept of the Second Impact Syndrome (SIS) (Saunders & Harbaugh, 1984). This condition occurs when an athlete sustains a head injury and subsequently receives a second head injury before full resolution of the first symptoms. The second impact may appear minor and it need not occur on the same day. Moreover, the athlete may not even appear injured, but shortly after the bout or game, he may collapse and lose consciousness. Respiratory failure ensues and death may occur (Cantu, 1992). In boxing, it is conceivable that a boxer could sustain a mild concussion, remain in a bout, and then receive a second head blow with more catastrophic consequences. A more likely scenario is the boxer who sustains a concussion in a fight and then fights again (possibly without clearance by physicians or in another jurisdiction) no more than one week later. The immediate cause of death in Second Impact Syndrome is typically brain swelling, increased intracranial pressure and subsequent herniation of either the uncus of the temporal lobe or the cerebellar tonsils through the foramen magnum causing brain stem failure. The apparent physiological mechanism is failure of the autoregulation of cerebral circulation, causing vascular engorgement (Saunders & Harbaugh, 1984).

Results of recent animal research suggests that there is a "critical period" for optimal recovery from a concussion (Prins, Lee, Cheng, Becker, & Hovda, 1996). This is related to the cerebral maturation of the brain, rather than chronological age. Thus, it is important for understanding the Second Impact Syndrome because this is a condition which is reported to occur in individuals no more than 21 years old. It suggests that children who engage in contact sports may be more at risk for the development of this catastrophic condition than adults. As it relates to boxing, this would suggest that amateurs and children who participate in Golden Gloves Boxing tournaments should be monitored closely and that ringside physicians need to clearly be educated about this condition and examine these young boxers after they have sustained a concussion and before they make a determination about when a fighter can return to fight again.

Neuropsychological Syndromes Associated with Boxing

Brain damage from boxing takes three major forms: acute neurologic injuries, groggy states and the postconcussion syndrome, and the punch-drunk syndrome or boxer's chronic traumatic brain injury (cTBI). Most of the research on acute neurologic injuries in boxing results primarily from studies examining professional boxers; those looking at amateur boxers are relatively new and less frequent, but they provide some important insights into who is likely to sustain chronic neuropsychological impairment and when this can be expected to emerge.

Acute neurologic injuries

The knockout is the most common acute neurologic injury in boxing. It is synonymous to a Grade 2 or 3 cerebral concussion and can be defined as "an impairment in neurologic function secondary to mechanical forces that results in either unconsciousness or at least a groggy or dazed state (Jordan, 1987). According to Critchley (1957) the knockout "entails the deliberate and violent production of a state of motor hypotonus and helplessness coupled with a severe-if short lived-disturbance of consciousness. The unconsciousness produced by the knockout blow is rather unusual, being as a rule very abrupt in onset, quite short in duration, and comparatively complete in "recovery." Although there are other causes of knockouts besides a direct blow to the chin, the classical KO usually results from a direct blow to the chin, usually from a rotational force, and the force of the blow is transmitted up and back to the base of the skull, affecting the cerebellum and causing imbalance and unsteadiness so that the boxer is unable to remain standing and falls to the mat.

Jordan et al. (1992) developed a severity rating scale for acute cerebral injury in boxing, which is highly analagous to Blonstein and Clarke's (1957) knockout classification system (Table 14.1). Grade 1 is where the boxer experiences transient neurologic impairment without loss of consciousness that resolves within 10 seconds (i.e., the boxer is not counted out and is allowed to continue); Grade 2 is where the boxer experiences transient neurologic impairment without loss of consciousness that does not resolve within 10 seconds (i.e., the boxer is counted out or the referee stops the bout); Grade 3 is where the boxer loses consciousness with complete recovery within two minutes; and Grade 4 is where the boxer is knocked out and has prolonged neurologic impairments lasting more than two minutes. Of note is the relationship between this classification system used in boxing and the ones established by Cantu (1986) and Kelly, Nichols, Filley et al. (1991) which classified concussion into three grades (they did not separate Grades 3 and 4).

Table 14.1 Severity rating scale for acute cerebral injury in boxing.

Grade	Symptoms
I	Transient neurologic impairment without loss of consciousness that resolves within 10 s (i.e., the boxer is not counted out and is allowed to continue)
II	Transient neurologic impairment without loss of consciousness that does not resolve within 10 s (i.e., the boxer is counted out or the referee terminates the bout)
III	Loss of consciousness with complete recovery within 2 min
IV	Loss of consciousness with prolonged neurologic impairment lasting more than 2 min

The incidence of KO's has been as high as six per every 100 bouts (Council on Scientific Affairs, 1983). It is important to note that these "knockouts" may be an underestimate of the true rate of concussive blows. Most studies have included the classical KO (where the fighter is unable to stand up for ten seconds) and the technical knockout (when a bout is stopped because one of the fighters is unable to continue for various reasons). Given the relative infrequency of the true knockout, the evidence would suggest that it is not the concussive blows to the head which are responsible for the brain damage seen in some boxers, but rather, the subconcussive head blows (Morrison, 1986). This will be discussed in greater detail in the section on "groggy states" and the postconcussion syndrome.

Intracranial hematomas can be demonstrated in boxers, especially with MRI, which is more sensitive than CT for imaging the consequences of brain trauma. For the most part, hematomas themselves are not the major cause of brain damage in boxers. Direct injury to the brain itself and resultant contusions, shear injuries, and cerebral edema account for most of the symptoms. When intracranial hematomas do occur, they are likely to be small and not of sufficient size to compress the brain and cause symptoms by themselves; however, the presence of a hematoma is a clear indication that a significant brain injury has occurred. Another occasional cause of acute brain injury in boxing is dissecting aneurysm of the carotid artery. Sudden flexion of the neck (especially in a tired boxer) can be sufficient to tear the intima of one or both carotid arteries, usually high in the neck near the base of the skull. The tear in the intima can allow blood to dissect under the intima, and the dissection can extend up into the brain. The carotid or middle cerebral artery is usually occluded and a hemispheric infarction results.

Groggy states and the postconcussion syndrome

Intermediate between the KO and the chronic manifestation of multiple head injuries is the "groggy state," more commonly referred to as the postconcussion syndrome. This is a condition where the boxer experiences persistent neurologic symptoms for many days or weeks after a fight. According to Critchley (1957), "as a result of severe battering sustained during a particular contest, the victim develops a mental confusion with subsequent amnesia, together with an impairment in the speed and accuracy of the motor skill represented by the act of boxing." The boxer who is groggy may continue to fight but in a more "automatic fashion" and he may appear to be "out on his feet". After the bout, the he may experience severe headaches, dizziness, imbalance, irritability, fatigue, poor memory, and dysarthria. Most often, the boxer is able to return to his previous level of functioning, but there is evidence to suggest that the accumulation of groggy states can lead to the development of the more chronic punch-drunk state.

Memory and concentration deficits are two of the most common complaints after mild head injury (Rimel, Giordani, Barth, Boll, & Jane, 1981). Studies have shown that memory impairments can occur as the result of a blow that fails to produce a loss of consciousness (Leininger, Kreutzer, & Hill, 1991; Levin, Mattis, Ruff et al., 1987a). Yarnell and Lynch (1973) identified postraumatic short-term memory deficits and delayed retrograde amnesia in football players. They coined the term "ding" amnestic states and felt that such states could prevent consolidation of short-term memories, despite adequate registration and recall ability. Several prognostic variables have been hypothesized to relate to the development of the post-concussion syndrome (Binder, 1986). The effects of a previous head injury is a critical one in that patients with a previous concussion have been shown to do more poorly on a complex serial addition task compared to persons concussed only once (Gronwall & Wrightson, 1975). The number of previous fights a boxer has fought has also shown a relationship to the degree of cortical atrophy on CT scan (Casson et al., 1982). Importantly, this was noted in professional boxers with a career of 20 or more fights. To date, no one has objectively counted the number of head blows incurred by a boxer in a fight and then correlated this to post-fight cognitive test performance. This is an arduous task as it may be difficult to define what constitutes an actual head blow.

Chronic traumatic brain injury

The ataxia, slurred speech, and slowness of thought which constitute Martland's (1928) original description of the punch-drunk syndrome calls to mind the characterization of boxers often depicted in films. In the medical literature, this syndrome has also been referred to as dementia pugilistica (Millspaugh, 1937), chronic progressive traumatic encephalopathy of boxers (Critchley, 1957), chronic traumatic encephalopathy (Mendez, 1995), and most recently, chronic traumatic brain injury (Jordan et al., 1997). The term chronic traumatic brain injury (cTBI) most accurately reflects the origin of the dysfunction (i.e., recurrence of head trauma over a period of time) as well as the fact that deficits can occur before the onset of a pure "dementia." In one of the more thorough investigations of chronic neurologic dysfunction in a randomly selected sample of boxers, Roberts (1969) estimated that only 17% of professional boxers experience the most severe form of this condition.

In general, reports of chronic neurologic dysfunction in amateur boxers include isolated signs and symptoms which are relatively mild in degree (Thomassen et al., 1979). Because of the standard use of head gear as well as shorter and fewer rounds, amateur boxing affords fewer opportunities for the head blows typically associated with persistent neurologic impairment. Kaste et al. (1982) found EEG abnormalities in 4 out of 7 amateur boxers despite their lack of symptoms and normal neurologic exam. Amateur boxers have shown neuropsychological deficits on tests of verbal memory immediately following a bout (Heilbronner, Henry, & Carson-Brewer, 1991); however, it is not known if these deficits persisted beyond the immediate post-match period or to what degree they existed before the fight. Levin et al. (1987b) found a trend toward deficient verbal learning in their sample of amateur boxers with low professional exposure (range = 0-10 bouts); however, performance at six month follow-up was similar to that of controls. In a well designed longitudinal investigation of amateur boxers, Stewart et al. (1994) found that neuropsychological test scores correlated with prior boxing exposure (e.g., number of fights and rounds fought). The methodological advantages of the Stewart et al. study, such as a large sample size, a prospective design, and the control of potentially confounding factors, give weight to these findings. These authors concluded that there may be a latency period before the neurobehavioral sequelae associated with head injury become evident, a hypothesis which is consistent with the theory that prior brain injury increases vulnerability to subsequent neuropathological processes (Cantu, 1992; Carlsson, Svardsodd, & Welm, 1987). Generally speaking, the majority of studies suggest that amateur boxing does *not* lead to the extent and degree of deficits typically associated with cTBI (Brooks, Kupsik, Wilson, S., & Ward, 1987; Butler et al., 1993; Casson et al., 1984; Murelius & Haglund, 1991).

Mild to severe clinical manifestations of cTBI have been observed in numerous investigations of professional boxers. Motor impairments can include dysarthria, cerebellar ataxia, parkinsonism, spasticity, and hyperreflexia (Jordan, 1987). Neuropsychiatric manifestations include personality changes, rage reactions, impulsivity, and childishness (Johnson, 1969; Mendez, 1995). Neuropsychological investigations have documented impairments in memory, speed of information processing, complex attention, and executive functioning (Casson et al., 1984; Drew et al., 1986; Johnson, 1969; Jordan et al., 1996; Kaste et al., 1982; Ross et al., 1987). Evidence also suggests that the presence of cTBI is positively correlated with the frequency and degree of boxing related injuries as measured by number of bouts, sparring exposure, and abnormalities on neuroimaging (Casson et al., 1984; Jordan et al., 1996; Ross et al., 1987).

High exposure to boxing in and of itself is not sufficient to cause cTBI. Factors such as a boxer's style and skills are undoubtedly significant variables in the development of chronic brain damage, yet very difficult to quantify and study systematically. Comorbid conditions (i.e., learning disorders, psychiatric disturbances, substance abuse) can also complicate the initial diagnosis of cTBI. As is the case with most dementing disorders, the neuropsychological deficits of cTBI are indistinguishable from other dementias in their advanced stages and research has also shown similarities in the symptomatology and neuropathology of cTBI and Alzheimer's disease (Rasmusson et al., 1995). But, some (Jordan et al., 1996) believe that the symptoms and neuropathology associated with cTBI of boxing are unique to this condition.

The documentation and measurement of exposure to cerebral trauma in boxing can be problematic and several methodological considerations in the study design should be considered (Table 14.2). Moreover, there are a number of important putative exposure variables that must also be investigated and correlated with neuropsychological impairment (Table 14.3).

A careful review of published studies to date reveals a number of methodological limitations such as lack of, or inappropriate, control groups, combining amateurs with professionals, and no measure or control for premorbid

Tables 14.2. Methodological considerations in the documentation and measurement of exposure to boxing-associated cerebral trauma.

Reliability of putative variables of boxing exposure in predicting trauma
Assessment of boxing-related cerebral trauma during sparring
Type of neurologic injury and the sample population of boxers
- Acute neurologic injury in active boxers
- Chronic neurologic injury in active boxers
- Chronic neurologic injury in retired boxers

Method of data collection
- Retrospective
- Prospective

Tables 14.3. Putative variables to measure boxing-related cerebral trauma.

Total number of fights
Number of knockouts experienced
Number of losses
Duration of boxing career
Fight frequency
Age of retirement from boxing
Age of initial participation in boxing

abilities. Further, boxers at various stages of their careers (some retired, others still active) are often included in studies on cognitive functioning without controlling for exposure to the sport, a variable shown to be associated with presence of impairment (Jordan et al., 1996; Jordan et al., 1997). As an example, a boxer with only one bout and another with as many as greater than one hundred bouts may be included in the same sample. Young active fighters may not have had enough boxing exposure to elicit objective deficits. By the same token, studies of active pugilists that include those with substantial careers may be misleading because of a selection bias against any who may have already retired secondary to boxing related impairment. Interpretation of neuropsychological test scores in professional boxers may be further complicated by the fact that, as a group, these individuals tend to have fewer years of formal education than other athletic controls and than the population in general.

Risk Factors Associated with CTBI in Boxers

Sports related head trauma, particularly the kind of repetitive trauma observed in boxers, is of increasing concern given accumulating evidence which suggests a possible association between a history of head trauma and the development of dementia later in life (Heyman et al., 1984; Mayeux et al., 1995; Mortimer, 1985; Nicoll, Roberts, & Graham, 1995). In fact, the concept of dementia pugilistica is often referred to as evidence in support of the hypothesis that head trauma is a risk factor for AD or dementia in general. Gedye et al. (1989) found that only a head injury severe enough to cause symptoms beyond the acute phase (i.e., with greater than momentary loss of consciousness) predicted dementia. Furthermore, more severe injuries were associated with an earlier age of onset of cognitive decline. Calne et al. (1986) posited that late life dementia results from the combined disability of damage sustained by injury with that of age-related neuronal loss. That is, in order to develop cTBI, a critical number or percentage of functional neurons must be damaged or experience cell death. A boxer who ends his boxing career and has experienced some neuronal loss may not exhibit signs of cTBI because there remains a critical number or percentage of functioning neurons. But, as he ages and experiences the normal neuronal dropout associated with aging, he may develop clinical signs of dementia because he has less than the critical level of functioning neurons. This would explain why, in many cases, cTBI appears after the end of a boxing career (Jordan, 1993).

Recent research indicates that genetic factors, more specifically the APOE genotype, may place some boxers at increased risk for the development of cTBI (Jordan et al., 1997). APOE-e4 is a genetic susceptibility factor for late-onset Alzheimer's disease (Roses et al., 1996). Evidence suggests that APOE-e4 individuals with a positive history of head trauma are at increased risk for dementia as compared to e-4 carriers with no prior head trauma (Mayeux et al., 1995). In the Jordan et al study (Jordan et al., 1997), all boxers with severe cTBI possessed at least one copy of the APOE-ε4 allele. A dose effect similar to that observed between APOE genotype and Alzheimer's disease has also been observed in non-boxing head trauma patients where all individuals homozygous for the e4 allele were severely disabled at 6 months follow-up (Teasdale, Nicoll, Murray, & Fiddes, 1997). These studies suggest that the presence of the APOE-ε4 allele may be prognostic of a poor outcome following head injury. Further research may uncover environmental factors other than boxing exposure that interact with genes and increase vulnerability to dementia.

A Review of Neuropsychological Studies on Boxers

Professional boxers

There are only a few published studies which have examined the neuropsychological functioning of professional boxers. One of the first published accounts using a multidisciplinary approach was a case series of 17 retired professional boxers using EEG's, AEG's (air-encephalograms), and psychological tests (Johnson, 1960). Results demonstrated that 11 of the boxers exhibited deficits in attention, concentration, memory, and learning ability. Johnson also described five psychiatric syndromes which occurred in boxers traumatic encephalopathy: a chronic amnestic state, dementia, morbid jealousy syndrome, rage reactions and psychosis. He concluded that "the neurological aspects of encephalopathy are due to local neuronal damage in the upper brain stem, and that it probably derives from the repeated rotational torque to which the brain stem is subjected in repetitive head blows in boxing." This is a view which is consistent with contemporary theories about the hypothesized cause of brain damage in some boxers. Three of the boxers in Johnson's study also had neuropathological changes which resembled those seen in Alzheimer's disease.

Kaste et al. (1982) evaluated 14 European boxers, all of whom had been at least national champions: 8 of them were amateurs and 6 were professionals. They looked at CT scans, EEG's, neurological exams, and neuropsychological tests, including some commonly used measures (e.g., subtests from the WAIS,

WMS, the Wisconsin Card Sorting Test, Trailmaking, Benton's Visual Retention Test, and the Purdue Pegboard). CT scans were abnormal in four of the six professionals and one amateur. Twelve of the boxers had "psychological test results which suggested brain injury" (e.g., a slower time than normal on Trailmaking). In the remainder of the tests, the average scores of the boxers did not differ from normal controls. Two professionals had definite deviations from normal: one performed below normal on all tests and the other one had low scores on tests reflecting slow and inflexible learning. Based upon the results, the authors concluded that, although intellectual performance eventually returns to normal after two concussions, the effects of repeated concussions are cumulative, and for each boxer there is a limit beyond which recovery is not complete. Again, this is consistent with contemporary views on boxing. This study was flawed by a failure to report mean scores, state criteria for test abnormality, and the authors did not conduct a statistical analysis of the data.

Casson et al. (1984) evaluated 13 former professional boxers, two active professionals, and three active Golden Gloves boxers. Eighty-seven percent of the former and active professionals had abnormal results on at least two of four tests (EEG, CT scan, neurological exam, neuropsychological tests) and all of the boxers had more than one abnormal neuropsychological test score. Boxers with abnormal CT scans had significantly higher mean impairment indices than those with normal CT scans, and boxers with abnormal EEGs had higher mean impairment indices than those with normal EEGs. The impairment index also correlated significantly with the number of professional fights, but not with the number of knockouts or episodes of amnesia. The authors supported the use of neuropsychological tests in the study of brain damage in boxers and they advocated the use of such tests on a periodic basis as a means by which to detect the early signs of encephalopathy at a potentially reversible stage.

Drew et al. (1986) compared 19 active professional boxers to 10 matched control athletes utilizing a complete neuropsychological test battery. Fifteen of the 19 boxers scored in the impaired range on the Reitan Impairment Index (compared to 2 of the controls) and boxers were more impaired than controls on all tests except Seashore Rhythm, Finger Tapping, and the Category Test. The authors concluded that both the number of professional bouts and number of professional losses plus draws correlated highly with boxers' deficits. Amateur bouts and amateur losses plus draws showed no significant correlations. The importance of this study is that it was the first to include a matched control group and it also eliminated the effects of one of the more confounding influences affecting neuropsychological test results by excluding any boxer who was known to have abused drugs or alcohol.

Jordan et al. (1996) looked at the relationship between a history of sparring and cognitive functions in 42 professional boxers. They included a fairly comprehensive battery of neuropsychological tests and they also used a questionnaire to assess the degree of boxing "exposure" in both competition and sparring. The boxers had an average of 10 professional fights and most of them engaged in only one sparring bout per day (ranging from 1 to 7 days per week). Seventeen boxers had CT scans that showed borderline brain atrophy: six of them had cavum septum pellucidum. In general, correlations between boxers' neuropsychological test performance and their age, amateur or professional boxing record, duration of career, and history of TKO's/KO's were nonsignificant. But, various indices of increased sparring exposure were inversely related to test scores, mostly reflected in dysfunction on tests measuring attention, concentration, and memory. The authors concluded that, sparring, not competition, is associated with poorer cognitive functions in professional boxers and that future studies should include an assessment of the amount of time and intensity of sparring. Neuropsychological tests measuring planning, attention and concentration, and memory were felt to be the most sensitive measures of brain damage in boxers and they correlated well with the focal abnormalities evident on CT scans.

Amateur boxers

There have been eight studies which have investigated the neuropsychological test performance of amateur boxers. Thomassen et al. (1979) compared 53 former champion amateur boxers with a control group consisting of 53 former football (soccer) players. The median length of a boxing career was 8 years, 11 years had passed since they retired, and the boxers engaged in an average of 10 fights per year. Subjective complaints, neurologic findings, and EEG changes were identical in the boxers and control group. Neuropsychological tests were felt to reveal more dysfunction (than the other medical tests), but after statistical corrections for education, age, and vocabulary, differences between the two groups were not significant, except for one subtest which showed slight motor dysfunction of the left hand in boxers. No relation between abnormal findings and "occupational exposure" during the boxing career could be demonstrated, not even by comparing three pairs of identical twins! The authors felt that the results from their study did not provide a basis for legislation against amateur boxing and that existing safety precautions protected the boxers against serious and permanent brain damage.

In a study of 20 active amateur boxers, McLatchie et al. (1987) used clinical neurological examinations, EEG's, CT scans, and neuropsychological tests with 20 active amateur boxers and they compared the neuropsychological test results to a control group of orthopedic outpatients with limb fractures. The neuropsychological tests they used were based upon the assumption that boxing may cause damage of the kind found in minor head injury (i.e., deficits in learning and memory, and various aspects of attention). Neurological abnormalities were noted in 7 of the boxers, 1 had an abnormal CT scan, and EEG's were abnormal in 8 of them. Of the boxers with EEG abnormalities, 4 had abnormal clinical exams. Nine of the 15 boxers had poor performance on two or more of the clinical neuropsychological measures and they performed more poorly on a word learning task and on the copy and immediate recall of a complex figure: they did not differ on any of the other measures. Boxers also had significantly faster movement times and slower complex reaction times compared to a group of university students. The authors suggested that neuropsychological tests were the best method for detecting neurological dysfunction in active amateur boxers, but they cautioned against attributing these abnormalities to solely to the effects of boxing.

Brooks et al. (1987) investigated the neuropsychological performance of 29 amateur boxers and 19 controls (11 of whom were prospective amateur boxers in training, but not sparring) matched for age, ethnicity, and education. A comprehensive battery of neuropsychological tests was utilized. Results revealed no evidence of significantly impaired neuropsychological test performance in boxers compared to controls. Within the boxing group, however, a variety of features of boxing history (e.g., number of KO's, duration of career) were examined as possible predictors of cognitive test performance. None of these features were significant predictors of lower cognitive performance in this sample of boxers. The authors opined that carefully controlled duration amateur boxing may indeed be neuropsychologically safe. In Scotland where the study occurred, if any boxer receives a severe blow to the head during sparring he is immediately stopped from boxing and sparring for 28 days. This is important in light of the findings of Jordan and colleagues (Jordan et al., 1996) which showed a relationship between sparring and cognitive test performance. On of the limiting factors of this, and other amateur studies, is subject self-selection, i.e., those boxers who refuse to participate may have a subjective awareness of impairments: those who participate are often younger and engage in boxing for shorter periods of time.

Levin and colleagues (1987b) compared the neurobehavioral functioning of 13 boxers with extensive amateur careers and a limited number of professional fights to a group of matched controls. Their results revealed more proficient verbal learning in controls, whereas delayed recall and other measures of memory did not differ between groups. Reaction time was faster in the boxers than controls, but no other differences were significant. There were no differences in scores between the boxers and controls nor in the magnitude of improvement from baseline to testing 6 months later, although boxers' reading scores at follow-up still tended to be lower than controls. This may reflect the effects of a premorbid learning disability, which is an important factor to consider given recent research which has documented a relationship between learning disability and performance on select neuropsychological measures following concussion in football players (Collins et al., 1999). Magnetic resonance imaging disclosed normal findings in the boxers. The authors concluded that young boxers may escape disabling brain injury provided that their total ring exposure is limited both in frequency and total duration.

In the first study designed to measure cognitive functions both within and between subjects following a bout, Heilbronner, Henry and Carson-Brewer (1991) tested 23 active, amateur boxers before and after a boxing match. They included a 20 minute screening battery that incorporated measures of new learning and memory, attention and concentration, thinking and motor speed, sequencing and cognitive flexibility. Compared to their pre-fight performance, boxers demonstrated significant deficits in verbal and incidental symbolic memory, but enhanced executive and motor functions after the fight. A comparison of test scores between winners and losers did not reveal any significant differences. Of note is the fact that the four boxers with the most extensive fight histories all demonstrated slower dominant hand tapping speed after the fight compared to their prefight speed and compared to the other boxers. This suggested a possible correlation between length of boxing career and neuropsychological impairment. Limitations of this study include a failure to calculate the number of subconcussive head blows and a lack of a matched control group of boxers who engaged in exercise for a time period equivalent to a three round boxing match.

Murelius and Haglaund (1991) also found differences in motor speed in their sample of amateur boxers with extensive boxing histories. In this retrospective study, cognitive functioning in former amateur boxers was compared to that of soccer players and track and field athletes. Boxers were divided into two groups based on their boxing exposure: high match boxers (mean number of bouts=59.6, range 25-230) and low match boxers (mean number of bouts=5.5, range 0-15). The only statistically significant difference between the groups was on nondominant finger tapping speed. These results are consistent with the results of Thomassen et al. (1979) as outlined above. Since most of the boxers tested reported that they often relied on their nondominant hand for throwing the majority of the punches, the findings were interpreted as likely reflecting a peripheral rather than central nervous system deficit.

In an effort to assess both the acute and long-term neuropsychological consequences of amateur boxing, Butler and colleagues (1993) examined cognitive functioning pre-bout, immediate post-bout, and two years following the event. Eighty-six amateur boxers and 78 athletic controls (31 water polo and 47 rugby players) underwent neuropsychological testing, neurologic and ophthalmic assessments. Cognitive testing consisted of tests from the British Ability Scales, a serial addition task, and immediate and delayed recall of words and visual stimuli. Participants in all groups showed significant improvements in the immediate post-test, and these improvements were maintained at follow-up at two years. Compared to the other athletes, boxers showed the greatest improvements on timed tasks, such as serial addition, visual scanning, and speed of information processing. Neither prior boxing exposure or number of head blows during the bout were associated with neuropsychological test performance. The authors acknowledged that practice effects likely contributed to the findings of improvement post bout. Based on the lack of differences between boxers and other athletic controls, the authors concluded that there are no significant cognitive deficits associated with amateur boxing.

The first prospective investigation of amateur boxers was conducted in six US cities from 1986-1990 to determine whether changes in central nervous system (as evaluated by neurologic exam, EEG's, brainstem auditory evoked responses, and a battery of neuropsychological tests) function over a 2 year interval were associated with amateur boxing (Stewart et al., 1994). A total of 484 boxers were examined at baseline and 81.2% were re-examined 2 years later. Results showed very few statistically significant odds ratios between exposure (defined by number of bouts, sparring years, and sparring with a professional boxer) and change in function. Significant trends were found between the total number of bouts incurred before the baseline exam and changes in memory, visuoconstructional ability, and perceptual/motor ability and no significant associations were found between more recent bouts (after the baseline visit) and any functional domains, nor between bouts or sparring and any other outcome measures. In general, this study provided supporting evidence than an increased number of bouts in the past is associated with diminished performance in selected cognitive domains, but none of the observed changes were felt to be clinically significant.

Summary

Studies on the neuropsychological/neurobehavioral effects of amateur boxing are in their relative infancy, especially when they are compared to those examining professional boxers. With time, improved methodology, and through an examination of critical "exposure" variables, greater insight into the potential effects of repeated subconcussive head blows on a boxer's neuropsychological abilities can be determined. There is not doubt that neuropsychological tests have proven to be the most sensitive measures of brain dysfunction in both amateur and professional boxers. Thus, as a discipline, clinical neuropsychology has demonstrated its sensitivity and its value in this particular arena of sport. We suggest that boxers should be tested longitudinally over an extended period of time or at least serially after repeated concussive or subconcussive head blows in order to monitor changes in their cognitive status before significant and irreversible damage becomes a reality. It is unlikely that a single boxing bout will lead to irreversible and permanent brain damage. But, specific variables such as the number and frequency of head blows, velocity of punches, etc., should by analyzed in order to gain a clearer understanding of whether or not there is a critical number of fights, knockouts, or punches from which a boxer's cognitive reserve may be compromised.

Future Directions

Neuropsychological tests have proven to be the most sensitive measure of brain dysfunction in studies of both amateur and professional boxers. Future studies aimed at identifying critical "exposure" variables may provide even greater insight into the potential neuropsychological effects of repeated subconcussive head blows. It is unlikely that in most cases, a single boxing bout will lead to irreversible and permanent brain damage. However, analysis of relevant factors such as the number and frequency of head blows and velocity of punches may help to gain a clearer understanding of whether or not there is a critical number of fights, knockouts, or punches which compromise a boxer's cognitive reserve.

There is great debate in the medical community regarding whether boxing should be banned. We recommend that the data obtained from neuropsychological studies on boxers be used to improve safety standards in the sport. Medical requirements for boxers set forth by the various boxing commissions vary a great deal from state to state. In New York, probably the strictest state in terms of medical requirements for active professionals, boxers must undergo serial CT scans, an EEG, and a neurologic exam in order to maintain their license. Given that neuropsychological testing has been shown to be sensitive to sports-related head injuries in cases where other medical exams (i.e., neuroimaging and neurologic exam) are unremarkable, serial assessments would serve as an objective measure to monitor changes in cognitive status throughout a boxer's career. Systematic monitoring of cognition in boxers would allow for appropriate interventions before significant and irreversible neurologic dysfunction becomes a reality.

Acknowledgement

Tables 14.1–14.3 are taken from B. Jordan (Ed.), Medical Aspects of Boxing, with permission from CRC-Press.

References

Adams, J.H., Graham, D.I., Murray, L.S., & Scott, G. (1982). Diffuse axonal injury due to nonmissile head injury in humans: an analysis of 45 cases. *Annals of Neurology, 12*(6), 557–563.

Binder, L.M. (1986). Persisting symptoms after mild head injury: a review of the post-concussive syndrome. *Journal of Clinical and Experimental Neuropsychology, 8*(4), 323–346.

Blonstein, J., & Clarke, E. (1957). Further observations on the medical aspects of amateur boxing. *British Medical Journal, I*, 362–364.

Brooks, N., Kupsik, G., Wilson, L.S.G., & Ward, R. (1987). A Neuropsychological study of active amateur boxers. *Journal of Neurology, Neurosurgery, and Psychiatry, 50*, 997–1000.

Butler, R.J., Forsythe, W.I., Beverly, D.W., & Adams, L.M. (1993). A prospective controlled investigation of the cognitive effects of amateur boxing. *Journal of Neunerology, Neurosurgery, and Psychiatry, 56*, 1055–1061.

Calne, D., Eisen, A., & McGreer, E. et al. (1986). Alzheimer's disease, Parkinson's disease, and motoneurone disease: A biotrophic interaction between aging and environment? *Lancet, ii*, 1067.

Cantu, R.C. (1992). Second Impact Syndrome: Immediate Management. *Physician and Sports Medicine, 20*, 55–66.

Carlsson, G.S., Svardsodd, K., & Welm, L. (1987). Long term effects of head injury sustained during life in three male populations. *Journal of Neurosurgery, 67*, 197–205.

Casson, I., Sham, R., Campbell, E., Tarlau, M., & DiDomenico, R. (1982). Neurological and CT evaluation of knocked-out boxers. *Journal of Neurology, Neurosurgery, and Psychiatry, 45*, 170–174.

Casson, I., Siegel, O., Sham, R., Campbell, E., Tarlalu, M., & DiDomenco, R. (1984). Brain damage in modern boxers. *Journal of the American Medical Association, 251*, 2663–2667.

Collins, M.W., Grindel, S.H., Lovell, M.R., Dede, D.E., Moser, D.J., & Phalin, B.R. et al. (1999). Relationship between concussion and neuropsychological performance in college football players. *Journal of the American Medical Association, 282*, 964–970.

Corsellis, J., Bruton, C., & Freeman-Browne, D. (1973). The aftermath of boxing. *Psychological Medicine, 3*, 270–303.

Council on Scientific Affairs. (1983). Brain injury in boxing. *Journal of the American Medical Association, 249*(2), 254–257.

Critchley, M. (1957). Medical aspects of boxing, particularly from a neurological standpoint. *British Medical Journal, 1*, 357–362.

Drew, R., Templer, D., Schuyler, B., Newell, T.G., & Cannon G. (1986). Neuropsychologic deficits in active licensed professional boxers. *Journal of Clinical Psychology, 42*, 520–525.

Enzenauer, R.W. (1994). Let's stop boxing in the Olympics and the US military. *Journal of the American Medical Association, 272*(23), 1821.

Estwanick, J.J., Boitano, M., & Ari, N. (1984). Amateur boxing injuries at the 1981 and1982 USA/ABF national championship. *Physicians Sports Medicine, 12*, 123–128.

Gedye, A., Beattie, B., Tuokko, H., Horton, A., & Korsarek, E. (1989). Severe head injury hastens age of onset of Alzheimer's disease. *Journal of the American Geriatrics Society, 37*, 970–973.

Gennarelli, T.A., Thibault, L.E., Adams, J.H., Graham, D.I., Thompson, C.J., & Marcincin, R.P. (1982). Diffuse axonal injury and traumatic coma in the primate. *Annals of Neurology, 12*(6), 564–574.

Gonzales, T.A. (1951). Fatal injuries in competitive sports. *Journal of The American Medical Association, 146*(16), 1506–1511.

Gronwall, D., & Wrightson, P. (1975). Cumulative effect of concussion. *Lancet, 2*, 995–997.

Haines, J.D., Jr. (1994). Let's stop boxing in the Olympics and the US military. *Journal of the American Medical Association, 272*(23), 1821.

Heilbronner, R.L., Henry, G.K., & Carson-Brewer, M. (1991). Neuropsychologic test performance in amateur boxers. *American Journal of Sports Medicine, 19*, 376–380.

Heyman, A., Wilkinson, W.E., Stafford, J.A., Helms, M.J., Sigmon, A.H., & Weinberg, T. (1984). Alzheimer's disease: a study of epidemiological aspects. *Annals of Neurology, 15*(4), 335–341.

Isherwood, I., Mawdsley, C., & Ferguson, F.R. (1966). Pneumoencephalographic changes in boxers. *Acta Radiol Diagn, 5*, 654–661.

Johnson, J. (1960). Organic psychosyndromes due to boxing. *British Journal of Psychiatry, 115*, 45–53.

Johnson, J. (1969). Organic psychosyndromes due to boxing. *British Journal of Psychiatry, 115*, 45–53.

Jordan, B. (1987). Neurologic Aspects of Boxing. *Archives of Neurology, 44*, 453–459.

Jordan, B. (1993). *Chronic neurologic injuries in boxing*. Boca Raton: CRC Press.

Jordan, B., Jahre, C., & Hauser, W. et al. (1992a). Serial computed tomography in professional boxing. *Journal of Neuroimaging, 2*, 181–185.
Jordan, B., Jahre, C., & Hauser, W.A. et al. (1992b). CT of 338 active professional boxers. *Radiology, 185*(2), 509–512.
Jordan, B., Matser, E., & Zimmerman, R. (1996). Sparring and cognitive function and professional boxers. *Physician Sports Medicine, 24*(5), 87–98.
Jordan, B., Relkin, N., Ravdin, L.D., Jacobs, A.R., Bennett, A. & Gandy, S. (1997). Apolipoprotein E e4 associated with chronic traumatic brain injury in boxing. *Journal of the American Medical Association, 276*, 136–140.
Jordan, B.D., & Campbell, E. (1986). Acute boxing injuries among professional boxers in New York State: A two-year survey. *Medicine and Science in Sports and Exercise, 17*, 212.
Kaste, M., Vikki, J., Sainio, K., Kuurne, T., Katevuo, K., & Meurala, H. (1982). Is chronic brain damage in boxing a hazard of the past? *Lancet, 2*, 1186–1188.
Kelly, J.P., Nichols, J.S., Filley, C.M., Lillehei, K.O., Rubinstein, D., Kleinschmidt-DeMasters, B.K. (1991). Concussion in sports: Guidelines for the prevention of catastrophic outcome. *Journal of The American Medical Association, 266*, 867–869.
Lampert, P.W., & Hardman, J.M. (1984). Morphological changes in brains of boxers. *Journal of the American Medical Association, 251*(20), 2676–2679.
Leininger, B.E., Kreutzer, J.S., & Hill, M R. (1991). Comparison of minor and severe head injury emotional sequelae using the MMPI. *Brain Injury, 5*(2), 199–205.
Levin, H.S., Mattis, S., Ruff, R.M., Eisenberg, H.S., Marshall, L.F., & Tabaddor, K. et al. (1987a). Neurobehavioral outcome following minor head injury: A three center study. *Journal of Neurosurgery, 66*, 234–243.
Levin, H.S., Lippold, S.C., Goldman, A., Handel, S., High, W.M., & Eisenberg, H.M. et al. (1987b). Neurobehavioral functioning and magnetic resonance imaging findings in young boxers. *Journal of Neurosurgery, 67*, 657–667.
Ludwig, R. (1986). Making boxing safer: The Swedish model. *Journal of the American Medical Association, 251*, 2696–2698.
Lundberg, G.D. (1986). Boxing should be banned in civilized countries–round 3. *Journal of the American Medical Association, 255*(18), 2483–2485.
Lundberg, G.D. (1994). Let's stop boxing in the Olympics and the United States Military. *Journal of the American Medical Association, 271*(22), 1790.
Martland, H. (1928). Punch drunk. *Journal of the American Medical Association, 91*, 1103–1107.
Mayeux, R., Ottman, R., Maestre, G., Ngai, C., Tang, M.X. , & Ginsberg, H. et al. (1995). Synergistic effects of traumatic head injury and apolipoprotein E epsilon 4 in patients with Alzheimer's Disease. *Neurology, 45*, 555–557.
McCown, I.A. (1959). Boxing Injuries. *American Journal of Surgery, 98*, 509.
McLatchie, G., Brooks, N., Gallbraith, Hutchinson, J.S.F., Wilson, L., Melville, I & Teasdale, E. (1987). Clinical neurological examination, neuropsychology, electroencephalography and computed tomographic head scanning in active amateur boxers. *Journal of Neurology, Neurosurgery, and Psychiatry, 50*, 96–99.
Mendez, M. (1995). The neuropsychiatric aspects of boxing. *International Journal of Psychiatry in Medicine, 25*(3), 249–262.
Millspaugh, J.A. (1937). Dementia pugilistica. *U.S. Naval Medical. Bulletin, 35*, 297.
Morrison, R.G. (1986). Medical and public health aspects of boxing. *Journal of the American Medical Association, 255*(18), 2475–2480.
Mortimer, J.A. (1985). Epidemiology of post-traumatic encephalopathy in boxers. *Minnesota Medicine, 68*(4), 299–300.

Murelius, O., & Haglund, Y. (1991). Does Swedish amateur boxing lead to chronic brain damage? *Acta Neurologica Scandinavica, 83*, 9–13.
Nicoll, J., Roberts, G., & Graham, D. (1995). Apolipoprotein E e4 allele is associated with deposition of amyloid B-protein following head injury. *Nature Medicine, 1*, 135–137.
Ommaya, A.K., & Gennarelli, T.A. (1974). Cerebral concussion and traumatic unconsciousness. Correlation of experimental and clinical observations of blunt head injuries. *Brain, 97*(4), 633-654.
Parkinson, D. (1982). The biomechanics of concussion. *Clinical Neurosurgery, 29*, 131–145.
Patterson, R.H. (1986). On boxing and liberty. *Journal of the American Medical Association, 251*, 2481–2482.
Payne, E.E. (1968). Brains of boxers. *Neurochirurgia (Stuttg), 11*(5), 173–188.
Prins, M.L., Lee, S.M., Cheng, C.L., Becker, D.P., & Hovda, D.A. (1996). Fluid percussion brain injury in the developing and adult rat: A comparative study of mortality, morphology, intracranial pressure and mean arterial blood pressure. *Developmental Brain Research, 95*(2), 272–282.
Rimel, R.W., Giordani, B., Barth, J.T., Boll, T.J., & Jane, J.A. (1981). Disability caused by minor head injury. *Neurosurgery, 9*, 221–228.
Roberts, A. (1969). *Brain Damage in Boxers*. London: Pitman Medical Scientific Publishing Co.
Roses, A., Einstein, G., Gilbert, J., & et al. (1996). Morphological, biochemical and genetic support for an apolipoprotein E effect on microtubular metabolism. *Annals of the New York Academy of Sciences, 777*, 146–157.
Ross, R., Casson, I.O., & Siegel, R. et al. (1987). Boxing Injuries: Neurologic, radiologic, and neuropsychologic evaluation. *Clinics in Sports Medicine, 6*, 41–51.
Ross, R., Cole, M., Thompson, J., & Kim, K. (1983). Boxers-computed tomography, EEG and neurosurgical evaluation. *Journal of the American Medical Association, 249*, 211–213.
Sammons, J.T. (1989). Why physicians should oppose boxing: an interdisciplinary history perspective. *Journal of the American Medical Association, 261*(10), 1484–1486.
Saunders, R.L., & Harbaugh, R.E. (1984). The second impact in catastrophic contact-sports head trauma. *Journal of the American Medical Association, 252*(4), 538–539.
Stewart, W., Gordon, B., Selnes, O., Bandeen-Roche, K., Zeger, S., & Tusa, R.J. et al. (1994). Prospective study of central nervous system function in amateur boxers in the United States. *American Journal of Epidemiology, 139*, 573–588.
Stiller, J.W., & Weinberger, D.R. (1985). Boxing and chronic brain damage. *Psychiatric Clinics of North America, 8*(2), 339–356.
Stritch, S.J. (1956). Diffuse degeneration of the cerebral white matter in severe dementia following head injury. *Journal of Neurology, Neurosurgery and Psychiatry, 19*, 163–185.
Teasdale, G., Nicoll, J., Murray, G., & Fiddes, M. (1997). Association of apolipoprotein E polymorphism with outcome after head injury. *Lancet, 350*, 1069–1071.
Thomassen, A., Juul-Jensen, P., Olivarius, B., Braemer, J., & Christensen, A.L. (1979). Neurological, elcetroencephalographic, and neuropsychological examination of 53 former amateur boxers. *Acta Neurologica Scandinavica, 60*, 352–367.
Unterharnscheidt, F. (1975). Injuries due to boxing and other sports. In P.J. Vinken, G.W. Bruyn, J.A.N. Corsellis (Eds.). *Handbook of Clinical Neurology*. New York: American Elsevier Publishing.
Unterharnscheidt, F., & Sellier, K. (1971). Boxing. Mechanics, pathomorphology and clinical picture of traumatic lesions of the CNS in boxers. *Fortschr Neurol Psychiatr Grenzgeb, 39*(3), 109–151.

Welch, M., Stiler, M., & Kroeten, H. (1986). Boxing injuries from an instructional program. *American Journal of Sports Medicine, 14*, 81–89.

Yarnell, P. R., & Lynch, S. (1973). The 'ding': amnestic states in football trauma. *Neurology, 23*(2), 196–197.

Chapter 15[1]

EQUESTRIAN SPORTS

Donna K. Broshek, Amy M. Brazil, Jason R. Freeman, and Jeffrey T. Barth

Brain Injury and Sports Concussion Institute,
Neuropsychology Assessment Laboratory,
Department of Psychiatric Medicine,
University of Virginia School of Medicine,
Charlottesville,Virginia

Historical Background

Although concern for safety in athletics dates back to Philostratus in the 3rd century A.D. when he warned athletes about the danger of high humidity in hot weather, there was little attention to equestrian safety until the development of the first jockey hat in England in 1963 (McLain, 1997). That same year, the first standards for equestrian headgear were published in Britain (Watt & Finch, 1996). Medical research on equestrian injuries appeared in the 1970s with the first articles published in British and Scandinavian medical journals in 1973 (McLain, 1997). Due to concern about the 19 equestrian related fatalities that occurred in 1982-1983, the Royal Society of Medicine founded the Medical Equestrian Association in 1984 (McLain, 1997). In 1986, the American Medical Equestrian Association (AMEA) was founded as a section of the American Medical Athletic Association, and in 1990, the AMEA was incorporated as an independent organization.

In the United States, there are over six and a half million horses and approximately 10,000 sanctioned equestrian events (Brooks & Bixby-Hammett, 1998). In addition, there are numerous unsanctioned local horse shows.

[1] Special thank you to Dr. Doris Bixby Hammett, Founder of the American Medical Equestrian Association, for her assistance in providing information and resourses for this chapter.

Data from 1992 revealed that more than 12,000 children and adolescents participate in the United States Pony Clubs and nearly a quarter million youths were active in 4-H horse programs (Brooks & Bixby-Hammett, 1998; Lamb, 2000). According to the American Horse Council, there are approximately 27 million riders over the age of 12 and the equestrian industry is a $12.3 billion business (excluding pari-mutuel betting) (Lamb, 2000).

Mechanisms of Injury in Equestrian Sports

Equestrian sports are the only sporting activity involving the cooperation (synergy/symbiosis) between two species (Hamilton & Tranmer, 1993). Part of the sport is anticipating and reacting to the spontaneous and at times unpredictable actions of the horse. Considering that the horse weighs approximately 1,000 to 2,500 pounds and reaches speeds up to 40 miles per hour, the unpredictable nature of the horse creates a risk for serious injury relative to other sports (Brooks & Bixby-Hammett, 1991; Hamilton & Tranmer, 1993). In addition, the rider's head is generally 9-10 feet above ground when mounted. Considering these factors, falling or being thrown from a horse can create tremendous velocity and impact force, resulting in central nervous system injury. The distance involved, along with the obtained velocity and rate of deceleration, can create enough energy to exceed the protective cushioning of the skull, resulting in significant intracranial injury (Brooks & Bixby-Hammett, 1991). Newtonian formulas have been applied to the study of mild head injury and sports concussion (Barth, Varney, Ruchinskas, & Francis, 1999; Varney & Roberts, 1999; Barth, Freeman, Broshek & Varney, 2001). These formulas indicate that the greater the velocity, the larger the masses involved, and the shorter the distance or time across which deceleration occurs during a sports related accident, the greater the potential for traumatic brain injury. Given the information presented above regarding the weight and speed of a horse, along with the rider's distance above the ground, it is clear that equestrian injuries, in which a rider is thrown or falls to the ground, have tremendous potential to cause significant traumatic brain injury.

"Double impact" injuries are one of the most lethal sports injuries and occur when a rider's head strikes the ground and is then kicked or trampled by the horse (Brooks & Bixby-Hammett, 1991). This is not to be confused with second-impact syndrome, described in other chapters in this volume. Crush injuries, which occur when the horse falls and/or rolls on the equestrian, are often fatal (Whitlock, 1999). Equestrian related injuries can also occur while managing or handling a horse or during equestrian sports. Head injuries may result from being kicked, crushed, or trampled by a horse while feeding, shoeing, grooming or otherwise engaging in routine equine management, particularly if the horse is startled (Brooks & Bixby-Hammett, 1998). Neurologic injuries may also occur during foaling. Sources of potential injury are described further below.

Most injuries result from falls or being thrown. When this is associated with subsequent trampling of the rider by a falling or undirected horse, the risk of catastrophic injury increases greatly. Indeed, the mechanism of these injuries is potentially one of the most lethal of all sports-related accidents. Unexpected falls have various causes related to both rider and horse. For example, an experienced rider may be thrown by a less experienced mount refusing to negotiate a complex jump. Alternatively, a less experienced rider may fall when a well-schooled horse takes a jump for which the rider is unprepared. In addition, the horse may lose its footing and fall while turning suddenly and thereby pin or crush the rider beneath it. Another source of potential injury is the rider's foot becoming caught in the stirrup or the rider holding or being entangled in reins after an unexpected dismount and being dragged, with repeated injury to the head, spine, or peripheral nerves (Brooks & Bixby-Hammett, 1998, p. 382).

Risk Factors for Injury in Equestrian Sports

Clearly there are numerous factors affecting the risk of injury, including traumatic brain injury. Inexperience on either the rider or the equine's part, or even unfamiliarity with one another, potentiates the risk for injuries. More importantly, equestrian sports are replete with capricious variables. Dependency on what may be an ephemeral symbiosis, the influence of outside stimuli on both rider and mount, and imperfect timing of highly coordinated, cooperative movements can have devastating consequences given the physics involved. Even aesthetics and appearance can play a role. The head-forward stance adopted in equestrian activities increases the risk of head and spinal injury (Brooks & Bixby-Hammet, 1991; Brooks & Bixby-Hammett, 1998). Most head injuries result from impact injuries, such as the head striking the ground or another object (e.g., tree, fence), although acceleration-deceleration injuries may occur as the rider is ejected from the horse. As a result, both focal and diffuse cerebral injury may result (Brooks & Bixby-Hammett, 1998). The use of headgear may reduce the risk of depressed or linear skull fracture, but rotational and/or acceleration-deceleration forces on the brain are not generally reduced by helmet use. Thus, even helmeted riders may sustain a head injury. Thankfully, however, 80-90% of equestrian related head injuries are cerebral contusions or concussions rather than more serious forms of brain injury (Brooks & Bixby-Hammett, 1991). A neurosurgeon with a practice in an equestrian community (Lexington, KY) estimates that one head injury occurs per 25 equestrian events (Brooks, 2000). An important safety advance is that protective equestrian riding helmets are now radiolucent (Brooks & Bixby-Hammett, 1998). Therefore, to protect the rider from further injury the helmet should not be removed from an unconscious rider until after X-rays have been obtained to rule out cervical fracture.

General Prevalence and Incidence Data

In a three-year review of Emergency Department records conducted at a Pennsylvania trauma center, 80% of equestrian related injuries were due to falls from a horse (Frankel, Haskell, Digiacomo, & Rotondo, 1998). Nearly 50% of the injuries were orthopedic, but closed head injury was the most common diagnosis requiring hospital admission. Approximately 25,710 individuals were estimated to require emergency room admissions in 1997 due to equestrian related injuries (Lamb, 2000). A telephone survey of this patient sample revealed that 36% had previous equestrian injuries, suggesting a risk of cumulative head injuries.

Across equestrian sports, there are differences in the injury rate depending upon the activity (see Table 15.1). Horse trials or events, which involve dressage, cross country, and show jumping phases, have been associated with a high rate of injury (Paix, 1999). Based on data collected in South Australia from 1990–1998, a 0.88% injury incidence rate per competitor per event was calculated for event riders (Paix, 1999). All of the injuries, which were predominately head and neck injuries, occurred during the cross-country phase and most occurred while jumping obstacles. There was a trend for increased injury rates as the difficulty level of competition increased. According to Paix (1999), cross-country equestrian events are "over 70 times as dangerous as horse riding in general" (p. 47). "Eventing" has been described as "one of the most dangerous equestrian sports" (Whitlock, 1999; p. 212). Rodeo, polo, and horse racing have a higher injury rate compared to recreational riding and dressage (Bixby-Hammett & Brooks, 1981).

Although data is available from several state trauma registries, the only comprehensive national figures on equestrian injuries are available through the National Electronic Injury Surveillance System (NEISS), a division of the United States Consumer Product Safety Commission (Hammett, 2000c). According to NEISS data provided by Dr. Hammett, there was a decrease in equestrian related injuries in 1995–1996, followed by an increase in injuries each year from 1997 through 1999. It is not clear if the increase in injuries is due to a greater number of individuals becoming involved in equestrian activities, a greater emphasis on seeking medical care after injury, or a true increased rate of injury (Hammett, 2000c). Although the lower trunk was most frequently involved, injuries to the head constituted the second most frequent injury type with 8,867 head injuries reported in 1999. According to NEISS figures, the largest percent of head injuries relative to the total number of equestrian related injuries occurred in 1998 with the next highest percentage of head injuries occurring in 1995 and 1999. For all years with available data, females have a greater number of horse related injuries than males and females had a higher rate of injury in 1999 than in any previous year since 1992. Injuries to the youngest riders have decreased (ages 0–24), but there has been an increase in injuries to older equestrians (ages 25–64).

Table 15.1. Descriptions of equestrian events/activities.

Dressage: Primarily a competitive discipline in which riders strive to reach different levels of mastery measured by various tests requiring fine movement of the horse. Tests demand a wide range of maneuvers from the simplest riding gaits to intricate and demanding airs and figures of *haute école* ("high school"). Performance of the required test elements, control of the horse, and horse and rider presentation are judged by a jury and points are awarded.

Show jumping: Horse-and-rider teams compete by jumping the same course with a specific number of fences. Fences vary in appearance, structure, and height (three to six feet in novice classes and six feet or higher in advanced classes). Competitions take place in arenas and the series of obstacles are designed for specific shows. Both course completion time and number of jumping faults are taken into account when determining scores.

Hunter trials: A form of competitive show jumping that focuses on speed and maneuverability. Course completion time is the only consideration when determining scores. Jumping faults are added to the time as a penalty.

Flat racing: A form of horse racing in which thoroughbreds are galloped over a "flat" course free of obstacles. The jockey rides crouched forward and out of the saddle.

Steeplechase (National Hunt racing): A form of horse racing in which horses race over a series of relatively easy obstacles – hurdles and fences – at top speed.

Eventing (horse trials; combined training events): An all-around test of horse and rider that incorporates numerous disciplines of competitive equestrian sport into a three- or four-day event. One or two days of a dressage test are followed by a day of speed and endurance testing that includes a steeplechase and cross-country section. During the final day, competitors complete a show jumping course.

Cross-country jumping: Competitions can be held on their own or in conjunction with combined training events. Horse-and-rider teams travel over a given distance (4 ½ miles as part of an eventing competition) and traverse a series of obstacles made of natural materials such as wooden fences and water-filled trenches. Although no obstacle is higher than four feet, they are daunting due to their positioning, how they are combined, and the drop on the landing side. Cross-country stages of eventing competitions must be completed before the maximum time limit and there is no advantage to be gained by arriving early. When held independently, horse-and-rider teams compete by completing the course in the least amount of time. Horses are expected to jump the obstacles without the least bit of hesitation.

Hunt Seat: A discipline extremely popular in the United States and rooted in the British sport of fox hunting. Riders use a hunt-seat saddle, which is a saddle with a seat that is designed for jumping and inclined slightly forward to provide close contact between horse and rider. Competitions are held in arenas and both flat and jumping classes are offered. Fences range from two to four feet in height, depending on the class.

Summary of Detailed Studies of Equestrian Related Head Injury

During a four-year period in the 1990s, 30 patients were admitted to a neurosurgery unit at the University of Kentucky Medical Center due to equestrian-related injuries (Kriss & Kriss, 1997). Of these, 24 admissions were due to head injury. Severe head injury with subsequent herniation was the cause of all fatalities. Sixty percent of the injuries were due to falling from or being ejected from a horse, while 40% of head injuries resulted from being kicked by a horse. Notably, 33% of the patients were injured as bystanders or while handling horses, leading the authors to advise the use of helmets around horses even when not mounted. None of the patients wearing a helmet sustained severe or fatal head injury.

A retrospective review of medical records at three University of Calgary hospitals revealed 156 equestrian-related nervous system injuries that occurred over a six-year period in equestrian sports activities (Hamilton & Tranmer, 1993). Of these injuries, 91% were head injuries and 11 patients died due to severe head trauma. Common injuries included depressed skull fractures, basal skull fractures, linear skull fractures, and hematomas (acute subdural, extradural, and intracerebral). Twenty-two injuries required neurosurgical intervention. Eight of the injuries were also associated with spinal cord injury. Of the 143 head injuries, mild head trauma accounted for 121 of these, most of which involved a brief loss of consciousness and were serious enough to warrant admission for further observation. During the same time period, the medical examiner's office in the same catchment area recorded 14 equestrian related deaths with 11 of those deaths due to severe head trauma.

Hamilton and Tranmer (1993) reported the vast majority of injuries (81%) in their sample occurred during recreational activity with farm or ranch work activity constituting 10.3% of the injuries. Nearly six percent of the accidents involved alcohol use and only two of those injured were wearing protective headgear. The primary mechanism of injury was falling or being thrown from the horse (81% of the total sample) with many patients sustaining additional injury from being kicked, crushed, or dragged by the horse. Being kicked by the horse was the primary source of injury in 18.6% of the accidents. Hamilton and Tranmer (1993) noted that their data likely underestimated the incidence of mild head injury since the majority of those patients would not have presented to a neurosurgical center.

Data gathered over a ten year period by a neurosurgeon with a practice in Lexington, Kentucky, a community rich in equestrian tradition, revealed 234 neurologic injuries with the majority (n=139) occurring during recreational riding (Brooks, 2000). Of those diagnosed with head injury (n=187), concussion (n=83) and cerebral contusion (n=90) were the most frequent injuries. Skull fracture (n=67) and intracranial hematoma (n=35) represented the more severe head traumas. Skull fractures typically occurred in those not wearing protective headgear or improperly fastened headgear. Those patients injured while grooming a horse most frequently sustained depressed skull fractures and none were wearing helmets. Notably, there were no deaths or skulls fractures in those equestrians wearing properly harnessed protective headgear. Some of these individuals, however, did sustain intracranial hematomas, suggesting that helmets provide protection against skull fracture, but do not fully protect against injuries secondary to forces of acceleration-deceleration. Fourteen of those patients who sustained head injuries were not riding at the time of injury, but were kicked in the head while foaling or grooming a horse. Six of these were fatal injuries. Again, none were wearing helmets.

According to data collected by the Justin Sportsmedicine Program, concussion accounted for the greatest number of serious injuries (38%) in professional rodeo athletes (Hammett, 1997). Nearly a third of the injuries sustained over a six-year period (54 event days) during the fixed obstacle cross-country phase were head and face injuries (Whitlock, 1999). Out of a total of 193 injuries and two fatalities, 20 equestrians were admitted to the hospital with head injuries. One of the fatalities resulted from a severe head injury that occurred when the horse fell on the rider.

An investigation into injuries at the University of Virginia Pediatric Emergency Department documented that 32 children under the age of 15 were evaluated for equestrian-related injuries during a two-year period (Bond, Christoph, & Rodgers, 1995). Ten patients were diagnosed with concussion with eight of them sustaining loss of consciousness. One child died following a basilar skull fracture and one child developed an intracranial hemorrhage. Neither of these two children was wearing a helmet. Helmet use was associated with less severe and decreased incidence of head injury.

Based upon a retrospective review of the New Mexico State Trauma Registry, horse-related injuries were the second leading cause of pediatric trauma admissions (n=8) in 1990 (Sapien, 2000). Five of the injuries were caused by horse kicks with the remainder due to falls from a horse. Notably, all of those children kicked in the head (n=4) sustained depressed skull fractures, prompting the physician author to recommend that children wear helmets whenever they are in proximity to horses, regardless of whether they are riding. Another interesting finding in this study was that half of the injured children were Native American, although Native Americans constitute only 10% of the state population. According to the author, Native Americans in rural New Mexico often are involved with the rodeo or livestock management, resulting in an increased risk for horse-related injuries for these children. Educational programs promoting equestrian safety should be tailored and promoted to this potentially high-risk group.

Still Unconvinced about the Value of Wearing Helmets?

A one-year prospective survey in the Oxford catchment area conducted in 1991 revealed that the incidence of equestrian related head injuries decreased nearly fivefold relative to a similar study conducted 20 years earlier (Chitnavis,

Gibbons, Hirigoyen, Parry, & Simpson, 1996). The reduction in injury severity was attributed to the increased use of protective riding helmets across that same time period, as well as improvements in the safety features of helmets.

A five-year study of equestrian injuries in young people was conducted through the United States Pony Clubs (USPC) in the 1980s (Bixby-Hammett, 1987). During the study period, the USPC had 46,531 members between the ages of six to 21 located in 47 states. Of the 160 accidents reported, 130 occurred during riding, 20 were associated with handling, and 10 were not equestrian related. Twenty two percent involved injury to the head or face with 9.9% associated with concussion or unconsciousness. Notably, the horse's behavior (e.g., bucking, refusing to jump) caused 76% of the accidents, highlighting the potential for injury in this collaborative, synergistic sport. In 1999, concussions accounted for 11% of the 81 injuries reported by USPC clubs (USPC Accident Study, 2000). On a positive note, some parents have reported that their children sustained either no or only minor head injury despite a shattered or cracked helmet while participating in USPC activities. USPC members are required to wear helmets when mounted on a horse.

Based on data available from the North Carolina State Medical Examiner, head injury was the cause of death in 60% of the equestrian related fatalities that occurred between 1987 and 1999 (Hammett, 2000b). In contrast to data from NEISS indicating that females have a greater rate of injury, the North Carolina data revealed that males had a significantly high rate of death from horse related activities (Hammett, 2000b; Hammett, 2000c). Nearly three quarters of the deaths occurred to equestrians mounted on a horse with the vast majority of those deaths (85%) due to falls from a horse (Hammett, 2000b). Of those who died from such a fall, head injury was the cause of death in 86% of the recorded cases. A particularly concerning finding is that in those individuals who had blood drawn, an elevated blood alcohol level was found in 43% of those over the age of 17 who died. While national equestrian head injury prevalence data is important, assessing details that are unique to different regions of the country (i.e., states) is important in identifying "at risk" populations as they suggest foci for prevention strategies.

Management Issues following Equestrian Related Head Injury

Another area of great concern is that equestrians who sustain a head injury and immediately return to riding are putting themselves at greater risk for further injury. A questionnaire was distributed to members of the Masters of Foxhounds Association in March of 2000 and asked them to reply if they had fallen and struck their head within the previous two years (Hammett, in press). Of the 197 members who returned completed questionnaires, 59.4% reported an alteration in consciousness after falling with a significant number experiencing confusion or disorientation from five to 30 minutes (25.6%), 30 minutes to one hour (18.8%), and longer than one hour (17.9%). A third of those who fell reported loss of consciousness (LOC) and only two-thirds of those with LOC sought evaluation by a medical professional. In the total sample, only one third of those who sustained a concussion or more severe head injury were evaluated at an emergency room. Over half (54.5%) of the injured equestrians experienced headache, double vision, dizziness, or nausea. The most concerning aspect of the study was that 7.7% of those with LOC returned to riding the same day. An additional 20% returned to hunting within a week and 8.9% reported persisting symptoms. For those individuals who sustained a concussion but did not lose consciousness, 17% returned to riding the same day and an additional 23% returned within one week.

From this data, it is clear that many riders who sustain head injuries, even those significant enough to cause LOC, are not seeking medical treatment or evaluation. As some of this unevaluated group resume riding that same day, they risk further injury, including head injury. This can have tragic and fatal consequences particularly for younger riders, even if the second head injury is mild in nature (i.e., second-impact syndrome – Saunders & Harbaugh, 1984; Schneider, 1973). The pathophysiology behind this process is reviewed in detail by David Hovda, Ph.D. in an earlier chapter.

Given that females appear to be at greatest risk for injury in equestrian activities (Chitnavis et al., 1996; Frankel et al., 1998; Hammett, 2000c; Hammett, in press), the lack of research examining the role of gender on outcome in traumatic brain injury (TBI) is particularly concerning (Farace & Alves, 2000; Kraus, Peek-Asa, & McArthur, 2000). A recent meta-analysis on gender differences in outcome after TBI found only nine studies that reported data by gender (Farace & Alves, 2000). One study was excluded due to biased methodology, resulting in eight studies that altogether contained 20 outcome variables reported separately by gender. Females demonstrated poorer outcome in 17 of the 20 variables (85%) with an average effect size of -0.15. It is clear that future studies should examine the role of gender as moderating variable.

A recent prospective study of patients with moderate and severe TBI revealed that the females had a mortality rate that was 1.28 times higher than that of males and that the females were more likely to die from their injuries (Kraus et al., 2000). The latter finding is in contrast to the data available from the North Carolina State Medical Examiner, which found that males have greater mortality in equestrian related accidents (Hammett, 2000b). Females have been noted to have a larger number of persisting symptoms one year after a mild brain injury (Rutherford, Merrett, & McDonald, 1979), a greater incidence of depression post mild TBI (Fenton, McClelland, Montgomery, MacFlynn, & Rutherford, 1993), and a greater likelihood of postconcussion syndrome (Bazarian et al., 1999). In contrast, other researchers have reported that females are more likely to return to school or work after TBI (Groswasser, Cohen, & Karen, 1998). These findings are particularly concerning considering the large percentage of females who sustain head injuries in equestrian related activities and who are potentially at risk for poorer outcome by virtue of their gender.

Case Studies of Equestrians with Head Injury

The three case studies presented below are individuals who were referred for neuropsychological evaluation and/or consultation within the past two years. All identifying information has been deleted or altered.

Case Study 1

Jane Doe is an 18 year-old female who was thrown forward from her horse while on a jumping course, striking her chin and the back left of her head, and cracking her helmet. She denied loss of consciousness or posttraumatic amnesia and reported that she got back on her horse and finished the competition. An MRI of her head and neck was normal. Notably, she was involved in a motor vehicle accident two months earlier in which she struck the right side of her forehead on the rearview mirror. She experienced no loss of consciousness or posttraumatic amnesia in that accident either, but presented to the emergency room several hours later due to headache, fatigue, and a "spacey" feeling. Ms. Doe was evaluated and released, but she indicated that her headaches persisted for three weeks after the accident.

On the day after her equestrian accident, Ms. Doe became confused on a familiar jumping course. She also experienced lapses in her attention and began taking shortcuts even for horse-related activities despite previous meticulousness. In addition, she had difficulty keeping track of her responsibilities at work. Due to these cognitive concerns and changes, she was referred for a complete neuropsychological evaluation approximately six weeks after her equestrian accident. On the Wechsler Adult Intelligence Scale-Third Edition (WAIS-III), Ms. Doe's verbal intellectual ability was in the very superior range and her nonverbal verbal intellectual ability was significantly lower, falling in the average range. Among other cognitive abilities, Ms. Doe demonstrated superior abstract reasoning, complex concept formation skills, complex processing speed, and mental flexibility. Her simple cognitive processing speed and rapid new problem solving skills were generally intact, with some mild deficits on the most speed-dependent tasks. Her memory and new learning for verbal and visual information was average to very superior, and she demonstrated well intact encoding, retention, and retrieval of new information. Ms. Doe's sensory and motor skills were intact. She demonstrated difficulty with written calculation on an aphasia screening exam, possibly due to mild inattention. On the MMPI-2, she endorsed significant depression and anxiety. Her mild attention difficulties were consistent with the sequelae of her mild head injury and emotional distress, but overall she appeared to have made a good recovery from her concussions.

Case Study 2

Ms. Jones is a 34 year-old healthy woman with a college degree who sustained a concussion when she fell from her horse. She reported that she was wearing a properly fastened helmet at the time. According to Ms. Jones, she lost consciousness for less than one minute, followed by a profound alteration of consciousness, including feelings of depersonalization and derealization. She was seen and released at the emergency room after a normal head CT scan. On the day following the accident, she experienced considerable dizziness, nausea, and headaches, and had difficulty watching television or reading. Ms. Jones returned to work as a computer technology consultant three days after her equestrian accident, but experienced persisting headaches and dizziness, which were exacerbated when scrolling through documents on a computer screen. She also noticed increased irritability, difficulty concentrating, significant fatigue, and word finding/substitution problems. These symptoms slowly resolved, although she continued to experience headaches, irritability, and occasional word finding deficits, along with depressed mood and crying episodes.

Due to her concerns about these persisting symptoms, Ms. Jones presented for a comprehensive neuropsychological evaluation four months after her injury. The results of the evaluation revealed high average verbal intellectual ability and average nonverbal intellectual ability on the WAIS-III. She also demonstrated average to above average nonverbal abstract reasoning and complex concept formation abilities, as well as new learning and memory for verbal information. Her recall of faces, both immediately and upon delay, was average, but her delayed recall of a complex geometric figure was mildly impaired. She made no errors on the sensory-perceptual examination and her motor performance was in the expected range. Her language skills, including naming ability, were intact. Ms. Jones had considerable difficulty on a serial addition task used to assess capacity and rate of information processing as well as sustained and focused attention (PASAT). She became overwhelmed and frustrated with this task, and made few attempts to respond. Her overall performance on the PASAT fell in the severely impaired range, which appeared to reflect her preexisting difficulty and anxiety with math and slightly reduced processing speed, rather than a severe impairment in her attentional abilities. Given her educational and occupational history, Ms. Jones' performance on tasks of processing speed and attention/concentration were lower than expected.

On the MMPI-2, her responses were guarded and her clinical profile revealed that she is extroverted and likely to be assertive. Although subclinical, she endorsed mild elevations on scales sensitive to depression and anxiety. Overall, the neuropsychological evaluation suggested that Ms. Jones continued to experience subtle and mild cognitive difficulties subsequent to her mild head injury. By self-report, she had already made a significant recovery at the time of the evaluation and her persisting symptoms were most problematic when she was fatigued. She was advised to reduce her workload and get adequate rest until her symptoms fully resolved, and to receive a follow up neuropsychological assessment if her symptoms continued beyond six months.

Case Study 3

Mr. Smith is a 50 year-old male who was fox hunting in a remote area when he was thrown from his horse. He was wearing a helmet at the time and the helmet stayed securely fastened. Upon impact, he lost consciousness. Due to the remote location, it took three hours for an ambulance to arrive. When emergency medical personnel initially evaluated him, he had a Glasgow Coma Scale score of five to eight. He was intubated and taken to a small regional hospital for further evaluation. A head CT scan revealed a subdural hematoma with right frontal contusion. Due to increased intracranial pressure, a craniotomy was performed and the subdural hematoma was evacuated. A repeat head CT scan two days later revealed significant edema and an extensive right frontal hemorrhagic contusion. He underwent a second craniotomy to remove nonviable brain tissue and shortly thereafter developed a wound infection. A few days later he was transported to a major tertiary care medical center where the wound was debrided and closed. He was also diagnosed with MRSA nosocomial meningitis/cerebritis and abscess.

Prior to his accident, Mr. Smith was a successful attorney who was described by his family as motivated, highly energetic, and strong willed. He had no known history of depression or anxiety. He did not recognize his family until three weeks after his injury. Five days later, he began to understand gestures, demonstrated increased attention, and he was able to follow basic commands shortly thereafter. Mr. Smith was diagnosed with expressive aphasia and left hemiplegia and he began working with an occupational therapist. The neuropsychology consult service was contacted nearly two months after the injury to assess his cognitive functioning, his emotional status, and to determine his readiness for rehabilitation. Brief bedside screening revealed that the patient was oriented to person, month, day, date, and year, but not to season. Although he was oriented to place on a formal mental status exam, he repeatedly confused his actual location with his hometown, which was several hundred miles away. Mr. Smith had mild difficulty following simple commands. For example, when asked to fold a piece of paper in half and place it on the floor, he folded it in half and then in half again. When he was asked to follow a simple command written on a sheet of paper, he read the command out loud. His most unusual error occurred when he was asked to copy a drawing of two intersecting pentagons. He responded tearfully, "two houses," and began sketching a row of house-like figures (non-intersecting figures). As is frequently the case with bedside screenings, multiple interruptions occurred during the administration of the Rey Auditory Verbal Learning Test (RAVLT) and the test was discontinued prior to the delayed recall trial. Nevertheless, his immediate recall was in the low average range and his recall after thc interference trial was slightly above average (.66 SD above the mean).

During a follow-up visit two days later, Mr. Smith's mood was labile and tearful. He reported that he was easily depressed and concerned about returning to his former level of functioning and his great difficulty controlling emotions. He and his family were given supportive education about the emotional sequelae of head injury and his behavior was normalized given his stage of recovery. Although Mr. Smith's performance on bedside testing clearly represented a decline from his premorbid level of functioning, his generally average performance on the RAVLT was a favorable prognostic indicator that he would be able to benefit from rehabilitation. The neuropsychology consult service recommended that Mr. Smith be transferred to a rehabilitation hospital close to home and that a comprehensive neuropsychological evaluation be conducted at that facility to facilitate treatment planning.

Summary of Clinical Cases

These three cases demonstrate the range of head injuries sustained by equestrians and the variability in neuropsychological performance. Notably, all three of these equestrians were wearing helmets at the time of injury and all three were thrown from their horse. The neurocognitive sequelae were complicated by emotional distress and/or lability. One of these patients commented that she believed her depression was due to her ignorance of head injury sequelae and that she had been told in the emergency room that she would be "fine" in a day or so. When her symptoms persisted, she became distressed, fearing that something was wrong was her, and resulting in increased depression and anxiety. Neither of the two individuals who presented for an outpatient evaluation had received any education about the normal recovery curve for mild head injury prior to their neuropsychology appointment. Clearly, education regarding the use of protective helmets, as well as informing head trauma victims and family about what to expect following injury are critical edification objectives.

The Role of Helmet Use in Reducing Head Trauma

Over the last decade, the equestrian community and the public at large have become aware of the need for proper head protection in equestrian sports, as well as other athletic events. The large number of head injuries sustained by riders has revealed the sports' inherent dangers. The three safety issues concerning equestrian helmets are: (1) the determination of which standards provide optimal protection, (2) the safety life spans of the respective products, and (3) the development of both educational and legal means of encouraging riders to practice safe riding with a focus on the use of properly fitted protective head gear at all times.

The latest innovations in protective helmets have introduced numerous smaller, lighter, and more ventilated models in comparison to their predecessors. Protective liners in helmets are designed to compress and absorb the impact of a fall or kick from the horse by minimizing the force of impact between the rider's brain and skull (Biokinetics & Associates Ltd., 2000). Sometimes, through the actual destruction of the helmet itself, the wearer's head is spared the trauma of the impact. Additionally, as Newtonian principles predict, the force of impact on the brain itself is reduced through helmet use as the force is distributed across the entire surface area of the helmet. This decreases the force on any one aspect or portion of the brain in blunt traumas (Barth, Freeman, Broshek, & Varney, 2001). One important factor in assuring maximum head protection is a proper helmet fit. A simple test to assure that a helmet fits properly is to fasten the helmet and have the rider move it up and down vertically with his/her hands (Jahiel, 2000). If the rider can feel his/her eyebrows move along with the helmet, the helmet is fastened securely. Proper use of the retention system in securing the helmet to the wearer's head, proper care for the helmet and a thorough inspection of the helmet prior to riding are additional habits which, when acquired, can help assure the effectiveness of the gear (Beel, 1998).

Standards for Equestrian Helmets

There exist three equestrian headgear standards developed through multiple series of performance tests which simulate the stresses the helmet systems undergo in the event of a head impact (Biokinetics & Associates Ltd., 2000). The two major components of these evaluations are impact and retention tests. Impact tests evaluate the ability of a helmet to reduce the amount of brain acceleration in an impact to a level that is acceptable based on predicted human tolerance. In these tests, helmets are attached to humanoid-shaped head forms, which are raised to certain levels and then released onto various surfaces, including a solid steel anvil, so that contact is made with the target test site of the helmet. Shock-sensing instrumentation imbedded at the center of the head form measures the acceleration transmitted through the helmet in an impact. Retention tests evaluate the ability of the helmet to remain in proper position upon the wearer's head in the event of an impact. Various contraptions have been designed to stress the retention systems of the helmets by testing the buckles, fasteners, stitching and webbing. Penetration resistance, peak deflection, lateral deformation, resistance to temperature extremes, and adequate coverage of the back of the head are other helmet features considered in the development of the standards. By assigning acceptable values for each of these attributes, each standard is designed to assure that the wearer is provided adequate protection. For a helmet to receive certification under one of the standards it must meet those values (Biokinetics & Associates Ltd., 2000).

In an attempt to determine which type of helmet standard provides the most adequate protection, a number of evaluations of the three standards available to riders in the United States and around the world have been conducted. Helmets that meet the American Standard for Testing Material (ASTM) F1663 requirements receive additional certification from the Safety Equipment Institutes (SEI), a compliance organization responsible for certifying industrial products. The ASTM certified helmets are most often considered products of the highest standard because they must pass the most severe impact and retention test requirements (Biokinetics & Associates Ltd., 2000). Australian/New Zealand (ASNZ) 3838 certified helmets rate equally with ASTM helmets in terms of providing the most head coverage. The ASNZ certified helmets, however, are less adequate with respect to retention strength and cold temperature conditioning. The real-world requirements necessary to deal with the Canadian winter climate were not met. The major deficit of the third standard, the European EN 1384, is that it lacks the steel anvil portion of the impact test and, therefore, relies on a less rigid penetration test to assess focused impact protection. Although not a standard in the regulatory sense, the British PAS 015, a product assessment specification based on the European standard, is the only standard deemed comparable to the ASTM standard. However, it is considered by some to be too restrictive in terms of design parameters.

In 1998, the Transport Research Laboratory conducted an in-depth comparison of the impact protection ability of the two standards at the request of the Mark Davies Injured Riders Fund (Transport Research Laboratory, 1998). Researchers found that the ASTM certified helmets provided superior impact protection and asserted that they therefore provide superior head injury protection. Biokinetics and Associates Ltd., an Ottawa-based firm, conducted a similar comparison of all three standards and the British PAS in 1999. Their report deemed the ASTM standard the toughest and PAS as the most thorough (Biokinetics & Associates Ltd., 2000).

Currently, there remain proponents for each of the two standards. The majority of equestrian associations in the United States, including racing organizations and the US Pony Club and 4-H clubs in most states, require use of ASTM approved helmets. 4-H Horsemanship programs in the majority of U.S. states include educational programs in addition to helmet policies (Lamb, 2000). Organizations like SAFE KIDS have supported these programs and policies by assisting 4-H youth in the purchase of new equestrian helmets. The American Association for Horsemanship Safety, the USPC and the Washington 4-H Foundation have collaborated on a video created by 4-H called "Every Time, Every Ride" (Malavase, 1998). The video is a valuable resource for educating riders, parents, and instructors as to the importance of wearing ASTM/SEI certified helmets in all equestrian sport disciplines. Other organizations such as the Canadian Equestrian Federation recommend helmets certified under the ASTM, the PAS or both (Biokinetics & Associates Ltd., 2000). The American Academy of Pediatrics, the American Medical Association through the Committee on Sports Medicine, Canadian Medical Association, and the American Medical Equestrian Association publicly recommend that approved, fitted and secured helmets be worn by all equestrians on every ride (AMEA, 2000). Other organizations requiring helmets for equestrian activities are listed in Table 15.2.

Table 15.2. Organizations Requiring or Recommending Helmets for Equestrian Activities

Organizations Requiring F1163/SEI Riding Helmets
American Riding Instructor Certification Program
Association for Horsemanship Safety and Education (1989)
Eastern Competitive Trail Ride Association
Endurance and Competitive Trail Riding Association (riding, 1992; driving, 1993)
Girl Scouts of America (1992) – all riding activities and camps
Horsemanship Safety Association (1991)
New York State Department of Health – camps with riding programs
New York State Horse Council – sponsored events
New York State V & T Law & Business Obligation Law (2000)
North American Horseman's Association – all insured facilities
North American Riding for the Handicapped Association
North American Singlefooting Horse Trail, Field & Pleasure Division
North American Trail Riding Conference (1991)
United States Pony Clubs (1990) – all activities except vaulting
U.S. Polocrosse Association (1991)
*4-H Club requirements vary by state

Organizations Recommending F1163/SEI Riding Helmets
American Horse Shows Association
American Morgan Horse Association
American Steeplechase and Hunt Association
Canadian Equestrian Federation
Racing Commissioners International
United States Combined Training Association

Organizations which Mention Helmets in Their Rules
American Quarter Horse Association
Appaloosa Horse Association
Intercollegiate Riding Association
International Arabian Horse Association
Paint Horse Association
U.S. Polo Association

Acknowledgement

Special thanks to Drusilla Malavase, Chairman, ASTM Subcommittee on Protective Headgear, and Dr. Doris Bixby Hammett, Founder, American Medical Equestrian Association, for providing this information.

Along with the steps taken by equestrian organizations to encourage helmet use, two U.S. states have enacted helmet use laws. New York's riding helmet bill, signed into law on September 7, 1999, requires that all riders under 14 years of age wear approved helmets and that horse providers make helmets available to those riders and all beginning riders at no extra cost to the rider (Pinsky, 2000). In addition, all riders regardless of age or experience are to be provided with helmet safety information and offered the use of protective headgear. The City of Plantation, Florida enacted a municipal ordinance that became effective April 1, 1999. It is similar to the New York law except it applies to riders under 16 years of age (AMEA, 1999).

Helmets Remain Underutilized

Despite legal and educational head injury prevention efforts, a large number of equestrians continue to ride without helmets. Western riders have traditionally been less willing to wear helmets because previously all

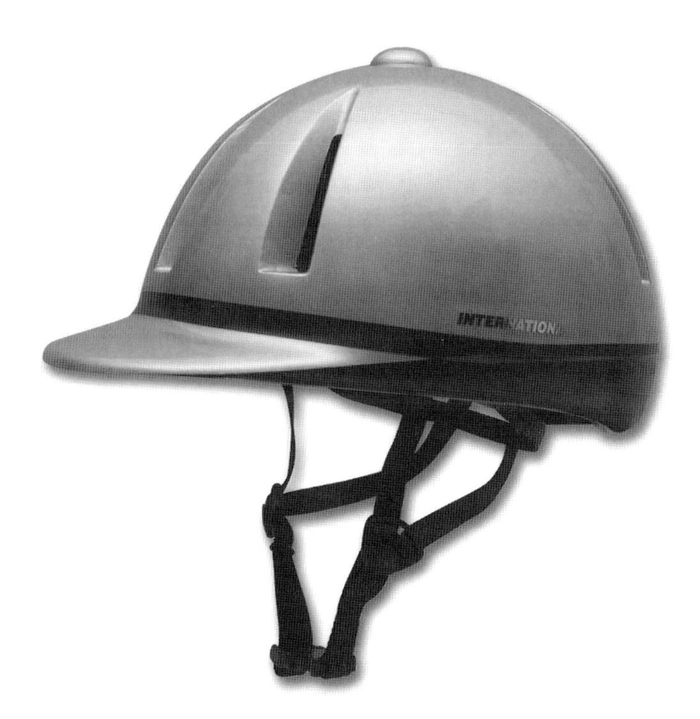

Figure 15.1. International Air-Lite Helmet meets visual standards for equestrian riding by preserving the traditional width, shape, top button, and flexible peak. This light weight, ventilated helmet is certified by SEI to ASTM F1163.95 standards. Photo and description provided courtesy of International Riding Helmets, Ltd.

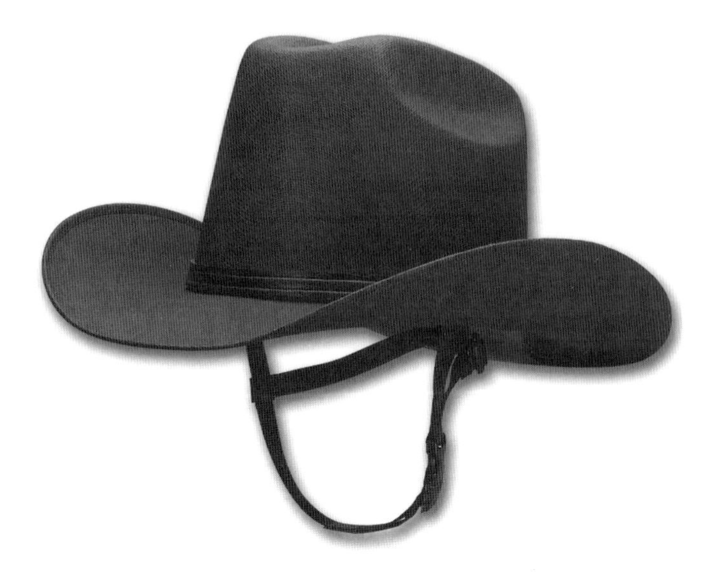

Figure 15.2. Sport Guard Western is the first authentic Western style safety helmet. The Western style hat has a protective safety helmet inside. Description and photo provided courtesy of International Riding Helmets, Ltd.

helmets were English style as seen in Figure 15.1 (Jahiel, 2000). A number of helmet manufacturers now produce western-style hat covers for ASTM/SEI approved helmets. International Riding Helmets, a New York-based helmet manufacturer, created the first authentic style western safety helmet respecting the traditional western styling and is shown in Figure 15.2. The fact that the majority of states where 4-H programs do not include helmet rules have Western riding as the prevailing discipline reflects the extent to which Western riding has maintained its status as a non-helmeted discipline (Lamb, 2000).

A 1993 study that investigated helmet use among equestrians in three counties of Washington State revealed that 40% of the respondents never wore a helmet and only 20% always wore a helmet (Condie, Rivara, & Bergman, 1993). Although the equestrians indicated that they felt safer wearing a helmet and recognized the role of helmets in reducing the incidence and severity of head injury, a large majority held negative attitudes about helmet use. Most respondents described helmets as uncomfortable, too hot, and "silly" looking. Interestingly, many of these equestrians reported wearing bicycle helmets for cycling, noting that everybody wears bicycle helmets. Adolescent respondents felt that equestrian helmets were for younger children and expressed concern about their appearance (i.e., did not want to look "silly"). Many of the equestrians felt that there was less need for safety helmets for experienced riders, with quiet horses, or on flat ground. The cost of equestrian helmets was also cited as a factor. Women, younger riders (<age 15), and English-style riders were more likely to wear helmets (Nelson, Rivara, & Condie, 1994). The "macho" image of Western-style riding was associated with minimal or nonexistent helmet use.

Some riders neglect to wear a helmet because of concern over increased body temperature in hot weather. A 1997 study in which 14 cyclists were observed while riding in a hot-dry or hot-humid environment reported that the use of a commercially available cycling helmet does not increase body temperature or the rider's perception of head or body temperature (Sheffied-Moore et al., 1997). The American Medical Equestrian Association stated that the study's findings are equally valid for helmeted equestrian riders (Hammett, 1999).

By wearing bicycle helmets in the place of certified equestrian helmets, riders sacrifice adequate head protection. A fall from a horse is very different than one from a bicycle; therefore, helmets used in the two sports cannot be substituted for each other. A fall from a horse is from a height greater than one from a bicycle and while bicycle falls are usually forward, most likely injuring the top and front of the rider's head, the back and sides of the head are equally vulnerable in equestrian sport accidents (www.horse-country.com/safety.html). Helmets are designed under standards based on the nature of the possible injuries a rider may sustain. Because equestrian helmets are the only helmets designed to withstand the mechanisms of kicks, falls and ejections, and the intensities of other horse-related injuries, there are no effective substitutes.

Addressing Limitations of Headgear for the Future

One issue regarding the role of headgear in equestrian injury protection that has perhaps not received sufficient attention is helmet life span as the standards process excludes aging tests. Neither the ASTM standard nor any other standard has an aging section (Malavase, 1997). Manufacturers use five years as a rule of thumb for helmet replacement. There is a chance, however, that helmets will sit on the shelf for an extended amount of time before purchase, allowing the rider to continue wearing the helmet beyond its life span. More extensive research into the aging of the plastics used in helmets is necessary, including the consideration of UV exposure. Intensive educational programs that inform riders of the importance of helmet life span issues would also optimize the benefit of protection. Riders must be informed that helmets are designed to withstand only one impact, after which they should be retired. Even if simply dropped, serious, undetectable, damage may occur that compromises the quality of protection. While auto racing helmets are not permitted on the track after five years and football players must have their helmets inspected and reconditioned every three years, equestrians are encouraged to inspect their helmets often and use common sense about replacement (Malavase, 1997). Along with additional education, action from the equestrian governances will be necessary to ensure that riders are not merely fastening on a false sense of security when buckling their helmets.

Recent advances and research in the field of equestrian head gear have allowed manufacturers to offer certified helmets in a variety of designs that meet the desires of riders participating in any form of equestrian sport. The fact that riders continue to participate without these certified helmets, under the assumption that helmets are uncomfortable or unstylish, is evidence that the riding community as a whole is unaware of the many innovative styles that are available. A survey published in a 1999 issue of the American Medical Equestrian Association newsletter reported that the majority of competitive hunter and jumper riders do not wear approved helmets due to concern about being penalized by judges for their appearance (Neal, 1999). Neal interviewed three American Horse Association Judges and found that judges do, in fact, prefer to see competitors wearing non-approved helmets at higher levels of competition. All competitive event riders surveyed, however, stated that they wear approved helmets and must do so according to regulations. Although there has been a significant rise in helmet use over the last decade, there is strong evidence supporting the need for additional educational, regulatory and, perhaps, legal action. One of the first steps in accurately compiling data on equestrian related head injury is to ascertain whether a helmet was worn and, if so, the type of helmet, the certification or protective standard for the helmet, and whether the helmet was properly fitted and fastened (Hammett, 2000a). According to Dr. Bixby-Hammett, helmet manufacturers have been receptive to input designed to improve helmet safety, but the burden falls upon the equestrian community to participate in research and apply the information and knowledge gathered through such studies.

Return to Riding after Head Injury – Summation

Although the old adage says "if you fall off a horse, get right back on again," this is the worst possible advice for an equestrian who has sustained a concussion or more severe head injury. The American Academy of Neurology has published guidelines to protect athletes from further serious and catastrophic injury following even mild sports related head injuries (1997). Other researchers in the area of head injury have suggested other guidelines, primarily based upon professional and expert consensus (e.g., Cantu, 1998b). Despite subtle differences among various guidelines, they each have classification of the severity of injury as the primary goal. This classification is generally derived from considering such variables as the length, if any, of loss of consciousness and/or post traumatic amnesia, as well as the presence and persistence of neurological symptoms, such as headache, dizziness, and nausea following the incident. These variables, and particularly their duration, are then used to establish the guidelines for how long an athlete should refrain from any activity that risks a second, even mild, head injury.

Why should this be of interest to the equestrian community? Foremost, premature risk for a second concussion prior to recovery from the first leaves the equestrian vulnerable to the devastating if not fatal "second-impact syndrome" (Cantu, 1998). Ensuring that the equestrian has fully recovered from a first head injury is the best protection against this syndrome. Consultation with neurologists and/or neuropsychologists to determine the severity of concussion, its impact on neurocognitive functioning, and the recommended time to refrain from activity is essential. Additionally, despite the relative infancy of this research and incomplete understanding of the mechanisms, there is evidence to suggest that a first head injury leads to increased risk for having a second or multiple head injuries. This emphasizes the importance of holding riders from premature eventing or practicing prior to full recovery from any concussion.

If an equestrian sustains more than one concussion, it is important to examine the factors contributing to such injury. Factors might include failure to wear an approved helmet, inappropriate use of a horse that is not adequately trained or capable of performing in a specific capacity, and/or riders attempting equestrian activities that are beyond their level of skill (Brooks & Bixby-Hammett, 1998). Individuals sustaining multiple concussions may need to limit or curtail their equestrian activities, although such advice is rarely followed (Brooks, 2000). Other important safety measures have been proposed by the International Eventing Safety Committee (2000), including medical coverage sufficient for on-site management of severe trauma, minimizing response times for medical personnel to reach injured equestrians on cross-country courses, random drug testing of competitors, and inspection of helmets at all three-day events.

The importance of educating the equestrian community about mild head injury cannot be emphasized strongly enough. Personnel should be on hand at all equestrian events who are capable of identifying and assessing concussion and making recommendations for further medical evaluation. Based on return to play guidelines for sports, equestrians should be counseled about how long they should refrain from riding in order to prevent further head injury. In addition, those individuals who sustain concussions would benefit from education about the normal recovery curves of head injury and should be advised to get adequate rest, minimize stress, and abstain from alcohol to optimize their recovery. Furthermore, any equestrian who experiences persisting symptoms after head injury and/or experiences multiple concussions should be referred for neurological and neuropsychological evaluations. Although research into this area is still early stage, one need not look farther than the sports pages, to see the concern about the influence of multiple concussions on future neurocognitive and neurological functioning.

References

AMEA. (1999). City of Plantation, Florida, requires ASTM SEI helmet when riding on public property. *American Medical Equestrian Association News, 10*(1), 6–8. Available: www.law.utexas.edu/dawson/amea/feb99nws.htm

AMEA. (2000). Equestrian helmet fact sheet. *American Medical Equestrian Association News, 11(1)*, 3–4. Available: www.law.utexas.edu/dawson/amea/feb00nws.htm

American Academy of Neurology: Practice parameter (1997). The management of concussion in sports (summary statement). *Neurology, 48*, 581–585.

Barth, J.T., Varney, R.N., Ruchinskas, R.A., & Francis, J.P. (1999). Mild head injury: The new frontier in sports medicine. In R.N. Varney & R.J. Roberts (Eds.), *The Evaluation and Treatment of Mild Traumatic Brain Injury* (pp. 81–98. Mahwah, NJ: L. Erlbaum.

Barth, J.T., Freeman, J.R., Broshek, D.K., & Varney, R.N. (2001). Acceleration-deceleration sports-related concussion: The gravity of it all. *Journal of Athletic Training, 36*(3), 253–256.

Bazarian, J.J., Wong, T., Harris, M., Leahey, N., Mookerjee, S., & Dombovy, M. (1999). Epidemiology and predictors of post-concussive syndrome after minor head injury in an emergency population. *Brain Injury, 13*(3), 173–189.

Beel, J. (1998). Head protection research laboratory. *American Medical Equestrian Association News, 9*(1),7–9. Available: www.law.utexas.edu/dawson/amea/feb98nws.htm

Biokinetics & Associates, Ltd. (2000). Equestrian headgear standards. *American Medical Equestrian Association News, 11*(3), 1–3. Available: www.law.utexas.edu/dawson/amea/sep00nws.htm

Bixby-Hammett, D.M. (1987). Accidents in equestrian sports. *American Family Physician, 36*, 209–214.

Bond, G.R., Christoph, R.A., & Rodgers, B.M. (1995). Pediatric equestrian injuries: Assessing the impact of helmet use. *Pediatrics, 95*, 487–489.

Brooks, W.H. (2000). Neurologic injuries in equestrian sport. In R.C. Cantu (Ed.), *Neurologic athletic head and spine injuries* (pp. 305–316). Philadelphia, W.B. Saunders.

Brooks, W.H., & Bixby-Hammett, D.M. (1991). Head and spinal injuries associated with equestrian sports: Mechanisms and prevention. In J.S. Torg (Ed.), *Athletic injuries to the head, neck, and face* (pp. 133–141). St. Louis: Mosby Year Book.

Brooks, W.H., & Bixby-Hammett, D.M. (1998). Equestrian sports. In B.D. Jordan (Ed.), *Sports Neurology* (2nd ed.) (pp. 381–391). Philadelphia: Lippincott-Raven Publishers.

Cantu, R.C. (1998). Second-impact syndrome. *Clinical Sports Medicine, 17*, 37–44.

Cantu, R.C. (1998). Return to play guidelines after a head injury. *Clinical Sports Medicine, 17*, 45–60.

Chitnavis, J.P., Gibbons, C.L.M.H, Hirigoyen, M., Parry, J.L., & Simpson, A.H.R.W. (1996). Accidents with horses: What has changed in 20 years? *Injury, 27*, 103–105.

Condie, C., Rivara, R.P., & Bergman, A.B. (1993). Strategies of a successful campaign to promote the use of equestrian helmets. *Public Health Reports, 108*, 121–126.

Farace, E. & Alves, W.M. (2000). Do women fare worse? A metaanalysis of gender differences in outcome after traumatic brain injury. *Neurosurgery Focus, 8*(1), Article 6. Available: www.neurosurgery.org/focus/index.html

Fenton, G., McClelland, R., Montgomery, A., MacFlynn, G., & Rutherford, W. (1993). The postconcussional syndrome: social antecedents and psychological sequelae. *British Journal of Psychiatry, 162*, 493–497.

Frankel, H.L., Haskell, R., Digiacomo, J.C., & Rotondo, M. (1998). Recidivism in equestrian trauma. *The American Surgeon, 64*, 151–154.

Grosswasser, Z., Cohen, M., & Karen, O. (1998). Female TBI patients recover better than males. *Brain Injury, 12*, 805–808.

Hamilton, M.G., & Tranmer, B.I. (1993). Nervous system injuries in horseback-riding accidents. *The Journal of Trauma, 34*, 227–232.

Hammett, D.B. (1997). Justin Sportsmedicine Program 15-year PRCA study of rodeo injuries. *American Medical Equestrian Association News, 8*(3), 1–3. Available: www.law.utexas.edu/dawson/amea/nov97nws.htm

Hammett, D.B. (1999). Responses to cycling with and without a helmet [editor's note]. *American Medical Equestrian Association News, 10*(1), 5-6. Available: www.law.utexas.edu/dawson/amea/feb99nws.htm

Hammett, D.B. (2000a). Editorial comment. *American Medical Equestrian Association News, 11*(2),17. Available: www.law.utexas.edu/dawson/amea/jun00nws.htm

Hammett, D.B. (2000b, October). *Horse related deaths: North Carolina 1978-1999 Medical Examiner Reports*. Paper presented at the American Medical Equestrian Association annual meeting, Painsville, OH.

Hammett, D.B. (2000c, October). *What the horse community can learn from the National Electronic Injury Surveillance System Figures*. Paper presented at the American Medical Equestrian Association annual meeting in Painsville, OH.

Hammett, D.B. (in press). Medical implications Masters of Foxhounds Association *Covertside* survey March 2000. *American Medical Equestrian Association News*.

International Eventing Safety Committee. (2000). Eventing. *American Medical Equestrian Association News, 11*(2), *18-19*. Available: www.law.utexas.edu/dawson/amea/jun00nws.htm

Jahiel, J. (2000). *Complete idiot's guide to horseback riding*. Indianapolis, Alphabooks.

Kraus, J. F., Peek-Asa, C., & McArthur, D. (2000). The independent effect of gender on outcomes following traumatic brain injury. *Neurosurgery Focus, 8*(1), Article 5. Available: www.neurosurgery.org/focus/index.html

Kriss, T.C., & Kriss, V.M. (1997). Equine-related neurosurgical trauma: A prospective series of 30 patients. *The Journal of Trauma: Injury, Infection, and Critical Care, 43*, 97-99.

Lamb, C. (2000). Equestrian helmet use in the National 4-H Program. *American Medical Equestrian Association News, 11*(3), 12-17. Available: www.law.utexas.edu/dawson/amea/sep00nws.htm

Malavase, D. (1997). *A helmet's lifespan*. Retrieved November 15, 2000 from the World Wide Web: http://www.horse-country.com/safety2.html

Malavase, D. (1998) How does equestrian headgear compare and what should I wear? *American Medical Equestrian Association News, 9*(3), 3–4. Available: www.law.utexas.edu/dawson/amea/nov98nws.htm

McLain, D. (1997). The development of equestrian sports medicine. *American Medical Equestrian Association News, 8*(3), 6–8. Available: www.law.utexas.edu/dawson/amea/nov97nws.htm

Neal, S. (1999, September). Approved vs. non-approved riding helmets in competition disciplines. *American Medical Equestrian Association News, 10*(3), 13–17. Available: www.law.utexas.edu/dawson/amea/sep99nws.htm

Nelson, D.E., Rivara, F.P., & Condie, C. (1994). Helmets and horseback riding. *American Journal of Preventive Medicine, 10*, 15–19.

Paix, B.R. (1999). Rider injury rates and emergency medical services at equestrian events. *British Journal of Sports Medicine, 33,* 46–48.

Pinsky, B.M. (2000). New York equestrian helmet legislation. *American Medical Equestrian Association News, 11*(1), 1–3. Available: www.law.utexas.edu/dawson/amea/feb00nws.htm

Rutherford, W.H., Merrett, J.D., & McDonald, J.R. (1979). Symptoms at one year following concussion from minor head injuries. *Injury, 10*, 225-230.

Saunders, R.L. & Harbaugh, R.E. (1984). The second impact in catastrophic contact-sports related trauma. *Journal of the American Medical Association, 252,* 538–539.

Schneider, R.C. (1973). Head and neck injuries in football. Williams and Wilkins (Eds.), Baltimore, MD.

Sapien, R. (2000). Pediatric horse-related injuries in New Mexico. *American Medical Equestrian Association News, 11*(2), 13–17. Available: www.law.utexas.edu/dawson/amea/jun00nws.htm

Sheffied-Moore, M., Short, K.R., Kerr, C.O., Parcell, A.C., Bollster, D.R., & Costill, D.L. (1997). Thermoregulatory responses to cycling with and without a helmet. *Medicine and Science in Sports and Exercise, 29*(6), 755–761.

Transport Research Lab. (1998). Equestrian helmet testing. *American Medical Equestrian Association News, 9*(1), 6–7. Available: www.law.utexas.edu/dawson/amea/feb98nws.htm

United States Pony Club Accident Study 1999. (2000, Fall). *USPC News*, 22–26.

Varney, N.R., & Roberts, R.J. (1999). Forces and accelerations in car accidents and resultant brain injuries. In R.N. Varney & R.J. Roberts (Eds.), *The Evaluation and Treatment of Mild Traumatic Brain Injury* (pp. 39–47). Mahwah, NJ: L. Erlbaum.

Watt, G. M., & Finch, C.F. (1996). Preventing equestrian injuries: Locking the stable door. *Sports Medicine, 22*, 187–197.

Whitlock, M.R. (1999). Injuries to riders in the cross country phase of eventing: the importance of protective equipment. *British Journal of Sports Medicine, 33,* 212–214.

SECTION III

METHODOLOGICAL ISSUES

EDITED BY

JEFFREY T. BARTH

Chapter 16

METHODOLOGICAL CONCERNS IN TRAUMATIC BRAIN INJURY

Stephen N. Macciocchi
Shepherd Center and Department of Rehabilitation Medicine, Emory University School of Medicine

Jeffrey T. Barth
Department of Psychiatric Medicine and Neurological Surgery
University of Virginia School of Medicine

Over the past fifteen years, research examining concussive injuries sustained during athletic endeavors has increased substantially (Macciocchi, Barth, & Littlefield, 1998). Attention devoted to athletic injuries resulted from recognition that concussions were associated with potential morbidity (Kelly & Rosenberg, 1997), but interest in athletic injuries was also fueled by a desire to study mild brain injury in populations and settings that allowed for methodologic precision and control. Clinicians disgruntled with the methodologic complexities, contradictory findings and slow progression of normal science in clinical populations turned to sports injuries as a less complicated methodological endeavor. As will become apparent, research examining mild brain injuries in sports has been vulnerable to many of the methodologic nuances that plagued mild brain injury research in general clinical populations (Dikmen & Levin, 1993; Macciocchi et al., 1998).

In clinical populations, empirical investigations have both helped and hindered a progression towards a sound scientific understanding of concussive injuries. Unfortunately, conflicting research findings are common, and debate about the severity and duration of post concussive symptoms as well as the potential for these injuries to cause permanent disability continues (Dikmen & Levin, 1993; Binder, Rohling, & Larrabee, 1997). While science may ultimately prevail and provide answers to questions that have thus far eluded definitive understanding, we are dependent on methodologically sound and interpretable research for answers. Accordingly, we will present a number of metholodologic issues facing persons undertaking research in mild traumatic brain injury – concussion in sports. Our chapter is focused on both consumers of research and persons with interest in actually executing research projects. For a number of reasons, most of us will not become actively involved in research, but we must still be able to assess the internal and external validity of studies. If we do choose to become involved in research, the need to employ sound methodology is patently obvious (Dikmen & Levin, 1993). In the succeeding sections of this chapter, we review a number of topics including causation, experimental designs, internal validity, statistical issues, and application of research findings.

Causation and Quasi Experimentation

Researchers and consumers of research are both interested in science as a means of enhancing understanding and decision making in situations where uncertainty exists. Since initial studies raised concerns that concussive injuries may have time limited or possibly permanent morbidity, researchers have labored to examine the causal relationship between concussion and neuropsychological functioning (Binder et al., 1997). Unfortunately, in clinical studies conducted outside the laboratory, causality is an elusive construct. In fact, philosophers have argued about the conditions required to determine causality for some time. In the positivist tradition, cause and effect must be contiguous, have temporal precedence and "constant conjunction" (Cook & Campbell, 1979). Therefore, concussive injuries must occur prior to and in close proximity to the symptoms associated with the injury. In addition, the symptoms (effect) should always and only be present when the injury (cause) is present (Cook & Campbell, 1979). There are other perspectives on causation, but in general there should be "covariation between presumed cause and effect" and cause temporally precedes effect, even if effect(s) are instantaneous (Campbell & Stanley, 1963, p. 31).

While the relationship between cause and effect may seem straightforward, in concussion research the concept of causation is not always given serious consideration. For example, some investigators consider the mere presence of post concussive symptoms (headache, dizziness, irritability, anxiety, and memory problems) as prima facie evidence of cerebral injury even though research has shown that such symptoms are not unique to concussion, but occur in equal frequency and severity in persons without histories of cerebral trauma (Gouvier, Uddo-Crane, & Brown, 1988; Lees-Haley & Brown, 1993; Ferguson, Mittenberg, Barone, & Schnieder, 1999). Because post concussive symptoms are not specific to cerebral trauma, the presence of these symptoms does not meet the "constant conjunction" requirement for causation. In any case, clinicians and researchers are principally interested in documenting the specific neurocognitive and neurobehavioral effects of concussive injuries in order to make decisions regarding medical management and reduction of morbidity in athletes. Consequently, studies must be designed to validate the relationship between presumed concussive injuries and the neurobehavioral and neurocognitive consequences of such injuries.

In order to accomplish this task, researchers empirically test the theory that concussive injuries have defined neuropsychological consequences that cannot be due to other factors such as a history of prior cerebral trauma, prior or concurrent extracranical injury, medical disorders, psychiatric disorders, substance abuse, learning disability, nonspecific test findings and/or motivation problems. Unless the research design permits exclusion of these and other alternative explanations, investigators cannot presume the concussion is associated with post injury symptoms. As expected, excluding plausible alternative explanations for post concussive symptoms is highly dependent on methodology. Unfortunately, many existing investigations of concussion utilize quasi-experimental designs which do not provide adequate controls for identifying and isolating the effects of concussions.

For our purposes, internal validity is defined as the extent to which "extraneous variables... in the experimental design produce effects" that would confuse or confound the experimenter's interpretation of the data (Campbell & Stanley, 1963, p. 5). These extraneous variables refer, but are not limited to history, selection, instrumentation, maturation and history – selection interaction. History simply relates to unique preinjury – premorbid factors athletes possess or have experienced that may bias interpretation of data. In other words, athletes may have unique histories effect experiemntal outcome. Selection refers to bias introduced by selectively as opposed to randomingly assigning participants. History – selection interaction addresses the potential influence of selection on promoting participant differences in history or premorbid functioning. Instrumentation refers to measurement bias and error. Finally, maturation addresses bias due to development or change of participants over time which is independent of injury. As mentioned previously, threats to internal validity are closely related to the design employed by investigators. Accordingly, we briefly discuss common experimental designs and then review specific threats to internal validity associated with these designs.

Experimental Designs

Because concussions are naturally occurring, unpredictable events, researchers are typically limited to quasi-experimental (non-randomized) designs (see Table 16.1). The quasi-experimental designs typically employed in concussion research include the posttest only design, the one group pretest-posttest design, the posttest only control group design and the nonequivalent control group design (Campbell & Stanley, 1963; Cook & Campbell, 1979). The posttest only design is a single sample design. Typically, the experimental group (athletes) is administered dependent measures (tests) after sustaining a concussion or at some arbitrary point in time following injury. Athletes' data are then compared to an established normative database in order to determine if neuropsychological impairment is present. The posttest only design is essentially clinical methodology and is vulnerable to several threats to validity including history, maturation, instrumentation and selection (see Table 16.1). Specific validity concerns are reviewed in more detail somewhat later, but in general, athletes selected for posttest only investigations may have preinjury histories of cognitive and emotional disorders which could be attributed to the injury even though these deficits were preexisting. In addition, athletes arbitrarily selected may have a disproportionate frequency of extracranial (muscoskeletal) injuries which may influence symptom reports or test performance. As expected, early research in mild brain injury using this design has been systematically and appropriately criticized (Dikmen & Levin, 1993).

More recently, posttest only designs have become more common, but researchers typically employ posttest only comparison (control) group designs which help to control for the effect of preinjury history, but not bias introduced by selection and interaction of history and selection (Cook & Campbell, 1979). In other words, a matched posttest control group compares athletes with injuries to players without injuries. Consequently, the likelihood that injured players individual histories may differentially affect outcome is constrained or limited (see Table 16.1). Nonetheless, posttest only control group designs also have problems. For example, investigators cannot match groups on all variables and if the players selected for each group differ on a significant factor such as intelligence or academic acheivement, then the groups are unbalanced and the design may not control for varibales known to affect neuropsychological test performance. Research using the posttest only and posttest control group designs are less common, but despite potential threats to internal validity, the data obtained from these studies is typically treated with more empirical respect than is warranted (Cook & Campbell, 1979).

A third design used by investigators is the single group pretest – posttest design. In a single group, pretest – posttest design, athletes are assessed prior to and following an injury, but no controls are utilized. In other words, investigators obtain preinjury and postinjury data on a group of athletes who sus-

Table 16.1. Quasi–experimental designs used in concussion research.

Experimental designs				
Sources of Invalidity	Posttest Only X O_1	Pretest Posttest O_1 X O_2	Posttest Control X O_1 - - - - - - - O_1	Non Equivalent Control O_1 X O_2 - - - - - - - O_1 O_2
History	–	–	+	+
Selection	–	–	–	+
Instrumentation	–	–	+	+
Maturation	–	–	?	+
History – Selection	–	–	–	+

X = injury O = measurement
Minus (–) represents design weakness. Plus (+) indicates design strength.
Question mark (?) indicates possible weakness.
Adapted from Campbell and Stanley (1963), and Campbell and Cook (1979).

tained a concussion. Changes in functioning presumably reflect the effects of concussion, but this design is vulnerable to threats from history, selection and to some extent instrumentation, which relates to the reliability and validity of dependent measures. Again, athletes may be selected for various reasons and not adequately represent the population of concussed players. Also, reliability problems intrinsic to repeated measures designs may be a problem depending on the tests and symptoms checklists utilized.

In contrast to the three designs previously mentioned, nonequivalent control group designs are stronger and more interpretable (see Table 16.1). Nonequivalent control or comparison group designs utilize pretest and post-test measurement with a matched control group for comparison purposes. In comparison (control) group designs, concussed athletes neuropsychological data are compared to controls with similar histories. The optimal design is one that can plausibly control for history and selection. For example, between group differences in premorbid cognitive ability is a threat to internal validity in all quasi-experimental concussion investigations. Therefore, in an attempt to control for history, some investigators have examined athletes' preinjury Scholastic Aptitude Test (SAT) scores to determine whether premorbid cognitive functioning might have affected post injury test performance (Collins, Grindell, Lovell, Dede et al., 1999). In other words, athletes with lower SAT scores may have less cognitive capacity, and consequently, evidence impairment on neuropsychological tests simply due to premorbid cognitive idiosyncrasies. Most importantly, if athletes who sustain injuries also have lower SAT scores, then history cannot be excluded as a rival plausible alternative. Unfortunately, in the absence of randomization, concussion research can never be considered truly "experimental", but appropriate use of quasi-experimental methodology may assist researchers in providing compelling support for their experimental findings. Currently, the nonequivalent comparison group design with preinjury and postinjury testing provides the strongest inference for association between concussions and post injury cogntive-behavioral symptoms/deficts.

Because research conducted with athletes has significant medical, economic and social implications, studies without credible defenses against threats to internal validity should be avoided. Retrospective studies attempting to document cumulative effects of concussion are problematic due to reliance on posttest only methodology (see Table 16.1). Prospective research examining the effects of concussive injuries in sports is less vulnerable to empirical challenges, but these studies should have both pretesting, posttesting and a thoughtfully constructed control group against which to compare test scores and symptoms. Under ideal circumstances, concussed players should be compared to players of similar age, duration of competitive athletics, cognitive capacity, medical, neurologic (head injury), psychiatric and academic histories who have not been head injured, but determining who has and who has not sustained a concussion premorbidly is not always a straightforward endeavor. For example, in certain sports such as football, concussions are common, but these injuries may not rise to the clinical threshold needed for diagnosis. Also, players typically accept certain injuries and may not report commonly experienced symptoms to medical staff. In other words, one can assume that a large number of football players have suffered concussions even though there may not be a formal medical history documenting these injuries. In any case, investigators must be concerned about the history and selection bias which can unbalance group comparisons independent of concussion. Constructing control comparison groups is a complicated process. Participants cannot be equated on all factors, but investigators should take particular care to equate participants on variables that would be expected to affect dependent measures in a significant and systematic manner.

History

Now that commonly used experimental designs have been briefly reviewed, specific threats to validity will be discussed. These threats are discussed in the context of the control group comparison designs since limitations of other designs significantly impair interpretability and scientific utility. In all neuropsychological, neurobehavioral and medical studies, history is critical. Most researchers recognize the importance of history, but face the challenge of controlling factors which are really not in their control. In other words, players are not randomly assigned to groups in concussion studies, which means that researchers must attempt to balance historically relevant threats to validity. Obviously some historical factors are more important than others, particularly, when neuropsychological tests are used as dependent measures. For example, athletes' medical, neurologic, cognitive and psychological histories may vary and should be documented when possible. Whether these factors can be "controlled" remains debatable, but various methods of accomplishing this task have been employed. One method is to match participants in different groups on relevant variables such as age, education, medical, cognitive and neurologic history. Players who sustain concussions are often compared with players with similar histories who have not sustained concussions, but possibly an orthopedic injury. The assumption is that this process contrasts individuals with statistically identical histories except for concussive injury. Logically, any differences observed between concussed players and controls on neuropsychological tests and symptom checklists should be due to concussive injuries.

While appealing, there are a number of problems with this approach. Studies with neuropsychological measures often match experimental (concussion) and control athletes on various demographics (age, gender, education and so on), but fail to consider other variables that may explain results in quasi-experimental studies. One variable that is conspicuously absent in most quasi-experimental comparison studies is a measure of general intellectual functioning, yet, there is ample evidence that intellectual functioning affects neuropsychological test performance (Chelune, 1982; Tremont, Hoffman, Scott & Adams, 1998). Many researchers presume that "controlling" for the education of participants also controls for variability in intellectual capacity, but this may not be the case. One only need consider the assumption that everyone who is a college graduate has the same IQ score or that all football players or soccer players are equal in intellectual or neuropsychological capacity. If you accept this premise, then ignoring the effect of intellectual or cognitive capacity on test performance makes sense. If not, then some attempt should be made to match participants used in control comparisons on a measure of intellectual/cognitive capacity such as reading skills (WRAT-III), vocabulary skills, abstract reasoning or SAT scores (Hinton-Bayre, Geffen, Geffen, McFarland & Friis, 1999) prior to injury. Because intellectual functioning and neuropscyhological functioning are highly correlated, some investiagtors may argue that matching subjects based on general intellectual functioning may obscure post concussive deficits, but neurocogntive impairment following concussion (attention – working memory) can be dissociated from other neuropsychological and intellectual skills and should not be affected by controling for general intellectual skills.

Most importantly, if players with lower preinjury intellectual or neurocognitive capacity are inadvertently, but systematically included in the concussion (experiemental) group, concussed players may evidence impairment relative to controls simply due to a history of intellectual impairment and associated deficts in attention and working memory rather than concussion (Chelune, 1982; Tremont et al., 1998). Alternatively, if athletes with pre-existing cognitive (intellectual) impairment are inadvertently and systematically assigned to control groups, the effect of concussion may be obscured in comparisons with concussed athletes. In other words, pre-existing impairment in the control group would result in the concussion group appearing unimpaired by comparison. Parenthetically, while one would not expect cognitive capacity to be correlated with vulnerability to concussion, there is one recent study that suggested an association between premorbid cognitive impairment (learning disability) and neurocognitive functioning following injury. In this study, Collins, Grindell, Lovell, Dede et al. (1999) found players who had a history of learning disability and two or more concussions performed worse than players with two or more concussions who did not have a history of learning disability. While these findings are interesting and merit further examination, the methodology used by the investigators was a posttest only design. The authors do comment on limitations of the findings, but do not address any specific threats to validity particularly the interaction of group assignment and concussion history (Collins, Gindall, Lovell, Dede, et al., 1999).

History – selection

All quasi-experimental designs comparing participants must not only deal with history, but the interaction of history and selection. For example, most current studies select participants for various reasons, often due to opportunity. In a recent study of soccer players, the basis for selecting athletes for the study was not documented, but the method section describes that 27.3% of the players studied suffered a concussion "not due to soccer play". This rate was twice the rate of "non sports" concussions in "matched" controls (Matser, Kessels, Lezak, Jordan, & Troost 1999). While the cause of "non sports" injuries in this study was not documented, it is plausible that history (non sports head injury) and selection interacted sufficiently to provide a plausible alternative to the authors assertion that soccer play results in cognitive impairment.

Obviously, a detailed premorbid history of sports related concussion and brain injury in general is necessary in all studies of cerebral trauma in sports. History is particularly relevant in posttest only control group designs such as the one mentioned, but most retrospective or prospective concussion research does not consider the severity of prior cerebral injuries because the clinical features of these disorders typically is unknown. Even if features of the injury are known, there are problems with assigning reliable severity indices. For example, most current guidelines used to rate injury severity recommend using presence and duration of unconsciousness and posttraumatic amnesia (Collins, Lovell, & McKeag, 1999), but despite these guidelines, grading systems may not reliably and validly predict neuropsychological impairment following injury. For example, current Practice Parameters published in 1997 imply a player with a Grade II injury (no unconsciousness/greater than 15 minutes confusion) would sustain less neuropsychological impairment than a player with a Grade III injury (loss of consciousness, no posttraumatic confusion), but there is no empirical evidence supporting this presumption. The presence of brief or extended posttraumatic confusion may in fact indicate the injury was more severe. In any case, the degree of post injury neuropsychological and neurobehavioral impairment related to specific injury grades (I-III) remains to be empirically determined.

While severity indices need empirical attention, a recent study suggests loss of consciousness may not be predictive of subsequent neuropsychological impairment (Lovell, Iverson, Collins, McKeag, & Marron, 1999). Therefore, using currently accepted injury grades to establish a basis for matching in control comparisons may be problematic even if injury "severity" is known. As an alternative, investigators may want to consider duration of posttraumatic amnesia or confusion as a more reliable indicator of injury severity. In fact, studies show that PTA does vary in concussive injuries (Macciocchi, Barth, Alves, Rimel, & Jane, 1996), but duration of PTA has not been systematically studied in concussive injuries. In any case, having the experimental (concussion) and control groups differ with respect to prior concussion or non sports related brain injury history is methodologically problematic, but the example of injury severity in the context of history-selection is just one problem. In the soccer study mentioned, the concussion group also had a history of significantly greater alcohol use than the control group which could further influence research results.

As a guideline, when planning or reviewing a study, consider how quasi-experimental control comparisons can be undertaken with special attention to history and selection. Document the relevant historical factors such as age, education, general intellectual functioning, medical history (neurologic, psychiatric, alcohol, drug, developmental), brain injury (frequency, severity, etiology). Define past and especially current injuries with as much precision as possible including presence/duration of unconsciousness and posttraumatic amnesia. Duration of posttraumatic-confusion appears to be quite important. For example, duration of posttraumatic amesia (confusion) has been shown to be highly related to outcome in more severe injuries (Dikmen, Machamer, Winn, & Temkin, 1995). Whether this holds true for concussive injuries remains to be seen. In any case, if participants are selected on the basis of opportunity, attempt to document the representativeness of the selected group. In small samples, groups with significantly different histories, particularly in areas that affect neuropsychological test performance or symptom reports, can substantially unbalance groups and lead to faulty inferences. While statistical methods such as analysis of covariance (ANCOVA) have been used to theoretically control for such differences among groups, ANCOVA may not effectively equate experimental and control groups depending on statistical relationships among covariates and dependent variables. When using ANCOVA, there must be a significant linear relationship between the covariate and the dependent measures, and the regression slopes for the covariates must be equivalent (Weinfort, 1998).

Instrumentation

In most studies, concussion is inferred from the presence of unconsciousness and/or posttraumatic confusion and typically validated by neuropsychological tests and symptoms. Unfortunately, neuropsychological tests and symptom checklists are prone to instrumentation problems. Consequently, selection and application of dependent measures is a concern in all investigations of concussion. On a positive note, neuropsychological tests are readily available and easily administered, but despite the availability and ease of administration, several problems associated with test application deserve mention. First, neuropsychological tests have variable reliability. Tests used in some studies are clearly more reliable than others (see Table 16.2). False positive or false negative findings can be the result of employing tests with low test-retest reliability. As such, investigators must balance theoretical and practical concerns. For example, the Trail Making Test (TMT) is widely used in clinical settings as well as research investigations of concussive injuries (Collins, Grindall, & Lovell et al., 1999; Macciocchi et al., 1996; Matser et al., 1999), but the TMT is known to have test-retest reliability in the questionable range in some studies (.50 –.60) and documented practice effects in others (Spreen & Strauss, 1998). Consequently, investigators should carefully consider the reliability of all instruments selected for studies.

A related issue involves the susceptibility of neuropsychological instruments to practice effects. Although there is limited literature regarding practice effects, many measures used in studies of concussion have been found to have prominent practice effects (Macciocchi, 1990; McCaffrey, Duff & Westervelt, 2000; Spreen & Strauss, 1998). In fact, some tests have practice effect sizes that equal or exceed effects of concussions on those same instruments (McCaffrey et al., 2000). In repeated measures designs, one solution to practice effects is use of alternate forms of the same test, but the extent to which this effectively reduces practice effects is questionable particularly when tests are administered numerous times over brief periods (Macciocchi et al., 1996; Macciocchi et al., 2001). Methodologically rigorous research indicates the most prominent cognitive impairment following concussion occurs during the few (1–5) days following injury (Collins, Grindell, & Lovell et al., 1999; Macciocchi et al., 1996). Therefore, research could be organized around an empirically derived model which minimizes or limits the number of actual assessments. An alternative approach employed by Hinton-Bayre, Geffen, Geffen, McFarland and Friis (1999) utilizes multiple preinjury assessments in order to obtain maximal performance prior to injury while limiting practice in subsequent postinjury assessments. In this approach, athletes are administered dependent measurers several times prior to entering a study. Consequently, athletes' optimal level of performance is reached prior to injury and a decrement in performance following injury would reflect change from this optimal level. This methodology has considerable promise because changes in performance would theoretically reflect genuine impairment in neuropsy-

Table 16.2. Ranges of reliability coefficients, standard error of measurement and practice effect sizes for neuropsychological tests commonly utilized in concussion research.

Test	Reliability	SEM	Practice Effect Size
$WCST_{PR}$	$.39 - .72_{1,5}$	$8.0 - 11.9_{5}$	$.30 - 1.0_{7}$
TMT_{B}	$.45 - .72_{1}$	$4.7 - 5.6_{1}$	$.20 - .73_{7}$
SDMT	$.72 - .80_{1}$	4.5 - 5.3	$.10 - .20_{7}$
DST	$.80 - .91_{1,4}$	$.90 - .95_{4}$	$.10 - .45_{7}$
PASAT	$.80 - 90_{1}$	$3.1 - 3.9_{1}$	$.40 - 1.3_{7}$
GPT	$.69 - .78_{2}$	$6.9 - 8.1_{2}$	$.10 - .35_{7}$
COWAT	$.70 - .88_{1,2}$	$5.1 - 6.2_{1,2}$	$.30 - .52_{7}$
$HVLT_{T/D}$	$.78_{3}$	$.95 - 2.1_{3}$	$.24 - .30_{3}$

Wisconsin Card Sort Test $(WCST)_5$ Trail Making; Test $(TMT)_1$ Symbol Digit Modalities Test; $(DSMT)_6$ Digit Span Test $(DST)_4$; Paced Auditory Serial Addition Test $(PASAT)_1$; Grooved Pegboard Test $(GPT)_2$; Controlled Oral Word Association Test $(COWAT)_1$; Hopkins Verbal Learning Test $(HVLT)_3$

1. Spreen and Strauss (1998); 2. Mitrushina, Boone and D'Elia (1999);
3. Benedict, Schretlen, Groninger and Brandt (1998); 4. WAIS–III/WMS–III Technical Manual (1997); 5. Heaton, Chelune, Talley, Kay and Curtis (1993);
6. Smith (1995); 7.McCaffery, Duff and Westervelt (2000)

* *Range of SEM based on lower and upper reliability coefficients and normative data for age-education-gender appropriate comparison groups 16–20.*

chological functioning post injury, but few studies using this approach have been published and further investigation is warranted.

Finding changes in neuropsychological functioning (test scores) over time may be due to factors other than practice including maturation. In other words, repeated measure designs must consider the interactions of subject selection and cognitive change or maturation during the study period. For example, athletes may mature cognitively at different rates over the course of a one to four year study, and differential maturation across groups may influence outcome (Daniel et al., 1999). Practice and maturation would of course not affect the study's outcome unless control and "experimental" (concussion) groups are unbalanced in a systematic manner with respect to maturation. Depending on the number of subjects, this may be more or less of a concern. Small samples give reason for concern due to a greater impact of imbalance or failure to match adequately, but the outcome could be affected in favor of a false positive or false negative finding.

The sensitivity and specificity of neuropsychological tests is also important. Neuropsychological instruments used in most studies of concussion are adequately sensitive to cognitive impairment, but the problem is specificity. Tests that are sensitive to subtle changes in cognition typically lack specificity (Spreen & Strauss, 1998). Impairment observed on neuropsychological tests could be related to medical illness, depression, hyposomnia, residual effects of alcohol intoxication, motivation and/or anxiety. Again, one assumes these factors will not systematically affect one group versus another, but this assumption may not be valid. For example, consider the base rate of headache immediately following concussion. Headache is one of the most common symptoms following concussion in sports (70%) as well as in general clinical populations (Alves, Macciocchi & Barth, 1993, Macciocchi et al., 1996). One can imagine how headache could affect sleep which in turn could affect test performance up to several days following injury. One cannot assume that impaired performance on neuropsychological tests is due to transient neurocognitive impairment secondary to cerebral trauma when other factors such as a headache may have a significant direct or indirect effect on test performance. Accordingly, attention to the alertness, energy and stamina of participants at the time of assessment appears prudent, and assessing players during optimal arousal periods may also be helpful.

Another instrumentation concern involves documenting symptoms using self-report checklists. While self-reported symptoms are an important component of research, particularly due to management concerns, there is empirical evidence that the self-report of persons with concussions may not be entirely accurate. Persons may either over or under report symptoms associated with trauma (Ferguson et al., 1999). Therefore, studies should seek to provide multiple indices of change (neurocognition and symptoms), and these measures should corroborate one another. For example, in a recent study, players with two or more concussions reported significantly more symptoms than athletes with no history of concussion, but concussed players evidenced significant differences on only two of seven neuropsychological tests (Collins, Grindell, Lovell et al., 1999).

A final instrumentation concern involves the pragmatics of the study. Often, there is limited time and resources. As such, constraints are placed on access to participants, duration of testing and other data collection. Test administration requires trained professionals, time and space. Most recently, computerized testing via the Internet has been available and this technique offers many advantages over more traditional methods. In addition, there are a number of practical concerns that can result in missing or incomplete data sets. In repeated measure designs, lines of communication with athletic staff and players must be established early in the study and addressed repeatedly as the research progresses. Moreover, athletes may not always respond favorably to being studied. Some athletes may attempt to circumvent the research process by not reporting injuries or avoiding testing. Athletes may also communicate with one another regarding tests which may or may not diminish test validity depending on the methodology employed (Hinton-Bayre, Geffen, Geffen, McFarland, & Friis 1999). Finally, while concussion research may have many positive effects on athletics, perceptions that concussion research may fundamentally alter the game can and do occur. Many sports, especially football have functioned with impugnity for many years. The intrusion of "science" into a sport may not be welcomed by some who do not want investigators altering the demeanor of the game which is another reason for researchers to have meticulous methodology supporting all claims of morbidity associated with concussion.

Statistical issues

In addition to validity issues, statistical concerns merit attention. Prior to beginning a study, researchers typically assess the theoretical magnitude of the effect they expect to observe. The effect size of the independent variable enables computation of the required sample size. Nevertheless, as sample size increases, so does statistical power and the probability of finding a significant difference between experimental and control groups. Simply finding a statistically significant difference between groups is often limited in value, especially if research is supposed to inform clinical practice. The relationship between clinical and statistical significance is important, but the effect size of the independent variable has theoretical value as well. For example, can we specify an effect size for various levels of injury severity? Do grade I, II, and III injuries produce increasing impairment that can be quantified? Of course, some of the problems noted previously suggest that the current grading system may require modification, but in general, more severe injuries should be associated with larger effects on dependent (neuropsychological) measures. In this regard, effect size (d) is technically the difference between group means (experimental minus control) divided by a pooled standard deviation of both groups (Weinfort, 1998). Effect sizes of .2 are considered "small" while effect sizes of .5 and .8 are considered "moderate" and "large" respectively (Cohen, 1977). The size of the effect is dependent on many factors, but in general, small effects suggest limited influence of the independent variable (concussion).

When examining most studies of concussive injury or mild brain injuries in general clinical populations, effect sizes are uniformly small and unimpressive (Binder et al., 1997). In some cases involving athletes, authors do not publish standard deviations so effect sizes cannot be computed (Matser, Kessels, Lezak, Jordan, & Troost, 1999), but in other cases, differences between concussion groups and controls are not particularly impressive. For example, in a recent study, the average effect size for a comparison of athletes with no concussions versus two or more concussions on nine test indices was approximately .2 (Collins, Grindell, Lovell et al., 1999). While one may argue such an effect is meaningful given the number of tests utilized, practice effects in controls can approach or exceed such effects. In another study, change scores were used and effect sizes were equally limited (Macciocchi et al., 1996). While finding statistical significance is meaningful, it is not the sine qua non of research. Investigators should determine effect sizes so that meaningful clinical information can be extrapolated. For example, players with larger injury effects may be managed differently or followed up in a more systematic manner. In fact, some researchers have argued that group studies obscure individual injury responses and have advocated the use of reliable change indeces (RCI) (Hinton-Bayre et al., 1999). RCI's are very similar to calculating effect sizes in that changes on tests or dependent measures are placed in the context of the observed standard deviation. The classic RCI is D divided by σ_{ED} where D is the difference in test scores $(X_1 - Y_1)$ and σ_{ED} is the standard deviation of the sampled measure. Typically an RCI greater than or equal to 1.96 is considered significant (Maassen, 2000).

In addition to placing an emphasis on effect size as well as statistical significance, researchers should consider other issues. For example, most neuropsychological studies employ multiple dependent measures. In such cases, corrections for the number of statistical tests undertaken must be employed. Some authors have used Bonferroni or other corrections which statistically holds alpha at the traditional .05. Statistical procedures such as Multivariate Analysis of Variance (MANOVA) are used to keep alpha levels at a nominal level, but when using a MANOVA, researchers should only interpret individual ANOVA's when the multivariate test is significant. Even when the overall MANOVA is significant, separate ANOVA's do not take into account the correlation between dependent measures (Weinfort, 1998). In any case, as the number of statistical tests increases, the probability of finding statistically significant differences between experimental and control groups by chance increases substantially. Actually, if six dependent measures are used without a correction procedure the overall alpha rises to .265 which is quite higher than the traditional $p<.05$ (Weinfort, 1998). Consequently, statistical conservatism should be considered in concussive research, particularly when numerous dependent measures are employed.

A final issue involves the specific statistics utilized. Many researchers use parametric statistics which require that data be randomly sampled, normally distributed and that experimental and control groups have homogeneous variance. Violation of these assumptions is believed to lead to an increase in Type I (finding a difference between groups when one does not exist) errors (Bordens & Abbott, 1999). Whether research in concussion typically violates these assumptions is questionable, but in most cases, participants are not randomly sampled and neuropsychological data are not normally distributed. As such, researchers may want to consider non-parametric comparative procedures such as the Wilcoxon or Kruskal Wallis depending on the study design (Bordens & Abbott, 1999). Actually, consultation with a statistical expert is prudent prior to initiation of any research. In addition, statistical procedures and the logic in applying these procedures should be clearly discussed in the results section so readers can understand the methods used to reach statistical conclusions.

Table 16.3. Research evaluation checklist.

Experimental Design:
- Posttest only
- Single group pretest-posttest
- Post test control group
- Non equivalent control group

Threats to Validity:
- History
- Selection
- Instrumentation
- Maturation
- Interaction History-Selection

Control Comparisons:
- Age
- Education
- Cognitive (Intelligence/Learning Disability)
- Medical History (Neurologic/Psychiatric)
- Injury History (Prior concussions/severity/frequency)
- Sports History (Duration/Cumulative Cranial/Extracranial Injuries)

Concussion Classification:
- Severity
- Frequency

Instrumentation:
- Tests (Reliability/SEM/Practice Effect Size)
- Symptoms (Reliability/Comprehensiveness)

Statistics:
- Type (Parametric versus non parametric)
- Appropriateness (Assumptions met)
- Dependent Measures (Number)
- Statistical Significance (Power/Alpha/N)
- Effect size (statistical versus clinical significance)

External Validity:
- Data/Interpretation
- Generalization

Summary

Attention has become increasingly focused on concussion in athletics. While data are currently being gathered, there is scientifically credible evidence that recovery from single concussions is usually rapid and complete presuming athletes do not suffer additional injuries (Macciocchi et al.,1996). While this tentative conclusion may be erroneous, the burden is on researchers to design and implement studies that provide interpretable and defensible data to the contrary. Studies with flawed methodology only complicate an already complex clinical and research problem. For example, most researchers are appropriately cautious when interpreting data, and criticizing one's own methodology is obligatory, but all too often researchers do not take their self criticism seriously. For example, in the soccer study cited earlier, the authors generally minimized threats to validity and concluded that soccer presents a "medical and public health concern" (Matser et al., 1999, p. 973). While their conclusion may in fact be accurate, a more adequately designed and executed study would certainly be more persuasive and helpful in addressing the concerns they express.

We have presented a number of issues relevant for designing and implementing studies of concussion (see Table 16.3). We intentionally avoided discussing specific measures or test batteries since this topic has been addressed in other chapters. We also avoided proposing specific designs, but we do recommend prospective pretest-posttest comparison group methodology unless randomized designs can be employed. In addition, established multiple assessment preinjury test baselines and reliable change estimates appear quite promising. Despite our attempt to address many of the problems facing researchers, there are other issues that arise from time to time depending upon the type of research being conducted. Most importantly, many issues remain to be investigated. First, we need to establish reliable and valid severity indices for concussions. Second, the neuropsychological consequences of single and multiple concussions must be firmly established and then the results should be replicated. Third, the short and long-term morbidity related to concussive injuries requires attention. Finally, models of concussion prevention need to be investigated. Unfortunately, none of the aforementioned issues are easily researched, but investigators would benefit from focusing on methodology as a primary consideration in all empirical efforts. In the final analysis, there is nothing more comforting than a reliable and valid scientific finding that stands the test of time.

References

Alves, W.A., Macciocchi, S.N., & Barth, J.T. (1993). Post concussive symptoms after uncomplicated mild brain injury. *Journal of Head Trauma Rehabilitation, 8*(3), 48–59.

Binder, L.M. Rohling, M., & Larabee, G.J. (1997). A review of mild head trauma. Part I: Meta analytic review of neuropsychological studies. *Journal of Clinical and Experimental Neuropsychology, 19*(3), 421–431.

Bordens, R.S. & Abbott, B.B. (1999). *Research design and methods.* London: Mayfield Publishing.

Campbell, D.T. & Stanley, J.C. (1963). *Experimental and quasi-experimental designs for research.* Chicago: Rand McNally College Publishing Company.

Chelune, G.J. (1982). A re-examination of the relationship between the Luria-Nebraska and the Halstead Reitan batteries: Overlap with the WAIS. *Journal of Consulting and Clinical Psychology, 50*(4), 578–580.

Cohen, J. (1977). *Statistical power analysis for the behavioral sciences.* San Diego: Academic Press.

Collins, M.W., Grindell, S.H., Lovell, M.R. Dede, D.E., Moser, D.J., & Phalin, B.R. et al. (1999). Relationship between concussion and neuropsychological performance in college football players. *Journal of the American Medical Association, 282*(10), 964–970.

Collins, M.W., Lovell, M.R., & McKeag, D.B. (1999). Current issues in managing sports-related concussion. *Journal of the American Medical Association, 282*(24), 283–285.

Cook, T.D. & Campbell, D.T. (1979). *Quasi experimentation; Design and analysis for field settings.* Boston: Houghton Mifflin.

Daniel, J.C., Olesniewitz, M.H., Reeves, D.L., Tam, D., Bleiberg, J., & Thatcher, R. et al. (1999). *Journal of Neurology, Neurosurgery and Psychiatry, 12*(3), 167–169.

Dikmen, S. & Levin, H.S. (1993). Methodological issues in the study of mild head injury. *Journal of Head Trauma Rehabilitation, 3*, 30–47.

Dikmen, S.S., Machamer, J.E., Winn, R., & Temkin, N.R. (1995). Neuropsychological outcome at 1-year post injury. *Neuropsychology, 9*(1), 80–90.

Ferguson, R.J., Mittenberg, W., Barone, D.F., & Schnieder, B. (1999). Post concussion syndrome following sports-related head injury; expectation as etiology. *Neuropsychology, 13*(4), 582–589.

Gouvier, W.D., Uddo-Crane, M., & Brown, L.M. (1988). Base rate of post concussive symptoms. *Archives of Clinical Neuropsychology, 3*, 273–278.

Hinton-Bayre, A.D., Geffen, G.M., Geffen, L.B., McFarland, K.A., & Friis, P. (1999). Concussion in contact sports: Reliable change indeces of impairment and recovery. *Journal of Clinical and Experimental Neuropsychology, 21*(1), 70–86.

Kelly, J.P. & Rosenberg, J.H. (1997). Diagnosis and management of concussive in sports. *Neurology, 48*, 575–580.

Lees-Haley, P.R. & Brown, R.S. (1993). Neuropsychological complaint base rates of 170 personal injury claimants. *Archives of Clinical Neuropsychology, 8*, 203–209.

Lovell, M.R., Iverson, G.L., Collins, M.W., McKeag, D., & Marron, J.C. (1999). Does loss of consciousness predict neuropsychological decrements after concussion? *Clinical Journal of Sports Medicine, 9*, 193–198.

Macciocchi, S.N. (1990). Practice makes perfect: Retest effects in college athletes. *Journal of Clinical Psychology, 5*, 628–631.

Macciocchi, S.N., Barth, J.T., Alves, W.A., Rimel, R.W., & Jane, J.A. (1996). Neuropsychological Functioning and Recovery Following Mild Head Injury in Collegiate Athletes. *Neurosurgery, 39*, 510–514.

Macciocchi, S.N., Barth J.T., & Littlefield L. (1998). Outcome after mild head injury. *Clinics in Sports Medicine, 17*(1), 27–36.

Macciocchi, S.N., Barth, J.T., Alves, W.A., & Littlefield, L. (2001). Multiple concussions and neuropsychological functioning in college football players. *Journal of Athletic Training, 36*(3), 303–306.

Maassen, G.H. (2000). Principles of defining reliable change indices. *Journal of Clinical and Experimental Neuropsychology, 22*(5), 622–632.

Matser, E.J.T., Kessels, A.G., Lezak, M.D., Jordan, B.D., & Troost, J. (1999). Neuropsychological impairment in amateur soccer players. *Journal of the American Medical Association, 292*(10), 971–973.

McCaffrey, R.J., Duff, K., & Westervelt, H.J. (2000). *Practitioners guide to evaluating change with neuropsychological assessment instruments.* New York: Kluwer Academic/Plenum.

Spreen, O. & Strauss, E. (1998). *A compendium of neuropsychological tests.* New York: Oxford University Press.

Tremont, G., Hoffman, R.G., Scott, J.G., & Adams, K. (1998). Effect of intellectual level on neuropsychological test performance: A response to Dodrill (1997). *The Clinical Neuropsychologist, 12*, 560–567.

Weinfort, K.P. (1998). Multivariate analysis of variance. In L. Grim & P. Yarnold (Eds.), *Reading and understanding multivariate statistics.* Washington, D.C.: APA Press.

Chapter 17

RELIABILITY, VALIDITY, AND THE MEASUREMENT OF CHANGE IN SERIAL ASSESSMENTS OF ATHLETES

Michael D. Franzen
Allegheny General Hospital

Robert J. Frerichs
University of Victoria

Grant L. Iverson
University of British Columbia

Introduction

Traditionally, neuropsychological assessment has been primarily used either in diagnosis or in the description of skills and deficits in a static temporal context. These characteristics are due to the early historical use of neuropsychological assessment in medical settings. As neuropsychological assessment moves into nontraditional settings, the temporal qualities of assessment results have assumed greater importance. This is particularly true when

Author Notes: A portion of this chapter is derived from the second author's dissertation.

assessment is used with athletes where diagnosis is rarely at issue. Instead the results are used to track the recovery from injury through the recovery of function and the prediction of capacity to perform behaviors outside the test setting. Here, the results of assessment are used to make decisions about the ability to return to play without risking further, and perhaps permanent, injury as well as the relation of test results to behavioral competence.

The reliability and validity of assessment instruments are not merely a function of the quality of the instruments themselves. Reliability is usefully conceptualized as the reliability of the use of an instrument in a particular setting (e.g., sideline and post-injury assessment) with a particular population, such as amateur and professional athletes. Similarly, it is better to conceptualize validity as being a quality of the application of the test results rather than a quality of the instrument itself (Franzen, 2000). Furthermore, the reliability and validity of a neuropsychological evaluation is always partly determined by setting and subject variables.

Competing demands and practical concerns influence the approach to neuropsychological assessment. For example, previously, neuropsychological evaluations were conducted in the luxury of practically unlimited time but with the constraint of requiring sufficient information from the evaluation to not only answer the clinical question but also provide convincing argument to the medical community regarding the utility and seriousness of this approach. It was not uncommon to utilize lengthy evaluations with multiple demands placed on the subjects. Currently, lengthy evaluations are relatively uncommon outside forensic evaluations or grant-supported investigations. As clinical neuropsychology moved into the realm of nontraditional settings and as managed care exerted its influence, there has been a dramatic reduction in evaluation time. Therefore, the issues of reliability and validity are more important in the choice of the evaluation instruments. An example of the nontraditional setting can be found in the current context, evaluating professional athletes for the purpose of baseline information as well as for the purpose of determining the possible effects of concussion and documenting recovery. The constraints of conducting a clinical neuropsychological evaluation are not unique to amateur or professional athletes, but the collection and configuration of constraints is unique and deserving of special consideration. The importance of these constraints relates to their impact on the reliability and validity of the assessment results.

This chapter presents an overview of the practical and methodological considerations relating to the reliability and validity of neuropsychological assessment in sports settings. We also provide a detailed review of the methodological issues associated with the measurement of change in clinical neuropsychology (the practical applications of change methodologies are illustrated in Chapter 18 in this volume by Iverson & Gaetz). We also will consider some basic characteristics, constraints, and limits as they apply to the task of evaluating athletes following concussion. One of the constraints is related to the characteristics of the subjects – the athletes themselves.

On one hand, there may be a wide range of cognitive skill level in amateur athletes, ranging from athletes with significant learning disabilities to the scholar\athlete. Generally speaking, because of the visual-spatial demands of most sports, there might be greater than average skill in this area with greater variability in the verbal areas. On the other hand, professional athletes might have less variability and a greater mean level of cognitive skill, in some areas, than the general population.

Certain subject variables known to influence test scores may be relatively uniform in athletes. These variables include age, gender, and physical health. This degree of consistency may result in attenuation of the variability of baseline scores. As a result, the presence of ceiling effects in the professional athlete is an area of concern because it will have deleterious effects on the accuracy of the estimates of both reliability and validity. If the chosen verbal memory instrument does not measure accurately in the high range then there can be moderate decrements in skill level without significant changes in score, leading us to overestimate the temporal reliability of the instrument. More importantly, this might cause us to overlook subsequent improvement following injury. The same ceiling effects may also result in underestimating the actual skill level of the athlete, adversely affecting estimates of validity. Therefore, it is extremely important to choose instruments that have been evaluated in the context of subject characteristics similar to those of the athlete population in question.

Another issue is that the time allotted for the evaluation is limited. The evaluation period may be only one-half hour. This one-half hour evaluation restricts what can be accomplished, obviating the use of a traditional test battery. In a given amount of time, there is a limit on the number of tests that can be completed. In devising a specific collection of tests, two approaches are available. The first approach is to use few items for each construct (skill) measured, but to assess several skill areas. Because of the small numbers of items for each skill area, there is decreased reliability in the measurement of each skill. Conversely, there may be an increased relation to molar predictions (validity), because a greater number of relevant skill areas have been assessed. Of course the limits on reliability will form a lower bound to the validity of the assessment.

The second approach would be to use a set of procedures that tapped or measured only a few skill areas, but did so with a greater number of items. Increasing the number of items used to tap each skill will increase the reliability of the measurement, but may decrease the validity of judgments made based on the obtained data. The skills tapped may not adequately reflect the target of predicting return to play or skill in the performance of sport-related tasks.

Reliability Issues

Reliability can be estimated using several methods. The methods are related to the hypothesized sources of error. For example, if an important source of error is thought to be a collection of situational variables such as mood, arousal, and energy level of the subject, the test may be administered twice to the same subjects over a standard period of time. The two obtained sets of test scores are then correlated, resulting in a test-retest reliability coefficient. Another relevant source of error is the effect of using items that do not share equal amounts of relation to the intended construct. In this case, the component items' correlation with each other will need to be evaluated by calculating an internal consistency reliability coefficient. Depending upon the setting, different sources of error and therefore different forms of reliability may possess differential importance. It is impossible to conduct measurement completely free of error, and the usual approach is to attempt to minimize the most conceptually relevant sources of error.

It is useful to think of error as multiple extraneous sources of influence on the measurement process. Conceptualizing the process in this manner allows us to accurately minimize the effects of variables obscuring the measurement process. For example, the serial assessment of athletes following injury and recovery from concussion can be affected by many potential sources of error. These include the effects of time, practice, and sufficient sampling from the universe of relevant items.[1]

When administering repeat assessments, knowledge regarding temporal stability and practice effects is required. Error in measurement over time originates from at least two basic areas. First, there may be instability in the scores due to fluctuations in variables, extraneous to the construct being measured, that influence scores. Second, there may be instability due to improved performance secondary to multiple exposures or experiences with the test (a practice effect). If practice effects are a concern, two possible approaches can be attempted. First, multiple forms of the same test can be used. For instance, the Hopkins Verbal Learning Test or HVLT (Brandt, 1991) has six different forms and the Trail Making Test (Reitan & Wolfson, 1985) has an alternate form as well (Franzen, Paul, & Iverson, 1996; McCracken & Franzen, 1992). Each form may have a different level of difficulty or dispersion (as measured by the standard deviation). As such, the raw scores cannot be directly compared and standardized scores such as z-scores or T-scores need to be developed for within subject comparisons using different forms of the test.

A second approach is to conduct research in order to determine the magnitude of the practice effect and subsequently remove this source of error from

[1] McCaffrey, Duff, and Westervelt (2000a, b) performed yeoman duty by cataloging various studies that presented test-retest data for a number of intellectual and neuropsychological instruments. These data are described in terms of subjects' characteristics such as diagnosis, gender, and age, and retest interval. For the purposes of this chapter, however, there are no data reported related to athletes.

the score. However, practice effects can vary as a function of the intertest intervals. Larger intervals may result in less of a practice effect. The interval used in research should be the same as that required by the clinical situation. Because the interval in a practical situation is dictated by the clinical situation, a range of research intervals may need to be obtained. For example, if the athlete is tested preseason in July and retested after an injury in December, we would not want to use a magnitude of practice effect that was generated by research that used a one-week interval. Another limitation of using this approach occurs in the context of multiple assessments. In those situations, using a test with multiple test forms may be more appropriate. Of course, practice effects might still occur with alternate forms of a test; if so, this would require additional study. Alternatively, whenever possible, preseason baseline evaluations may be conducted serially until further practice effects are minimized. Hinton-Bayre, Geffen, and McFarland (1997) demonstrated that if athletes are given two baseline preseason administrations of several speed of processing tests, that practice effects were diminished. Relatedly, Connor, Franzen, and Sharp (1988) found that the practice effects of the Stroop Color Word Test (Golden, 1978) were maximal between the first and third administrations, and became minimal after that time.

Historically, reliability issues have carried less weight for neuropsychologists than have validity issues. It was generally considered that if a test was valid, the reliability issues would be minimized or obviated. This is a view that was born as much out of ignorance as out of convenience. Reliability and validity estimation are highly related in that both are attempts to increase the veridicality and utility of a measurement process. However, demonstrating reliability does not ensure validity. A test with perfect temporal reliability or internal consistency reliability may have no relation to the construct under consideration. However, reliability estimates can provide the lower limit to validity estimates. If a test results in different scores depending upon the time of day, its validity in predicting a construct that is conceptualized as being stable (for instance IQ) is limited.

Validity Issues

The validity of a test is actually an estimate of the validity of decisions made on the basis of the test scores or of the accuracy of the interpretation of the test. In order to judge the validity of tests used in evaluating athletes with concussions, we need to ask ourselves, to what end are the results being used? Basically, the test needs to be a valid index of cognitive impairment following concussion. The tests can be selected following a review of the literature regarding mild head injury, although some additional work in cross-validating the tests for use with athletes will be needed. Sensitive tests appear to be those of sustained attention, memory (especially delayed recall), abstract problem solving, and procedures that are sensitive to speed of information processing and general cognitive efficiency such as the Stroop Color Word Test, Trail Making Test, or the Digit Symbol subtest of the Wechsler Adult Intelligence Scale-Revised (WAIS-R; Wechsler, 1981). It is also important to consider whether the test consistently measures the same construct across different occasions (Richter et al., 1997).

Neuropsychologists need to consider the potential alternate uses for test data and then develop the empirical background necessary to allow for responsible use. Two general areas of test use will engender their own sets of validity issues (as well as their associated ethical concerns). These areas involve the return to active participation in sport and the relation of test scores to athletic performance. Both of these areas are related to the growing concern among clinical neuropsychologists regarding ecological validity. As in other areas of clinical neuropsychological assessment, the ecological validity of the assessment of athletes will have to address both the issues of verisimilitude, the similarity to the target task or skill, and veridicality, the actual empirical relation to prediction of real life behaviors or skills (Franzen & Wilhelm, 1996). Tasks of motor coordination and visual-motor integration might have greater verisimilitude to specific sports-related behaviors, and certain cognitive problem solving skills may have greater veridicality to performance on the field. The ecological validity of neuropsychological assessment needs to be better developed in terms of empirical accuracy and in terms of understanding the ethical dilemmas associated with it. Clearly, predicting the return to active participation involves some of the same issues as predicting the return to work for the average individual with mild traumatic brain injury. In particular, a statement must be made regarding the athlete's ability to perform relative to previous levels, or at least, at a level consistent with competitive play. However, the relation of neuropsychological test scores to athletic performance is beyond the limits of this chapter. At present, no predictor of sports performance is greater than performance on the practice field.

From a clinical standpoint, the most important use of neuropsychological data in this setting is to predict when an athlete can reasonably return to play. Although mild head injury usually shows good improvement, repeated head trauma might have cumulative effects. In addition, there may be a critical period of recovery during which additional injury could result in severe consequences. Therefore, the validity of inferences regarding return to play, based on neuropsychological test data and symptom inventories, is worthy of considerable study. The decision to return to play, to sit out the season, or to retire from the sport is complex and requires accurate information.

Measurement of Change Issues

The measurement of change is an important issue that has attracted the attention of many different researchers and methodologists. An early and influential book was edited by Chester Harris (1963), following a conference on the topic. It wasn't until nearly thirty years later that a subsequent book was edited on the topic, again the consequence of a conference (Collins & Horn, 1991). Yet a second volume of papers (Collins & Sayer, 2001) provided an overview of the advances made in the recent past. The focus of these papers is primarily on the measurement of change in "group" data in experimental rather than clinical settings. However, there is value in examining the concepts and methods. For example, Osgood (2001) briefly discusses the use of individual growth curves and latent curve models. Differential structural equation modeling of change in a single individual may seem like overkill and unnecessary complication. However, the use of this methodology is greatly simplified by the availability of computer programs. Furthermore, latent trait analysis may help examine whether the tests are actually measuring the same construct at different times. For example, is Digit Span measuring focused cognitive processing immediately following a concussive injury but measuring simple attention six months post-injury? This methodology was used to examine the use of the Beck Depression Inventory in measuring change in depressed subjects in light of the possibility that the total scores on the BDI may reflect different constructs at different levels and times in treatment (Richter et al., 1997).

It is instructive to examine other approaches used by psychologists and researchers in the measurement of change. Because researchers have examined the measurement of change most intensively, much of the theory and applications have pertained to measurement of change in "group" data. Of course, the clinical perspective is to measure change in the individual. Despite this basic difference in perspective, there is much to be gained from surveying the measurement of change in other areas. One of the most universally vexing factors is the Law of Initial Values or LIV (Jamieson, 1995). The LIV has been found to apply in almost every biological and social system that has been subject to repeat measurements. The proposed theoretical reasons for the ubiquitous presence of LIV include the conservative nature of most systems and the notion that the measured value of any multiply determined variable will partly depend on values of the influential factors at some time prior to the measurement instance, and by extension, would be partly dependent upon values of the measured variable at a time prior to the measurement instance. In simple but poetic language, the past is prologue to the present.

The relation among successive measurement values is conceptualized as an autocorrelation. The behavioral literature, the psychophysiological literature, and the econometric literature have proposed various methods of reducing the influence of the autocorrelation. These proposals include residualizing the autocorrelation function or using simple arithmetic to calculate moving averages across various time intervals. Unfortunately, both of these methods require a greater number of observations than are usually found in sports concussion data. However, the conceptual considerations alert the sports neuropsychologist to the notion that the two measurements used to determine if change has occurred are actually drawn from a universe of possible observa-

tions and measurements, all of which are related to each other.
The following section contains a detailed review of methods used to measure change in clinical psychology and neuropsychology. This literature has evolved over many years. To date, there has been very little application of these methodologies to sports neuropsychology, so the vast majority of this review relates to the psychotherapy literature and the clinical neuropsychology literature.

Methods for Measuring Change

Over the past decade, various statistical methods have been proposed to minimize or account for the errors and biases inherent in multiple assessments. The following review will focus on those methods designed to measure change over two occasions (i.e., test-retest designs). Change, arguably, is most meaningfully examined through the collection of multi-wave data employing more than two measurements (Rogosa, 1988; Rogosa, Brandt, & Zimowski, 1982; Speer, 1999; Speer & Greenbaum, 1995), but there are instances when this is neither feasible nor appropriate (Hageman & Arrindell, 1999a). The test-retest design remains common in the neuropsychological literature and pertinent to clinical practice. Sports neuropsychology is one of the few areas where data on multiple measures over several brief intervals are collected. Nonetheless, it is important to review carefully the variety of methods for studying change using two-wave data, before the field advances to the more complex area of considering multiple evaluations.

Simple difference method

The difference in observed scores between pretest and posttest is the most obvious and simple measure of change. It is also the most maligned. Difference scores have been frequently criticized as poor indicators of change due to low reliability and their tendency to correlate negatively with initial status (Cronbach & Furby, 1970; Linn & Slinde, 1977; Lord, 1963). Under certain circumstances, it has been shown that the reliability of the difference score tends to decrease as the pretest-posttest correlation increases. The implication is that the use of neuropsychological measures with high test-retest reliability may not yield reliable difference scores. The second criticism implies that persons with low (or high) scores on a certain measure are more likely to exhibit large (or small) difference scores. This relation would appear to "give an advantage to persons with certain values of the pretest score" (Linn & Slinde, 1977, p. 125) making the use of difference scores untenable.

Rogosa (1988; Rogosa et al., 1982) has challenged both criticisms and defended the use of the difference score as an unbiased estimate of true change. He argued that difference scores are not intrinsically unreliable; they are only unreliable if there is little variability in change rates across persons. The reliability of a difference score is quite respectable so long as there are individual differences in true change within the population of interest. Furthermore, Rogosa viewed the negative correlation between initial status and change (r_{X1D}) as an irrelevant artifact arising from errors of measurement. The correlation between an observed pretest score and observed change (both of which are subject to measurement error) provides an inadequate and biased estimate of the population correlation between initial *true* score and *true* score change (i.e., the correlation of real interest). He summarily argued: "in no way is the negative bias of r_{X1D} a fundamental problem with the use of the difference score as a measure of individual change" (Rogosa et al., 1982, p. 734).

Several measures of change (to be discussed) are linear transformations of the difference score involving a standard error term. For the difference score to be used as an indicator of "significant" or diagnostic change requires a cutoff point. Matarazzo, Carmody, and Jacobs' (1980) rule of thumb exemplifies this approach. These authors suggested that a change of at least 15 points in IQ must be evident before interpreting a change as "potentially" clinically important. One of the main drawbacks to this approach is that cutoff scores often are arbitrarily chosen. If they are derived empirically, cutoff scores may vary as a function of the sample from which they are derived. Another disadvantage of simple difference scores is that they do not account for measurement errors or practice effects.

Standard deviation method

A second approach to define change in cognitive functioning is the standard deviation (SD) method in which a person is considered to have deteriorated if his/her difference score is more than one SD below the group mean pretest score on a certain measure. The use of one SD as the criterion for cut-off appears to be arbitrary since it is not clearly informed by any sound psychometric consideration. In practice, the SD method has been used to assess neuropsychological change following temporal lobectomy and cardiac surgery (Hermann & Wyler, 1988; Mahanna et al., 1996; Phillips & McGlone, 1995; Shaw et al., 1986). It has also been used to classify cognitive change in persons with and without dementia (Bieliauskas, Fastenau, Lacy, & Roper, 1997). Though the method is simple, there is little consistency in how the approach is applied. Some researchers treat a significant decline on a single test as evidence of change whereas others operationalize change as a decline of one SD on 20% of all measures administered. The SD method for detecting change in test-retest scores can be criticized for its failure to account for measurement errors in the observed scores and the effects of practice.

Reliable change indices

The SEM has been advocated as an acceptable method for estimating the significance of test-retest changes in the individual (Edwards, Yarvis, Mueller, Zingale & Wagman, 1978; Shatz, 1981), despite cautions about its appropriate use (Brophy, 1986; Charter, 1996; Dudek, 1979). Jacobson,

Follette, and Revenstorf (1984) proposed a reliable change index (RCI), which was based on the SEM, as a means to evaluate psychotherapeutic change in individuals over time. The RCI was created to ensure that observed test score change is statistically reliable (this was one part of their criteria for clinically significant change). Reliable change refers to a difference in observed test scores that exceeds the amount of variation that could be reasonably attributed to measurement error. The RCI was originally defined as: RCI = $X_2 - X_1$ / SEM. The SEM = $SD\sqrt{1-r_{12}}$ where SD is the pretest or normal control group standard deviation and r_{12} is the test-retest reliability coefficient.

The use of the RCI assumes that the true score of the individual remains constant from time one to time two. RCIs are based on a fixed-alpha strategy, and therefore their interpretation is similar to null hypothesis testing. After the alpha level is set, the critical z-score(s) are determined to mark the fixed boundaries of reliable change. For $\alpha = .05$ (two-tailed), the RCI must exceed 1.96 for the change to be deemed a statistically reliable improvement. A decrement in performance is identified as statistically reliable if the RCI is less than –1.96. RCI scores falling between these two critical cutoff points represent no reliable change; this amount of change is expected to occur by chance 95% of the time. A more lenient RCI of ±1.645 ($\alpha = 0.10$, two-tailed) is also common.

Speer (1992) attempted to improve Jacobson et al.'s (1984) RCI by correcting for the effects of regression to the mean. In accordance with the methods of Edwards et al. (1978) and Nunnally (1967), a regression adjustment was made to the numerator of the RCI by replacing the observed pretest score with an estimate of the individual's true initial score (which is always closer to the mean). One limitation of the method proposed by Speer is that it does not account for practice effects. It has also been criticized for using an improper standard error term (i.e., the SEM) and for ignoring the unreliability inherent in the measurement of the posttest score (Hageman & Arrindell, 1993).

The RCI, as defined in most current research, no longer employs the SEM in the denominator (Jacobson & Revenstorf, 1988; Jacobson, Roberts, Berns, & McGlinchey, 1999; Jacobson & Truax, 1991). The formula was amended following Christensen and Mendoza's (1986) suggestion that the standard error of difference (S_{diff}) between two observed test scores was the more appropriate error term. The S_{diff} refers to the distribution of difference scores that one would expect from the same person on the same test as a function of measurement error alone (i.e., when no real change has occurred). It has been defined as $\sqrt{2(SEM_1^2)}$, where the SEM from time one is squared before it is multiplied by two. By this definition, the S_{diff} is always larger than the SEM (by a factor of 1.414) and it therefore results in a more stringent criterion for change.

In light of recent confusion in the literature (see Abramson, 2000; Hinton-Bayre, 2000; Temkin, Heaton, Grant, & Dikmen, 2000), it should be noted that there are several methods for computing the S_{diff}. The most common method (Christensen & Mendoza, 1986; Jacobson & Truax, 1991) provides an approximation of the S_{diff} because it assumes that the standard deviations of the test scores are equivalent at both time 1 and 2. The S_{diff} has alternatively been defined and applied as $\sqrt{SEM_1^2 + SEM_2^2}$ (Anastasi, 1988; Franzen & Iverson, 2000; Hageman & Arrindell, 1993; Iverson, 1998, 1999, 2001; Iverson, Sawyer, McCracken, & Kozora, 2001). The practical impact of using one method over another has not been systematically investigated. However, mathematically, it is clear that the implications for the computed S_{diff} are negligible if the test and retest standard deviations are very similar. However, if they differ, the S_{diff} will be affected. We recommend the use of the "true" S_{diff} formula, rather than the more commonly computed "estimated" S_{diff}.

The simplicity of the original reliable change formula, as provided in Jacobson and Truax (1991), has made it popular in both the psychotherapy and neuropsychological literature (Hinton-Bayre, Geffen, Geffen, McFarland, & Friis, 1999; Jacobson et al., 1999). Although this method yields important categorical information (i.e., reliable improvement, no reliable change, or reliable decrement), it is not meant to explicitly measure the relative magnitude of individual change. Furthermore, it is not amenable for use in making comparisons among different measures because the index is expressed in the units of a specific measure. The method does account for errors due to the unreliability of the measure, but it does not make specific adjustments for practice effects or regression to the mean (Hsu, 1989; Hsu, 1995; Speer, 1992).

There have been several attempts to improve the reliable change methodology. Chelune and colleagues proposed a correction that accounts for practice effects. Their correction simply involves subtracting a constant value from the observed difference score (Chelune, Naugle, Luders, Sedlak, & Awad, 1993). The constant is typically the mean amount of group improvement or decrement over a specified interval in a control sample. This approach subsequently has been employed in several neuropsychological studies (e.g., Hermann et al., 1996; Ivnik et al., 1999; Kneebone, Andrew, Baker, & Knight, 1998) and has been largely viewed as an appropriate means to measure individual change in cognitive abilities. The main limitation of this method is that practice effects associated with any specific measure are assumed to be uniform for all people. This assumption is likely incorrect since practice effects, as previously mentioned, are also determined by the test-retest interval and the characteristics of the persons who comprise the reference sample.

Hsu (1989; 1999), like Speer (1992), proposed an alternate reliable change formula to correct for the effects of regression to the mean. His modification changed the raw change score in the original equation into a "residualized gain" score to take into account an individual's level of performance relative to the group mean. The standard error term relevant to a residual change score is the standard error of prediction (SEP). Accordingly, the S_{diff} (technically, the estimated S_{diff} ; Iverson, 1998) in the denominator of the formula was replaced with the SEP. A criticism of the method proposed by Hsu is that the relevant group mean to which test scores are supposed to regress toward may not be known or easily determined. Nunnally and Kotsh (1983) have addressed this issue and recommend using the general norms that exist for a specific measure when an individual's group membership is in question. Hageman and Arrindell (1993), in contrast, have suggested that reference need only be made to the observed pretest and posttest means.

Hageman and Arrindell (1993; 1999a; 1999b) have proposed two different refinements of the reliable change methodology. The first, named RC_{ID} (for "improved difference" score) modifies the numerator substantially by accounting for regression to the mean due to measurement unreliability. The reliability term used to estimate measurement error is the reliability of the difference score (r_{DD}). In the denominator, the S_{diff} term is retained but is calculated based on separate SEMs for the pretest and posttest. This differs from Jacobson and Truax's (1991) method in which a single SEM value is assumed for both the pretest and posttest score distributions. For the calculation of the pretest and posttest SEMs, Hageman and Arrindell (1993) recommended the use of Guttman's (1945) reliability coefficients. These coefficients represent the lower bounds of the reliability of a measure calculated from a single sample.

The latest index from Hageman and Arrindell (1999a; 1999b), named RC_{INDIV}, is unique in that it does not employ a fixed-alpha strategy like other reliable change indices. It instead uses a phi-strategy introduced by Cronbach and Gleser (1959) in which the risk of being misclassified as "improved" or "deteriorated" is set to a maximum allowable value (e.g., 5%). There is an important distinction between the phi-strategy and the more popular alpha-strategy used in decision-making. The fixed-alpha strategy assumes that the true difference is zero (i.e., no real change from time 1 to time 2) and a sufficiently large difference score will result in the rejection of the null hypothesis and infer that true change has occurred. The traditional question addressed is therefore: "Given an individual for whom the true difference is zero, how likely is it that we will interpret a difference". The RC_{INDIV} based on the phi-strategy answers a slightly different question: "Given an individual with an observed difference, how likely are we to be correct in classifying the difference?" (McGlinchey & Jacobson, 1999, p. 212). An $RCI_{INDIV} > 1.65$ indicates a statistically reliable change at the individual level with a maximum 5% chance of misclassifying the direction of change. The RC_{INDIV} creators claim it is more sensitive than other RCIs to declining scores, but the use of the phi-strategy for decision-making is neither well-known nor widely applied. The utility of this approach needs to be adequately tested in clinical research.

Regression-based change scores

Linear regression models have been used to evaluate change on neuropsychological tests (e.g., McSweeny, Naugle, Chelune, & Luders, 1993; Salinsky, Storzbach, Dodrill, & Binder, 2001; Sawrie, Chelune, Naugle & Luders, 1996; Sawrie, Marson, Boothe & Harrell, 1999; Temkin, Heaton, Grant, & Dikmen, 1999). The simplest model is to use time one scores to predict time two scores (i.e., simple linear regression, where Y = a + bX, and "a" equals the point where the regression line crosses the Y-axis and "b" equals the slope of the line). If you imagine athletes test scores on the X-axis and retest scores on the Y-axis, then conceptually the retest scores are regressed on the test scores, and the regression equation is written Y = a + bX, where Y is the predicted retest score and X is the time one score. If additional variables, other than initial score, are related to the retest score, then multiple regression can be used. Multiple regression, in contrast to simple regression, involves generating an equation that includes the pretest score in addition to any other relevant variables that may influence test performance. Age, education, gender, and overall cognitive status are common examples of variables that might influence cognitive test performance. Application of the multiple regression equation allows one to generate an expected time two score for an individual (i.e., predicted X_2 = (beta weight * X_1) + (beta weight * V_1) + ... + (beta weight * V_n) + constant).

The advantage, of course, of linear regression is that this approach accounts for both practice effects and regression to the mean. However, linear regression has certain statistical assumptions that frequently are violated in sports concussion data. Homoscedasticity, analogous to homogeneity of variance in ANOVA, assumes an equal variation in Y's across the entire range of X's. Thus, for each value of the time 1 variable, the retest variable is assumed to have a normal distribution, and the mean of this distribution is the predicted retest score (i.e., Y). Moreover, the standard deviation of Y is assumed to be the same for every value of X. Another assumption of linear regression relates to the term "linear"; that is, the mean values of Y corresponding to the various values of X fall in a straight line. Fortunately, regression is fairly robust to violations of some of its underlying assumptions such as the assumption of homoscedasticity; nonetheless, researchers should consider the nature of their data carefully with regard to the assumption of linearity of regression prior to employing these models.

Crawford and Howell (1998) introduced a new, and more technically accurate, regression method for comparing predicted and obtained scores. This newer method addresses the error that arises from the use of sample coefficients to estimate population regression coefficients. In McSweeney et al.'s (1993) approach, the regression equation is specific to the sample and therefore represents an optimal fit of the sample data. It is assumed that the sample is representative of the population and that the derived equation may be used to accurately predict posttest scores for individuals who were not in the original sample. A failure to adjust the regression equation to reflect the estimation of population regression coefficients might increase the likelihood that discrepant scores would be identified as significantly changed. This error would be magnified for pretest scores that are further from the mean pretest score. The new method accounts for this potential error by multiplying a correction factor to the SEE for each individual case. It should be noted that the authors recommended the use of the t-statistic, rather than the z-statistic, when working with samples rather than populations. A $t_{\alpha/2}$ (df = N – 2) is therefore used to replace the $z_{\alpha/2}$ value (e.g., 1.96 or 1.64) used in other methods to demarcate the bounds of reliable change.

Crawford and Howell (1998) employed hypothetical neuropsychological data to examine the impact of using the unadjusted and technically correct regression methods. Their examination suggested that the unadjusted method systematically yielded narrower confidence intervals than those obtained using the correct method. For sufficiently large sample sizes (i.e., N > 100) and pretest scores that were not extreme (i.e., > 2 SDs), the differences between the two approaches were modest. The authors recommend using the technically correct method for use with smaller samples. Crawford and Howell's (1998) correct method is beginning to be applied in clinical neuropsychological research (e.g., Graves, 2000).

The strength of regression approaches in change measurement is that they control for practice effects, regression to the mean, and any other test-retest confound observed in the normal population for a particular measure (McSweeney et al., 1993). By factoring out the variance of the pretest from the posttest, this approach essentially serves to equate individuals who differ in their baseline performance. Another advantage is that regression-based change scores may be expressed as continuous variables in terms of a common metric (e.g., z-scores or T scores), thus facilitating comparison of scores among different measures. This differs from the limited categorical information yielded by reliable change indexes (i.e., reliable improvement, no change, or reliable decline).

As previously noted, the regression methods described above are not appropriate when the assumptions of multiple regression are violated. The relation between the pretest and posttest scores should be linear and homoscedastic and the predictor(s) should be measured without error (Pedhazur, 1982). The assumption of classical test theory regarding the fallibility of measurement is inconsistent with the assumption of regression analysis. McSweeney et al. (1993) recommended that this method should not be used when the data for change are not normally distributed. As well, measures prone to floor or ceiling effects are not amenable for use with regression methods. Finally, one needs to consider the appropriateness of the regression equation for use with a specific individual. The accuracy of the regression equations may be compromised when applied to individuals whose scores or characteristics are outside of the range of the reference sample from which the equation was derived. It is not clear how robust regression methods are to violations of these assumptions.

Comparing Methods of Change Measurement

A variety of methods have been proposed over the last decade to assist clinicians in determining the significance of changes in test scores. With each proposal, there has been considerable debate as to the "right" way to address errors and biases in measurement and the proper standard error term that should be used. It is surprising that few attempts have been made to directly compare these methods. This may, in part, reflect the fact that at least two of the methods have been introduced only very recently (i.e., Crawford & Howell, 1998; Hageman & Arrindell, 1999b). Jacobson et al. (1999) acknowledged the current state of the literature and concluded "less mathematical wrangling and more empirical testing is needed" (p. 306) to determine the utility of different change scores.

Speer and Greenbaum (1995) were one of the first researchers to examine the relation among different RCIs. They compared the formulas reported in Jacobson and Truax (1991), Speer (1992), and Hsu (1989) with hierarchical linear modeling (HLM) using multi-wave data from 73 outpatients on a scale of general well-being. With the exception of the formula by Hsu, there was considerable agreement (ranging from 78% to 81%) among the various methods in terms of the proportion of cases classified as "improved" and "not improved." The HLM method was quite liberal and was more likely than the other methods to classify a change as improved. The HLM method failed to identify a single case as significantly deteriorated. The other methods were slightly more conservative and yielded similar classifications for reliable change. Hsu's method, in contrast, had the lowest agreement with the other methods; it generated the lowest improvement rate and the highest deterioration rate. Speer and Greenbaum (1995) favored the HLM method, but recommended use of the Jacobson and Truax (1991) method in situations in which there are only two testing occasions.

Kneebone et al. (1998) examined methods for change using neuropsychological test data. These researchers compared the reliable change method that corrects for practice effects to the SD method in 50 patients following coronary artery bypass grafting. RCIs were calculated using a 90% confidence interval based on the initial and follow-up data of 24 control participants (7-day test-retest interval). The neuropsychological battery included the California Verbal Learning Test (CVLT; Delis, Kramer, Kaplan & Ober, 1987), Purdue Pegboard (Tiffin, 1968), word fluency measures (Benton & Hamsher, 1978), Trail Making Tests, Digit Symbol subtest from the WAIS-R, and the Boston Naming Test (BNT; Kaplan, Goodglass, & Weintraub, 1983). Test-retest reliability coefficients over the one-week interval ranged from 0.67 to 0.94. The results of the study revealed that the RCI method with correction for practice classified more patients as showing post-operative decline than the SD method on 7 of the 11 neuropsychological measures (including word fluency, Trail Making Parts A and B, BNT, and the Digit Symbol subtest). The SD method classified more individuals as deteriorated on the three main indices of the CVLT. The investigators interpreted these differences as the failure of the SD method to account for practice effects and measurement unreliability.

Bruggemans,Van de Vijver, and Huysmans (1997) also examined neuropsychological test data from persons who had cardiac surgery. These investigators compared the SD, RCI without practice correction, RCI with practice correction, and a regression-based method using data from a sample of 63 patients seen over four occasions. In addition, they included a complex method for measuring change that involved controlling for error and practice effects by matching each patient with a group of control participants on the basis of pretest scores. With the exception of the SD method, critical values for determining reliable deterioration were based on $z > 1.645$ ($\alpha = 0.05$, one-tailed) for all methods. The battery of measures included the Rey Auditory Verbal Learning Test (RAVLT; Lezak, 1995; Rey, 1964), subtests from the Wechsler Memory Scale –Revised (WMS-R; Wechsler, 1987), word fluency (Benton & Hamsher, 1978), Trail Making Test, the Stroop Interference test, and the Symbol Digit Modalities Test (Smith, 1982). A different pattern of results emerged between the lower reliability learning and memory measures ($r = 0.45$ to 0.79) and higher reliability fluency, attention, and psychomotor measures ($r = 0.76$ to 0.92). In measures with lower reliability, the use of the SD method (which does not correct for measurement error) resulted in an overestimation of deterioration rates relative to the other methods. There were few differences among the two RCIs and the regression-based change scores under these conditions. For highly reliable measures, the failure to correct for practice effects resulted in an underestimation of deterioration rates using the SD method and the RCI. These findings are consistent with the results of Kneebone et al. (1998) who also reported inflated deterioration rates when using the SD method on measures of memory but an underestimation of deterioration in other cognitive domains.

Temkin et al. (1999) compared RCI methods with and without correction for practice, simple linear regression-based, and stepwise multiple regression-based change scores using two-wave neuropsychological data from 384 neurologically stable adults. The sample included 37 adults over the age of 65 years. Test-retest intervals varied substantially from 2.3 to 15.8 months (mean = 9.1 months). The neuropsychological measures were indices from the original WAIS (Wechsler, 1955) and the Halstead-Reitan Neuropsychological Test Battery (HRB; Reitan & Wolfson, 1993). These researchers evaluated the four methods on the basis of (a) the width of the prediction interval yielded by each method, and (b) the accuracy with which each model fit an expected normal distribution of scores (in which 5% of cases were expected to show a significant improvement and 5% a significant deterioration). The authors concluded that the RCI method with no correction for practice was the least accurate because it consistently yielded the widest prediction intervals and classified more cases than expected as improved and fewer cases as deteriorated. The RCI with a correction for practice yielded equally wide prediction intervals as the RCI without correction, but improved classification accuracy. The best method by their evaluation criteria was the multiple regression-based method that incorporated baseline test performance and additional demographic variables. But overall, this more complex multivariate method did not substantially improve classification accuracy over that of either the simple linear regression method or the RCI with correction for practice.

In a follow-up study, Heaton and colleagues compared the RCI with correction for practice, simple regression, and multivariate regression methods in a samples of healthy controls (n = 124), patients believed to have stable schizophrenia (n = 69), and in small samples of patients in acute recovery from traumatic brain injury (n = 23) or diverse neuropathological conditions (n = 10) (Heaton et al., 2001). WAIS VIQs and PIQs; the Halstead Impairment Index and Average Impairment Rating; and individual scores from the Category Test, Trails B, and the Tactual Performance Test (time per block) were compared. These researchers demonstrated clearly that the standard errors of difference between time one and time two varied considerably based on level of performance at time one (consistent with the findings of Temkin et al., 1999). Therefore, different S_{diffs} were calculated based on whether the subject had low initial performance or average or greater initial performance. They also demonstrated larger-than-expected misclassification rates on retest, in both directions, for patients with presumed stable schizophrenia, suggesting that normative data for change need to be generated for both healthy controls and clinical groups. The authors concluded that the more sophisticated regression-based methods did not outperform the RCI with correction for practice. Thus, they recommended continued use of the latter, with the caveat that it is necessary to consider carefully the initial level of performance. Different confidence intervals will apply to different baseline neuropsychological test scores.

Conclusions

The comparison studies reviewed above differ in terms of the measures that were used, the sample studied, the test-retest interval, and the specific change methods that were examined. It is therefore difficult to draw firm conclusions, but it may be worthwhile to comment on the emerging patterns and trends. The findings across the studies suggest that the SD method is inferior to the reliable change and regression-based methods. This is consistent with hypotheses based on measurement theory since the SD method employs an arbitrary criterion for change and fails to account for a single error or bias. The original reliable change method represents an improvement over the SD method but lacks the improved accuracy of methods that adjust for practice effects. Finally, the reliable change method that corrects for practice appears to be as accurate in classification as the more complex regression models (Heaton et al., 2001; Temkin et al., 1999).

A major limitation of the studies that have compared methods for measuring change involves their evaluative standards. The common (and reasonable) focus among these studies has been the proportion of cases classified as improved or deteriorated by each method. However, simply looking at the classification differences between two methods (e.g., Kneebone et al., 1998) does not adequately address whether either method actually captured "real" change (unless it is assumed that *all* cardiac surgery patients show substantial declines across a broad range of cognitive abilities). Comparing the observed improvement and deterioration rates to the pattern that is expected on the basis of chance alone (e.g., 5% to show improvement and 5% to show deterioration) also provides only limited evidence in support of a method's usefulness in change measurement. Consider Temkin et al.'s (1999) study. How much can be learned about the utility of different methods for detecting cognitive change when the sample is comprised of "neurologically stable" individuals who presumably did not evidence "real" change? An important test of a method's utility might involve examining a group of individuals for whom clinically significant change has been well documented. Of course, clinically significant change could be operationalized in a variety of ways; but the point is that a reasonable index of clinically meaningful change would be a useful yardstick for evaluating change methods than what has been employed to date.

The real world significance of statistically reliable change is an important issue that has not been thoroughly investigated (Kazdin, 1999). The RCI, for example, assesses whether an observed change exceeds that which might be reasonably attributed to measurement error but it does not specifically address how rare or abnormal a difference score is in the population. Research is needed to determine exactly what reliable change (as defined using different methods) on one or more neuropsychological tests actually means. Is reliable change related to a diagnostic change? Or is reliable change common among certain populations? Adopting clinical significance as a comparative standard may help answer these questions. It should be noted that such a standard not only provides a means by which to compare methods for measuring change, it may also serve to establish the validity of neuropsychological instruments for the purpose of measuring change. A frequent finding of reliable change on certain tests in the absence of clinically meaningful change, or a failure to observe reliable change when clinically significant change was deemed to have occurred, may suggest that the instrument is inappropriate for documenting change.

The reliable change methodology has only recently been applied to sports neuropsychology (Hinton-Bayre et al., 1999). These researchers applied the formula from Jacobson and Truax (1991) to small samples of athletes with concussions versus uninjured controls. This elegantly written paper is an important step for the field. These data are limited, however, because (a) the original formula uses and estimated S_{diff}, as opposed to the actual S_{diff}, which assumes that the dispersion in retest scores is the same as the dispersion in baseline scores; (b) the sample sizes were very small which reduces the accuracy of the reliability and dispersion estimates, (c) their was no correction for practice effects applied to the formula, and (d) there was no consideration of baseline level of performance in relation to the test-retest difference scores.

These methodological limitations are not unique to this study, of course. Many apply to the majority of studies relating to reliable change. They are mentioned here, as a means of summarizing what has been discussed in this chapter, to encourage advancements in the methodologies as applied to sports neuropsychology.

The measurement of change is a complex undertaking that is receiving increasing attention in both the clinical and experimental literature. The fact that it had historically received scant attention despite almost universal recognition of its challenge is an index of the difficulties involved. Sports neuropsychologists involved with sideline and return-to-play evaluations cannot ignore these issues. Many of the issues are shared with the field of measurement of change in general, although some issues are unique to athletes and situational demands. This area of research eventually will provide essential information to advance the clinical practice of evaluating athletes following concussions.

References

Abramson, I.S. (2000). Reliable change formula query: A statistician's comments. *Journal of the International Neuropsychological Society, 6*, 365.

Anastasi, A. (1988). *Psychological testing* (6th ed.). Upper Saddle River, NJ: Prentice Hall.

Benton, A.L., & Hamsher, K. (1978). *Multilingual Aphasia Examination manual.* Iowa City: University of Iowa Press.

Bieliauskas, L.A., Fastenau, P.S., Lacy, M.A., & Roper, B.L. (1997). Use of the odds ratio to translate neuropsychological test scores into real-world outcomes: From statistical significance to clinical significance. *Journal of Clinical and Experimental Neuropsychology, 19*, 889–896.

Brandt, J. (1991). The Hopkins Verbal Learning Test: Development of a new memory test with six equivalent forms. *The Clinical Neuropsychologist, 5*, 125-142.

Brophy, A.L. (1986). Confidence intervals for true scores and retest scores on clinical tests. *Journal of Clinical Psychology, 42*, 989–991.

Bruggemans, E.F., Van de Vijver, F.J.R., & Huysmans, H.A. (1997). Assessment of cognitive deterioration in individual patients following cardiac surgery: Correcting for measurement error and practice effects. *Journal of Clinical and Experimental Neuropsychology, 19*, 543–559.

Charter, R.A. (1996). Revisiting the standard errors of measurement, estimate, and prediction and their application to test scores. *Perceptual and Motor Skills, 82*, 1139–1142.

Chelune, G.J., Naugle, R.I., Luders, H., Sedlak, J., & Awad, I.A. (1993). Individual change after epilepsy surgery: Practice effects and base-rate information. *Neuropsychology, 7*, 41–52.

Christensen, L., & Mendoza, J.L. (1986). A method of assessing change in a single subject: An alteration of the RC Index. *Behavior Therapy, 17*, 305–308.

Collins, L.M. & Horn, J.L. (Eds.). (1991). *Best Methods for the Analysis of Change.* Washington, D.C.: American Psychological Association.

Collins, L.M. & Sayer, A.G. (2001). *New Methods for the Analysis of Change.* Washington, DC: American Psychological Association Press.

Connor, A., Franzen, M.D., & Sharp, B.S. (1988). The effect of practice and instruction on Stroop performance. *International Journal of Clinical Neuropsychology, 10*, 1–4.

Crawford, J.R., & Howell, D.C. (1998). Regression equations in clinical neuropsychology: An evaluation of statistical methods for comparing predicted and obtained scores. *Journal of Clinical and Experimental Neuropsychology, 20*, 755–762.

Cronbach, L.J., & Furby, L. (1970). How should we measure "change" – or should we? *Psychological Bulletin, 74*, 68–80.

Cronbach, L.J., & Gleser, G.C. (1959). Interpretation of reliability and validity coefficients: Remarks on a paper by Lord. *Journal of Educational Psychology, 50*, 230–237.

Delis, D.C., Kramer, J.H., Kaplan, E., & Ober, B.A. (1987). *California Verbal Learning Test.* San Antonio, TX: Psychological Corporation.

Dudek, F.J. (1979). The continuing misinterpretation of the standard error of measurement. *Psychological Bulletin, 86*, 335–337.

Edwards, D.W., Yarvis, R.M., Mueller, D.P., Zingale, H.C., & Wagman, W.J. (1978). Test-taking and the stability of adjustment scales. Can we assess patient deterioration? *Evaluation Quarterly, 2*, 275–291.

Franzen, M.D. (2000). *Reliability and Validity in Neuropsychological Assessment.* (2nd ed.) New York: Kluwer Academic/Plenum Press.

Franzen, M.D., Paul, D., & Iverson, G.L. (1996). Reliability of alternate forms of the Trail Making Test. *The Clinical Neuropsychologist, 10*, 125–129.

Franzen, M.D. & Iverson, G.L. (2000). Wechsler Memory Scales. In G. Groth-Marnat (Ed.), *Neuropsychological Assessment in Clinical Practice: A Practical Guide to Interpretation and Integration* (pp. 195–222). New York: John Wiley & Sons.

Franzen, M.D. & Wilhelm, K.L. (1996). Conceptual foundations of ecological validity in neuropsychological assessment. In R.J. Sbordone & C.J. Long (Eds.), *Ecological Validity of Neuropsychological Testing* (pp. 91–112.). Del Ray Beach, FL: St Lucie Press.

Golden, C.J. (1978). *Stroop Color and Word Test: A manual for clinical and experimental use.* Chicago: Stoelting.

Graves, R.E. (2000). Accuracy of regression equation prediction across the range of estimated premorbid IQ. *Journal of Clinical and Experimental Neuropsychology, 22*, 316–324.

Guttman, L. (1945). A basis for analyzing test-retest reliability. *Psychometrika, 10*, 255–282.

Hageman, W.J.J.M., & Arrindell, W.A. (1993). A further refinement of the reliable change (RC) index by improving the pre-post difference score: Introducing RC(ID). *Behaviour Research and Therapy, 31*, 693–700.

Hageman, W.J.J.M., & Arrindell, W.A. (1999a). Clinically significant and practical! Enhancing precision does make a difference. Reply to McGlinchey and Jacobson, Hsu, and Speer. *Behaviour Research and Therapy, 37*, 1219–1233.

Hageman, W.J.J.M., & Arrindell, W.A. (1999b). Establishing clinically significant change: Increment of precision and the distinction between individual and group level of analysis. *Behaviour Research and Therapy, 37*, 1169–1193.

Heaton, R.K., Temkin, N., Dikmen, S. Avitable, N., Taylor, M.J., & Marcotte, T.D. et al. (2001). Detecting change: A comparison of three neuropsychological methods using normal and clinical samples. *Archives of Clinical Neuropsychology, 16*, 75–91.

Hermann, B.P., Seidenberg, M., Schoenfeld, J., Peterson, J., Leveroni, C., & Wyler, A.R. (1996). Empirical techniques for determining the reliability, magnitude, and pattern of neuropsychological change after epilepsy surgery. *Epilepsia, 37*, 942–950.

Hermann, B.P., & Wyler, A.R. (1988). Neuropsychological outcome of anterior temporal lobectomy. *Journal of Epilepsy, 1*, 35–45.

Hinton-Bayre, A. (2000). Reliable change formula query. *Journal of the International Neuropsychological Society, 6*, 362–363.
Hinton-Bayre, A.D., Geffen, G.M., Geffen, L.B., McFarland, K.A., & Friis, P. (1999). Concussion in contact sports: Reliable change indices of impairment and recovery. *Journal of Clinical and Experimental Neuropsychology, 21*, 70–86.
Hinton-Bayre, A.D., Geffen, G.M., & McFarland, K.A. (1997). Mild head injury and speed of information processing: A prospective study of professional rugby league players. *Journal of Clinical and Experimental Neuropsychology, 19*, 275–289.
Hsu, L.M. (1989). Reliable changes in psychotherapy: Taking into account regression toward the mean. *Behavioral Assessment, 11*, 459–467.
Hsu, L.M. (1995). Regression toward the mean associated with measurement error and the identification of improvement and deterioration in psychotherapy. *Journal of Consulting and Clinical Psychology, 63*, 141–144.
Iverson, G.L. (1998). Interpretation of Mini-Mental State Examination scores in community-dwelling elderly and geriatric neuropsychiatry patients. *International Journal of Geriatric Psychiatry, 13*, 661–666.
Iverson, G. (1999). Interpreting change on the WAIS-III/WMS-III following traumatic brain injury. *Journal of Cognitive Rehabilitation, 17*, 16–20.
Iverson, G.L. (2001). Interpreting change on the WAIS-III/WMS-III in clinical samples. *Archives of Clinical Neuropsychology, 16*, 183–191.
Iverson, G.L., & Gaetz, M. (in press).
Iverson, G.L., Sawyer, D.C., McCracken, L.M., & Kozora, E. (2001). Assessing depression in Systemic Lupus Erythematosus: Determining reliable change. *Lupus, 10*, 266–271.
Ivnik, R.J., Smith, G.E., Lucas, J.A., Petersen, R.C., Boeve, B.F., Kokmen, E. et al. (1999). Testing normal older people three or four times at 1- to 2-year intervals: Defining normal variance. *Neuropsychology, 13*, 121–127.
Jacobson, N.S., Follette, W.C., & Revenstorf, D. (1984). Psychotherapy outcome research: Methods for reporting variability and evaluating clinical significance. *Behavior Therapy, 15*, 336–352.
Jacobson, N.S., & Revenstorf, D. (1988). Statistics for assessing the clinical significance of psychotherapy techniques: Issues, problems, and new developments. *Behavioral Assessment, 10*, 133–145.
Jacobson, N.S., Roberts, L.J., Berns, S.B., & McGlinchey, J.B. (1999). Methods for defining and determining the clinical significance of treatment effects: Description, application, and alternatives. *Journal of Consulting and Clinical Psychology, 67*, 300–307.
Jacobson, N.S., & Truax, P. (1991). Clinical significance: A statistical approach to defining meaningful change in psychotherapy research. *Journal of Consulting and Clinical Psychology, 59*, 12–19.
Jamieson, J. (1995). Measurement of change and the law of initial values: A computer stimulation study. *Educational and Psychological Measurement, 55*, 38–46.
Kaplan, E.F., Goodglass, H., & Weintraub, S. (1983). *The Boston Naming Test.* (2nd ed.). Philadelphia: Lea & Febiger.
Kazdin, A. (1999). The meanings and measurement of clinical significance. *Journal of Consulting and Clinical Psychology, 67*, 332–339.
Kneebone, A.C., Andrew, M.J., Baker, R.A., & Knight, J.L. (1998). Neuropsychologic changes after coronary artery bypass grafting: Use of reliable change indices. *Annals of Thoracic Surgery, 65*, 1320–1325.
Lezak, M.D. (1995). *Neuropsychological assessment* (3rd ed.). New York: Oxford University Press.
Linn, R.L., & Slinde, J.A. (1977). The determination of the significance of change between pre- and posttesting periods. *Review of Educational Research, 47*, 121–150.

Lord, F.M. (1963). Elementary models for measuring change. In C. W. Harris (Ed.), *Problems in measuring change* (pp. 21–38). Madison, WI: University of Wisconsin Press.

Mahanna, E.P., Blumenthal, J.A., White, W.D., Croughwell, N.D., Clancy, C.P., Smith, L.R. et al. (1996). Defining neuropsychological dysfunction after coronary artery bypass grafting. *Annals of Thoracic Surgery, 61*, 1342–1347.

Matarazzo, J.D., Carmody, T.P., & Jacobs, L.D. (1980). Test-retest reliability and stability of the WAIS: A literature review with implications for clinical practice. *Journal of Clinical Neuropsychology, 2*, 89–105.

McCaffrey, R.J., Duff, K., & Westervelt, H.J. (2000a). *Practitioner's guide to evaluating change with neuropsychological assessment instruments*. New York: Kluwer Academic/Plenum.

McCaffrey, R.J., Duff, K., & Westervelt, H.J. (2000b). *Practitioner's guide to evaluating change with intellectual assessment instruments*. New York: Kluwer Academic/Plenum.

McCracken, L.M. & Franzen, M.D. (1992). A principal components analysis of the equivalence of two forms of the Trails test. *Psychological Assessment: A Journal of Conculting and Clinical Psychology, 4*, 235–238.

McGlinchey, J.B., & Jacobson, N.S. (1999). Clinically significant but impractical? A response to Hageman and Arrindell. *Behaviour Research and Therapy, 37*, 1211–1217.

McSweeney, A. J., Naugle, R. I., Chelune, G. J., & Luders, H. (1993). T scores for change: An illustration of a regression approach to depicting change in clinical neuropsychology. *The Clinical Neuropsychologist, 7*, 300–312.

Nunnally, J.C. (1967). *Psychometric theory*. New York: McGraw Hill.

Nunnally, J.C., & Kotsch, W.E. (1983). Studies of individual subjects: Logic and methods of analysis. *British Journal of Clinical Psychology, 22*, 83–93.

Osgood, D.W. (2001). Application of multilevel models to the measurement of change. In L.M. Collins & A.G. Sayer (Eds.) *New methods for the analysis of change* (pp. 97–104). Washington, DC: American Psychological Association.

Pedhazur, E.J. (1982). *Multiple regression in behavioral research: Explanation and prediction* (2nd ed.). Fort Worth, TX: Harcourt Brace College Publishers.

Phillips, N.A., & McGlone, J. (1995). Grouped data do not tell the whole story: Individual analysis of cognitive change after temporal lobectomy. *Journal of Clinical and Experimental Neuropsychology, 17*, 713–724.

Reitan, R., & Wolfson, D. (1985). *The Halstead-Reitan Neuropsychological Test Battery*. Tempe, AZ: Neuropsychology Press.

Reitan, R.M., & Wolfson, D. (1993). *The Halstead-Reitan Neuropsychological Test Battery: Theory and clinical interpretation* (2nd ed.). Tucson, AZ: Neuropsychology Press.

Rey, A. (1964). *L'examen clinique en psychologie*. Paris: Presses Universitaires de France.

Richter, P., Werner, J., Bastine, R., Heerlein, A., Kick, H., Sauer, H. (1997). Measuring treatment outcome by the Beck Depression Inventory. *Psychopathology, 30*, 234–240.

Rogosa, D. (1988). Myths about longitudinal research. In K.W. Schaie, R.T. Campbell, W. Meredith & S.C. Rawlings (Eds.), *Methodological issues in aging research* (pp. 171-209). New York: Springer.

Rogosa, D., Brandt, D., & Zimowski, M. (1982). A growth curve approach to the measurement of change. *Psychological Bulletin, 92*, 726–748.

Salinsky, M.C., Storzbach, D., Dodrill, C.B., & Binder, L.M. (2001). Test-retest bias, reliability, and regression equations for neuropsychologial measures repeated over a 12-16 week period. *Journal of The International Neuropsychological Society, 7*, 597–605.

Sawrie, S.M., Chelune, G.J., Naugle, R.I., & Luders, H.O. (1996). Empirical methods for assessing meaningful neuropsychological change following epilepsy surgery. *Journal of the International Neuropsychological Society, 2*, 556–564.

Sawrie, S.M., Marson, D.C., Boothe, A.L., & Harrell, L.E. (1999). A method for assessing clinically relevant individual cognitive change in older adult populations. *Journal of Gerontology: Psychological Sciences, 54B*, P116–P124.

Shatz, M.W. (1981). WAIS practice effects in clinical neuropsychology. *Journal of Clinical Neuropsychology, 3*, 171–179.

Shaw, P.J., Bates, D., Cartlidge, N.E.F., French, J.M., Heaviside, D., Julian, D.G. et al. (1986). Early intellectual dysfunction following coronary bypass surgery. *Quarterly Journal of Medicine, 225*, 59–68.

Smith, A. (1982). *Symbol Digit Modalities Test manual – revised*. Los Angeles: Western Psychological Services.

Speer, D.C. (1992). Clinically significant change: Jacobson and Truax (1991) revisited. *Journal of Consulting and Clinical Psychology, 60*, 402–408.

Speer, D.C. (1999). What is the role of two-wave designs in clinical research? Comment on Hageman and Arrindell. *Behaviour Research and Therapy, 37*, 1203–1210.

Speer, D.C., & Greenbaum, P.E. (1995). Five methods for computing significant individual client change and improvement rates: Support for an individual growth curve approach. *Journal of Consulting and Clinical Psychology, 63*, 1044–1048.

Temkin, N.R., Heaton, R.K., Grant, I., & Dikmen, S.S. (1999). Detecting significant change in neuropsychological test performance: A comparison of four models. *Journal of the International Neuropsychological Society, 5*, 357–369.

Temkin, N.R., Heaton, R.K., Grant, I., & Dikmen, S.S. (2000). Reliable change formula query: Temkin et al. reply. *Journal of the International Neuropsychological Society, 6*, 364.

Tiffin, J. (1968). *Purdue Pegboard examiner's manual*. Rosemont, IL: London House.

Wechsler, D. (1955). *Manual for the Wechsler Adult Intelligence Scale*. New York: Psychological Corporation.

Wechsler, D. (1981). *WAIS-R manual*. New York: Psychological Corporation.

Wechsler, D. (1987). *Wechsler Memory Scale – Revised manual*. San Antonio, TX: Psychological Corporation.

Chapter 18

PRACTICAL CONSIDERATIONS FOR INTERPRETING CHANGE FOLLOWING BRAIN INJURY

Grant L. Iverson
University of British Columbia and Riverview Hospital

Michael Gaetz
University of British Columbia

The assessment of change is the *sine qua non* of clinical neuropsychology. One of the primary functions of the neuropsychologist, in both research and clinical practice, is to determine if the athlete has experienced a decline in functioning following concussion and then an improvement during recovery. The assessment of change occurs in two domains: subjectively experienced and reported symptoms, and measured cognitive and neurobehavioral abilities.

This chapter provides practical information regarding interpreting change in concussed athletes. There are three major sections. Several fundamental issues and challenges associated with the assessment of change in athletes are described in the first section. The reliable change methodology is discussed

Author Notes: The data used to illustrate the interpretation of change methodologies for this chapter were graciously provided by Michael Collins, Ph.D. and Mark Lovell, Ph.D. (collegiate football database), David Goodman, Ph.D. (British Columbia Junior Hockey League), and Ruben Echemendia, Ph.D. (Penn State University Soccer).

in the second section. Three specific postconcussion symptom inventories are presented in the third section, with detailed information regarding their clinical use.

Fundamental Issues and Challenges

There are five fundamental issues and challenges that complicate the interpretation of change in sports neuropsychology: (a) initial level of performance, (b) practice effects, (c) regression to the mean, (d) measurement error, and (e) response set. These factors are discussed in the following sections.

Conceptualizing initial level of performance

The profession of clinical neuropsychology has a long history of over-interpreting and over-pathologizing change. The most obvious, persistent, and pervasive example is the use of the term "impaired." It is extremely common for researchers to state that a specific group of patients has impaired cognitive abilities because, as a group, they had statistically lower scores than a group of control subjects. This often occurs when the effect sizes for these differences are small or modest. Moreover, it is frequently the case that the mean scores for the patient group on various neuropsychological tests, although lower than the control group, still fall in the average or low average classification range; thus, they represent a presumed lowering, decline, diminishment, or decrement in performance, but not an impairment.

Although it can be argued that the term impairment simply refers to a negative change in function, for most people the term carries much more serious connotations. This is a particularly important issue when working with athletes, or others, who have sustained concussions. As a profession, we must guard against iatrogenesis (i.e., health care providers making the problem worse). It is quite possible that by over-pathologizing an injury, the health care provider can inadvertently make the athlete worse. Focusing, dwelling, and worrying about symptoms of concussion, and "brain damage", can magnify them and protract the recovery period. Having stated this, it is important to accurately detect change that has occurred, and to determine whether this is a statistically and/or clinically meaningful change. Detection of clinically meaningful change is important because athletes function in an environment where subsequent injuries can occur, making it necessary to address the issue of cumulative effects. The need to detect subtle changes when they occur, without over-pathologizing these changes, adds to the complexity of assessing athletes.

When considering the effects of a concussion on neuropsychological test performance, it is important to properly conceptualize and explain initial level of performance. Initial levels of performance can affect practice effects, regression to the mean, and relations among test scores. Therefore, a basic conceptualization of initial level of performance is provided below.

Table 18.1. Normative scores and classification ranges in neuropsychology (M = Mean (average), SD = (Standard deviation).

Descripto/ Classification Range	Scaled Scores M=10, SD=3	Standard Scores (IQs) M=100, SD=15	T–Score M=50, SD=10	Percentile Rank
Severely Impaired	<1	<55	<20	<.13
Moderately Impaired	1	55–59	20–23	.13–.35
Mildly Impaired	2–4	60–69	24–29	.38–1.9
Borderline	5–6	70–79	30–36	2–9
Low Average	7	80–89	37–43	10–24
Average	8–12	90–109	44–56	25–75
High Average	13	110–119	57–63	76–90
Superior	14–15	120–129	64–69	91–97
Very Superior	16–19	130+	70+	98+

Standardized tests yield scores that fall within certain classification ranges. The following classification ranges and their corresponding percentile rank ranges are commonly used, although not universally accepted: Mildly Impaired < 2nd percentile; Borderline 3rd – 9th percentile; Low Average 10th – 24th percentile; Average 25th – 75th percentile; High Average 76th – 90th percentile; Superior 91st – 98th; Very Superior > 99th percentile. Thus, if an individual obtained a score at the 42nd percentile, this would mean that his performance was equal to or exceeded 42% of his same-aged peers in the general population, and that his score would fall in the Average classification range.

Different normative scores and their corresponding descriptors (i.e., their classification ranges) are illustrated in Tables 18.1 and 18.2. It is important to note that there is not precise agreement in our profession as to where exactly the cutoffs should fall between certain classification ranges (e.g., some may call a percentile rank of 9 low average instead of borderline, because it corresponds to an IQ of 80). There is also disagreement as to the three "impaired" classification ranges. The system below is similar to the more traditional IQ classifications corresponding to mild, moderate, and severe mental retardation.

When interpreting test scores, three basic psychometric principles are often minimized or overlooked by psychologists. First, scores are not exact. They contain measurement error. When a score is reported, this represents an estimate of the person's true ability. Second, the more tests that are given, the more likely the person is to score in the extreme ranges (high or low). Third, variability in test performance across a battery of tests is the rule, not the exception. In other words, it is very common for "normal" (i.e., non brain injured) individuals to obtain scores ranging from the borderline classification range to the high average classification range.

Table 18.2. Comprehensive table of normative scores (T-scores, IQ scores, Scaled Scores, z-scores, and percentile ranks).

Classification	T	IQ[1]	SS[2]	%ile	−z | +z	%ile	SS[2]	IQ[1]	T	Classification
	19			.10	3.10	99.90			81	
Severe Impairment		54		.11	3.07	99.89		146		
	20	55	1	.13	3.00	99.87	19	145	80	
		56		.17	2.93	99.83		144		
	21			.19	2.90	99.81			79	
Moderate Impairment		57		.21	2.87	99.79		143		
	22	58		.26	2.80	99.74		142	78	
		59		.31	2.70	99.69		141		
	23			.35	2.73	99.65			77	
		60	2	.38	2.67	99.62	18	140		
	24	61		.5	2.60	99.5		139	76	Very Superior
	25	62		.6	2.53	99.4		138	75	
		63		.7	2.47	99.3		137		
	26	64		.8	2.40	99.2		136	74	
Mild Impairment		65		1.0	2.30	99.0		135		
	27			1.1	2.33	98.9			73	
		66		1.2	2.27	98.8		134		
		67	3	1.4	2.20	98.6	17	133		
	28	68		1.6	2.13	98.4		132	72	
	29	69		1.9	2.07	98.1		131	71	
	30	70	4	2.3	2.00	97.7	16	130	70	
	31	71 - 72		3	1.82 - 1.95	97		128 - 129	69	
	32 - 33	73 - 74		4	1.70 - 1.81	96		126 - 127	67 - 68	
Borderline	34	75 - 76	5	5	1.60 - 1.69	95	15	124 - 125	66	
		77		6	1.52 - 1.59	94		123		Superior
	35	78		7	1.44 - 1.51	93		122	65	
	36	79		8	1.38 - 1.43	92		121	64	
		80	6	9	1.32 - 1.37	91	14	120		
	37	81		10	1.26 - 1.31	90		119	63	
				11	1.21 - 1.25	89				
	38	82		12	1.16 - 1.20	88		118	62	
		83		13	1.11 - 1.15	87		117		
	39	84		14	1.06 - 1.10	86		116	61	
				15	1.02 - 1.05	85				

Table 18.2 (Continued).

	40	85	7	16	.98 - 1.01	84	13	115	60	
Low Average				17	.94 - .97	83				
	41	86		18	.90 - .93	82		114	59	High Average
		87		19	.86 - .89	81		113		
				20	.83 - .85	80				
	42	88		21	.79 - .82	79		112	58	
				22	.76 - .78	78				
		89		23	.73 - .75	77		111		
	43			24	.70 - .72	76			57	
		90	8	25	.66 - .69	75	12	110		
				26	.63 - .65	74				
	44	91		27	.60 - .62	73		109	56	
				28	.57 - .59	72				
				29	.54 - .56	71				
		92		30	.52 - .53	70		108		
	45			31	.49 - .51	69			55	
		93		32	.46 - .48	68		107		
				33	.43 - .45	67				
	46	94		34	.40 - .42	66		106	54	
				35	.38 - .39	65				
				36	.35 - .37	64				
Average		95	9	37	.32 - .34	63	11	105		
	47			38	.30 - .31	62			53	Average
		96		39	.27 - .29	61		104		
				40	.25 - .26	60				
				41	.22 - .24	59				
	48	97		42	.19 - .21	58		103	52	
				43	.17 - .18	57				
				44	.14 - .16	56				
		98		45	.12 - .13	55		102		
	49			46	.09 - .11	54			51	
		99		47	.07 - .08	53		101		
				48	.04 - .06	52				
				49	.02 - .03	51				
	50	100	10	50	.00 - .01	50	10	100	50	

[1]M=100, SD=15; [2]M=10, SD=3

Table B.5 of the WAIS-III Administration and Scoring Manual (Wechsler, 1997) can be used to illustrate variability in normal subjects on cognitive tests (p. 211). If six Verbal subtests are given, 90.3% of the population will have a one standard deviation difference (i.e., three points between highest and lowest scaled scores) and 31.3% will have a two standard deviation difference. Therefore, if their highest scaled score on the six subtests was 12, the lowest would be six, corresponding to the 75th and 9th percentiles, respectively. If five Performance subtests are given, 37.5% of the normal population shows a two standard deviation split between the highest and the lowest subtest. The more tests you give, the greater the proportion of the normal population who show large splits between scores. For example, if you give the 11 subtests that comprise the index scores, 71.4% will show a two standard deviation high-low split, and 17.6% will show a three standard deviation split. Thus, it is apparent that intersubtest scatter (i.e., "inconsistency") is normal in the general population, even among intercorrelated tests such as the Verbal subtests of the WAIS-III.

Practice effects

Practice effects are a systematic source of bias in test scores. They are relevant for performance-based measures, such as speed of information processing, reaction time, or memory. Practice effects are not relevant to self-reported concussion-related symptom inventories. The importance of practice effects can be seen in a study of collegiate football players who sustained a single concussion and who were evaluated with neuropsychological tests at pre-season, 24 hours post-injury, 5 days post-injury, and 10 days post-injury (Macciocchi, Barth, Alves, Rimel, & Jane, 1996). These researchers compared a large sample of concussed athletes (N = 183) to matched, non-injured controls on the Digit Symbol subtest of the Wechsler Adult Intelligence Scale-Revised (WAIS-R). The average total raw scores for the players with concussions were 58.7, 59.3, 66.3, and 71.5 for pre-season, 24 hours post-, 5 days post-, and 10 days post-injury, respectively. The athlete controls obtained the following scores for the same intervals: 59.4, 63.9, 70.8, and 73.8. Concussions essentially diminished the normal practice effect, as seen in the comparison of pre-season mean scores to the 24-hour post-injury scores (i.e., 58.7 – 59.3). Similar patterns were seen on the Paced Auditory Serial Addition Test and the Trail Making Test. Therefore, in this study, concussion was not associated with major declines on performance-based measures. Rather, subtle declines occurred, and largely resolved within 10 days. These subtle declines can be very difficult to detect, especially within the context of potentially poorly understood practice effects.

It is important to study practice effects at the interval of interest. For example, from preseason to date of injury may be anywhere from days to 30 weeks. Choosing an interval, such as 8–12 weeks might be appropriate for understanding the effects of practice on immediate, post-concussion test scores. However, this is not sufficient, because athletes are often examined serially to track recovery. Therefore, we need to know practice effects at weekly intervals for approximately one month to adequately interpret the performances of athletes during the normal recovery period (notably, most athletes are recovered in less than two weeks).

It is difficult to predict whether a practice effect is present in the majority of athletes, at specific intervals, without proper data. Clinical judgment will be inadequate under most circumstances, because the presence or absence of practice effects does not always make intuitive sense. To illustrate, the preseason data from 126 collegiate football players were compared at preseason and postseason on the Trail Making Test, Digit Symbol subtest of the WAIS-R, Controlled Oral Word Association Test (FAS version), and the grooved pegboard. There was a presumed practice effect for Trails A ($p = .03$) and for Trails B ($p = .008$), but not the other measures. During the second season, on average the players performed Trails A 1.2 seconds faster and Trails B 4.0 seconds faster. This is a very small effect size for practice for Trails A and a relatively small effect size for practice for Trails B.

The distribution of test-retest difference scores for Trails B is presented graphically in Figure 18.1. Practice effects are fairly evenly distributed for the total sample, with the distribution shifted to the right by approximately four seconds. However, examining this distribution alone can be misleading because level of performance at time one is very important for predicting performance at time two. To illustrate, the distributions of Trails B test-retest difference scores are presented graphically in Figure 18.2 for three subgroups of athletes based on their time one scores: (a) the 20% who performed the fastest ($n = 25$), (b) the 60% in the middle of the distribution ($n = 77$), and

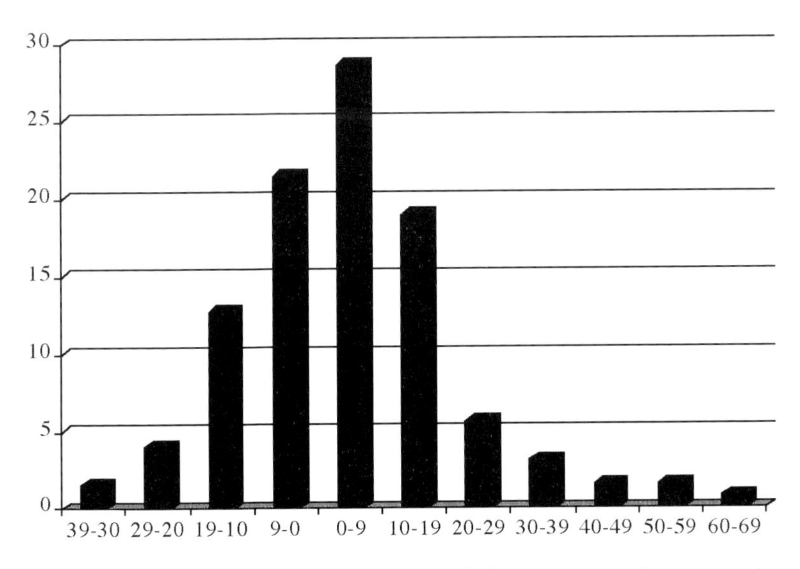

Figure 18.1.Distribution of Trails B test-retest difference scores for the total sample.

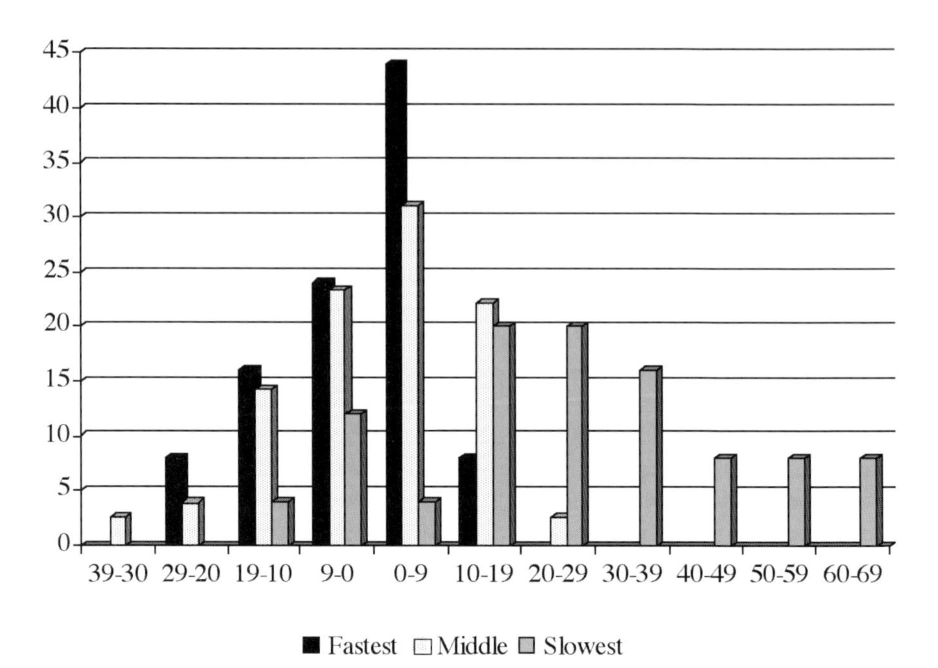

Figure 18.2. Distributions of Trails B test-retest difference scores for fast, medium, and slow subsamples.

(c) the 20% who performed the slowest (n = 24). Players who perform the fastest at time one tend to perform, on average, slightly slower at time two. However, those athletes who perform poorly at time one (i.e., 62 seconds or more) are much more likely to perform faster at time two. On average, this group performed 23 seconds faster on retest. The distribution of test-retest difference scores is shifted right. Therefore, from a practical perspective, it is important to consider where an athlete was at baseline to adequately gauge the possible effects of practice and the interaction between practice and the effects of a concussion.

Regression

Regression and measurement error are very important to consider for both performance measures and symptom measures. In regards to regression, if a person obtains an extreme score on a test he likely will obtain a score closer to the mean on retesting. That is, an extreme score is statistically more likely to become less extreme, rather than more extreme, on retesting. Therefore, by correcting scores for regression to the mean, we are less likely to "over-interpret" change (e.g, spontaneous recovery or response to treatment). Regression and practice can have a simultaneous impact on a test score. Imagine an athlete who scores below the 10th percentile on a pre-season memory test and then takes the test again following a concussion, 3 weeks into the season. Both regression and practice could have a positive impact on his performance, while the concussion might be exerting a negative influence. In theory, the net effect could be a post-concussion test score that is essentially identical to the pre-season score. Under these circumstances, the neuropsychologist could misinterpret this test and assume that there has been no change in his ability resulting from the immediate effects of the concussion.

Regression certainly can complicate the interpretation of concussion symptom inventories. Imagine athletes who endorse unusually high or low symptoms pre-season (i.e., their baseline of subjectively experienced headaches, irritability, and concentration problems). The low symptom endorsers are statistically more likely to have higher scores and the high symptom endorsers are statistically more likely to have lower scores. This would obviously complicate the interpretation of their scores on a self-report measure following a concussion.

To illustrate this issue, a sample of 76 collegiate football players who completed a 20-item postconcussion symptom inventory (described in detail in a later section of this chapter) at preseason and postseason was divided into thirds on the basis of their season one scores (i.e., total scores equal to 3 or less, 4 to 11, or 12 or greater). Test-retest difference scores were created by subtracting the season one score from the season two score. Therefore, negative scores reflect higher preseason scores. The average test-retest difference scores were as follows: (a) low group mean = 2.4 (Median = 1.0; Interquartile Range = 0 – 4.5; Range = -2 – 14); (b) medium group mean = 6.2 (Median = 1.0; Interquartile Range = -3 – 14; Range = -11 to 46); and (c) high group mean = -9.6 (Median = -8; Interquartile Range = -14 – 4; Range = -50 – 21). These data illustrate that if an athlete begins with a high score (i.e., the "high group"), then he is statistically very likely to score lower on retest (i.e., 80% of this group scored 4 or more points lower on retest). In contrast, athletes who begin with low scores (i.e., 3 or less) are more likely to have higher scores on retesting (56% had higher scores). The test-retest difference scores for the middle group are relatively evenly distributed.

Measurement error

Measurement error is closely related to test reliability. Reliability relates to the consistency or stability in test scores. According to classical test theory, it has been viewed in terms of the relationship between "true" scores and obtained scores. Obtained scores are believed to contain an error component, which influences the consistency or stability of a particular score. Thus, reliability may be viewed as the ability of an instrument to reflect an individual score that is minimally influenced by error. Reliability should not be considered a dichotomous concept; rather it falls on a continuum. One cannot say an instrument is reliable or unreliable, but more accurately should say it possesses a high or low degree of reliability for a specific purpose, with a specific population (Franzen, 1989, 2000).

Most reliability estimates are reported in terms of correlation coefficients. These coefficients measure the degree of association between two or more variables. Common estimates of association are internal consistency, alternate forms, and test-retest measures. Internal consistency measures the internal structure of a test and is influenced by how well the test actually taps the psychological construct it purports to measure. Internal consistency is further influenced by the nature of the construct itself. Heterogeneity in the construct is inversely related to the internal consistency of a test designed to measure it. Thus, reliability estimates based on internal consistency estimates should be evaluated in light of the aforementioned issues.

Test-retest reliability is influenced by error resulting from situational variables (Franzen, 1989, 2000). This reliability estimate is greatly influenced by the stability of the construct of interest. If the construct varies systematically in the same way for every individual, the resultant correlation coefficient would be unaffected. However, under most circumstances, it can be assumed that situational and temporal factors will introduce considerable variability into the construct being assessed. Consequently, stability estimates will be attenuated.

Response set: Minimization and under-reporting of symptoms

The neuropsychologist must be alert to the possibility that symptom inventories with athletes might not be fully accurate. Unlike the magnification of PCS symptoms that can occur with medical-legal assessment, the response tendency of some athletes is biased toward minimization or under-reporting of symptoms. The reasons for this response bias are numerous. There might be a desire to be a "team player," putting the needs of the team ahead of the individual. There might be practical considerations, such as the reality in sport that the longer you are inactive, the greater the probability that your position on the roster will be assumed by a non-injured player. In addition, young male athletes in particular often present themselves outwardly as "invincible."

This response set has very practical implications for return-to-play decisions. Accurately determining when it is safe for players to return to active participation in their sport is important for obvious reasons. First, players who return too early may be at risk for further injury. Contact sports in particular require the ability to "read and react" to plays, in order to be an effective participant, and more importantly, to avoid further injury. In addition, subtle problems with judgment that might occur following concussion may make some players over-aggressive, extending themselves beyond their normal range of ability. This scenario can lead to anecdotal reports of a player having the "game of his life" following a concussion, possibly due to the subtle changes in judgment and reductions in inhibition he would normally experience. Most importantly however, is the risk of cumulative injury, even in athletes who are very young. The possible cumulative effects of concussion have recently been reported using neuropsychological testing (Collins et al., 1999; Iverson, Gaetz, Lovell, Collins, & Maroon, 2002; Matser, Kessels, Lezak, Jordan, & Troost, 1999) and physiological indices of brain function

(Gaetz, Goodman, & Weinberg, 2000). Proper assessment and treatment of the first concussion may allow for more complete recovery since a player who returns to play prior to the cessation of acute post-concussion symptoms might be at risk for further injury. Although this has not been demonstrated experimentally, a player who experiences dizziness, attention deficits, and slowed reaction times is at greater risk of further injury since balance, the ability to attend and anticipate play development, and the ability to react appropriately, are necessary to avoid potentially dangerous body contact.

Section Summary

In summary, there are numerous factors that neuropsychologists must be aware of when assessing post-concussion change in athletes using self-report inventories or performance-based measures. It is important to consider carefully the effects of practice, regression to the mean, and the reliability and validity of what is being measured. Although self-reported symptom inventories are less susceptible to some of these factors compared to performance-based measures, there are additional factors to consider when using symptom inventories with athletes. Specifically, post-concussion changes observed in athletes may be qualitatively and quantitatively different than other situations of MTBI assessment (e.g., medical-legal evaluations). In athletes, the clinical or research goal is to accurately document subtle changes from baseline (i.e., within subject) in order to determine the severity of injury and when it is safe to return to play. Obviously, these issues are very different from those related to the assessment of MTBI in a medical-legal context, where symptom reporting might be complicated by many factors including depression, anxiety, life stress, chronic pain, substance abuse, litigation stress, exaggeration, and malingering. Athletes on the other hand often minimize symptoms, are rarely involved in litigation, and are highly motivated to recover quickly. Therefore, the neuropsychologist assessing post-concussion change in athletes must be aware of factors related to all psychological assessment, as well as those specific to the assessment of the athlete.

Reliable Change Methodology

The reliable change methodology has been discussed extensively in the psychotherapy literature (e.g., Hageman & Arrindell, 1993; Hsu, 1989; Jacobson & Revenstorf, 1988; Jacobson, Roberts, Berns, & McGlinchey, 1999; Jacobson & Truax, 1991; Ogles, Lambert, & Masters, 1996; Speer, 1992; Speer & Greenbaum, 1995). Several years later it was employed in clinical neuropsychology (e.g., Chelune, Naugle, Luders, Sedlak, & Awad, 1993; Heaton et al., 2001; Iverson, 1998, 1999, 2001; Temkin, Heaton, Grant, & Dikmen, 2000) and sports neuropsychology (Hinton-Bayre, Geffen, Geffen, McFarland, & Friis, 1999; Iverson, Lovell, Collins, & Norwig, 2002). In the chapter by Franzen, Frerichs, and Iverson in the present book, several technical issues relating to reliable change were reviewed. The reader is encouraged to review that section of the chapter.

The reliable change methodology is applied systematically to several post-concussion inventories in the next section of this chapter. Therefore, we will review the basic principles here. The standard error of the difference (S_{diff}) can be used to create a confidence interval (i.e., a prediction interval in the statistical literature) for test-retest difference score. The formula for calculating the S_{diff} is printed below.

$SEM_1 = SD\sqrt{1-r_{12}}$ Standard deviation from time 1 multiplied by the square root of 1 minus the test-retest coefficient.

$SEM_2 = SD\sqrt{1-r_{12}}$ Standard deviation from time 2 multiplied by the square root of 1 minus the test-retest coefficient.

$S_{diff} = \sqrt{SEM_1^2 + SEM_2^2}$) Square root of the sum of the *squared* SEMs for each testing occasion.

Note that the formula for the S_{diff} includes the SEM for time one and time two. The formula, as originally printed in Jacobson and Truax (1991), was incorrect. Unfortunately, nearly every study has utilized the incorrect formula in the psychotherapy and neuropsychology literature, including the most recent studies (e.g., Temkin et al., 2000). This formula should be considered an "estimated S_{diff}" (Estimated $S_{diff} = \sqrt{2(SEM_1^2})$; Hageman & Arrindell, 1993; Iverson, 1998, 2001), not the actual S_{diff}. This formula represents an "estimated" standard error of difference because the SEM for time one is prorated instead of using the SEM for time two. This formula can be used out of necessity, when subjects have not undergone follow-up testing (e.g., Iverson, 1998, 2001). Under these circumstances, the S_{diff} is estimated from a single testing session.

The confidence interval for the test-retest difference score is obtained by multiplying the S_{diff} by a value from the *z*-distribution. Multiplying by a value of 1.64, for example, results in a change score in either direction that would be unlikely to occur by chance ($p < .05$ in each tail). Multiplying by a value of 1.28 forms a .80 confidence interval ($p < .10$ in each tail).

The reliable change methodology allows the clinician to reduce the adverse impact of measurement error on test interpretation. To represent clinically significant improvement, the change score must be statistically reliable. However, the converse is not true; *a statistically reliable change does not necessarily guarantee a clinically meaningful change*. For example, if an athlete endorsed a very large number of severe concussion symptoms on an inventory, and then obtained a score that showed statistically reliable improvement five days later, yet the score still fell in the moderate-to-severe symptom range, this change score may not be interpreted as clinically meaningful.

Chelune and colleagues (1993) realized that the reliable change methodology, as applied to neuropsychological test scores, was less accurate when practice effects were present. These researchers made the important innovation to correct the confidence interval for the average practice effect in the sample.

For postconcussion inventories, however, practice effects are not an issue. Instead, regression to the mean must be considered carefully. The reliable change methodology, in its standard form, does not control for regression (Hageman & Arrindell, 1993; Speer, 1992). To illustrate this concept, imagine an athlete who obtains an extreme score on a concussion inventory. If he was retested after one week, and his baseline score was corrected for regression to the mean, he would require a relatively larger change to be classified as "improved", and a relatively smaller change to be classified as deteriorated (as compared to the Jacobson and Truax method of non-correction for regression).

A method for determining whether regression to the mean is present in a data set is to correlate the baseline score with the baseline-retest difference score (Speer, 1992). If this correlation is significant, regression likely is present (although this method is not universally accepted because both the baseline and retest raw scores are fallible and there correlation is not necessarily an accurate estimate of the true correlation of interest, i.e. baseline true score and retest true score). If regression is present, then athletes' scores can be "corrected". Instead of using the obtained scores, the practitioner or researcher can use the *estimated true score*. The estimated true score is calculated by subtracting the "population mean" (e.g., a large sample of collegiate football players) from the actual score. This difference score is multiplied by the test-retest reliability coefficient. This product is added to the population mean, and this final sum is considered the estimated true score. The confidence interval for measurement error is then surrounded around the estimated true score. The estimated true score contains a correction for regression to the mean. Therefore, extreme "obtained" scores will have to show relatively *greater* improvement, and *less* deterioration, to be considered reliably changed.

Application of reliable change with correction for practice

The application of the reliable change methodology appears relatively straightforward, once you get beyond the mathematical haggling that has occurred for the past decade. However, basic considerations regarding stability of the construct of interest, measurement error, and dispersion remain critically important. To illustrate, Trails A and B scores are presented for two groups of athletes for preseason and postseason test administrations in Table 18.3. Three issues will be discussed. First, note that the SEM for Trails B in both the football players and soccer players is smaller for time two than time one. This is because the standard deviation for time two is smaller than for time one in both groups. This illustrates the importance of using the proper S_{diff} formula, which takes into account the SEM from test and retest, as opposed to prorating the SEM from time 1 (as is usually done in the literature). Second, note that the S_{diffs}, especially for Trails B, vary between the football players and the

Table 18.3. Comparison of reliable change statistics in collegiate football players and soccer players.

Statistic	Football Players Trails A	Football Players Trails B	Soccer Players Trails A	Soccer Players Trails B
$Mean_1$	20.4	52.1	23.0	46.7
$Mean_2$	19.1	46.9	19.7	41.6
SD_1	6.1	21.9	7.4	14.9
SD_2	5.6	16.4	6.1	9.4
Test-retest (r_s)	.47	.59	.49	.39
SEM_1	4.5	14.0	5.3	11.7
SEM_2	4.1	10.5	4.4	7.3
S_{diff}	6.0	17.5	6.9	13.7
Average practice effect	1.2	5.2	3.2	5.2
.80 Confidence interval	6.5 – 8.9	17.2 – 27.6	5.7 – 12.1	12.4 – 22.8
.90 Confidence interval	8.7 – 11.1	23.5 – 33.9	8.2 – 14.6	17.3 – 27.7
Percentage improved (.80 CI)	7.1%	7.9%	5.3%	7.9%
Percentage declined (.80 CI)	8.7%	7.9%	5.3%	7.9%
Percentage improved (.90 CI)	4.7%	5.5%	2.6%	5.3%
Percentage declined (.90 CI)	6.3%	3.9%	5.3%	0%
No Correction for Practice				
Percentage improved (.80 CI)	13.4%	11.0%	13.2%	10.5%
Percentage declined (.80 CI)	7.1%	3.9%	5.3%	0%
Percentage improved (.90 CI)	4.7%	7.9%	5.3%	7.9%
Percentage declined (.90 CI)	5.5%	1.6%	2.6%	0%

soccer players. This illustrates the importance of having reliable change data on subtypes of athletes. Finally, note that correcting the confidence intervals for practice results in fewer athletes being classified as improved and more classified as declined (as a general rule). The methodology rarely results in a perfectly normal distribution, however, with 10% and 5% of subjects falling in the tails of the .80 and .90 confidence intervals.

Interpreting Change on Postconcussion Symptom Inventories

Trainers, coaches, team physicians, and neuropsychologists rely heavily on subjectively experienced, self-reported, postconcussion symptoms for making decisions regarding medical management and return to play. This is a complex area of inquiry for numerous reasons, such as the (a) base rate of these symptoms in non-injured athletes, (b) subjective nature of the symptoms, (c) response tendency of some athletes to minimize symptoms, and (d) unknown reliability and validity of scales used to document these symptoms.

The primary purpose of this section is to discuss, in detail, the clinical use of postconcussion symptom inventories with athletes. Three symptom inventories are presented, with an emphasis on their reliability, clinical utility, and interpretation of change.

Rivermead symptom checklist

The Rivermead Symptom Checklist, hereafter referred to as the Rivermead, is printed as Appendix 6 in Wrightson and Gronwall's (1999) book on mild head injury. The Rivermead is a 16-item questionnaire that instructs subjects to rate themselves on a Likert-type scale regarding the degree to which they are experiencing PCS symptoms. Examples of symptoms include physical complaints such as "headaches" and "nausea and/or vomiting", cognitive complaints such as "poor concentration" and "forgetfulness, poor memory", and emotional complaints such as "feeling depressed or tearful" and "being irritable, easily angered". In addition, there is a section at the bottom of the questionnaire that asks "Are you experiencing any other difficulties?" Subject's are instructed to rate each symptom on a scale from 0–4, with 0 being "not experienced at all" and 4 being "a severe problem". For the hockey players presented below, at baseline they were asked to respond to the questionnaire regarding their symptoms over the last 24 hours.

The Rivermead is an appropriate choice to document change in PCS symptoms because it covers the majority of symptoms while being easy and quick to administer. Weaknesses of the Rivermead include a brief reporting interval of symptoms over the past 24 hours "compared with before the accident." It was discovered through its use that episodic complaints, such as those associated with the flu or acute headache, would elevate PCS scores. In addition, there is limited information about each symptom. For instance, the frequency, intensity, and duration of each symptom are measured and rated with other inventories.

Baseline data were collected from the British Columbia Junior Hockey League (BCHL) over a two-year period. The subjects' ages ranged from 15-20 years. The baseline testing was performed on site in each of the 14 communities with teams in the BCHL.

Reliability of the Rivermead in Hockey Players

The internal consistency reliability of the scale was estimated using Cronbach's alpha (α = 0.89). The split-half reliability was .88. The test was administered to all the athletes at the beginning of each season. The one-year test-retest reliability coefficients for 113 subjects were .24 (p = .011; Pearson) and .23 (p = .017; Spearman). The very low test-retest correlation after 12 months is probably due to the "state" nature of the assessment. Athletes are instructed to rate these symptoms based on the past 24 hours. This would obviously make the ratings highly susceptible to situational factors. The test-retest reliability is affected further by restriction in range and skewness in these score distributions.

Interpretation of the Rivermead in Hockey Players

When interpreting the Rivermead in a young hockey player, the first step is to determine whether the endorsement of symptoms is normal or unusual. In this sample of 113 young men, their average score was 6.5 (SD = 6.8) and their

Table 18.4 Classification ranges for raw scores and corresponding percentile rank ranges for a sample of 113 young men from the British Columbia Junior Hockey League.

Classification	Raw Scores	Percentile Ranks for Players
Low	0	0 – 14%
Normal	1 – 10	25 – 75%
Unusual	11 – 15	76 – 90%
High	16+	>90%

median score was 4. Classification ranges for raw scores and corresponding percentile rank ranges are provided in Table 18.4. These percentile ranks were not force-normalized; they reflect the natural score distribution.

The second step in the interpretation process is to examine the individual item scores. The percentages of players who endorsed each symptom during preseason assessment as at least a mild or moderate problem are presented in Table 18.5. The symptoms are organized in descending order so that it is apparent which symptoms are the most frequently endorsed, in the absence of concussion. As seen in this table, at least mild levels of fatigue, frustration, dizziness, and irritability are fairly common in athletes. It is important to appreciate that postconcussion symptoms are non-specific; they occur in daily life and are magnified by stress, fatigue, depression, and pain. Therefore, clinicians should consider carefully a host of factors when interpreting these symptom inventories.

The third step in the interpretation process is the consideration of change. It is becoming increasingly common to have preseason assessments on players. Thus, their postconcussion symptom reporting can be compared to their preseason baseline.

Standard errors of measurement and the standard error of difference are less meaningful for the interpretation of change on the Rivermead in these hockey players because the preseason scores separated by one year were minimally correlated. It is possible that the scores would have a higher correlation if the retest interval were shorter (e.g., days or weeks). However, in this situation, the raw frequency distributions were examined to estimate change scores. Specifically, year two scores were subtracted from year one scores to create a difference score. The raw, natural (i.e., not normalized) distributions of difference scores, accompanied by their corresponding percentile ranks, are presented in Table 18.6. A negative difference score means that the year two score was higher and a positive difference score means that the year one score was higher. An increase in postconcussion symptoms is represented in negative values and a decrease is represented in positive values. Therefore, a postconcussion score that is 13 points higher than a baseline score has a base rate of 5% in nonconcussed athletes (–13 in the second column of the table).

Table 18.5. Percentages of preseason symptoms reported by a sample of 113 young men from the British Columbia Junior Hockey League.

Symptom	Mild Problem or Greater	Moderate Problem or Greater
Frustrated or impatient	16.8	6.2
Upset by bright light	15.9	1.8
Headaches	15.0	2.7
Irritable	14.2	4.4
Fatigue	12.4	3.5
Poor concentration	11.5	3.5
Feelings of dizziness	10.6	2.7
Forgetful, poor memory	9.9	2.7
Taking longer to think	9.7	.9
Poor sleep	8.8	4.4
Blurred vision	8.8	1.8
Sensitivity to noise	5.3	.9
Depressed or tearful	5.3	2.7
Restlessness	5.3	1.8
Nausea and/or vomiting	1.8	.9
Double vision	0	0

Table 18.6. Natural distributions of difference scores, accompanied by their corresponding percentile ranks.

Percentile Rank	Total Sample	Total 3 or less	Total 4-10	Total 11-14	Total 15+
5	–13	–14	–17	–10	–3
10	–9	–9	–11	–9	–2
16	–6	–7	–9	1	–1
25	–3	–5	–5	3	4
50	1	–1	1	7	13
75	5	1	5	8	15
84	8	1	6	9	18
90	11	2	7	10	20
95	15	3	8	11	22
Mean	1.0	–2.6	–.7	5.3	11.5
Median	1.0	–1.0	1.0	7.0	14.0
SD	8.3	5.5	8.1	5.1	8.4
N	113	55	27	14	17

It is very important for neuropsychologists to note that the magnitude and base rates of difference scores are very much influenced by the magnitude of the baseline score. This is illustrated clearly in Table 18.6. Athletes who begin with low normal scores (i.e., 3 or less) on the Rivermead require larger change scores to be confident that the change was not due to measurement error. For example, a change score of –14 corresponds to the 5th percentile in this subgroup. In contrast, athletes with baseline scores in the high range (i.e., 15 or greater) have a fundamentally different distribution of difference scores. For this group, a change score of –3 points corresponds to the 5th percentile. To assume someone from this group is getting better requires a change score of 20 points (90th percentile). This is because athletes with high baseline scores are expected, due to regression and other factors, to have lower retest scores.

Interpretation in concussed players

The subjects shown in Table 18.7 are 14 players monitored at baseline, immediately following their injury, at two-weeks, and at one month. Generally speaking, there are two main patterns. First, are those who initially report low-normal scores, high scores following concussion, with a subsequent return to lower levels. The pattern for these subjects is relatively straightforward regarding interpretation, and very consistent with the natural course of recovery from concussion. Specifically, reliable change from baseline must be determined, followed by whether this change is clinically meaningful.

Second, there are players who do not report substantial change. Within this group, there are two subsets, those who are initially high and remain high (subjects 7 & 9), and those who are initially low and remain low (subjects 5, 6, & 10). Regarding interpretation, these patterns of responding are obviously more challenging. Subjects with high levels of symptoms at baseline should be questioned as to the cause of the symptoms. Reasons for high baseline reports could be acute illness, a recent concussion, or a chronic medical condition

Table 18.7. Rivermead scores for 14 concussed junior hockey players.

	Preseason		24 Hours		Two Weeks		One Month	
Subject	Score	Classification	Score	Classification	Score	Classification	Score	Classification
1	0	Low	20	High	31	High	0	Low
2	2	Normal	35	High	19	High	4	Normal
3	8	Normal	32	High	22	High	26	High
4	0	Low	36	High	0	Low	1	Normal
5	3	Normal	4	Normal	4	Normal	0	Low
6	1	Normal	9	Normal	1	Normal	3	Normal
7	34	High	35	High	21	High	19	High
8	5	Normal	14	Unusual	8	Normal	0	Low
9	25	High	38	High	18	High	18	High
10	2	Normal	5	Normal	4	Normal	5	Normal
11	9	Normal	28	High	11	Unusual	3	Normal
12	7	Normal	25	High	16	High	11	Unusual
13	7	Normal	20	High	11	Unusual	0	Low
14	8	Normal	42	High	3	Normal	0	Low

such as migraine headaches. Psychological distress, particularly in the form of depression, but also anxiety, usually results in elevated scores on this type of questionnaire. Therefore, it can be very difficult to disentangle concussion-related from other-related symptoms in athletes who endorse a large number of symptoms. At the opposite end of the spectrum, those subjects who do not report any symptoms following a concussion may be genuinely experiencing low levels of symptoms, or they might be minimizing symptoms. These subjects should be monitored throughout the recovery process to ensure an appropriate amount of time is allowed for recovery and return to play.

One subject (#3) did not fit either of the global patterns. His baseline score was in the normal range and his subsequent three assessments were all in the high range. This athlete should be followed carefully over a longer interval, because his recovery is atypical and protracted. Additional co-morbid factors that might be influencing symptom endorsement should also be investigated (e.g., psychological distress, life problems, medical problems, substance abuse).

In addition, there may be a shift in the symptom profile over time. For instance, a concussed player may initially report problems related to cognition, and physical problems such as headache and dizziness. Over time, physical and cognitive symptoms may decrease, and symptoms reflecting emotional problems may emerge. This appears to be the case with subject #3, as shown in Table 18.8. With the persistence of symptoms such dizziness, nausea,

Table 18.8. Individual symptom scores from the first three athletes presented in Table 18.7.

Symptom	Unusual / Abnormal: ≤ 10%	Preseason	24 Hours	Two Weeks	One Month
Headaches	3	0 (0) 1	2 (3) 4	3 (2) 2	0 (0) 1
Feelings of dizziness	2	0 (0) 2	1 (3) 3	2 (2) 1	0 (0) 3
Nausea and/or vomiting	2	0 (0) 0	0 (1) 2	2 (0) 2	0 (0) 3
Sensitivity to noise	2	0 (0) 0	1 (0) 2	2 (0) 1	0 (0) 2
Poor sleep	2	0 (2) 2	2 (3) 1	3 (0) 1	0 (0) 3
Fatigue	3	0 (0) 0	2 (3) 2	2 (2) 2	0 (0) 3
Irritable	3	0 (0) 0	2 (2) 3	1 (2) 1	0 (0) 1
Depressed or tearful	2	0 (0) 0	0 (2) 1	1 (0) 1	0 (0) 4
Frustrated or impatient	3	0 (0) 0	1 (3) 3	1 (2) 1	0 (1) 1
Forgetful, poor memory	2	0 (0) 0	2 (3) 2	2 (2) 2	0 (1) 2
Poor concentration	3	0 (0) 0	2 (3) 1	3 (2) 1	0 (1) 1
Taking longer to think	2	0 (0) 1	2 (3) 3	3 (2) 2	0 (1) 1
Blurred vision	2	0 (0) 0	1 (3) 1	1 (1) 1	0 (0) 0
Upset by bright light	2	0 (0) 0	0 (0) 2	1 (0) 1	0 (0) 1
Double vision	1	0 (0) 0	0 (0) 1	1 (0) 1	0 (0) 0
Restlessness	2	0 (0) 2	2 (3) 1	3 (2) 2	0 (0) 0
Total Score	16	0 (2) 8	20 (35) 32	31 (19) 22	0 (4) 26

fatigue and poor sleep, there was a dramatic increase in the self-reported depression at one-month. This might be an example of secondary depression that results from persistent symptoms in an athlete.

To further illustrate the progression of symptoms over a one-month period, individual symptom scores from the first three athletes presented in Table 18.7 are presented in Table 18.8. In the second column of Table 18.8, the item scores corresponding to the 10th percentile in non-concussed players are presented. In general, all three athletes had preseason scores that were normal. Immediately following their concussions, they had a large increase in symptoms, and their total scores were in the abnormal range. At the item level, the three athletes endorsed 4, 11, and 10 symptoms in the abnormal range, respectively. At two weeks post injury, all three continued to have total scores in the abnormal range. At the item level, they endorsed 10, 4, and 4 symptoms, respectively. By one-month post injury, two of the athletes had recovered and the third reported 7 symptoms in the abnormal range.

British Columbia postconcussion symptom Iinventory-short form (BC-PSI-Sf)

The BC-PSI-Sf is an unpublished, 16-item measure designed to assess the frequency and severity of postconcussion symptoms (see Appendix A). The test was based on ICD-10 (World Health Organization, 1992) criteria for postconcussion syndrome, and requires the test taker to rate the frequency and intensity of 13 symptoms (e.g., headaches, fatigue, sensitivity to noises, and poor concentration), and the effect of three life problems on daily living (i.e., greater present versus past effects of alcohol consumption, worrying and dwelling on symptoms, and self-perception of brain damage). The three life problems are rated on a scale from one to five, where 1 = “not at all” and 5 = “very much.”

The 13 psychological symptoms are rated on a six-point Likert-type rating scale that measures the frequency and intensity of each symptom in the past two weeks. Frequency ratings range from 0 = “not at all” to 5 = “constantly.” Intensity ratings range from 0 = “not at all” to 5 = “very severe problem.” To score the BC-PSI-Sf, the two ratings are multiplied together (how often x how bad) to create a single score for each item. These product-based scores are then converted to item scores that reflect both the frequency and intensity of symptom endorsement (range = 0 to 4). Item product scores convert to item total scores as follows: 0-1 = 0, 2-3 = 1, 4-6 = 2, 8-12 = 3, and 15+ = 4. While item scores of 3 or higher are considered to be “clinically meaningful”, scores from 1 to 2 reflect a mild endorsement of the symptom (i.e., the frequency and severity of the symptom is considered to be sub-clinical). At this stage of test development, scores of three or higher are referred to as “clinically endorsed” symptoms, while scores of 1 to 2 are referred to as “non-clinically endorsed” symptoms.

In an initial study (Iverson & Lange, in press), the BC-PSI-Sf and the Beck Depression Inventory-Second Edition (BDI-II; *Beck, Steer, Ball, & Ranieri,*

1996) were administered to 104 community volunteers with no history of traumatic brain injury. Endorsement rates for specific symptoms ranged from 35.9% to 75.7% for any experience of the symptoms in the past two weeks, and from 2.9% to 15.5% for the experience of more severe, "clinically significant" symptoms. The BC-PSI-Sf total score was moderately correlated with the BDI-II total score [r (102) = .76, p < .01]. This study illustrated that the presence of postconcussion-like symptoms: (a) are not unique to mild head injury and are commonly found in healthy individuals, and (b) are highly correlated with depressive symptoms.

Examination of the BC-PSI-Sf in a heterogeneous community sample

In this section, symptom endorsement rates and psychometric properties of the BC-PSI-Sf are reported. Participants were 87 healthy community volunteers from British Columbia, Canada (40% male and 60% female). Their average age was 24.2 years [SD = 8.7, Interquartile range (IQR) = 19.7 – 24.4, Range = 16 – 71] and their average education was 15.2 years (SD = 2.3, IQR = 13 – 16, Range = 12 – 23). The ethnic breakdown of this sample was 30% Caucasian, 57% Asian, 5% East Indian, and 8% "other" ethnicities. Participants did not have a prior history of an Axis I psychiatric disorder, neurological condition, significant substance abuse, or treatment for mental health problems by a psychiatrist, psychologist, or medical practitioner. Moreover, these subjects scored less than 17 on the BDI-II. A cutoff score of 17 is reported in the manual as the most sensitive and specific to depression.

A sample of 21 community volunteers was analyzed separately because they had BDI-II scores of 17 or greater. This sample was 71.4% female and 28.6% male. Their average age was 22.1 years (SD = 5.6) and their average education was 14.4 years (SD = 2.1).

When interpreting the BC-PSI-Sf, the first step is to determine whether the endorsement of symptoms is normal or unusual. In this sample of 87 community volunteers, their average score was 5.9 (SD = 6.0) and their median score was 4. Classification ranges for raw scores and corresponding percentile rank ranges are provided in Table 18.9. These percentile ranks were not force-normalized; they reflect the natural score distribution.

The percentages of subjects who endorsed each symptom by group are presented in Table 18.10. It is clear from this table that mild levels of these

Table 18.9. Classification ranges for raw scores and corresponding percentile rank ranges for the BC-PSI-Sf.

Classification	Raw Scores	Percentile Ranks
Low	0	0-16%
Normal	1 – 9	25 – 75%
Unusual	10 – 12	76 – 90%
High	13+	>90%

Table 18.10. Percentage of subjects who endorsed each symptom by group.

	Healthy Community Controls		Community Subjects with Suspected Mental Health Problems	
Symptoms	Mild Endorsement	Clinical Endorsement	Mild Endorsement	Clinical Endorsement
Headaches	21.8	2.3	47.6	4.8
Dizziness/light-headed	14.9	2.3	57.1	19.0
Nausea/feeling sick	14.9	0	57.1	19.0
Fatigue	40.2	6.9	81.0	47.6
Extra sensitive to noises	18.4	1.1	28.6	9.5
Irritable	42.5	5.7	71.4	42.9
Sad/Down in the dumps	31.0	2.3	85.7	52.4
Nervous or tense	25.3	2.3	71.4	38.1
Temper problems		28.7	8.0	57.1
28.6				
Poor concentration	34.5	5.7	90.5	66.7
Memory problems	23.0	5.7	76.2	42.9
Difficulty reading	16.1	3.4	66.7	33.3
Poor sleep	35.6	6.9	61.9	33.3
Total Score [M (SD) IQR]	5.9 (6.0) 1 – 9		21.7 (8.4) 15 – 25	
BDI-II Score [M (SD) IQR]	5.9 (4.2) 2 – 8		23.0 (5.8) 18 – 26	
Sample Size	87		21	

symptoms are common in healthy controls and very common in persons with suspected mental health problems. The clinical endorsement of these symptoms is relatively rare in healthy subjects but common in those with suspected mental health problems.

The internal consistency reliability of the scale was estimated using Cronbach's alpha ($\alpha = 0.80$). Some of the healthy control subjects completed the BC-PSI-Sf a second time, 2 – 6 days later (n = 52, 60% of original sample). The test-retest reliability was r = .61 (Spearman). The standard deviations for test and retest were 4.33 and 4.82, respectively. Therefore, the SEM for time one was 2.68 and the SEM for time two was 2.99. The standard error of difference was 4.01. To create an 80% confidence interval, the S_{diff} should be multiplied by 1.28 and to create a 90% confidence interval, it should be multiplied by 1.64. This results in .80 and .90 reliable change difference scores of 5.13 and 6.58, respectively. Therefore, test-retest difference scores would need to exceed these values in order to assume statistically reliable improvement or decline.

The BC-PSI-Sf requires a modification in the instructions for use with athletes. At baseline (preseason) it is appropriate to give the test as is. However, during post-concussion follow-up, the athlete should be instructed to complete the scale based on his or her experiences over the past 24 or 48 hours.

Research is needed on this scale with athletes before it can be recommended for clinical use, except in those rare cases involving persistent postconcusssion symptoms (e.g., several months in duration).

Postconcussion scale

The Postconcussion Scale (Appendix B) is a 20-item scale designed to measure the severity of symptoms in the acute phase of recovery from concussion (Lovell & Collins, 1998). This scale has been used with large samples of collegiate football players (Collins et al., 1999).

Reliability

The internal consistency reliability of the scale was estimated using Cronbach's alpha ($\alpha = 0.87$) in a sample of 200 collegiate football players. Test-retest reliability was estimated using a Spearman nonparmetric coefficient ($r = .55$) in a sample of 76 young men who were tested at the beginning and end of a season. The standard error of measurement, using the standard deviation and internal consistency estimates from the total sample, is 4.17.

Interpreting single test scores

When interpreting this inventory in young athletes, the first step is to determine whether the endorsement of symptoms is normal or unusual. In this sample of 200 young men, their average score was 10.5 (SD = 11.6) and their median score was 7. Scores falling between 1 and 14 are normal, whereas scores of 25 or greater are very high (see Table 18.11). The percentile rank ranges are based on the natural distribution of total scores for the 200 athletes.

The confidence intervals, for single test scores, are 5.3 points (.80) and 6.8 points (.90). So, if an athlete obtained a score of 10 on the inventory, you could be 80% sure that his "true score" fell between 5 and 15.

Individual symptoms also can be interpreted on this scale. The cumulative frequencies of symptom endorsements are presented in Table 18.12. As seen in this table, scores in the moderate-severe classification ranges are rare for non-injured athletes, with the exception of fatigue (18%) and trouble falling asleep (9.5%). It is not possible to have a uniform cutoff for unusual or rare scores in non-injured athletes because the baseline scores across symptoms

Table 18.11. Classifications, raw scores, and percentile ranks based on a sample of 200 young male athletes for the Postconcussion Scale.

Classification	Raw Scores	Percentile Ranks for Players
Low	0	0 – 12.5%
Normal	1 – 14	25 – 75%
Unusual	15 – 24	76 – 90%
High	25+	>90%

Table 18.12. The cumulative frequencies of symptom endorsements for the Postconcussion Scale.

Symptom	None 0	Mild 1	Mild 2	Moderate 3	Moderate 4	Severe 5	Severe 6
Headache	100	40.5	20.5	**10.0**	4.5	.5	.5
Confusion/Disorientation	100	14.0	5.5	2.5	.5	0	0
Difficulty Remembering Incident	100	18.0	**9.0**	4.0	.5	.5	0
Nausea	100	17.5	10.5	**6.0**	1.0	0	0
Vomiting	100	**3.5**	1.0	1.0	.5	0	0
Dizziness	100	20.5	11.5	**7.0**	2.5	1.0	.5
Balance Problems	100	14.0	**5.5**	4.0	1.0	0	0
Fatigue	100	57.0	39.0	26.0	18.0	**7.5**	2.0
Trouble Falling Asleep	100	44.0	27.0	16.5	**9.5**	3.0	.5
Sleeping More Than Usual	100	28.0	18.0	12.0	**6.0**	2.5	1.5
Drowsiness	100	40.5	26.0	10.5	**4.5**	.5	0
Sensitivity to Light/Noise	100	15.5	**10.0**	6.5	2.5	.5	0
Irritability	100	24.0	15.0	**10.0**	2.5	1.0	1.0
Sadness	100	20.5	13.5	6.5	5.0	3.0	1.5
Nervousness	100	31.5	19.0	10.5	**5.0**	3.0	1.0
Numbness or Tingling	100	14.0	**8.0**	6.0	3.5	2.0	1.5
Feeling Slowed Down	100	26.5	16.5	**7.5**	2.0	.5	.5
Feeling Like "In a Fog"	100	11.5	**5.0**	2.0	.5	0	0
Difficulty Concentrating	100	26.0	17.5	**10.0**	4.0	1.0	0
Difficulty with Memory	100	20.0	**9.5**	6.5	2.0	1.0	0

vary considerably. Baseline scores falling at or below the 10th percentile are unusual; thus, they are bolded in the table. Mild levels of vomiting, balance problems, and feeling like one is "in a fog" are rare, whereas moderate levels of nausea, dizziness, excessive sleep, drowsiness, and nervousness are rare.

A simplified interpretation system for individual symptoms is presented in Table 18.13. Raw scores that are "unusual" (at or below the 10th percentile) or "rare" are presented for each symptom.

Interpreting change on the postconcussion scale

The confidence interval for test-retest difference scores was computed for data derived from the 76 athletes who completed the scale twice, using the following formula: $S_{diff} = \sqrt{SEM_1^2 + SEM_2^2}$), resulting in an Sdiff = 11.52. Therefore, the .80 confidence interval would be 14.8 points and the .90 confidence interval would be 18.9 points. In general, an athlete's score would have to improve or decline by 15 points to be 80% sure that this change was not due to measurement error.

It is important to reiterate that reliable change scores vary based on the level of the baseline score. If the baseline score is high, regression to the mean will usually be present. Smaller changes are necessary for reliable decline and

Table 18.13. A simplified interpretation system for individual symptoms on the Post-concussion Scale.

Symptom	Unusual	Rare	
	≤ 10%	≤ 5%	≤ 1%
Headache	3	4	6
Confusion/Disorientation	2	3	4
Difficulty Remembering Incident	2	3	5
Nausea	3	4	4
Vomiting	1	1	3
Dizziness	3	4	5
Balance Problems	2	3	4
Fatigue	5	6	--
Trouble Falling Asleep	4	5	6
Sleeping More Than Usual	4	5	6
Drowsiness	4	4	5
Sensitivity to Light/Noise	2	4	5
Irritability	3	4	6
Sadness	3	4	--
Nervousness	4	5	6
Numbness or Tingling	2	4	--
Feeling Slowed Down	3	4	6
Feeling Like "In a Fog"	2	2	4
Difficulty Concentrating	3	4	5
Difficulty with Memory	2	4	5

larger changes are necessary for reliable improvement. If the baseline score is low, it is very difficult to interpret improvement (because the score cannot change by much; e.g., a score going from 3 to 1), and relatively smaller changes are necessary to detect decline.

To illustrate, the 76 athletes who completed the scale twice were divided into binary groups: "normal" (time one scores of 14 or less; n = 56) and "abnormal" (time one scores of 15 or greater; n = 18). The raw distribution of test-retest difference scores was examined and cutoff points were selected at the 10th and 5th percentiles in each tail. For athletes who begin with normal scores, their total scores must increase by 16 or more points or decrease by 6 or more points to be 90% sure that the player is more symptomatic or less symptomatic, respectively. In contrast, for athletes who begin with unusually high scores, they must drop by 22 or more points or increase by only one point to be 90% sure that the player is less symptomatic or more symptomatic, respectively. Clearly, these issues are complex and require detailed study before practitioners will be adequately informed regarding how to interpret change.

The scores from three soccer players followed for one month are presented in Table 18.14. By one-month post injury, all three athletes reported total scores of zero, so these results are not shown. Note that two rows are blank

Table 18.14. Tracking recovery of symptoms in three concussed soccer players.

Symptom	Unusual / Abnormal: ≤ 10%	Baseline	2 hours	48 hours	1 week
Headache	3	6 (0) 0	5 (2) 3	2 (2) 3	0 (1) 0
Confusion/Disorientation	2	---	---	---	---
Difficulty Remembering Incident	2	---	---	---	---
Nausea	3	0 (0) 0	6 (0) 0	2 (0) 0	0 (0) 0
Vomiting	1	0 (0) 0	0 (0) 0	0 (0) 0	0 (0) 0
Dizziness	3	0 (0) 0	4 (2) 1	0 (1) 1	0 (0) 0
Balance Problems	2	0 (0) 0	3 (1) 2	0 (1) 1	0 (0) 0
Fatigue	5	0 (0) 0	6 (4) 2	2 (4) 3	0 (0) 0
Trouble Falling Asleep	4	3 (0) 0	0 (0) 0	2 (0) 4	0 (0) 0
Sleeping More Than Usual	4	0 (0) 0	5 (0) 0	0 (0) 0	0 (3) 0
Drowsiness	4	0 (1) 0	5 (3) 4	2 (4) 4	0 (1) 1
Sensitivity to Light/Noise	2	0 (0) 0	4 (0) 3	0 (0) 5	0 (1) 0
Irritability	3	0 (0) 0	6 (0) 2	2 (0) 1	0 (0) 0
Sadness	3	0 (0) 0	5 (1) 2	0 (2) 0	0 (0) 0
Nervousness	4	0 (1) 0	4 (2) 0	0 (2) 0	1 (0) 0
Numbness or Tingling	2	0 (0) 0	2 (0) 0	0 (0) 0	0 (0) 0
Feeling Slowed Down	3	0 (0) 0	5 (3) 5	2 (4) 4	0 (1) 0
Feeling Like "In a Fog"	2	0 (0) 0	6 (1) 5	2 (3) 4	0 (0) 0
Difficulty Concentrating	3	0 (0) 0	6 (1) 4	2 (1) 5	0 (0) 0
Difficulty with Memory	2	0 (0) 0	6 (1) 2	2 (2) 3	0 (0) 1
Total Score	25+	9 (2) 0	78 (21) 35	20 (26) 38	1 (7) 2

See Appendix B for a description of how the scale used with the collegiate football players differs from the version used with these soccer players. The sensitivity to light/noise item was coded with the highest value recorded for either item on the revised version of the scale.

because these athletes received a different version of the scale as compared to the football players presented previously. The changes to the scale are detailed in Appendix B. From baseline to immediately post injury, there was a dramatic increase in symptoms. At 48 hours post injury, the first athlete had a major decline in symptoms but the other two athletes remained constant. However, by one-week post injury, all three athletes had largely recovered. It is possible that the first athlete's symptom reporting reflected both the biological effects of the concussion and a psychological reaction, in that high levels of irritability, sadness, and nervousness were reported within two hours of injury. This athlete, however, also appears to have sustained the most severe concussion as indicated by the levels of headache, nausea, dizziness, feeling in a fog, and difficulty concentrating. Therefore, from a purely academic perspective (e.g., if studying the phenomenology of symptom experiences in the acute recovery period), it would be difficult to separate the "psychology" from the "biology" in this case.

Conclusions & Directions for Future Research

The determination of change on neuropsychological tests and on self-report concussion symptom inventories is complex. The psychologist must consider carefully the potential confounding influences of (a) initial level of performance, (b) practice effects, (c) regression to the mean, (d) measurement error, and (e) motivation (e.g., minimization of postconcussion symptom reporting to hasten return to play). Frankly, the single most important factor to consider when interpreting test-retest differences on a performance-based measure or on a self-report inventory is level of baseline performance. The effects of practice and regression vary in relation to baseline level.

We presented a rather simplistic approach for interpreting change on the three postconcussion symptom inventories. In general, either the reliable change methodology or a simple examination of the natural distribution of change scores was applied. More complex analyses were conducted but not reported. For example, for two of the inventories, we computed estimated true scores in an attempt to reduce the effects of regression (Speer, 1992). We also utilized the elaborate computational formula reported by Hageman and Arrindell (1993); this approach is quite sophisticated and represents a clear psychometric advancement over the traditional reliable change methodology. In addition, linear regression models were employed whereby retest scores were regressed on test scores, in an attempt to control for factors relating to initial level of performance and regression to the mean. We did not report the findings from these various analyses for three practical reasons. First, the two inventories that were employed with athletes are largely "state" measures of symptoms. They are influenced by numerous factors including stress, fatigue, depression, and transient health problems. When an athlete reports high preseason levels of symptoms, this might be due to situational factors. We would expect his score to drop after resolution of some of these factors. Because the test-retest interval for these two measures was long (i.e., preseason for two consecutive years or preseason to postseason), it was quite possible that temporal and situational factors substantially reduced the reliability of the difference scores. Therefore, the systematic study of shorter retest intervals is needed for self-report inventories designed to measure acute symptoms and initial recovery patterns following concussion in athletes. Second, the computations based on the methodologies not included in this chapter resulted in very few practical differences in conceptualizing change on these inventories. In other words, the results were quite similar to the methods included in the chapter. More importantly, these other methods also were adversely impacted by the long retest interval and the state nature of the symptom reporting. Finally, because of the aforementioned methodological limitations we wanted to reduce chapter length and reader fatigue, realizing that the presentation of numerous methods was largely academic and had limited practical application for these data, at present, in sports neuropsychology.

An important and obvious future direction in sports neuropsychology is to create test-retest normative databases for athletes for both performance-based and self-report measures. Sample sizes in excess of 200 will be necessary to adequately study change in high versus low scoring athletes. Different statistical methodologies likely will prove more or less effective for conceptualizing change in persons with low, average, or high baseline levels of performance. If very large databases become available (e.g., more than 500 collegiate football players), then the raw test-retest score distributions simply can be examined to determine the normal range for test-retest difference scores at various levels of baseline performance.

The serial assessment of athletes is challenging. The following is a list of considerations for the sports neuropsychologist engaged in this practice.

- Scores are not exact estimates of functioning or ability, all contain measurement error and some contain substantial measurement error.
- Variability on neuropsychological testing within a single session is very common. The more tests that are given, the more likely you will see intertest variability.
- Test-retest variability is commonly due to measurement error, situational factors, and practice effects. Unusual test performances are common and can be difficult to explain. For example, when the first author evaluated an athlete with multiple concussions in the post-acute recovery period (more than four months post) who obtained a scaled score of 4 (2nd percentile) on the WAIS-III Letter-Number Sequencing subtest during an initial examination and then a score of 10 (50th percentile) less than two weeks later.
- If baseline testing is conducted, and an athlete endorses a high number of symptoms, he or she should be canvassed to identify factors relating to this symptom reporting. Retesting will likely be necessary following resolution of these factors, if transient, to get a better estimate of baseline functioning.
- Immediately following concussion, athletes often report a large number of symptoms on a postconcussion inventory. There typically is rapid resolution of these symptoms over the next several days, and sometimes weeks. Knowing normal and abnormal symptom score ranges for athletes is helpful for interpreting the clinical significance of the symptom reporting patterns, irrespective of the reliability of the measures. As a general rule, statistically reliable change is a necessary precursor for inferring clinically meaningful change; however, reliable change alone does not mean that practically meaningful change has occurred (e.g., if the athlete reports reliably less severe symptoms at five days post-injury than one day post, but is still scoring in the "abnormal" range).
- When interpreting a neuropsychological test score or a concussion inventory score, the most important consideration is baseline level of performance. High scores are likely to be lower and low scores are likely to be higher upon retesting. The confidence intervals for test-retest difference

scores for baseline performances that fall in the average range are more evenly distributed.

- It is important to avoid over-interpreting or over-pathologizing neuropsychological test scores. Be careful not to inadvertently make the impact of the injury worse for the athlete. It is common to have concerns about "brain damage." Athletes who focus, dwell, and worry about their symptoms are at increased risk for protracted recovery patterns.
- Of course, it is also important not to minimize concussions. These injuries, unlike orthopedic injuries, cannot be seen. There is a tendency on the part of coaches, trainers, and athletes to ignore or minimize the injury. Thus, the sports neuropsychologist must consider carefully whether response bias might be affecting an athletes symptom reporting.
- There is very little research evidence to support the notion that we can detect changes on neuropsychological tests that are directly attributable to the effects of a concussion after three months post injury. This is because most of these injuries have resolved, at least functionally, before then. Moreover, neuropsychological tests, with their inherent measurement error and situational influences, typically are not sensitive to subtle medium-term effects from these injuries. Baseline, pre-injury testing increases the likelihood that the neuropsychologist will make valid and accurate inferences regarding test performances derived from evaluations occurring after the typical recovery period. The absence of pre-injury data increases the likelihood of interpreting natural variability in test scores as injury-related, or of misunderstanding premorbid abilities levels and thus misinterpreting post-injury test scores.

Considerable research is needed to enhance the reliability, validity, and accuracy of serial assessments with athletes. At present, this is largely a clinical process that is poorly informed with empirical data. In due course, because of the unique applications of neuropsychology with athletes, we predict that advancements in sports neuropsychology will be used to inform clinical practice in mainstream neuropsychology.

References

Beck, A.T., Steer, R.A., Ball, R., & Ranieri, W.F. (1996). Comparison of Beck Depression Inventories-IA and -II in psychiatric outpatients. *Journal of Personality Assessment, 67*, 588–597.

Chelune, G.J., Naugle, R.I., Luders, H., Sedlak, J., & Awad, I.A. (1993). Individual change after epilepsy surgery: Practice effects and base-rate information. *Neuropsychology, 7*, 41–52.

Collins, M.W., Grindel, S.H., Lovell, M.R., Dede, D.E., Moser, D.J., Phalin, B.R. et al. (1999). Relationship between concussion and neuropsychological performance in college football players. *Journal of the American Medical Association, 282*, 964–970.

Franzen, M.D. (1989). *Reliability and validity in neuropsychological assessment*. New York: Plenum Press.

Franzen, M.D. (2000). *Reliability and validity in neuropsychological assessment*. (2nd ed.) New York: Kluwer Academic/Plenum Press.

Gaetz, M., Goodman, D., & Weinberg, H. (2000). Electrophysiological evidence for the cumulative effects of concussion. *Brain Injury, 14*, 1077–1088.

Hageman, W.J.J.M., & Arrindell, W.A. (1993). A further refinement of the reliable change (RC) index by improving the pre-post difference score: Introducing RC(ID). *Behaviour Research and Therapy, 31*, 693–700.

Heaton, R.K., Temkin, N., Dikmen, S. Avitable, N., Taylor, M.J., Marcotte, T.D. et al. (2001). Detecting change: A comparison of three neuropsychological methods using normal and clinical samples. *Archives of Clinical Neuropsychology, 16*, 75–91.

Hinton-Bayre, A.D., Geffen, G.M., Geffen, L.B., McFarland, K.A., & Friis, P. (1999). Concussion in contact sports: Reliable change indices of impairment and recovery. *Journal of Clinical and Experimental Neuropsychology, 21*, 70–86.

Hsu, L.M. (1989). Reliable changes in psychotherapy: Taking into account regression toward the mean. *Behavioral Assessment, 11*, 459–467.

Iverson, G.L. (1998). Interpretation of Mini-Mental State Examination scores in community-dwelling elderly and geriatric neuropsychiatry patients. *International Journal of Geriatric Psychiatry, 13*, 661–666.

Iverson, G. (1999). Interpreting change on the WAIS-III/WMS-III following traumatic brain injury. *Journal of Cognitive Rehabilitation, 17*, 16–20.

Iverson, G.L. (2001). Interpreting change on the WAIS-III/WMS-III in clinical samples. *Archives of Clinical Neuropsychology, 16*, 183–191.

Iverson, G.L., Gaetz, M., Lovell, M.R., Collins, M., & Maroon, J. (2002). Cumulative effects of concussion in amateur athletes. *Archives of Clinical Neuropsychology, 17*, 769.

Iverson, G.L., & Lange, R.T. (in press). Examination of "postconcussion-like" symptoms in a healthy sample. *Applied Neuropsychology.*

Iverson, G.L., Lovell, M.R., Collins, M.W., & Norwig, J. (2002). Tracking recovery from concussion using ImPACT: Applying reliable change methodology. *Archives of Clinical Neuropsychology, 17*, 770.

Jacobson, N.S. & Revenstorf, D. (1988). Statistics for assessing the clinical significance of psychotherapy issues: Issues, problems, and new developments. *Behavioral Assessment, 10*, 133–145.

Jacobson, N.S., Roberts, L.J., Berns, S.B., & McGlinchey, J.B. (1999). Methods for defining and determining the clinical significance of treatment effects: Description, application, and alternatives. *Journal of Consulting and Clinical Psychology, 67*, 300–307.

Jacobson, N.S. & Truax, P. (1991). Clinical significance: A statistical approach to defining meaningful change in psychotherapy research. *Journal of Consulting and Clinical Psychology*, *59*, 12–19.

Lovell, M. R., & Collins, M. W. (1998). Neuropsychological assessment of the college football player. *Journal of Head Trauma Rehabilitation, 13*, 9–26.

Macciocchi, S. N., Barth, J. T., Alves, W., Rimel, R. W., & Jane, J. A. (1996). Neuropsychological functioning and recovery after mild head injury in collegiate athletes. *Neurosurgery, 39*, 510-514.

Matser, E.J.T., Kessels, A.G., Lezak, M.D., Jordan, B.D., & Troost, J. (1999). Neuropsychological impairment in amateur soccer players. *Jama, 282*, 971–973.

Ogles, B.M., Lambert, M.J., & Masters, K.S. (1996). *Assessing outcome in clinical practice*. Boston: Allyn and Bacon.

Speer, D.C. (1992). Clinically significant change: Jacobson and Truax (1991) revisited. *Journal of Consulting and Clinical Psychology, 60*, 402–408.

Speer, D.C., & Greenbaum, P.E. (1995). Five methods for computing significant individual client change and improvement rates: Support for an individual growth curve approach. *Journal of Consulting and Clinical Psychology, 63*, 1044–1048.
Temkin, N.R., Heaton, R.K., Grant, I., & Dikmen, S.S. (2000). Reliable change formula query: Temkin et al. reply. *Journal of the International Neuropsychological Society, 6*, 364.
Wechsler, D. (1997). *WAIS-III Administration and Scoring Manual.* San Antonio, TX: Psychological Corporation.
Wrightson, P. & Gronwall, D. (1999). *Mild head injury: A guide to management.* Oxford University Press.

Appendix A. BC-PSI-Sf Protocol

The following is a list of psychological symptoms that you may have experienced. Please rate each symptom or problem in regards to how often it happens and how bad it is. **Consider your experience with these symptoms or problems over the past two weeks, including today.**

How Often *(Frequency)*	How Bad *(Intensity)*
0 = Not at all	0 = Not at all
1 = 1-2 times	1 = Very mild problem
2 = Several times	2 = Mild Problem
3 = Often	3 = Moderate problem
4 = Very often	4 = Severe problem
5 = Constantly	5 = Very severe problem

Psychological Symptoms & Life Problems	How Often	How Bad
Headaches	________	________
Dizziness/light-headed	________	________
Nausea/feeling sick	________	________
Fatigue	________	________
Extra sensitive to noises	________	________
Irritable	________	________
Sad/Down in the dumps	________	________
Nervous or tense	________	________
Temper problems	________	________
Poor concentration	________	________
Memory problems	________	________
Difficulty reading	________	________
Poor sleep	________	________

Does alcohol affect you more than in the past?

1	2	3	4	5
Not at all		Somewhat		Very Much

Do you find yourself worrying and dwelling on the symptoms above?

1	2	3	4	5
Not at all	S	omewhat		Very Much

Do you believe you have damage to your brain?

1	2	3	4	5
Not at all		Somewhat		Very Much

Copyright © 1998, 2001, Grant L. Iverson, Ph.D.; Reprinted with Permission

Appendix B. The Postconcussion Scale

Directions: After reading each symptom, please circle the number that best describes the way you have been feeling **today**. A rating of **0** means you have **not** experienced this symptom today. A rating of **6** means you have experienced **severe** problems with this symptom today.

Symptom	None	Mild		Moderate		Severe	
Headache	0	1	2	3	4	5	6
Confusion/Disorientation	0	1	2	3	4	5	6
Difficulty Remembering Incident	0	1	2	3	4	5	6
Nausea	0	1	2	3	4	5	6
Vomiting	0	1	2	3	4	5	6
Dizziness	0	1	2	3	4	5	6
Balance Problems	0	1	2	3	4	5	6
Fatigue	0	1	2	3	4	5	6
Trouble Falling Asleep	0	1	2	3	4	5	6
Sleeping More Than Usual	0	1	2	3	4	5	6
Drowsiness	0	1	2	3	4	5	6
Sensitivity to Light/Noise	0	1	2	3	4	5	6
Irritability	0	1	2	3	4	5	6
Sadness	0	1	2	3	4	5	6
Nervousness	0	1	2	3	4	5	6
Numbness or Tingling	0	1	2	3	4	5	6
Feeling Slowed Down	0	1	2	3	4	5	6
Feeling Like "In a Fog"	0	1	2	3	4	5	6
Difficulty Concentrating	0	1	2	3	4	5	6
Difficulty with Memory	0	1	2	3	4	5	6

Note that a revised version of this scale has made several significant changes: (a) the "confusion/disorientation" and "difficulty remembering incident" items were dropped; (b) the single item "sensitivity to light/noise" has been converted to two items; (c) the "fatigue" item has been changed to "low energy"; (d) the "difficulty with memory" item has been changed to "difficulty remembering"; (e) "nervousness" has been changed to "nervous/anxious", and (f) an item called "more emotional than usual" has been added.

Chapter 19

SPECIAL CONSIDERATIONS AND IMPLICATIONS OF NEUROPSYCHOLOGICAL TESTING IN PROFESSIONAL ATHLETES

Elizabeth Kozora
National Jewish Medical and Research Center
University of Colorado Health Sciences Center, USA

Don Gerber
Craig Hospital Englewood, Colorado, USA

Introduction

Neuropsychological evaluation provides a sensitive tool for measuring the effects of concussion, and in sports-related head injuries, this has led to rapid and innovative development across clinical and research domains. Working with athletes can raise unique challenges in terms of assessment procedures, interpretation frameworks, and information transfer. In addition, gaining the cooperation of key personnel and working within the culture of the team becomes extremely important for the consultant. This new and exciting role is shaped by a well-defined neuropsychology discipline, yet demands constant adaptation and problem solving in the complex sports world. This chapter attempts to outline situations and challenges consultants face using information gathered directly from neuropsychologists working in this area.

As a brief overview, the chapter will begin with a discussion of neuropsychological research and clinical projects currently in use by the National Football League (NFL) and National Hockey League (NHL). The "working relationship" a neuropsychologist acquires with the athletic organization is considered a "key" component of successful interactions and some basic approaches and difficulties will first be addressed. Next, specific mechanisms of the "baseline" assessment and "post-concussive" work-ups utilized in these projects will be explored. Circumstances that affect cognitive test performance of the athlete may be multifactorial, therefore the following factors will also be examined: physical limitations of the testing situation, language differences, acceptance and emotional impact of testing on the athlete, player interactions and celebrity status, and impact of neurobehavioral symptoms on cognition. Finally, the use and transfer of neuropsychological data in clinical and research domains will be reviewed.

To better identify assessment concerns of professional athletes, a survey regarding practice issues and perceived responses from the sports community was sent to 38 neuropsychologists currently involved in protocols with professional hockey and football teams. Twenty-seven responses (71%) were returned, and the data from this survey will be presented throughout the chapter and referenced as the Sports Testing Survey. The respondents are neuropsychologists from both the NFL and NHL programs and the differences in these protocols (i.e. clinical and/or research) will have some influence in overall responses. The neuropsychologist's perspective likely differs from the team members and future studies involving professional players, coaches, trainers and physicians would be essential to broaden our understanding in this area.

Review of Development and Initiation of Neuropsychological Testing Protocols in Professional Sports (NHL and NFL)

Neuropsychological evaluation has emerged as a sensitive approach to quantifying specific changes in brain function following mild head injury (Levin, Eisenberg, & Benton, 1989). This methodology has been applied to sports concussion and frequently aims to quantify potential decline in cognition following an injury. "Baseline" cognitive scores are typically obtained on players before the season, and following a concussion, tests are re-administered and compared to baseline to assess change and potential decline.

The risk of sustaining a concussion has been estimated to be from 8.4% to 44.8% for professional athletes in football (Delaney & Drummond, 1999). At the professional level, the National Football League (NFL) has been conducting concussion research since 1996. The current research is a product of the NFL subcommittee on mild traumatic brain injury. At this time, team participation in the research is voluntary and involves approximately 22 teams. The NFL program consists of baseline screening of the athletes including a concussion history, symptom checklist (i.e. player rating of symptom severity such as dizziness and nausea) and cognitive testing. The neuropsychological screening battery takes approximately 30 minutes and the selected tests measure complex information processing, attention, learning and memory and fine motor skills (Lovell & Collins, 1998). The baseline data are anonymously entered into a database. Any athlete who subsequently sustains a concussion is re-evaluated against their baseline data within 24 to 48 hours post injury. Serial re-evaluation (until the athlete's symptoms and test performance normalizes) has also been recommended.

The incidence of concussion in hockey has been estimated between 18 to 28% (Biasca, Simmen, Bartolozzi, & Trentz, 1995). Since 1997, the National Hockey League (NHL) has conducted a league wide concussion research project. The project consists of pre-season baseline screening of every athlete, which is similar to the NFL studies (concussion history, concussion symptom checklist and neuropsychological screening of attention, speed of processing and memory (Lovell & Collins, 1998). Players sustaining concussions are re-evaluated within 24-48 hours of a concussion, and serial re-evaluation every 5 to 7 days until symptoms and test scores normalize has been recommended. At present, at least 1,400 athletes have completed baseline evaluation. Additionally, a number of post-concussive evaluations have been administered and are being analyzed.

Fitting In with the Team

There are many practical considerations that must be addressed in order to conduct successful long-term neuropsychological research with athletic teams. Bartolic (Bartolic, 1999) noted that the "successful execution of research programs will depend on multiple factors including, the adequacy of advanced planning and organization, the quality of the relationships developed with key personnel inside athletic organizations, flexibility of the research team members in obtaining neuropsychological test data from players, and calculated efforts to avoid disruptions of normal team operations."

An essential first step is to establish working relationships with key personnel within the athletic organization. It is important to recognize that the athletes, trainers, physicians, coaches and owners may question the need for concussion research because sport concussion has been customarily considered to be a transient phenomenon without significant sequelae. Additionally, these individuals are likely to be unfamiliar with neuropsychological assessment procedures and to be wary of introducing them into their sport. At a practical level, they are also likely to be concerned about any disruptive effects that the research may have on normal team operations. The role of the neuropsychologist within the operations of the organization is also likely to be a concern. The role may be exclusively research or may be a combination of research and clinical responsibilities. The context of the project, e.g. mandatory versus voluntary participation, will influence the role of the neuropsychologist within the organization. For example, the National Hockey League (NHL) requires mandatory participation in the concussion research with league-wide protocols. The neuropsychologist's role within this project is primarily research, although individual teams may expand the role to include some clinical responsibilities. The National Football League (NFL) has a voluntary concussion research program. The neuropsychologists role will vary dramatically from team to team, depending on individual arrangements with the team. All of these potential barriers must be anticipated, understood and addressed if we are to advance knowledge of the neuropsychological effects of sport concussion (Barth et al., 1989).

Introducing the research projects to key personnel within the athletic organization is a critical first step to establishing working relationships. There are a variety of approaches that the neuropsychologists may take. Respondents in the Sports Testing Survey reported that 70% met with the medical staff, 85% met with the team trainer, 44% provided copies of the consent form or research protocol or examples of tests, 26% provided additional educational materials (i.e. such as research articles) and 15% did other (i.e. team contacted the neuropsychologist). The degree of concern that the organizations medical staff has about concussions will influence their interest in pursuing research and clinical programs. At the onset of the projects, the neuropsychologists perceptions of the medical staff's concern about concussions were that 7% had no concern, 23% had limited concern, 48% were concerned, and 22% were extremely concerned. Over time, there appeared to be a shift of the medical staff's concern about concussion, at least as perceived by the neuropsychologist; 4% reporting no concern, 7% indicating limited concern, 59% reporting concern, and 30% reporting extreme concern. Results indicate a shift over time toward increased interest about concussion (medical impact, treatment, return to play, etc.) by the medical staff for their players.

At the onset of their particular involvement with the NFL/NHL teams, the respondents of the Sports Testing Survey indicated that 4% of the athletic organizations were extremely reluctant, 11% were reluctant, 19% were hesitant, 44% were willing and 22% were fully accepting and endorsing. Over time, the neuropsychologists perceived a change in the athletic organization's level of involvement: none of the respondents felt the teams were extremely reluctant, 4% felt the teams were reluctant, 11% were hesitant, 33% were willing and 52% were fully accepting and endorsing. The length of each project was not assessed, however, the NHL protocol has been in existence for the past three years, and some of the NFL protocols have been in place longer. These results suggest that overall, the teams were perceived as more involved and accepting after involvement with the project. The survey respondents saw their roles with their specific teams as: 56% researcher and data collector, 93% as diagnostician, 41% as problem solver and 15% as other. The NHL study was mandated as a "research" project but consultants are likely to have several roles. Whether or not the respondents were in the NFL or NHL, a large proportion saw their role as "diagnostician".

In summary, the survey results suggest that athletic organizations are concerned about concussions and that they appear to become more concerned over time. However, the reasons for this shift are not clear and likely multifactorial. It is possible that participation in concussion research heightens awareness of the problems associated with concussion. It is also possible that positive and informative interactions with the consultant increase the favorability of the project. If the protocols are initiated without disrupting the mechanics of the team and improve the overall health and protection of the athletes, the testing may become a valuable addition for the entire organization Finally, it is important to recognize that there has been increasing media attention to the effects of sport concussion that are changing perceptions about it. Although athletic organizations are somewhat hesitant about initiating neuropsychological research, they appear to become more comfortable with it over time.

Baseline Testing of Professional Athletes

A test battery for a mild head injury in sports should be constructed based on test sensitivity, brief duration, and inclusion of tests that have "face validity" (Levin & Jordan, 1993). The battery used in both the NFL and NHL study appears to match this criteria in that the tests are sensitive, the battery is quite brief (approximately 30 minutes) and tests offer face validity for mild head injury by including measures of reaction time, attention and memory. The batteries in the NFL/NHL studies differ slightly but are similar in content. Both batteries include a consent form and a background history (i.e. demographics and educational level, history of learning disability, number of years in sports, head injury and possible neurological evaluations). A language survey for players who are not primarily English speaking is available for the NHL study (i.e. time frame of English exposure and rating scales of verbal and written proficiency). The neuropsychological batteries typically include a general Orientation Scale (name, date of birth etc.), a Neurobehavioral Symptoms Checklist (rating severity of items such as headache, dizziness, nausea etc.), and tests of simple attention, learning, memory and fluency (Lovell & Collins, 1998).

Both the batteries used in the NHL and NFL (as well as multiple college and high school studies) utilize the "baseline" approach in order to specifically address cognitive change for the individual. While comparing performance on cognitive tests to normative peers is a standard neuropsychological practice, comparing the athlete against his own preconcussion baseline appears to provide the most sensitive method for detecting subtle cognitive changes from concussion. Establishing a preseason baseline is important because athletes vary considerably in their cognitive abilities, making it difficult to discern if any subtle deficits that are identified on post-concussion testing are attributable to the concussion or to other unrelated factors. Preseason baseline screening enables the athlete to act as his own control. Baseline screening is recommended whenever possible and is being used at the high school, college and professional levels. The mechanics (i.e. who introduces the player to baseline testing, how is it carried out) differ across teams.

In the Sports Testing Survey, the information presented to players regarding the nature of baseline testing was provided primarily by the consulting neuropsychologist (88%) and neuropsychology staff (17%). The trainer also provided information on the testing in 73% of the surveys returned. Only 31% of the team physicians and 4% of the coaches were involved in the dissemination of this initial information. These results indicate that in addition to the neuropsychology staff, the trainer for each team is a major source of information to the players. The "mechanism" for providing information to the players was examined and oral verbal explanations were the most frequent (96%) followed by written materials (62%). In addition, 12% reported information was provided indirectly through consent forms and 4% indicated that examples of the tests were utilized. It is not clear from the survey which approach would be the most beneficial, but it does suggest that verbal (oral and written) explanations are the most common. In terms of the actual administration of tests, most (88%) of the neuropsychologists test their athletes, 38% are tested by technicians, 54% by graduate students, 12% post-doctoral students, and 15% other (neurologist trained in psychology; predoctoral interns).

In summary, baseline neuropsychological testing at the beginning of a season is an essential component of all the NFL/NHL sports concussion programs. Introducing the concept of "baseline testing" with players and athletic organizations requires planning. Although the neuropsychologist is providing a majority of this information, the trainer's knowledge and ability to communicate the project will be essential for a successful project. This would suggest that preparing the trainer for this role could be critical. It is likely that the trainer's "endorsement" of the project will affect overall cooperation of the players, which will ultimately lead to the successful integration of the neuropsychologist into the team mechanisms. The impact of "source" and "type" of introductory information regarding baseline testing is not known. However, if this is presented clearly and efficiently, this material may contribute to the player's overall level of understanding, trust and cooperation with the project. A large proportion of the players in professional sports (particularly NHL) may have different language backgrounds and the dependence on English language could be problematic (see Language Differences below). Although only a small percent utilized examples of the tests to facilitate understanding, this could provide another valuable avenue of education. Other approaches might include having the information printed in several languages or players having access to as individual who can explain the study in their own language. Although a majority of the neuropsychologists are involved in the baseline testing (88%), both graduate students and technicians are also responsible across teams for a number of these evaluations. Given the large-scale nature of these projects the development of "team" approaches to baseline testing appears useful.

Post-Concussive Testing of Professional Athletes

For a single, uncomplicated concussion, a brief neuropsychological screening administered within 24-48 hours post injury provides basic information about the athlete's symptoms and cognitive functioning. The NFL/NHL protocols require a detailed post concussive interview, neurobehavioral symptoms checklist, and re-testing (using alternate versions whenever possible) of attention, processing speed and memory. The athlete's follow-up test results are compared to baseline numbers and symptoms. If cognitive deficits or persistent symptoms are identified, then follow-up testing within five to seven days is useful to monitor recovery and/or track ongoing problems. Symptoms and scores should normalize before the athlete returns to play. Athletes who have sustained multiple concussions or who have sustained concussions with persisting symptoms may require more extensive evaluation as part of the medical work-up.

The number of post-concussive evaluations performed per team neuropsychologist was requested in the Sports Testing Survey. Only 23 of the 27 sites reported on this frequency, therefore the actual incidence is not available. To better acknowledge the experience of the neuropsychologists in this survey, it should be noted that each of the sites conducted an average of 10 post-concussive evaluations ranging from 0 to 30 at individual sites. Additionally, an average of 3.5 post concussive evaluations were performed by neuropsychologists from different teams (range 0–10), indicating that it is not uncommon for follow-ups to be completed out of state and by consultants on the opposing team. These results would suggest that most of the neuropsychologists involved in this survey have experience in testing athletes following post-concussive events.

Ninety-six percent of the neuropsychologists in the Sports Testing Survey indicated they were directly involved in the testing of the athlete following a concussion. Only 8% of technicians, 12% graduate students and 12% post-doctoral level students were identified as involved in this aspect of testing. A large proportion (88%) of the respondents indicated that the evaluation is performed between 24 and 48 hours after the injury; the timeline recommended by prior studies. However, 23% reported administering the battery in less than 24 hours following the event, 31% more than 48 hours after the event and 12% over 72 hours later. These results indicate that despite the guidelines, post-concussive evaluations are not always performed at the suggested times, and the impact of this variability may be important. Protocols for the research components of the NFL/NHL batteries typically request "re-assessment" one week following the concussion if test results are "not normal". However, when the neuropsychologists were surveyed, only 29% reported that they always perform this follow-up evaluation, 55% report this occurs some of the time, and 17% indicated that they never do this testing to assure normalization. The reasons for variability in follow-up times are not clear. It is likely that the players (and medical personnel) are reticent to participate in retesting once they are asymptomatic and less concerned with the immediate effects of the head injury.

In summary, large-scale projects require extensive resources to effectively conduct evaluations. Assuring consistency of test administration from pre to post concussive testing is necessary to adjust to the diverse backgrounds of professional athletes. The survey indicates that neuropsychologists are performing a majority of the follow up evaluations. This may have some interesting implications if that neuropsychologist did not do the baseline testing and "nonstandard" approaches were utilized. Modifications should be anticipated and integrated into the protocols. Results at this time would suggest the need to begin identifying and recording these "nonstandard" administrations in order to assure "identical" testing parameters. It is not uncommon for some of the neuropsychologists to contact the initial test examiner regarding specific players or to interview the examiner on behavioral comments. It may be useful to encourage the actual documentation of procedures when modifications have been used so that this information is properly transferred to the next test situation. Interestingly, the survey indicates that a number of players have been tested by neuropsychologists at "another site". These numbers most likely represent the NHL protocol (it has been designed to accommodate players in other cities). The "impact" of a player being evaluated by an examiner from the "opposite" team is unknown. This protocol is routine for players in the NHL leagues, and because the medical staff routinely examines and treats players from "opposing" teams, this approach may be familiar and less threatening than expected. Although a majority of the tests are performed at the "recommended" time point of 24 to 48 hours, over a quarter indicate that testing is done before 24 hours, or after 48 hours. The potential impact of this in terms of research and clinical findings will need to be examined.

Circumstances that Affect Cognitive Test Performance of the Athlete

Heaton & Heaton (1981) indicate that "the goal of testing is to obtain the best performance the patient is capable of producing". For athletes, this would refer not only to follow-up post-concussive evaluations but their initial baseline-testing situation. If the player's baseline scores are not accurate due to any potential factors (i.e. failure to understand instructions, poor effort, and anxiety), then comparison of scores at follow-up may be quite flawed. Similarly, there may be factors associated with the player's performance at follow-up (i.e. anxiety about career, return to play decisions), which could interfere with getting the best test results and again impact interpretation. Most neuropsychologists would agree with Dr. Lezak's (1995) comment that the "quality of performance can be exceedingly vulnerable to external influences or changes in their internal state". She points out that maximum effort is essential for valid assessment and that "interpretation of test scores and of test behavior is predicted on the assumption that the demonstrated behavior is a representative sample of the patient's true capacity in the area"(p. 140). We can apply this principle to testing with athletes and suggest that if the player is not highly motivated to perform well, or if other factors interfere with obtaining optimal test results at baseline and/or follow-up, then accurate comparisons of test results and interpretation following a concussion may be jeopardized. If the goal is to help players "do their best so that the difference between what they can do and how they actually perform is negligible" (Lezak, 1995), then the neuropsychologist must be aware of circumstances that could interfere. These factors might include poor conditions of the environment at testing, high levels of anxiety or distress, language differences, celebrity status, player interactions, and interference via neurobehavioral symptoms.

Physical Conditions of Testing

The testing of athletes both at baseline and following a concussive event rarely conform to the "standard" office visit with which most neuropsychologists are familiar. "In the ideal testing situation both optimal and standard conditions prevail" (Lezak, 1995). Optimal conditions have been defined as those circumstances that allow a patient to perform his or her best on tests. Standard conditions refer to as actions by the test administrator that "ensure that each administration of the test is as much like every other administration as possible, so that scores obtained on different test administrations can be compared" (Lezak, 1995). How we define the "optimal" physical condition for testing athletes is not clear and likely does not adhere to our "standard" appointment.

The Sports Testing Survey asked respondents where they performed tests and whether distractions were noted. Fifty-eight percent noted that testing was performed in the locker room area, 50% during team physicals in a medical office, 27% were done via individual appointments at another facility, and 23% at another site (i.e. the neuropsychologists office). Surprisingly, 44% of the respondents indicated that there were no distractions at the time of testing for their athletes. However, other distractions were noted such as noise

(48% of responses), lack of privacy (16%), inadequate testing space such as lack of tables or small rooms (16%) and additional factors (13%) such as being rushed through the evaluations by the trainer. The question of "being rushed" was not specifically asked about in the Sports Survey, however, as the survey suggests about half of the players were tested during team physicals. This would indicate, based on the "typical" team physical prototype, that players are required to rotate through multiple medical stations (i.e. general physicals, fitness, orthopedics, optometry, etc.) as well as the neuropsychological exam in a short period. Not only are time pressures a concern, but the effect of other exams (i.e. eyes dilated for the optometrical exam) could have indirect effects on this testing situation which minimize that "optimal" testing standard one strives for.

In summary, the survey suggests that distractions and time constraints may be unidentified factors modifying test administration. Distractions for the neuropsychologist might be different for those of the players; for example, players may actually be more comfortable being tested in a room near the playing site or the locker room where sights, sounds and personnel are familiar to the player. What seems distracting to the examiner (i.e. noises of the athletic facility) may actually be reassuring to the player. Similarly, being seen in a doctor's office or medical center may have a negative effect on the player who suddenly sees themselves in a foreign environment with different "rules" of behavior (i.e. the sick role). Clearly the impact of this arrangement is not directly available but it may be worthwhile in the future to "survey" the players regarding such issues in order to maximize the "optimal" condition for this population.

Language Differences

Differing ethnic backgrounds and languages are clearly a descriptive component of players in professional sports. Although the exact proportions are not known, it is likely that in the NHL a large percentage of the players have a primary language other than English. For example, on one team the recorded primary language use was 51% English, 17% French, 12% Russian, 6% Czech, 5% Swedish, 3% German, 3% Finnish, 3% Slovakian and 1% Latvian. The impact of language and ethnic differences in test administration and scoring is a controversial area (Artiola, Fortuny, & Mullaney, 1998; Harris, 2002) and these differences may have direct implications on the testing situation with athletes. Typically, "highly standardized test administration is necessary when using norms of tests that have a fine-graded and statistically well standardized scoring system" (Lezak, 1995). However, by comparing the player to his own baseline testing, the critical nature of "standardization" may have more to do with consistency in test administration, and in the accuracy and detailed nature of recording and scoring individual player responses. A reasonable goal is to expose the player to an "identical" situation from baseline to follow-up for accuracy in test-score comparison. Additionally, assuring adequate comprehension of test demands and expectations is expected. It should be noted that the NHL battery was developed to be composed primarily a non-language-based tests to accommodate the high frequency of non-English speaking participants. However, there were not standard instructions regarding modifications, when to discontinue, and how to assure comprehension both of the consent form and test instruction.

In the Sports Testing Survey, respondents were questioned regarding their responses to language differences. Responses would suggest that neuropsychologists approached this several ways. Fifty-two percent reported that they administered "nonverbal testing" only, 52% reported that they modified the test instructions, 52% indicated that they assured that the player understood words and 14% chose other (i.e. use of translators; converting symptom checklist into other foreign languages). All the players were tested despite language differences. Multiple implications from these results regarding standardization and "validity" of test administration and interpretation are raised.

The results from the Sports Testing Survey indicate that over half of the neuropsychologists modify the test instructions in some way. Recommendations for ensuring standardization of modifications (which assure adequate comprehension) appear necessary. In addition, it may be useful to examine scoring and interpretation of these nonstandard procedures. Most information regarding nonstandard testing occurs in rehabilitation with disabled individuals. Caplan & Schecter (1995) write, "it is clear that clinicians have long wrestled with the question of whether the risk and losses entailed by jettisoning standard procedures are offset by the value of modifications that may restore construct or ecological validity". In a review of individual with various sensory and physical disabilities, modifications have included pantomiming instructions, multiple choice formats, enlarging stimulus materials, and using point response modes. In some literature these modifications "did not appear to produce significant changes in performance", however, there has been no empirical evidence to reject or support this to date (Caplan & Shecter, 1995). In addition, the impact of "language" differences and nonstandard modifications raises concern for the interpretation of results required of the neuropsychologists, particularly if they are testing a player who was baselined by another examiner using non traditional techniques. According to Standard 11.23 in the 1999 Standards for Educational and Psychological Testing "If a test is mandated for persons.....users should identify individuals whose disabilities or linguistic background indicates the need for special accommodations in test administration and ensure that these accommodations are employed". A reasonable goal might be to identify various environmental modifications that would allow the player to perform at their optimal level and for the neuropsychologist to feel confident in his or her ability to interpret this data.

Participation of the Athletes: Acceptance and Behavioral Responses to Testing

The behavioral and emotional "impact" of performing tests on athletes both at baseline and during post concussive events has never been systematically explored. Anxiety levels for each player will likely differ at baseline and post-concussive evaluation times due to various factors. For example, baseline testing has little "direct" relevance on a player's career and therefore may be less stressful. Baselines conducted in a group setting may also increase anonymity and reduce overall anxiety. On the other hand, individuals who have had prior concussions could feel threatened at this initial examination. Post concussive cognitive results could have an impact on their future participation for that day, week or career and may also exacerbate anxiety. Regardless of the situation, the obtained scores ultimately affect the interpretation, and recognizing anxiety or behavioral distress at each time point should be considered. At baseline, players who have been exposed to testing in the past for ranking purposes (i.e. use of the Wonderlic in football players to determine team selection) are likely to have a more negative attitude than players who have never been "selected" into competition based on these scores. For example, psychological and intellectual testing has occurred in professional football since the early 1970s and results on individual players have been published in newspaper articles in the player's home town (Armstrong, 1997). Players at post concussion could be vulnerable to a host of fears (i.e. brain damage, ineligible to participate in practice for the next game), which may increase their anxiety and potentially increase or decrease their motivation. Some studies suggest that high anxiety can produce slowing of verbal responses and deficits in motor speed (Buckelew & Hannay, 1986; King, Hannay, Masek, & Burns, 1978). However, not all studies indicate that anxiety interferes with cognitive performance, and interactions are probably complicated by multiple individual and test factors. Although the testing situation is complex, for athletes it is likely that they are uncomfortable and competitive in a new situation, and fears of failure are common. Awareness of these issues and recommendations for reducing fear and discomfort may be useful.

Results from our Sports Testing Survey indicate at the initiation of the project none of the players were extremely reluctant, however, 22% were reluctant, 11% were hesitant, 59% were willing and 7% were fully accepting at the onset of the project. After participating in the program for some time, none of the players were extremely reluctant, 4% were reluctant, 7% hesitant, 78% willing, and 15% were seen as fully accepting. Perceptions regarding the players concern about mild head injury at the beginning of the project were gathered and 11% thought the players had no concern, 41% thought there was limited concern, 41% reported concern, and none reported extreme concern (7% said they didn't know). In contrast, the current perceptions of players reaction to head injury indicate that 4% appear to have no concern, 30% have limited concern, 59% report concern and 4% demonstrate extreme concern (4% don't know). In general, the shift demonstrates (from the neuropsychologists perspective) increased interest and concern by the players regarding "mild concussion".

We also asked the Test Survey respondents if they thought that a player's "concern" about the test results interfered with the evaluation process. Forty six percent of the neuropsychologists answered yes, 50% no, and 4% were not sure. Some of the respondents indicated that the players had concerns about how their results could effect contract negotiations or future trades to other teams. Others noted that players feel pressure to return to play and are hesitant to acknowledge post-concussive symptoms or problems. Finally, there was some evidence that players were worried about "brain damage" after several concussions, and that highly "publicized" athletes who had sustained concussions had increased anxiety in players from other teams. In the Sports Testing Survey, approximately 19% of the players were rated as showing no overt anxiety or distress at the time of testing. Mild overt discomfort was noted 35% of the time and moderate discomfort 12% of the time. None of the consultants felt that severe distress was observed during any evaluation. Twenty-seven percent of the respondents indicated that players were reporting discomfort that was not observable. One of the respondents indicated that the evaluation is discontinued if there is overt concern and anxiety about the test results. Neuropsychologists report a variety of strategies to reduce anxiety. Based on the survey, educational informative data was used to increase the comfort level of the player during post-concussive testing in 100% of the responses; 28% report use of research oriented information, 36% used sports-related topics, 60% used humor and 16% utilized another approach (i.e. talking with the player about themselves, hobbies, home life, etc.).

Overall, the results from the survey indicated increased acceptance in the testing program by the players over time. This suggests that once the players are familiar with the mechanics and use of tests, they may feel increased comfort with the neuropsychologist. The survey does suggest that anxiety is notable and it may be important to utilize specific efforts to decrease anxiety. It should be noted that the Sports Testing Survey results are based on responses from the participating neuropsychologists and may reflect their own increased comfort working in the parameters of the team. Continued studies involving the player's perspective are necessary to provide a clear understanding in this area. Level of anxiety was not seen as a component for half of the neuropsychologists, but in the other half mild anxiety and discomfort of the player was noted. It may, therefore, be important to take special efforts to reduce player anxiety in order to assure long term success of the project. The approach to minimize this discomfort by the consultant was reportedly educational and informative, however humor and use of sport-related topics also occurred frequently.

Effect of Player to Player Interactions and Celebrity Status

Potential "communication" between players regarding the specific tests could affect reliability and validity. For example, during baseline testing it may not be uncommon to have players talking about tests, and even challenge other player regarding their memory of specific items on a list. The media may also play into these issues indirectly by questioning the players about their experience. For example, in one team, two players who had recently been through post-concussive neuropsychological evaluations were observed talking about specific tests in a locally televised show. During follow-up, again, the potential for player interactions cannot be determined although the prescribed use of alternate test versions likely inhibit possible contamination.

Approximately half (56%) of the respondents in the Sports Testing Survey indicated that "suspected conversations" between the players did not appear to interfere with test reliability and validity. Another 26% indicate yes and 19% were not sure. Some respondents indicated that they specifically asked players not to talk about the tests, but it is unlikely that this occurred across all teams as a standard format. When asked if the celebrity status and public forum of the player affected the evaluation process, 44% of the neuropsychologists reported that it had no apparent effect. However, 37% reported it had a mild effect, 11% reported a moderate affect and 7% reported a significant effect. These results suggest that only about half of the neuropsychologists felt that the status and public interest of the player affected the evaluation process, and typically this effect was mild.

Overall, it does not appear that player to player interaction and celebrity status of the players has a significant effect on the neuropsychological evaluation. The effect of "celebrity status" was felt to exist, but what "effect" was not clear. Continued evaluation of this area is recommended. Results from the survey would suggest that media contact and information that players release to the public should be approached with caution. Additionally, the neuropsychologist should make some attempts to assure that any reference to neuropsychological procedures and/or results in any media format are reported with accuracy and within the bounds of ethical parameters.

The Impact of Neurobehavioral Symptoms on Testing

The decision to return to play after a concussion is largely driven by the athlete's symptom presentation. Athletes' awareness of their symptoms and their willingness to report them are critical aspects of the clinical decision-making process. Since athletes regularly play with symptoms, they may feel ready to return to play after a concussion, even while symptomatic. Neuropsychological screening during this time period, especially when comparisons are made to the athlete's own baseline, provides a sensitive means to measure the acute effects of concussion for both research and clinical purposes. However, it must be recognized that there are factors, other than direct concussion effects, that could influence test performance, and must be considered when interpreting test results. A primary concern is potential direct negative effect of symptoms on test performance, e.g. the disruptive effect of pain. Headache, dizziness, and nausea are common symptoms after a sport concussion (Barth et al., 1989; Maddocks, Dicker, & Saling, 1995). Anxiety about the injury and the evaluation must also be considered in the neuropsychological interpretation. Research on the effect of symptoms such as pain, headache, and emotional distress on neuropsychological testing have primarily focused on chronic conditions and have yielded mixed results. The effects of acute symptoms following sports concussion in relation to cognitive function have not been adequately studied and remain controversial. This is an important line of research that may be addressed by simultaneously collecting data on injury variables, symptom ratings and test scores.

Sports Testing Survey respondents were asked what percent of the time they felt the players were reporting all of their post-concussive symptoms (i.e. headache, dizziness, nausea, etc.). Interestingly, 4% report never, 12% report players report symptoms one fourth of the time, 12% report symptoms half of the time, 64% report symptoms three fourths of the time, and 8% always report their symptoms. They were also asked what percent of the time they felt that symptoms interfere with testing and 21% reported never, 67% reported symptoms appear to interfere about one fourth of the time, and 13% report symptoms interfere half of the time. None of the respondents felt that symptoms interfered all of the time. One respondent indicated that they do not test until the athlete is asymptotic.

In summary, it is important for the neuropsychologist to obtain accurate symptom reporting following a player's concussion. In order to do this, it may be necessary to educate the athlete about the need for this information and to address any concerns about the use or misuse of this data. Next, it is important for the neuropsychologist to determine the significance of symptoms and to determine if they are interfering with obtaining reliable test results. The responding neuropsychologists reported that symptoms appeared to interfere with test performance about a fourth of the time. The survey did not differentiate which symptoms seemed to be most problematic. This will be an important issue for future research. At this point, it is common practice for neuropsychologists to evaluate individuals who are symptomatic. When symptoms appear to interfere with some of the testing, information should be incorporated into the interpretation, and limitations of the data acknowledged. Asking athletes to immediately identify any symptoms that they perceive as interfering with their test performance may help to better differentiate the effects of their symptoms. The relationship between acute symptoms and cognitive functioning following concussion is not clear, however it is common practice for neuropsychologist to evaluate individuals who are symptomatic. There is, however, disagreement on this point and in fact, it has been suggested that the neuropsychological screen be delayed until the athlete is asymptomatic. Further research will be needed to make a determination of this association and to provide guidelines.

Use of the Data

The data generated by the neuropsychological evaluation can be used in multiple ways (i.e. research and clinical) and potentially disseminated to multiple sources (i.e. player, team doctor, trainer, media). Heil (Heil, 1993) notes that athletes have the right to know the results of psychological testing and to whom the information will be provided. It has been suggested that psychologists working with athletes should preface the feedback with an explanation of the limitations inherent in testing, be concise, emphasizing a few key points, provide clear feedback, avoid the use of psychological jargon, balance positive and negative aspects of feedback, place feedback in a situational context and provide an opportunity for the athlete to ask questions (Nideffer, 1981).

Results from Sports Testing Survey indicate that the results of the post-concussive evaluation are primarily given to the team doctor (77%), however, 50% of the neuropsychologists said they give feedback directly to the trainer. None of the respondents reported giving this information to the coach or any other team staff member. This suggests that this information, whether it is research or clinically based, is going primarily to the team's physician and trainer. Efforts should be focused on educating these professionals about the uses and limitations of neuropsychological testing. Additionally, obtaining proper releases and assuring confidentiality are essential to protect the player and guarantee ethical handling of this data. Survey results further indicate that feedback to the player always occurred in 42% of the evaluations, 51% report giving feedback some of the time and 4% never gave feedback. One respondent indicated that feedback was fairly informal and occurred at the end of the session. Other neuropsychologists may give feedback over the phone, or arrange for test results to go through the team physician. Respondents also indicated that the team's medical staff requested feedback, and that more than half of the teams (56%) requested feedback immediately. The rest require feedback between 4 and 24 hours post testing. When questioned about frequency of writing a clinical report or a letter regarding post-concussive testing, 44% reported they always write either a report or letter, 16% write a report some of the time and 36% never write a report or letter.

In addition to test results, the neuropsychologist may contribute information used in "return to play" decisions. In fact, 28% of the survey respondents indicate that they always make return to play recommendations and another 21% make recommendations some of the time. Finally, 48% of the respondents indicated they never make return to play recommendations. This finding suggests that more than half of the neuropsychologists are providing information or advise on return to play. With regards to other medical work-ups

8% indicate they always provide recommendations, 84% report providing recommendations some of the time, and 8% never provide recommendations. One respondent indicated that since they work with a neurologist they don't have to make any other recommendations.

In summary, survey results suggest that in professional sports, results of post-concussive evaluations are being distributed primarily to the team physician 77% of the time. Additionally, 50% of the time feedback goes to the trainer. As indicated earlier, this places the trainer in a pivotal role and they should be informed on limitations of test data. Survey results further indicate that consultants are being asked to make extremely rapid interpretations of the test data as well as return to play recommendations. This suggests that an experienced neuropsychologist who can adapt to changing roles and time pressures will be necessary in the sports arena. Feedback directly to the player appears to occur in most cases and continued guidelines and recommendations might be useful.

Conclusion

This chapter has identified and explored issues a consulting neuropsychologist might encounter in working with professional athletes. As with the introduction of any new method into long established organizations, there are challenges, novel adaptations and practical issues that need to be addressed to assure success. Athletic organizations are likely to be unfamiliar with neuropsychological procedures and will probably be wary of the protocols at baseline and follow-up. Education of the key personnel (i.e. trainer and team doctor) is highly recommended to alleviate major problems. Quality working relationships with these key individuals appear essential in the overall mechanics of these projects. As the organization becomes familiar with the use of neuropsychological information and the consultant, there is likely to be increased acceptance. Trainers appear to have the most contact at the initiation of protocols and education as well as trainer endorsement will be critical to the success of baseline and post concussive testing with athletes. For the neuropsychologist, consistency in test administration at baseline and during follow-ups is challenging and necessary. Given the cultural diversity in the athletic organizations, it may be necessary to modify and apply nonstandard procedures in a consistent matter. Attention to special circumstances is recommended. For example, non-optimal and unfamiliar test conditions for the neuropsychologist, language differences, limited time frames, pressure to provide data and varying levels of acceptance across players should be anticipated and addressed. The public arena of professional sports also creates new demands on the neuropsychologist and media attention heightens the need for sensitivity and confidentiality. A neuropsychologist that is flexible, appreciative of the players perspective, works well within a team, and is prepared for careful handling of sensitive issues will likely thrive in the sports world. In spite of challenges, the launching of two large-scale professional head injury studies providing pre and post information on concussion will provide valuable data not only for sports but also for the general population.

References

Armstrong, J. (1997, April 13). NFL Mind games. *The Denver Post*, pp. 10C.

Artiola, I., Fortuny, L., & Mullaney, H. (1998). Assessing patients whose language you do not know: Can the absurd be ethical? *Clinical Neuropsychologist, 12*(1), 113–126.

Barth, J.T., Alves, W.M., Ryan, T.V., Macciocchi, S.N., Rimel, R.W., Jane, J.A. et al. (1989). Mild head injury in sports: Neuropsychological sequelae and recovery of function. In H. Levin, H. Eisenberg & A. Benton (Eds.), *Mild Head Injury* (pp. 257–276). New York: Oxford University Press.

Bartolic, E.I. (1999). Neuropsychological evaluation and testing: Research at the high school level. In J. Bailes, M. Lovell & J. Maroon (Eds.), *Sports Related Concussion* (pp. 188–195). St. Louis: Quality Medical Publishers, Inc.

Biasca, N., Simmen, H.P., Bartolozzi, A.R., & Trentz, O. (1995). Review of typical ice hockey injuries. Survey of the North American NHL and Hockey Canada versus European leagues. *Unfallchirurg, 98*(5), 283–288.

Buckelew, S.P., & Hannay, H.J. (1986). Relationships among anxiety, defensiveness, sex, task difficulty, and performance on various neuropsychological tasks. *Perceptual and Motor Skills, 63*(2 Pt 2), 711–718.

Caplan, B., & Shechter, J. (1995). The role of nonstandard neuropsychological assessment in rehabilitation: History, rationale, and xxamples. In L.A. Cushman & M.J. Schere (Eds.), *Psychological Assessment in Medical Rehabilitation* (pp. 359–391). Washington, DC: American Psychological Association.

Delaney, J.S., & Drummond, R. (1999). Has the time come for protective headgear for soccer? *Clinical Journal of Sport Medicine, 9*(3), 121–123.

Harris, J.G. (Ed.). (2002). Ethical decision making with individuals of diverse ethnic, cultural and linguistic backgrounds. In S. Bush & M. Drexler (Eds.), *Ethical Issues in Clinical Neuropsychology* (pp. 223–241). Lisse, The Netherlands: Swets and Zeitlinger.

Heaton, R., & Heaton, S. (1981). *Testing the impaired patient*. New York: John Wiley & Sons.

Heil, J. (1993). *Psychology of Sport Injury*. Champaign, IL.

King, G.D., Hannay, H.J., Masek, B.J., & Burns, J.W. (1978). Effects of anxiety and sex on neuropsychological tests. *J Consult Clin Psychol, 46*(2), 375–376.

Levin, H., & Jordan, B. (1993). *Neuropsychological Assessment of Brain Injury*: CRC Press.

Levin, H.S., Eisenberg, H.M., & Benton, A.L. (1989). *Mild Head Injury*. New York: Oxford University Press.

Lezak, M.D. (1995). *Neuropsychological assessment* (3rd ed.). New York: Oxford Press.

Lovell, M.R., & Collins, M.W. (1998). Neuropsychological assessment of the college football player. *Journal of Head Trauma Rehabilitation, 13*(2), 9–26.

Maddocks, D.L., Dicker, G.D., & Saling, M.M. (1995). The assessment of orientation following concussion in athletes. *Clinical Journal of Sport Medicine, 5*(1), 32–35.

Nideffer, R.M. (1981). *The Ethics and Practice of Applied Sport Psychology*. Ithaca, NY.

Chapter 20

COMPUTERIZED ASSESSMENT OF SPORTS-RELATED BRAIN INJURY

Kenneth Podell
Henry Ford Health System

Introduction

Sports-related concussion has become an increasingly prevalent clinical problem over the past few years. It has finally been recognized as a legitimate and serious medical condition that requires appropriate and full medical attention. The injury of a number of recent high profile professional athletes whom have suffered concussions has heightened awareness among both health care professionals and the public alike and has made it one of the most important clinical issues in sports medicine. Although increasingly common, concussions, by nature, are elusive and difficult to detect. Unfortunately, there is no current single litmus test that accurately and reliably detects the presence of a concussion. More often than not, concussed patients can have normal neurological examinations and negative neuroimaging results, yet may have the lingering aftereffects of the injury.

Since the detection of sports-related concussions is so difficult, it follows that determining when an athlete can return to play (e.g., when they have recovered from the concussion) is equally as perplexing and difficult to determine. The goal of the treating professional should be to avoid returning the athlete to the playing field before he/she has recovered fully. Prior to sports-related concussion becoming a high profile issue, players often returned to play before fully recovering from their injury. This was apparently particularly prominent at the professional level. While it can be argued that the professional athlete should be free to assume risks of participating in his/her sport, with younger athletes, the goal has always been to provide conservative treatment that limits the cumulative effects of multiple concussions (Cremona-Meteyard & Geffen, 1994; Cantu, 1992), and reduces the possibility of second impact syndrome (Cantu & Voy, 1995; McCrory, 1998).

Given the concerns reviewed above, it follows then that one of the most challenging components of sports-related concussion is developing sensitive and reliable tests that detect the presence of concussion (Collins & Hawn, 2002; Lovell & Collins, 1998). This will not only promote the better detection of the injury, but also help make more appropriate return-to-play decisions. This is where Neuropsychology, as a field, has made one of its greatest contributions. In fact, it appears that sports neuropsychology is emerging as a new sub-specialty within the field of neuropsychology.

Neuropsychologists have traditionally specialized in detecting cognitive and behavioral changes associated with central nervous system dysfunction. One of the most sensitive ways of detecting the presence of sports-related concussion, is through the measurement of subtle cognitive changes from baseline after a suspected concussion (Lovell, 2001, Maroon et al., 2000). This includes the evaluation of attention/concentration, reaction time, memory and speed of information processing. The newfound importance of neuropsychology in athletics has recently been highlighted by a consensus body of The First International Symposium on Concussion in Sport (2001). This panel was sponsored by the International Olympic Committee, the Federation Internationale de Football Association (FIFA) Medical Assessment and Research Centre and the International Ice Hockey Federation, and recently published their recommendations in three concurrent journal publications. The following statement indicates the central importance of neuropsychological assessment;"...neuropsychological testing is one of the cornerstones of concussion evaluation and contributes significantly to both the understanding of the injury and management of the individual (p. 8)." (Aubry et al., 2002).

The utilization of traditional neuropsychological assessment strategies is discussed elsewhere within this text. In summary, traditional "paper and pencil" assessment has proven to be very useful, but has practical and logistical limitations. First, the time and labor-intensive nature of these neuropsychological procedures has limited their adoption by non-professional athletic organizations. Second, the issue of test reliability over time has been raised as a limiting factor (see Collie, Darby, & Maruff, 2001). Although generally sensitive to the effects of concussion, traditional neuropsychological tests have not bee able to detect subtle changes in reactions time or processing speed due to limitations and errors inherent in how the data are acquired (e.g. via a stop-watch).

These factors provide a strong rationale for using more objective and accurate measures for detecting the effects of sports-related concussion. In the absence of objective concussion management criteria, over 20 opinion based concussion management guidelines have been developed that focus on grading severity of sports-related concussions (see Collins & Hawn, 2002; Collins, Lovell, & McKeag, 1999). Many of these guidelines have recommended periods of abstinence from play based upon arbitrary standards developed by individuals or panels of experts. These guidelines were largely developed without objective criteria or evidence to substantiate their ratings and recommendations and may over or underestimate the recovery time needed for a given individual. Thus, several authors have recommended the use of psychometric measures to objectively quantify the presence of, and recovery from, concussions, and computerized assessment may hold the key to practical neuropsychological assessment in this sports-concussion population (Brukner, 1996; Collins, Grindel, Lovell, et al., 1999; Echemendia & Julian, 2001; Echemendia et al., 2001; Grindel, Lovell, & Collins, 2001; Hinton-Bayre et al., 1999 Lovell & Collins, 1998). It should be emphasized that, at the current time, the use of computerized neuropsychological assessment in sports is in its infancy and we have much to learn and develop.

Historical Background

Before reviewing the literature on computerized assessment in mild traumatic brain injury (mTBI) and sports-related concussion, it might be useful to explain and define a few terms and concepts that will be utilized. First, reaction time (RT) simply refers to how long it takes the subject to respond to a stimulus or give an answer. RTs are typically measured in milliseconds (msec.) and obviously, a slower reaction time (higher value) reflects a relative decline in performance. Simple reaction time (SRT) refers to a response to a sensory stimulus with minimal or no higher order cogniture processing. For example, the subject might be instructed to press a space bar when they see a letter or number on the computer screen. Therefore, SRT simply measures how fast a subject reacts to stimuli. Complex RT tasks require the subject to process information and make a decision before responding. For example, was the current number in the sequence of numbers shown earlier? Here, RT reflects speed of information processing. Another measure often used to assess speed of processing is "throughputs" (i.e., efficiency; see Daniel et al., 1999). This refers to the number of correct responses per unit of time. Thus, the higher the number the quicker the RT and the better the rate of information processing.

Traumatic brain injury

As mentioned previously, one of the main advantages of computerized assessment is the ability to accurately measure RT. Thus, some of the earlier studies of mTBI evaluated the changes in RT as a function of TBI severity. Prolonged RT is considered a hallmark finding in traumatic brain injury. Deficits in both simple and complex reaction time have been found consistently. The literature indicates that the RT's in patients with mTBI were slower, less accurate, less efficient, and more variable over time than for control subjects. (Gronwall & Sampson, 1974; Hugenholtz, Stuss, Stethem et al., 1988; Jakobsen,

Baadsgaard, Thomsen & Henriksen, 1987; Stuss et al., 1989; Stuss, Ely, & Hugenholtz, 1985; Van Zomeren & Brauwer, 1987; Van Zomeren, 1981). As pointed out by Bleiberg, Halpern, Reeves and Daniel (1998), the difference in reaction time between patients with traumatic brain injury and healthy controls was in the range of 30 to 110 msec. It has been hypothesized that the slowness in RT is related to decrements in stimulus encoding (such as in SRT) and response selection (complex RT) (Van Zomeren & Brauwer, 1987).

As described by Bleiberg et al., (1998), evaluating group means for RT alone may not adequately describe the RT deficits found in patients with TBI. It has been demonstrated that not only is mean RT slower in patients with TBI, but that they are more likely to show greater variability within and across time periods. For example, patients with TBI are more likely to show greater variability (e.g., greater standard deviation of scores) in their individual RTs than healthy controls (Segalowitz & Dywan, 1997; Stuss et al., 1989; Stuss, Pogue, Buckle, & Bondar, 1994; Van Zomeren & Brauwer, 1987). Similarly, patients with TBI may also demonstrate greater deficits in sustained attention (ability to maintain level of performance over time within a session) and across testing sessions (Bleiberg et al., 1997; Stuss et al., 1989).

The effects of prolonged RT in TBI patients can persist for several weeks and months (Hugenholtz et al., 1988; Jakobsen et al., 1987; MacFlynn, Montgomery, Fenton, & Rutherford, 1984; Bohnen, Jolles, Twijnstra, Mellink, & Wijnen, 1995). Van Zomeren (1981) indicated that SRT shows maximal recovery within the first year with significant TBI. However, this might not be the case with complex RT tasks, as suggested by the work of Bohnen et al. (1995), whose group of patients with mTBI demonstrated deficits, on average, 21 months post injury, and Van Zomeren (1981) who demonstrated continued recovery of complex RT two years after injury. Finally, the question of practice effect has been raised as possibly accounting for the improvement in complex RT measures in patients with TBI (see Gronwall, 1987). Van Zomeren (1981) showed that there is no significant practice effect on SRT in healthy control subjects tested on five consecutive days. Healthy control subjects, however, demonstrated a consistent practice effect on a more complex (force choice) RT task (although this practice effect was only demonstrated between the first and second test days, without appreciable improvement between the following test days). Practice effects on other complex RT computerized tasks were also found in a study by Daniel, et al. (1999).

Sports-related concussion

In general, the results from the few studies that have evaluated RT in sports-related concussions mirrors those found in TBI. The one caveat may be that presently there is no consistent body of research indicating the duration of prolonged (impaired) reaction time in sports-related concussions. Several studies have demonstrated prolonged and variable reaction time in acutely concussed athletes. For example Warden et al., (2001) demonstrated increased SRT one hour post-concussion, relative to baseline, in acutely concussed military cadets, and lasting at least four days after the concussion occurred. Interestingly, the authors also reported that performance on more complex RT and memory tasks did not show any decrements. Similarly, Makdissi et al. (2001) found prolonged and more variable SRT in Australian Rules Footballers, but did not find deficits on other complex cognitive tasks. In contrast, others have found impairment in computerized tasks of complex RT, speed of information processing, and memory (Bleiberg et al., 1997).

Utility of Computerized Assessment in Sports-related Concussion

There has been ample evidence to date showing that traditional paper-and-pencil tests are sensitive to the effects of sports-related concussion (Collins et al., 1999; Lovell & Collins, 1998; Echemendia & Julian, 2001). The question then becomes is there a true need for using computerized assessment for sports-related concussion evaluations? The answer, at least in the opinion of several researchers and clinicians in this area is an emphatic yes (Bleiberg et al., 1998; Erlanger et al., 2001; Maroon et al., 2000). Some of the advantages that computerized assessment offer over traditional paper-and-pencil tests is the ability to measure reaction time in milliseconds, cost effectiveness in administration, and the ability to perform group administrations. Speed and cost-effectiveness have become very real and practical issues, and the ability to rapidly assess large groups of athletes simultaneous has played an integral role in neuropsychology's newfound prominence in sports-related concussion evaluations. For example, the ability to assess a large number of subjects at once (e.g., group administration) has promoted the acceptance of baseline neuropsychological assessment in athletic departments where coaches require efficient use of time by the medical and athletic training staff. Similarly the cost-effectiveness of computerized assessment has made this type of assessment accessible and affordable to high schools,organizations, and clubs that do not have a large budget to pay for individual assessments.

It has been demonstrated that cognitive processes such as speed of information processing, simple and complex RT, working memory and new learning are vulnerable cognitive processes following concussions. Therefore, the challenge has been to develop appropriate computer software that will be able to measure all of these cognitive processes in a user-friendly environment. Other factors that must be considered in developing the paradigms used in the design of the computer programs include: 1) ease and efficiency of administration that enables non-neuropsychologists (e.g., the athletic trainer) to administer the program, 2) the utilization of an "user-friendly" interactive assessment environment, 3) the ability to generate multiple, equivalent forms of the same test or to randomly generate stimuli, 4) rapidly generate useful data, and 5) the potential to administer in multiple languages.

To date, four computer programs are being used to evaluate sports-related concussion: The Automated Neuropsychological Assessment Metrics (ANAM), Immediate Post-Concussion Assessment and Cognitive Tests (ImPACT©; ImPACT Applications, Corp.), The Concussion Resolution Index (CRI™, Headminder, Inc.), and CogSport (CogState Ltd.). ANAM and ImPACT© are Window-based programs, while the CRI™ and CogSport are internet-based. See table one for a summary of the programs' features.

ANAM

ANAM (Reeves, Throne, Winter, & Hegge, 1989) was initially designed as both a clinical and research tool that could be used when repeated measures were required. It consists of self-contained modules (see Table 20.2) that draw from a large pool of stimuli using pseudorandomization of stimuli. This allows for repeated administration. ANAM is flexible, allowing the user to "fine-tune" and reconfigure the number of modules used, as well as the number of trials for a particular module. Test instructions are incorporated through separate ASCII files, and thus can be written for different languages.

ANAM has been used in a variety of studies that have evaluated the cognitive effects of pharmacological agents (Bleiberg, Garmoe, Cederquist, et al., 1993), and more recently traumatic brain injury (Bleiberg et al., 1997) and sports related concussion (Bleiberg et al., 1998; Daniel et al.,1999). In fact, Bleiberg et al., (2000) has recommended a "concussion optimized" ANAM (Table 20.1) based upon the factor analysis of ANAM modules and a few traditional paper-and-pencil neuropsychological tests often used to assess concussion. The authors reported that their data indicated that ANAM modules assess such constructs as cognitive efficiency (i.e., speed of processing), working memory, and susceptibility to interference. They also indicated that this particular configuration of ANAM takes less than 10 minutes to administer.

Using ANAM, Bleiberg et al., (1997) demonstrated that mildly concussed patients show slowed RT along with greater variability within and between closely repeated testing sessions. However, when looking specifically at 14 sports-related concussions in military cadets only simple RT, and not the more complex modules from ANAM, was significantly impaired relative to baseline, even when an additional memory module was added (Warden et al., 2001). The authors suspect that practice effect for the more complex modules of ANAM (Daniel et al., 1999), but not for simple RT, may have accounted for this finding.

ANAM is more of a generic program that has found a wide range of applications. Research conducted to date shows that it is a reliable program with acceptable construct and content validity and clearly is sensitive to at least the acute effects of concussion. Directions can easily be programmed for different languages. However, since it was not specifically designed for use in sports-related concussion it does not facilitate the collection of demographic and concussion-event related information. In addition, it does not assess concussion symptomatology, does not generate a report, nor display

Table 20.1. Summary of Sports-Concussion Computerized Neuropsychological Testing Software.

Program	Platform	Cognitive Measures	Administration Time	Repeatable Forms	Detailed Data Report	Decision Making Method
ANAM	Windows/DOS	Simple & Complex RT, Processing Speed, & Spatial Processing	10 minutes[1]	Randomization of stimuli	No	Neuropsychologist using statistical formulas
CRI™	Internet based requiring Macromedia flash player	Simple & Complex RT, & Processing Speed,	20-25 minutes	Multiple Equivalent Forms	Yes	Statistical Modeling[2]
CogSport	Windows 95 or higher or Mac OS 8.6 or higher; requires internet access for data transmission	Simple & Complex RT, Problem Solving, Learning & Memory	15-18 minutes	Multiple Equivalent Forms/ Randomization	Yes	Neuropsychologist using statistical formulas
ImPACT©	Windows 95 or NT or higher; uses internet/ e-mail for data transmission	Simple & Complex RT, Processing Speed, Learning & Memory, & Impulse Control.	20 - 22 minutes	Multiple Equivalent Forms/ Randomization	Yes	Neuropsychologist using statistical formulas

[1]Adminsitration time depends upon the number of modules used.
[2]Report generated immediately.

Table 20.2. Subtests from The Automated Neuropsychological Assessment Metrics (ANAM)[1].

1. Simple Reaction Time. The subject presses a mouse button as fast as possible when a large symbol (asterisk-like) appears at varying time intervals on the computer screen.

2. Sternberg Memory. A subject must remember a string of six letters presented on the screen. After indicting that they memorized the string it disappears and letters appear individually and the subject must indicate if they were part of the string just memorized.

3. Math Processing. The subject must solve three-step, single digit math problems (addition or subtraction) and then decide, by pressing the left or right mouse button, if the solution was less than or greater than five.

4. Spatial Processing. The subject must determine if two bar graphs would be identical if presented in the same orientation. One is presented vertically; the other is rotated 90 degrees either clock-wise or counter clock-wise.

5. Matching To Sample. A 4 X 4 red-and-white block design is presented briefly. The subject must then choose one of two designs that match the previously presented design.

[1]Descriptions adapted from Bleiberg et al., 2000.

data acquired in earlier evaluations. Results are interpreted by a qualified neuropsychologist.

CRI™

The Concussion Resolution Index or CRI™ is a Web-based computerized program that can be administered on Internet ready computers (see Erlanger et al., 2001 for a more detailed description). It was designed to compare post-concussion results to previous baseline performance. The test consists of six subtests and takes from approximately 20 to 25 minutes to administer and can easily be administered by an athletic trainer (see Table 20.3). It is reported to measure cognitive skills susceptible to concussion such as memory, simple and complex reaction time, speed of information processing, and decision making. Alternate forms are used for multiple testing. It also queries about post-concussive symptoms and records pertinent demographic information, medical history, and details regarding the concussion being evaluated.

Erlanger et al. (2001) reports normative data consisting of 414 athletes (52% males) at the high school, college, and club levels with roughly equal number of subjects above and below 18 years of age (means and standard deviations for age are not provided). The authors also report moderate correlations (ranging from 0.46 to 0.70) between the various CRI index scores

Table 20.3. Subtests included in Concussion Resolution Index™ (Headminder, Inc.)[1]

Processing Speed Index
1. Animal Decoding – subject inputs the number keyed to animal pictures.
2. Symbol Scanning – complex visual scanning where the subject must determined if an identified set of symbols are embedded in a group of distractors.

Simple Reaction Time Index
1. Reaction time – athlete presses the space bar as quickly as possible in response to a visual cue.
2. Cued Reaction Time – the athlete presses the space bar as quickly as possible when the target shape appears immediately after a "cue" shape.
3. Error Index – total number of false positive and false negative responses made during the Reaction Time and Cued Reaction Time tests.

Complex Reaction Time Index
1. Visual Recognition 1 & 2 – when presented with a series of pictures, some of which repeat, the athlete presses the space bar when the picture repeats (reaction time is measured).
2. Error Index - total number of false positive and false negative responses made during these two tasks.

[1]Descriptions taken from Erlanger et al., 2001.

and standard paper-and pencil neuropsychological tests (e.g., Symbol Digit Modality Test, Grooved Pegboard, WAIS-III Symbol Search subtest, and Trail Making Test Part A).

Issues of test-retest reliability have been studied by the developers (HeadMinder Concussion Resolution Index Professional Manual, 2002).A two-week test-retest interval was performed and correlations of 0.79 and 0.90 for Processing Speed Index, 0.72 and 0.73 for the Simple Reaction Time Index, and 0.65 and 0.72 for the Complex Reaction Time Index were found for athletes under and over 18 years of age, respectively. For the high school population, using the same test-retest time interval, correlations were 0.79 for the Processing Speed Index, 0.72 for the Simple Reaction Time Index, and 0.65 for the Complex Reaction Time Index.

The CRI™ was designed to compare intra-individual differences between baseline (preferably preseason) and post-concussion assessments. Consistent with others, the CRI™ (Erlanger et al., 2001) used a reliable change index (RCI) to determine significant score change, which has been successfully used in other studies of cognitive deficits in sports-related concussions (Hinton-Bayre et al., 1999). The CRI™ also corrects for practice effects when using RCI (see Temkin, Heaton, Grant, & Dikmen, 1999). CRI™ uses a one-tailed test with alpha=.05 given that one is only interested in worsening of performance. This too is consistent with RCI use in neuropsychological testing. Borderline performance was set with an alpha from .06 to .15. Error scores, which typically have a skewed distribution, were analyzed by looking at cut-off values for error differences (more post-concussion errors than baseline errors) based upon the normative sample. Following the same criteria used in their RCI, cutoffs were based upon fewer than the 5th percentile (significant) and 15th percentile (borderline) of their normative sample.

Unique to the CRI™ is the use of a traffic light symbol in its computer-generated report of data comparisons. The CRI™ does not offer a clinical interpretation, but provides return to play recommendations based upon multiple regression formulas. A red light indicates significant decline (based upon RCI) in at least one of the indexes and/or at least three "neurophysiologic symptoms" (post-concussive symptoms) and indicates that the athlete may not have yet recovered from their concussion. A yellow light would imply no significant declines, but rather borderline performance on at least one of the indexes and/or 1-2 "neurophysiologic symptoms" and suggests the need to look at other variables or factors in making a return-to-play decision. A green light indicates non-significant changes on cognitive tests and no report of "neurophysiologic symptoms". Erlanger et al., (2001) aptly point out that self-report symptoms alone are enough to trigger a red or yellow light, even if cognitive functioning showed no change relative to baseline.

Erlanger et al. (2001) describes their initial "field-trial" and report data for 26 concussed athletes. Twenty-three of the 26 concussed athletes were classified as red (n=16) or yellow (n=7). The authors point out that 3 of these cases were classified based solely on their cognitive performance (i.e., no increase in self-report symptoms). They further report that at the time of the second post-concussion evaluation 12 athletes were categorized as either red (n=7) or yellow (n=5). The authors further describe details about the performance of the concussed athletes.

Erlanger et al. (2001) report that the Complex Reaction Index was the most sensitive CRI™ cognitive index with a mean effect size of z= -1.44. The Simple Reaction Time Index had a mean effect size of z= -1.39 and the Processing Speed Index had a mean effect size of z=0.06. They point out that there was substantial variability in the effect sizes (e.g., large range), which is not uncommon in a concussed population, as cognitive abilities oscillate during the acute recovery of concussion (Bleiberg et al., 1997; Echemendia et al., 2001).

The initial study performed with the CRI suggests that it has reasonable reliability and construct validity. It is designed specifically for use in sports-related concussion and collects pertinent data regarding demographics and concussion-event details. It is designed to store and compared multiple test sessions for the same individual and produces a detailed report. Its determination of red, yellow, or green light status is statistically based only.

Table 20.4. Description of Subtests used in CogSport (CogState, Ltd.)[1].

Psychomotor Functions - Simple reaction time.
Decision Making - Choice and complex reaction time.
Problem Solving – Divided attention, working memory and dynamic monitoring.
Learning and Memory – Matching, incidental matching, and associate learning

[1]Descriptions taken from CogSport website.

CogSport, Ltd

CogSport is a web-based computerized program specifically designed to assess cognitive changes associated with sports-related concussions. It takes 15-18 minutes to administer. It reportedly measures various cognitive domains through several tasks using a series of playing cards as the stimuli (see Table 20.4 for a description of the subtests used). It has been designed for serial administration (e.g., multiple forms/stimuli randomization) and stores data for future comparison. The program is free to download but data must be submitted with a data generated report returned. While not specifically stated, it appears that the submitted data is analyzed by a qualified neuropsychologist.

It takes into account practice effects in its comparison to baseline performance (method not specified, but it does describe using an "optimized baseline" for comparison to any post-concussion assessment). This may represent taking the best of two baselines, which has been advocated by some – see Hinton-Bayre, Geffen, & McFarland, 1997). In a recently published study, Makdissi et al. (2001) administered CogSport twice and Trail Making Test (TMT) and Digit Symbol Substitution Test (DSST) as baselines to 240 Australian Rules footballers. Six players were assessed 72 hours following a concussion and matched to seven controls. Results indicated no change in DSST and TMT, but increased variability in RT (mainly due to an increase in the number of slow responses) was found.

This initial pilot study indicated CogSport's sensitivity in detecting RT variability in concussed athletes. However, the study did not appear to utilize all of the test components reportedly assessed by CogSport. Thus, a more definitive study would be needed to assess the full utility of CogSport.

ImPACT©

ImPACT© is a freestanding Windows-based application that runs on individual computers or network systems. ImPACT© was designed specifically for use with athletes with minimal language dependence and can be administered in either Spanish or English, with other language versions currently being developed. It consists of five sections: demographics/history, concussion symptom inventory, computerized neuropsychological testing, current concussion details, and comments and takes approximately 20 minutes to administer. The demographics/history section records detailed information about an athlete's general history, educational background, including self-report of learning disability – which has been found to be a critical factor in sports-related concussions (Collins et al., 1999), and prior concussion history. The neuropsychological testing section consists of seven modules. The section on current concussion details is a screen that is completed by a health care practioner (usually the athletic trainer) and details facts about the on-field concussion (soon to be available with use of a PDA). The comments section is used to note any irregularities that might have occurred during the administration of ImPACT©. See Table 20.5 for a description of the neuropsychological tests used in ImPACT©.

Table 20.5. Subtests and Modules used in ImPACT©[1](ImPACT Applications, Corp.)
.

Symptoms – self-report rating on 22 concussive symptoms, via a 7-point Likert-type scale.

Module 1 (Word Discrimination) – This module evaluates attentional processes and verbal recognition memory utilizing a word discrimination paradigm.

Module 2 (Design Memory) – This module evaluates attentional processional design recognition utilizing a discrimination paradigm.

Module 3 (X's and O's) – This module measures spatial working memory, as well as a choice RT (the distractor task for the working memory component). A screen appears with randomly placed X's and O's with three of the stimuli randomly highlighted in yellow. This is immediately followed by a force choice RT task. After the distractor task the subject must recall the spatial location of the previously highlighted items.

Module 4 (Symbol Matching) – This module evaluates visual processing speed, learning and memory through visual paired associate learning and recall.

Module 5 (Color Click) – This module represents a choice reaction time task modeled after The Stroop Test.

Module 6 (Three letters) – This module assess verbal working memory and processing and is modeled after Brown-Peterson trigram working memory paradigm.

Module 7 (Delayed memory) – Using a force choice paradigm of a target and distractor word (different from immediate recall), the subject must identify the words and designs presented approximately 20 minutes earlier in modules 1 and 2.

---

[1]Descriptions adapted from Maroon et al, 2000.

The seven modules that comprise the neuropsychological testing section were designed to assess various aspects of cognition susceptible to the effects of concussion, which include verbal and non-verbal working memory, choice reaction time, speed of information processing, and susceptibility to interference. The variables from these modules are combined to make up memory, reaction time, and processing speed indexes. All subjects receive the same stimuli at baseline. For post-concussion assessments there are four additional sets of stimuli for the word and design memory tests. The stimuli for all other modules are randomly generated.

Initial studies evaluating the test-retest reliability indicate that ImPACT© is a stable measure with good consistency, even across multiple administrations (Lovell et al., 2001; Lovell et al., 2002). For example, in an initial study, ImPACT© was administered four times, 2 to 8 days apart, to 24 high school athletes. The memory index yielded test-retest correlation coefficients ranging from 0.66 to 0.85 between test sessions 1-2, 2-3, and 3-4. Test-retest correlation coefficients for the processing speed index across the same assessment comparisons ranged from 0.75 to 0.88. The reaction index had test-reliability correlation coefficients ranging from 0.62 to 0.66. While the reaction time index was highly consistent across all of the testing sessions, the memory and processing reactions tended to show some slight variability in that the correlation between time 1-2 was slightly weaker than between time 2-3 and time 3-4. It appears that performance on these indexes improved after the first testing session with little after that. This would be consistent with the literature on tests of higher order cognitive processes that have shown improvement on some of the more complex cognitive tasks used in sports-related cognitive assessments between the first two testing sessions only, with none after that. In fact, some authors use this evidence to advocate the use of two baselines in order to eliminate any practice effect when comparing post-concussions results to baseline scores (Hinton-Bayre et al., 1997; Hinton-Bayre et al., 1999; Makdissi et al., 2001).

Baseline data has been collected on over 10.000 high school and college students. Post-injury concussion performance has been measured in over 500 high school and college athletes and has demonstrated the ability to separate injured from 50 age-matched control subjects who suffer from grade 1 (mild) concussions (Lovell, 2001).

Based on initial findings, ImPACT© appears to be a promising program that has shown good test-retest reliability and high sensitivity in documenting the presence of concussion in athletes. It is a user-friendly battery and the generated report displays all of the subject's data (baseline and all post-concussion testing sessions). A detailed report with tables and graphs (and previous test scores) is generated. The data are easily collated and sent via e-mail or fax and are interpreted by a qualified neuropsychologist.

Recent research using ImPACT has shown its sensitivity in detecting sports-related concussion and differential recovery patterns in high school and collegiate athletes (Field, Collins, Lovell et al., 2003; Lovell, Collins,

Iverson et al., 2003) and the relationship between on-field markers of concussion and post-concussive symptoms and neuropsychological deficits (Collins, Iverson, Lovell et al., 2003; Collins, Field, Lovell et al., 2003).

Interpretation of Data

The computerized neuropsychological programs described above differ in how the test data is analyzed and interpreted. ImPACT©, CogSport, and CRI™ are based upon comparing baseline to post-concussion data. Both ImPACT© and CogSport utilize the expertise and experience of a qualified neuropsychologist to interpret the test data using statistical methods. CRI™ immediately produces a computerized report (the traffic light system) that is based solely upon statistical modeling, without the interpretation or recommendations of a neuropsychologist.

Whether the test data needs to be interpreted by a neuropsychologist is a matter for continued debate and beyond the scope of this chapter. It is clear, however, that concussion represents a complex medical disorder and neuropsychological assessment represents an important tool in making return to play decisions. In keeping with new international directives for return to play decisions (Aubry et al., 2002), neuropsychological test results should be interpreted within the context of the athlete's overall medical care. Neuropsychological testing should not be utilized in a vacuum to make return to play decisions.

Computerized versus Paper-and-Pencil Testing

There is much debate about the use of computerized versus paper-and-pencil testing in sports-related concussion. The initial studies evaluating the effects of sports-related concussion used traditional paper-and-pencil neuropsychological testing (Barth et al., 1983; Collins et al., 1998; Hinton-Bayre et al., 1997; Hinton-Bayre et al., 1999; Lovell & Collins, 1998; see Echemendia & Julian, 2001 for a review). However, more recent studies using computerized assessment are starting to show extremely good sensitivity and effects (such as RT) that are not possible with paper-and-pencil testing. While both methods of assessment play a role in evaluating concussed athletes, there are clear advantages and disadvantages to both.

Traditional neuropsychological assessment (i.e., paper-and-pencil assessment) is predicated on the fact that it is done one-on-one between the patient and neuropsychologist/psychometrist. This allows for detailed observation of the patient, tight control over the testing environment, and assurance of optimal patient effort. Traditional neuropsychological tests were never designed with group administration in mind. In sports-related concussion assessment, however, the reality of the situation demands evaluating a large number of athletes quickly and cost effectively; two things that are not possible with paper-and-pencil testing. The use of computerized assessment allows one to perform group assessment that does not require a specially qualified technician for administration. This clearly cuts down on the time and cost of administration; two critical factors to contend with when doing sports related assessments. For example, all of the computerized programs cited above, take less than 25 minutes to administer. They can all be administered in a school's computer lab, thus can assess several athletes at a time. For example, a team's athletic trainer can group administer the test twice within a 60-70 minute time frame. Therefore, the time it takes to baseline an entire team is a function of the number of computers available, which is a huge advantage when attempting to make neuropsychological assessments available to all athletic populations.

There are several other advantages to computerized assessment. Probably one of the most important advantages is the ability to accurately and reliable measure reaction time and processing speed. Standard computer technology allows for millisecond accuracy in recording reaction time.The importance of this advantage becomes clear with reliable differences between concussed and non-concussed subjects ranging around 100 msec (see Bleiberg et al., 1998). The use of a stopwatch by an individual clearly cannot obtain the same level of accuracy and reliability in reaction time measurement, and traditional reaction time devices are bulky and can be expensive.

Computer assessment allows for randomization of stimuli that typically is not found with paper-and-pencil testing. Alternate forms in paper-and-pencil testing does, however, help to minimize practice effects. Computer assessment also allows for very fast and reliable scoring and report generation. This allows for immediate feedback from the test findings, as well as reducing the cost of the assessment, as technician time is not required for scoring, and most human error in scoring is eliminated. Computerized assessment also allows for very rapid data gathering, compilation and storage, all of which improves efficiency, reduces errors, and is very cost-efficient. The fact that these tests can be supervised by the athletic trainer, means that the computerized tests can be administered when needed (e.g., on the road or in a locker room) without the constraint of having to schedule testing with a neuropsychologist or technician.

While there are several advantages to computerized assessment, it is not perfect and still has some drawbacks. When conducting group administrations, or having a non-neuropsychologist supervise the testing, it is difficult to be sure if a player was completely motivated and put forth his/her best effort. Athletes, when not being supervised in a one-on-one fashion, as they would be with formal paper-and pencil testing, will occasionally not try or do their best. The majority of the time that this happens is during baseline testing. This complicates one's ability to then assess any post-concussion effect in that particular athlete. Others have mentioned that cost is a factor that may limit the use of computerized assessments. However, computerized assessments are highly cost-effective, especially relative to the costs incurred with face-to-face, paper-and-pencil testing. Computers are becoming more and more common at all levels of athletic competition, thus making them much more readily available to an ever-growing number of athletes. This is particularly relevant at the high school level where finding the funds for a concussion safety program is difficult. Computerized assessment has allowed many high school programs to participate in sport-concussion safety programs, which they would not have been able to afford if they had to depend upon paper-and-pencil testing._

The computerized assessment techniques described within this chapter have been shown to play a very critical role in helping to make return-to-play decisions following a concussion. It is clear, however, that at this point in time, there continues to be a place for traditional neuropsychological testing in working with athletes. In fact, some authors have advocated combining computerized assessment programs with traditional paper-and-pencil testing (see Echemendia & Julian, 2001) for assessing sports-related concussions. Moreover, athletes that have a prolonged post-concussive disorder may require a more extensive neuropsychological evaluation using more lengthy and detailed procedures. Yet it is important to recognize that traditional paper-and-pencil neuropsychological testing can no longer be the sole method used to assess large group of athletes in a time and cost-effective manner.

Summary

Assessment of sports-related concussion is critical in the medical management and good health of athletes. Sports-related concussion assessment has thrust neuropsychology to the forefront of this area of health-care in that neuropsychological assessments are considered a corner stone in detecting the effects of concussions and an integral part of making return-to-play decisions (Aubry et al., 2001). Research over the past few decades has consistently demonstrated that variable and slowed reaction time is particularly sensitive to the effects of concussion. The advent of new computerized programs designed to assess reaction time, working memory, speed of information professing, and anterograde memory have demonstrated good sensitivity in detecting concussions and are being used to assist physicians and athletic trainers make better return-to-play decisions, while helping to ensure the health and safety of athletes.

References

Aubry, M., Cantu, R., Dvorak, J., Johnston, K., Kelly, J., & Lovell, M.R. et al. (the concussion in Sport (CIS) Group). (2002). Summary and agreement statement of the first International Conference on Concussion in Sport. *British Journal of Sports Medicine*, *36*, 6–10.

Barth, J.T., Macciocchi, S.N., Giordani, B., Rimel, R., Jane, J.A., & Boll, T.J. (1983). Neuropsychological sequelae of minor head injury. *Neurosurgery, 13*(5), 529–33.

Bleiberg, J., Garmoe, W., Cedaerquist, J., Reeves, D., & Lux, W. (1993). Effects of D-amphetamine on performance consistency following brain injury: A double-blind placebo crossover case study. *Neuropsychiatry, Neuropsychology and Behavioral Neurology, 6*, 245–248.

Bleiberg, J., Garmoe, W.S., Halpern, E.L., Reeves, D.L., & Nadler, J.D. (1997). Consistency of within-day and across-day performance after mild brain injury. *Neuropsychiatry, Neuropsychology, and Behavioral Neurology, 10*(4), 247–253.

Bleiberg, J., Halpern, E.L., Reeves, D., & Daniel, J. C. (1998). Future directions for the neuropsychological assessment of sports concussion. *Journal of Head Trauma Rehabilitation, 13*(2), 36–44.

Bleiberg, J., Kane, R.L., Reeves, D.L., Garmoe, W.S., & Halpern, E. (2000). Factor analysis of computerized and traditional tests used in mild traumatic brain injury research. *The Clinical Neuropsychologist, 14*(3), 287–294.

Bohnen, N.I., Jolles, J., Twijnstra, A., Mellink, R., & Wijnen, G. (1995). Late neurobehavioral symptoms after mild head injury. *Brain Injury*, 9, 27–33.

Brukner, P. (1996). Sports medicine: Concussion. *Australian Family Physician, 25*, 1445–1448.

Cantu, R.C. (1992). Second impact syndrome: Immediate management. *Physician Sportsmedicine, 23*, 27–34.

Cantu, R.C. & Voy, R. (1995). Second impact syndrome: A risk in any sport. *Psysician Sports Medicine, 23*, 27–36

Collie, A., Darby, D., & Maruff, P. (2001). Computerised cognitive assessment of athletes with sports related head injury. *British Journal of Sports Medicine, 35*, 297–302.

Collins, M.W., Grindel, S.H., Lovell, M.R., Dede, D., Moser, D, Phalin, B. et al. (1999). Relationship between concussion and neuropsychological performance in college football players. *Jama, 282*, 964–970.

Collins, M.W. & Hawn, K.L. (2002). The clinical management of sports concussion. Current *Sports Medicine Reports, 1*, 12–22.

Collins, M.W., Lovell, M.R., & McKeag, D.B. (1999). Current issues in managing sports-related concussion. *Journal of The American Medical Association, 282*, 2283–2285.

Collins, M.W., Field, M., Lovell, M.R., Iverson, G.L., Johnston, K.M., Maroon, J.C. et al. (2003). Relationship between postconcussion headache and neuropsychological test performance in high school athletes. *American Journal of Sports Medicine, 31*, 168–173.

Collins, M.W., Iverson, G.L., Lovell, M.R., McKeag, D.B., Norwig, J., Maroon, J.C. (2003). On-field predictors of neuropsychological and symptom deficit following sports-related concussion. *Clinical Journal of Sports Medicine, 13*, 222–229.

Cremona-Meteyard, S.L., & Geffen, G.M. (1994). Persistent visuospatial attention deficits following mild head injury in Australian rules football players. *Neuropsychologia*, *32*, 649–662.

Daniel, C., Olesniewicz, M.H., Reeves, D.L., Tam, D., Bleiberg, J., Thatcher, R. et al. (1999). Repeated measures of cognitive processing efficiency in adolescent athletes: Implications for monitoring recovery from concussion. *Neuropsychiatry, Neuropsychology, and Behavioral Neurology*, *12*, 167-169.

Echemendia, R.J. & Julian, L.J. (2001). Mild traumatic brain injury in sports: Neuropsychology's contribution to a developing field. *Neuropsychology Review, 11*, 69–88.

Echemendia, R.J., Putukian, M., Mackin, R.S., Julian, L., & Shoss, N. (2001). Neuropsychological test performance prior to and following sports-related mild traumatic brain injury. *Clinical Journal of Sports Medicine, 11*, 23–31.

Erlanger, D.M., Kutner, K.C., Barth, J.T., & Barnes, R. (1999). Neuropsychology of sports-related head injury: Dementia Pugilistica to post concussion syndrome. *The Clinical Neuropsychologist, 13*, 193–209.

Erlanger, D., Saliba, E., Barth, J. Almquist, J., Webright, W., & Freeman, J. (2001). Monitoring resolution of post-concussion symptoms in athletes: Preliminary results of a web-based neuropsychological test protocol. *Journal of Athletic Training, 36*, 280-287.

Field, M., Collins, M.W., Lovell, M.R. Maron, J.C. (2003). Does age play a role in recovery from sports-related concussion? A comparison of high school and collegiate athletes. *Journal of Pediatrics, 142*, 546–553.

Grindel, S.H., Lovell, M.R., & Collins, M.W. (2001). The assessment of sport-related concussion: The evidence behind neuropsychological testing and management. *Clinical Journal of Sport Medicine, 11*, 134–143.

Gronwall, D. & Sampson, H. (1974). *The psychological effects of concussion.* Auckland: Oxford University Press.

Gronwall, D. (1987). Advances in the assessment of attention and information processing after head injury. In H.S. Levin, J. Grafman, & H.M. Eisenberg (Eds.), *Neurobehavioral recovery from head injury* (pp. 355–371). New York: Exfpord University Press.

Hinton-Bayre, A.D., Geffen, G.M., Geffen, L.B., McFarland, K.A., & Friis, P. (1999). Concussion in contact sports: Reliable change indices of impairment and recovery. *Journal of Clinical and Experimental Neuropsychology, 21*, 70–86.

Hinton-Bayre, A.D., Geffen, G., & McFarland, K. (1997). Mild head injury and speed of information processing: A prospective study of professional rugby league players. *Journal of Clinical and Experimental Neuropsychology, 19*, 275–289.

Hugenholtz, H., Stuss, D.T., Stethem, L.L., Richard, M.T. (1988). How long does it take to recover from concussion? *Neurosurgery, 22*, 853–857.

Jakobsen, J., Baadsgaard, S.E., Thomsen, S., & Henriksen, P.B. (1987). Prediction of post-concussional sequelae by reaction time test. *Acta Neurol Scand, 75*, 341–345.

Lovell, M.R. (2001). *New developments in sports related concussion.* The First International Concussion Conference, Vienna, Austria.

Lovell, M.R., & Collins, M.W. (1998). Neuropsychological assessment of the college football player. *Journal of Head Trauma Rehabilitation, 13*, 9–26.

Lovell, M.R., Collins, M.W., Fu, F.H., Burke, C.J., Maroon, J.C. Podell, K. et al. (2001). Neuropsychological testing in Sports: Past, Present and Future. *British Journal of Sports Medicine, 35*, 367.

Lovell, M.R., Collins, M.W., Maroon, J.C., Cantu, R., Hawn, K.L., Burke, C.J. et al. (2002). Inaccuracy of symptoms reporting following concussion in athletes. *Medicine and Science in Sports and Exercise*, 34, 1680.

Lovell, M.R., Collins, M.W., Iverson, G.L., Field, M., Maroon, J.C., Cantu, R., Podell, K. et al. (2003). Recovery from mild concussion in high school athletes. *Journal of Neurosurgery, 98*(2), 296–301.

MacFlynn, G., Montgomery, E.A., Fenton, G.W., & Rutherford, W. (1984). Measurement of reaction time following minor head injury. *Journal of Neurology, Neurosurgery, and Psychiatry, 47*, 1326–1331.

Makdissi, M., Collie, A., Maruff, P., Darby, D.G., Bush, A., McCrory, P. et al. (2001). Computerised cognitive assessment of concussed Australian Rules footballers. *British Journal of Sports Medicine, 35*, 354–60.

Maroon, J.C., Lovell, M.R., Norwig, J., Podell, K., Powell, J.W., & Hartl, R. (2000). Cerebral concussion in athletes: Evaluation and neuropsychological testing. *Neurosurgery*, *47*, 659–672.

McCrory, P.R. (1998). Second impact syndrome. *Neurology*, *50*, 677–683.

Reeves, D.. Thorne, R., Winter, S., & Hegge, F. (1989). The United Tri-Service Cognitive Performance Assessment Battery (UTC-PAB). Report 89-1. San Diego, CA: US Naval Aerospace Medical Research Laboratory and Walter Reed Army Institute of Research.

Segalowitz, S.J., Dywan, J., Unsal, A. (1997). Attentional factors in response time variability after traumatic brain injury: An ERP study. *Journal of International Neuropsychological Society*, *3*, 95–107.

Stuss, D.T., Stethem, L.L., Hugenholtz, H., Picton, T., Pivik, J., & Richard, M.T. (1989). Reaction time after head injury: Fatigue, divided and focused attention and consistency of performance. *Journal of Neurology, Neurosurgery and Psychiatry*, *52*, 742–748.

Stuss, D.T., Ely, P., Hugenholtz, H.H., Richard, M.T., LaRochelle, S., Poirter, C.A. (1985). Subtle neuropsychological deficits in patients with good recovery after closed head injury. *Neurosurgery*, *17*, 41–47.

Stuss, D.T., Pogue, J., Buckle, L., Bondar. (1994). Charaterization of stability of performance in patients with traumatic brain injury: Variability and consistency on raction time test. *Neuropsychology*, *8*, 316–324.

Temkin, N.R., Heaton, R.K., Grant, I. & Dikmen, S. (1999). Detecting significant change in neuropsychological test performance: A comparison of four models. *Journal of the International Neuropsychological Society*, *5*, 357–369.

Van Zomeren, A.H. (1981). *Reaction time and attention after closed head injury.* Lisse: Swets & Zeitlinger.

Van Zomeren, A.H. & Brauwer, W.H. (1989). Head injury and concepts of attention. In H.S. Levin, J. Grafman, & H.M. Eisenberg (Eds.), *Neurobehavioral Recovery from Head Injury* (pp. 398–415). New York, NY: Oxford University Press.

Warden, D.L., Bleiberg, J., Cameron, K.L., Ecklund, J., Walter, J., Sparling, M.B. (2001). Persistent prolongation of simple reaction time in sports concussion. *Neurology*, *57*, 524-526.

Warden, D.L., Bleiberg, J., Cameron, K.L., Ecklund, J., Walter, J., Sparling, M.B., et al., (2001). Persistent prolongation of simple reaction time in sports concussion. *Neurology*, *57*, 524-526..

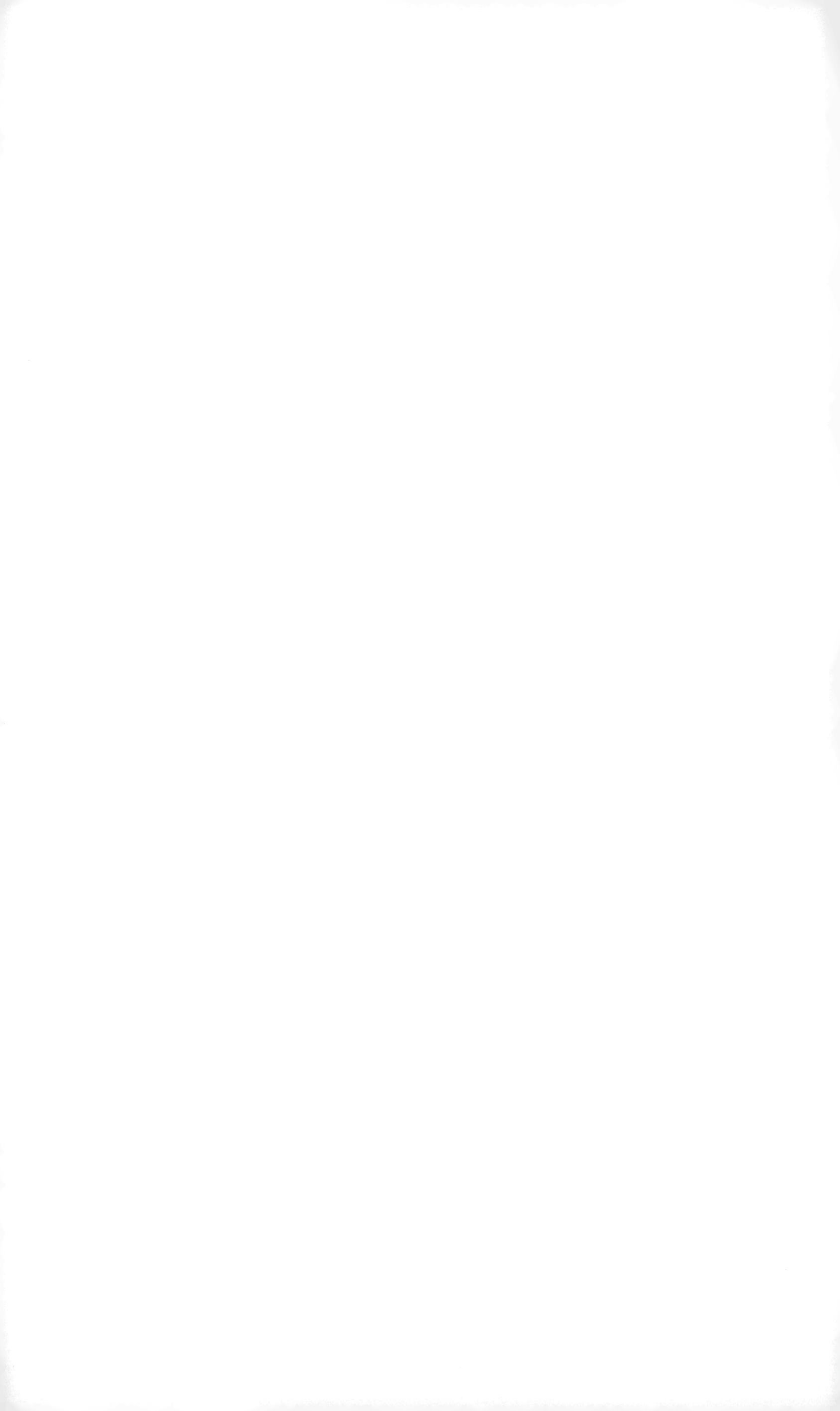

SECTION IV

SPECIAL TOPICS

EDITED BY

RUBEN J. ECHEMENDIA

Chapter 21

CONSULTATION WITH SPORTS ORGANIZATIONS

W. Gary Snow
Private Practice, Toronto

Kenneth C. Kutner
Weill Medical College of Cornell University
Consultant, New York Football Giants

Ronnie Barnes
Head Athletic Trainer
New York Football Giants

Introduction

Within the past 10 years, athletic associations and government organizations have begun to utilize neuropsychologists to assist in the return-to-play decision-making after a sports-related head injury has occurred. The large number of athletes at all levels of competition (from high school through professional teams) coupled with the frequency of concussions in sports will provide numerous future opportunities for neuropsychological consultation.

The clinical contributions which neuropsychologists have and will continue to make to the diagnosis and treatment of concussion in the individual athlete is a matter dealt with by other chapters in this volume. This chapter is intended to be more practically oriented and focuses on consulting with organizations, rather than with the individual athlete. The chapter raises a number of issues which the would-be consultant to such organizations should address, with some specific recommendations.

What Types of Sports Organizations Might Use Neuropsychological Services?

There are several types of sports-related organizations. First, at the youngest levels of competition, there are those organizations whose primary purpose is not sports, but where sports are nevertheless an important part of the organization's focus. High schools and colleges provide examples of this type of organization. Although success in sports is presumably not the primary goal of these academic institutions, their sports activities may nevertheless be governed in part by other organizations (such as school boards, athletic conferences, or national athletic associations) which also provide some opportunities for consultation. Second is the free-standing sports organization whose focus is exclusively on sports. Individual teams and leagues (both professional and nonprofessional) provide examples of this type.

In professional sports, there are also opportunities to consult to players' associations or unions. Although the mandate of such organizations primarily focuses on typical union-management issues, like many unions they may interpret the welfare of their members in the widest possible fashion, and may therefore be interested in ensuring that sports concussion programs both meet the health needs of the players and do not limit their rights to continue making a living in their chosen field.

Finally, neuropsychologists may consult to government bodies as well. For example, in Ontario, Canada, neuropsychological assessments of boxers who have been knocked out (or sustained a technical knockout) are mandatory before the boxer is allowed to box in the province again. In this program, the neuropsychologist is consulting, not to a sports organization (or even to an individual boxer), but to the Office of the Athletics Commissioner, which is part of the province's Ministry of Consumer and Commercial Relations.

Who is the Client?

Neuropsychologists are accustomed in health care settings to viewing the individual they are assessing as the client. In consulting to sports organizations, the player may be only one of several clients. The neuropsychologist needs to be clear as to whether the client includes the team, the league, the athletic conference, or some other body. Although the welfare of the player is paramount in such consultations, sports organizations may not always be mindful of the neuropsychologist's ethics and value system. Furthermore, even the player may subordinate personal welfare to other issues, such as the good of the team, the future of his/her career, and financial welfare.

In deciding who the various clients are in a given consulting role, the neuropsychologist may find it helpful to answer questions such as the following: Who wants my opinion? Who is paying for my opinion? Who will receive the results of my evaluation? What limitations are there in terms of release of information? How will my evaluation results be utilized? Is the ultimate decision about issues such as return-to-play mine, or does it belong to someone else (e.g., team physician, coach, government employee)?

Who Are the Other Potential Clients?

For a neuropsychologist to be effective in this type of consultation, it is important to identify all of the potential clients with whom one will, or may, interact.

If one is consulting to a team, the key personnel will include the coach or position coaches, the trainers, and the team physician. In many circumstances the neuropsychologist will have limited contact with the coaching staff. At the level of college and professional athletics, ultimate decisions about return-to-play will typically be made by the team physician in consultation with the trainer and others. Team trainers can play a unique and important role in any concussion monitoring program (please see section on Athletic Trainers).

At the collegiate and younger levels, parents will also be an important potential influence with respect to return-to-play issues. Some parents may respond to their children's injuries by overprotectiveness. Others may, for a variety of reasons, pressure their children to returning to play prematurely. The neuropsychologist, of course, needs to be aware of legal obligations with respect to the need to keep parents informed, but also cognizant of any legal restrictions which might keep him/her from discussing matters with parents. Neuropsychologists can also play an important role in educating parents about the effects of concussions, and can help parents to make reasonable decisions about the advisability of their child's returning to play.

When an athlete turns professional, there will be other potential clients. These will include personnel such as agents, the athlete's manager/trainer (in sports such as boxing, for example) and the player's spouse/partner. Each of these individuals may have different personal, or financial, concerns when the player suffers a concussion. It is necessary for the neuropsychologist to be aware of these issues.

In addition, it is probably helpful for the neuropsychologist to keep in mind how concussions may critically affect family members. Family members can be a key source of support for a player who is recovering from a concussion. However, family members may have their own emotional needs which arise from issues such as their concern about the player's current well-being, fears about reinjury when the athlete returns to competition, or difficulties in dealing with the emotional consequences of mild brain injury (such as irritability, depression, anxiety, or lack of self-confidence). Players who have persistent postconcussional symptoms may become withdrawn and be less interested in socializing, and family members need to understand these consequences, and learn how to communicate with the player and to seek additional help as needed.

One final constituent at the professional level is the team owner(s). As a person who is, or may be, paying for the neuropsychologist's services, the owner may feel entitled to receive confidential information about the players. It is of course imperative that the neuropsychologist clarify issues with respect to confidentiality with all team personnel prior to undertaking any concussion monitoring program (see chapter on ethics).

When one moves to the level of leagues, conferences, or players' associations, the neuropsychologist may deal less with individual issues, and may focus more on issues such as program development and evaluation. It is nevertheless crucial for the neuropsychologist in such cases to identify who the client is, and to understand her/his role clearly.

What Does the Neuropsychologist Need to Understand About the Sport to Which They Are Consulting?

Understand the player's "job"

Neuropsychologists typically understand the issues involved when a patient, for example, has sustained a mild brain injury in a motor vehicle accident. The risk, however, for an athlete for returning to training and competition is quite different than the risk incurred by a patient who sustained a mild brain injury in a motor vehicle accident for returning to normal activities of daily living. In addition, the risk levels for return to competition vary with the sport. For example, the risk of brain injury in boxing will be substantially higher than that in baseball.

We would also argue that it is important for the neuropsychologist to have a good general overview of what is required both in training and in actual competition. Just as a neuropsychologist who makes a decision about an individual's ability to return to work after brain injury needs to know something about the nature of the job the individual was performing, similarly the neuropsychologist who makes decisions about return-to-play needs to know what will be required of the athlete during training and during actual competition.

Understand the factors that will affect return-to-play decisions

Many of these issues are touched on elsewhere in this chapter and will not be reiterated here, other than to note that there will be a number of individuals on the team, and among the players' friends and family, who may place pressure on the individual with respect to return to competition. The neuropsychologist should have a thorough understanding of most well accepted return-to-play criteria and their scientific/medical bases.

There is also a silent constituency in sports at the collegiate and higher levels – the public. Alumni and fans can place varying degrees of pressure upon a player with respect to return to competition. Athletes in the more visible sports face unique psychosocial problems that do not characterize the typical individual with a concussion. For example, a trip to the store or restaurant may be interrupted by approaches from fans with concerns about the player's recovery (or ill-advised comments about the player's courage) – issues the average individual with a mild brain injury doesn't have to face.

What is the Service the Neuropsychologist Offers?

The neuropsychologist who wishes to consult to sports organizations needs to be clear about what services will be offered. Most neuropsychologists will think first in terms of assessment. Player monitoring programs fit easily within an assessment model which is familiar to most neuropsychologists.

Although such programs are conceptually easy for most neuropsychologists to design, there are, nevertheless, important decisions to be made with respect to test selection (the need for measures with alternate forms and small practice effects is key) and domains to be assessed. The neuropsychologist will also need to establish whether to assess only neuropsychological functioning, or to include measures of symptom reporting. A player monitoring program is probably significantly enhanced if the neuropsychologist can work with a physician who will monitor the player's medical status as well. Some more details of the practical issues in such programs are described below.

Although direct assessment is crucial in such programs (and provides an important vehicle for demonstrating the utility of neuropsychological consultation), there are other services the neuropsychologist can provide.

For example, any program which assesses players provides opportunities for research. From a clinical perspective, even the development of normative data may be useful both for the neuropsychologist and for the profession. As well, the development of a large data set (which is possible with some of the larger leagues or collegiate sports conferences) may permit the neuropsychologist to address issues which have clinical relevance beyond the sports organization. Within the next decade such programs will provide far more data about issues such as the recovery from concussion, the effects of multiple concussions, and the relationship between symptom recovery and neuropsychological recovery. Sports organizations may not be interested in the more esoteric theoretical research questions which interest our profession, but they will be interested in data which enable them to better predict successful return-to-play and to identify players who may be slower to recover and pose a risk for return-to-play.

In some cases, the role of the neuropsychologist may not be in the direct implementation of a program, nor even in assessing the players. The neuropsychologist might choose to consult to an organization which is designing such a program, while leaving the implementation to other individuals. For example, the neuropsychologist might advise a governmental body about the design of such a program, expecting that other neuropsychologists would then implement the program. In other cases, the neuropsychologist may consult to some other body (such as a player's association or union) about a program, providing advice about issues such as comprehensiveness, fairness, and general ethical matters.

It is crucial for the neuropsychologist to be clear about her/his role, and not to apply reflexively models (and expectations) from a health care setting when the expectations (and purposes) of the sports organization may be substantially different.

What Factors Need to be Considered in Concussion Monitoring Programs?

Baseline assessment is key

The neuropsychologist who designs a concussion monitoring program needs to begin by deciding whom and when to test. In clinical practice, it is rare to see individuals who have been tested prior to the onset of their illnesses. In sports consultation, the neuropsychologist may be able to (and, in our opinion should) test individuals before they have had a concussion. Given the subtle deficits which can characterize mild brain injury, baseline assessment can be crucial in determining whether an athlete has recovered from a concussion or not (see Chapter 16 in this volume).

Some sports organizations will only agree to have the neuropsychologist perform baseline examination on a subgroup of their athletes. The neuropsychologist needs to be clear in such cases about her/his mandate. The neuropsychologist should also be aware that, if a pilot program based on testing a subgroup of athletes is successful, this may allow the neuropsychologist to successfully argue for the necessity of testing all players.

Baseline assessments are best conducted as early as possible in training camp

Usually, it is best to complete baseline assessments prior to the season or on the first day that the team reports. It is important to schedule the assessments so that they do not interfere with the athlete's team meetings, weight lifting, practice or other critical appointments. The less a baseline assessment program conflicts with other aspects of training camp, the more likely it will be successful. This assessment is typically coordinated with the team trainer.

Testing should be done on site

It is important that exams be conducted not only at the team's convenience, but at the player's convenience as well. At both the collegiate and the professional level, athletes have a number of demands on their time, and it is important that the program be designed with the convenience of the player in mind.

Athletes may be able, either individually or as a group, to travel to the neuropsychologist's office, however, this will not work well in most cases. At the high school and collegiate level, athletes can usually be examined on school grounds. The neuropsychologist can usually easily obtain a classroom, nurse's office or other suitable space for performing the evaluations. While space is readily available at the collegiate level, it may not be convenient for the team. Generally, college teams would like to have their athletes examined in their training facility, which may not provide an ideal testing environment. Nevertheless, particularly for baseline assessments, finding space in the team's facilities will facilitate compliance with the program.

Testing of the player who has had a concussion may be performed at team facilities, but for reasons of confidentiality, and for player comfort, post-concussion assessments may be better performed in the neuropsychologist's office.

Use a concussion grading system designed specifically for sports

Multiple grading systems and recommendations for return-to-play for sports-related head injury have been established (American Academy of Neurology, 1997; Cantu, 1988; Kelly et al., 1991; Torg, 1982). The use of such grading systems may enable the neuropsychologist to determine whether there are, in fact, different outcomes associated with different grades of concussion. Furthermore, players (and family members) will learn about such systems, and may expect that the neuropsychologist be familiar with, and use such terminology.

Neuropsychological assessment should target abilities and symptoms

The neuropsychologist will typically not have time to assess issues of sports performance and mental health of athletes. Sports performance matters are probably best addressed by clinicians trained in sports medicine and sports psychology. Efforts to become involved in this area may reduplicate services already performed by other team consultants.

Test batteries should be short

Clearly, it would be ideal to obtain a comprehensive baseline examination. However, time and cost constraints will preclude the neuropsychologist from performing 5-8 hour baseline examinations on each athlete. In most cases teams will not allot more than 30 minutes per athlete. It is highly unlikely that teams will implement a program which is based on a comprehensive neuropsychological battery on all players. At the same time, the neuropsychologist obviously has an obligation to ensure that the amount of time allocated for assessment is sufficient to permit a reasonable assessment of abilities that will be useful for providing the types of advice required. Computerized assessments may be one answer to this quandary (see chapter on computer assessment).

Be clear about the information to be released and its format

Specifically, the neuropsychologist needs to determine if there will be a written report or not. Attention needs to be paid to the nature of the opinions that will be rendered in the report (will there be a recommendation regarding return-to-play, or merely a comment about recovery to baseline levels) and whether the report will be oral or written. (For the protection of both the neuropsychologist and the player we would recommend that the neuropsychologist provide some written report. The absence of a written report may lead to some subsequent needless controversy about what the neuropsychologist recommended, and written reports may protect both the player and the neuropsychologist). It is also important to have a clear understanding about who will have access to the neuropsychologist's report.

Consider the need for further testing

Some athletes after concussion will have symptoms which do not recover as quickly as one would predict given the typical recovery course following mild brain injury. In such cases, further testing may be warranted. In many cases the team neuropsychologist will feel comfortable in conducting such testing. However, if symptoms persist, the player may feel the need for a second opinion. The neuropsychologist should be prepared for this possibility, and for the possibility that another neuropsychologist may wish to obtain copies of raw data, both from baseline testing and from postconcussion assessments.

Arrange for a backup for the service

Concussion assessment programs typically require that the player be assessed soon after the concussion. The neuropsychologist needs to have a plan for ensuring that assessments are conducted even when she/he is out of town.

Know when to consult with a colleague

The ethical and professional issues involved in sports consultation can differ in a number of ways from those encountered in other aspects of clinical practice. It is particularly important that neuropsychologists who do not have expertise in sports-related head injuries know when to consult with those who do, and preferably to identify these individuals before problems arise.

What Other Services Might a Neuropsychologist Provide?

Education about the effects of concussions

Although neuropsychological assessment post concussion will probably play the central role in many sports consultation programs, neuropsychologists should not overlook the importance of other types of interventions. One of the key roles a neuropsychologist can play is in educating players, their families, and athletic personnel about the effects of concussions. For example, neuropsychologists can provide information to players and to teams which can normalize the experience of mild brain injury, and also provide information about the expected recovery time frame. Some research has indicated in other samples of individuals with mild brain injuries that education soon after the injury can reduce the number of symptoms the individual may report subsequently (Mittenberg et al., 1996). Although the effects of concussion are probably becoming more widely appreciated in athletic circles, players may nevertheless need reassurance that the sequelae of a concussion do not imply a psychiatric problem, as well as reassurance that their recovery (or the slowness thereof) is not the fault of some character deficiency on their part. Players need to know about the generally benign consequences of such injuries, but also need enough information to enable them to seek further assistance when recovery is prolonged.

Teams, parents, and players may also need information about the potential harm of returning a player to competition too soon. The neuropsychologist does not need to be an alarmist, but it is important to help everyone involved with a player to understand that the potential effects of waiting for symptom improvement outweigh any benefits of an impetuous decision to return to play. Some recent work has questioned the existence of Second Impact Syndrome (McCrory & Berkovic, 1998). Nevertheless, some athletes do face a risk of reinjury if they return to play too soon. In a sport such as boxing, there is a real risk of further brain injury each time the boxer steps into the ring. If the boxer is still recovering from a recent concussion, self defense in the ring will be diminished, which may increase the risk of reinjury. As well, the lingering effects of concussion may be misperceived as signs of poor motivation or lack of courage, and players need to understand the impact which a too-quick return-to-play may have, not just on their health and the way they are perceived, but also on their actual effectiveness at their sport.

Classroom intervention

Apart from the need for education about the effects of concussion, the neuropsychologist consulting to programs where there are student athletes may be able to provide some input into the effects of the concussion on the student athlete's academic program. Just as one wants to be careful about the physical effects of allowing the player to return to competition too quickly, one also wants to ensure that the student not return to full class participation too soon. Athletes may need help (particularly if they have preexisting learning disabilities) in understanding how the concussion affects their classroom performance. The neuropsychologist should be prepared to advise players and faculty about the effects of concussion on classroom performance, and the types of steps which may need to be taken (such as short term reduction in curricular load) to reduce the effects of concussion.

Treatment

Many neuropsychologists will limit their role to assessment of players with concussions. Some will feel that intervention is appropriate. Issues of conflict of interest aside, neuropsychologists should of course follow current scientific research and standards of practice in conceptualizing recommendations for cognitive or psychological treatment of sports-related head trauma. At this time, there is little scientific basis for using cognitive remediation to improve recovery from concussions. However, for some players, the psychological sequelae of concussion may include problems such as irritability, depression, or anxiety. Not all neuropsychologists will feel comfortable in treating such symptoms, but at a minimum the neuropsychologist should be able to identify those players who need such help and provide them with appropriate referrals.

What Does the Neuropsychologist Need to Know About Interacting with Athletes?

It is logical to assume that positive neuropsychologist-athlete interactions will increase the chance that the clinician will have an ongoing role with the team. This is especially true at the collegiate and professional levels. Understanding the athlete's perception of and reaction to the assessment process will increase the chance that they will have a positive experience with the neuropsychologist.

Make sure the player understands your role

It is often helpful to approach the athlete by correcting potential misperceptions and/or imparting useful information regarding the purpose of obtaining baseline and follow-up assessment. Athletes may perceive the assessment process as measuring their personality or intelligence. They may view the neuropsychologist as a "shrink" who is going to analyze them and divulge personal information to the coach and other team staff members. Athletes who have not experienced academic success may perceive these tests as being on a pass/fail basis. Collegiate and professional athletes may view the tests as being important to their status with the team. Therefore, it is important for the neuropsychologist to provide a clear explanation to individual athletes.

Be clear about confidentiality

Discussing confidentiality early will likely facilitate the assessment process. It is important for the neuropsychologist to be clear with everyone about who will get access to test results, and about how these will be communicated. It is particularly important that players understand this process.

Consider and reduce the effects of test anxiety

Athletes tend to be quite competitive and performance-oriented. They will often bring these characteristics to their approach to neuropsychological assessment. Although they have a good understanding of what characterizes excellent performance in their sport, they have little or no understanding of how they are doing on neurocognitive tasks. This factor results in anxiety for some athletes. Again, clear discussion of the testing format by the neuropsychologist will serve to reduce or eliminate this concern.

Understand how your recommendations affect the player
Interaction with the athlete who has sustained a concussion requires full understanding of her/his perceptions as well as of the potential ramifications of being removed from play due to a post concussion syndrome. One should keep in mind that athletes are accustomed to playing with injuries. Their competitive nature will likely push them to play despite ongoing concussion-related sequelae. Most athletes have continued to play with injuries in the past and will question why they cannot return to play when they are "physically capable." Starting athletes who are removed from the active roster will be concerned that they may be replaced by their back-ups. Many athletes worked hard to earn the starting role and will not easily give it up. Professional athletes may feel concerned if they are held from play due to a concussion since inability to play may affect incentive clauses in their contracts. Furthermore, a player who is in the last year of a contract may worry about the impact of injury on the negotiation process for, and eventual terms of, a new contract.

Return-to-Play Recommendations

The role of a consulting neuropsychologist in athletics is to provide accurate baseline assessment, meaningful post-concussion assessment and follow-up consultation. At a minimum, the clinician needs to be able to determine if the athlete has neurocognitive sequelae of the injury. In most cases, it is not the direct responsibility of the neuropsychologist to either clear an athlete or pull him/her from play. Rather, this responsibility typically falls in the hands of the team physician and/or athletic director (or, alternatively, a government employee). The neuropsychologist's role is to provide information about the athlete's condition, which will be used by the physician or trainer in their decision making.

Although it is often tempting for the neuropsychologist to want to address a number of safety and risk issues, for both political and professional reasons the neuropsychologist is wise to remain within his/her area of expertise. For example, the neuropsychologist might want to be judicious about making clinical decisions regarding an athlete's risk for developing second impact syndrome. At this time, neuropsychological test correlates of this condition have not been studied. In a similar vein, physical symptoms of nausea, dizziness, diplopia and headache are best addressed by the team physician.

At the same time, the neuropsychologist needs to be clear about what decisions he/she is making. There may be circumstances in which the neuropsychologist has primary input into return-to-play decisions. In other circumstances the neuropsychologist may not have the ultimate responsibility regarding return-to-play but may nevertheless have an implicit veto or input in such decisions.

Athletic Trainers

Athletic trainers probably have their most important role on the medical staff of collegiate and professional teams. The certified athletic trainer is the primary care health professional providing care on a daily basis to individuals in the athletic setting.

Athletic trainers graduate from degree programs specializing in athletic training, kinesiology, and sports medicine. Over 70 percent of all certified athletic trainers have earned advanced degrees including doctorates. Their academic preparation includes at minimum a baccalaureate degree that includes competencies in risk management and injury prevention, pathology of injuries and illness, assessment and evaluation, acute care of injury and illness, pharmacology, therapeutic modalities, therapeutic exercise, general medical conditions and disabilities, nutrition, health care administration, psychosocial intervention and referral, and professional development and responsibilities.

Athletic trainers work under the direction of a team physician and coordinate the daily routine medical care of the athletes they serve. In the absence of a physician, an athletic trainer is the first health care professional to evaluate the athlete's medical condition. Athletic trainers serve as triage agents to physician specialists and other health care professionals including neuropsychologists.

Because of the important role which the athletic trainer plays in the athlete's health, the importance of an effective ongoing liaison with the trainer is paramount.

The Team Physician

The team physician will, like the athletic trainer, be a person with whom the neuropsychologist will want to develop a good working relationship. The team physician often makes the final decision about whether the athlete has recovered sufficiently to return to competition. Despite the contributions which neuropsychology has made to the understanding of the effects of mild brain injury, many team physicians are skeptical concerning the need for neuropsychological assessment. Without a good relationship, the recommendations of the neuropsychologist may be disregarded, and the success of a concussion monitoring program may be jeopardized. The neuropsychologist should be prepared to educate the team physician about the role which neuropsychological evaluation can play, and to demonstrate how such assessment may make the physician's role easier (for example, by quantifying cognitive loss and documenting cognitive recovery). The neuropsychologist needs to appreciate the pressures and responsibilities of the physician's role. It is important to develop clear expectations about the role of each professional. A clear process about how to communicate findings to the player and coach, and how to keep each other informed, will also facilitate the success of such programs.

The Media

Be prepared to deal with the media

Neuropsychologists have recently been featured in the media during coverage of post concussion syndrome in athletes. The media provides an excellent format to inform the general public about sports-related head injury as well as to feature the field of clinical neuropsychology. It is likely that neuropsychologists who consult at the collegiate and professional level will eventually be interviewed by the media. It is better to be prepared for this possibility before the press calls.

The neuropsychologist who speaks to the press needs to be clear about the reason for doing so

Professionals are no different than anyone else and can enjoy seeing their names in the papers or their pictures on television. Neuropsychologists will often welcome the opportunity to educate the public and can see the media as a useful vehicle for such education. However, in every contact with press, the neuropsychologist should be clear about whether speaking to the media is necessary or desirable.

Player confidentiality is paramount

When dealing with the media about a specific player, the neuropsychologist needs to be careful. The agenda of the press may be quite different from that of the neuropsychologist. The neuropsychologist may be interested in talking about the general effects of concussion, while the reporter is interested in a story about whether a particular star athlete is going to have to retire. Even if the player explicitly consents to the release of information to the media, the neuropsychologist may want to reflect about (and counsel the player about) the wisdom of such disclosure.

Be clear about the reporter's role

The reporter is after a story. Your agenda may not matter to them. The reporter may even have a particular slant they are trying to develop (such as player concern about injury management, incompetence of medical staff, etc.)

Know the media policy of the organization you consult to

Many of the larger sports organizations have a designated public relations or media expert. The neuropsychologist should route all media requests through this individual before agreeing to being interviewed or responding to questions regarding athletes from the specific organization.

Consider how your comments will affect the player and the team

Good rapport helps us obtain the best possible results from the people we assess. Players read the papers and watch television and even if they don't, their friends and family do. The neuropsychologist needs also to be aware of the possibility of being misquoted, or quoted out of context. It's easier to say "no comment" than it is to correct a misquote.

Legal Issues

Be aware of your professional and financial liability

The neuropsychologist will, in most cases, be a consultant to the organization and not an employee. It will therefore be important to carry liability insurance and to regularly review the amount of coverage one has. There is always a risk, no matter how slight, that a player may be reinjured soon after a neuropsychologist has indicated that they are ready to return to play. At younger levels, one may have to contend with second-guessing by the player's parents, and there is always a risk of lawsuits (or complaints to governing bodies) in such cases.

Understand the financial impact of your decisions

At the professional level, there can be substantial amounts of money riding on the neuropsychologist's decision. Teams may not sell as many tickets if a key player is injured; a player may lose negotiating room in contract talks if the neuropsychologist recommends against a return to play. Indeed, in some sports (such as boxing) the athlete won't be paid at all if they can't compete. The neuropsychologist needs to realize that keeping the player out of competition may cost someone money, and potentially large sums of money. The neuropsychologist should not let matters of financial impact affect return-to-play decisions.

Be aware of the possible future ways your data may be used

It is important to realize that athletes are no different than any other client the neuropsychologist sees. Data obtained on a player during a baseline (or post-concussion) assessment may at some future point be deemed relevant to some matter the neuropsychologist did not even consider at the time the athlete was originally tested. Such issues might include matters such as custody and access (Is the athlete allegedly too impaired to be a good parent?), criminal charges (Did the player commit a crime because of diminished capacity caused by brain injury?), or even personal injury (Did the team expose the player to an unacceptable level of risk because of its management of brain injuries?). Such events may seem improbable but the neuropsychologist is well advised to consider these possibilities.

Develop a policy about how to handle data when players retire
Many jurisdictions will have regulations governing the retention of records and whether or when they can be destroyed. Sports concussion programs will, in the ordinary course of events, obtain data on a number of individuals who never suffer a concussion. The neuropsychologist will need to develop a policy about what happens to such data when the player retires. Although there might be some benefit in maintaining the data for possible clinical use in the future, there may also be arguments for protecting player confidentiality through a process of making the data anonymous after the player's career is over.

Remuneration

Get paid for what you do
Some neuropsychologists have provided consulting services to sports organizations pro bono. This has generally been the case for two reasons. First, a good deal of assessment has been done for research rather than clinical purposes. Second, many organizations do not have the budget to cover the cost of assessments.

It is likely that billing of services will become more common as neuropsychologists become more involved with sports organizations. The authors are not aware of any neuropsychologist who is employed full time by a sports organization. Consultants who bill for services do so on a per diem or per assessment basis. Some may provide their services as part of their duties within a larger organization (such as a university or hospital).

It is, of course, necessary to keep in mind that to get paid for a service, one needs to convince someone that the service is valuable. It is likely that some of the psychologists who have been providing services on a pro bono basis have done so with the expectation that such services will one day be reimbursed. Indeed, we would argue that it is important that neuropsychologists develop the expectation that such services should be paid for, since they are both valuable for protecting athletes, and involve professional risk and responsibility. Thus, any neuropsychologist who provides advice to a player or a team about issues such as return-to-play is making a clinical decision that can, under the worst of circumstances, have devastating consequences for a player. In the event that the neuropsychologist makes a decision that a player is capable of returning to competition, and an accident happens, there is some risk that the neuropsychologist could be sued for giving bad advice. Under such circumstances, it is unlikely that the fact that the service was provided pro bono will enter into the decisions made with respect to liability, and the neuropsychologist who practices in this area needs to keep such issues in mind. Even in the case where the neuropsychologist recommends against a return to play, and the team does not heed his/her advice, if there is a subsequent injury to the player, questions of liability may still arise. There may be some who feel that the enhancement of their reputation through association with a given team or league is payment enough, and there may indeed be some who would pay for the privilege of such an association. We do not recommend this as a routine course of action for neuropsychologists.

In setting fees for such services, the neuropsychologist needs to keep in mind that the value she/he ascribes to neuropsychological services may not be the same value that the client ascribes. The neuropsychologist should therefore have a clear understanding of the minimum amount of money that is necessary for funding the program, and for paying the neuropsychologist for her/his time. Baseline testing programs (even for 30-minute batteries) are not inexpensive when one considers the cost of technician services and the cost of test materials or computer programs. Even if the neuropsychologist does the testing themselves, it is important to realize that there are other services that might reimburse them more for their time, and that they are therefore sacrificing some income if they agree to do services for free or cheaply.

Be clear about who pays for what

In a concussion monitoring program, both baseline and post concussion assessments may be paid for by the same organization. In some cases, the baseline assessment may be paid for by the organization (such as the league), but the post concussion assessment may be paid for by someone else (such as the parent, player, or team). Services for follow-up assessment may be covered by the school or its insurance. At the collegiate level, services for baseline assessment are typically billed to the sports organization. Follow-up assessment services may be covered by the team's health insurance or the team itself. At the professional level, services are usually billed directly to the team. It is recommended that consultants carefully conceptualize and discuss billing of services during the initial presentation or soon thereafter.

How do I Begin?

There are two ways to become a consulting neuropsychologist for a team or league. First, one can be recruited by the sports organization. Second, the neuropsychologist can initiate contact with an organization in an effort to become one of their consultants. Contact can be initiated directly with a member of the organization or one of their consultants, such as the team physician. In either case, it is quite beneficial to prepare a plan or format for the initial meeting. This will assist the neuropsychologist in providing an organized, salient, and informative initial presentation. Appendix A provides a partial list of sports organizations, which may provide background information that can be used in preparation of the initial presentation.

It is suggested that one consider four issues in development of the initial presentation. First, impart information about why neuropsychological services are needed for their team. Be clear about how this will benefit the league and the player. Second, discuss your suggested plan for keeping an athlete out of play and return-to-play decision making. Third, discuss remuneration issues and be clear about whether services will be billed or provided pro bono. Finally, discuss logistics of completing baseline as well as post-concussion assessments.

Summary

Opportunities for neuropsychological consultation to sports organizations will only increase in the future. Such consultation will allow neuropsychologists to demonstrate their expertise, and the benefit of their skills, in an area which is not characterized by the turmoil within the current health care system. On a personal level, sports neuropsychology permits one to interact with healthy, normal, and highly motivated individuals. Such consultation also provides a unique opportunity to address questions of theoretical and practical importance to neuropsychology. Sports neuropsychology will also be a fertile ground for evaluating new tests and testing practices. For example, computerized neuropsychological assessment would appear to be particularly suited to an environment where rapid screening of large numbers of individuals is required.

To be prepared to capitalize on such opportunities, neuropsychologists need to ensure that they understand the unique needs of sports organizations, and how they are different from other institutions. Neuropsychologists also need to be prepared to demonstrate the practical utility of their skills to an audience which may be initially skeptical, and to demonstrate how a better appreciation of the neuropsychological sequelae of concussion can not only protect the player, but also enrich the organization. Some organizations may initially be shortsighted in their perspective about such matters, seeing only how the team may be affected by keeping a player out of competition. However, with time, such organizations may come to appreciate the protection they are afforded by basing decisions about return to play on actual data, rather than some less reliable criteria. Indeed, in the long run, if we are successful in such consultations, sports organizations may feel that it is as essential to have a team neuropsychologist, as it is to have a team physician.

References

American Academy of Neurology. Quality Standards Subcommittee. (1997). Practice parameter: The management of concussion in sports (summary statement). *Neurology, 48*, 581–585.

Cantu, R.C. (1988). When to return to contact sports after a cerebral concussion. *Sports Medicine Digest, 10*, 1–2.

Kelly, J.P., Nichols, J.S. Filley, C.M., Lillehei, K.O., Rubinstein, D. & Kleinschmidt-DeMasters, B.K. (1991). Concussion in sports: Guidelines for the prevention of catastrophic outcome. *Journal of the American Medical Association, 266*, 2867–2869.

McCrory, P. & Berkovic, S. (1998). Second Impact Syndrome. *Neurology, 50*, 677–693.

Mittenberg, W., Tremont, G., Zielinski, R.E., Fichera, S., & Rayls, K.R. (1996). Cognitive-behavioral prevention of postconcussion syndrome. *Archives of Clinical Neuropsychology, 11*, 139–145.

Torg, J.S. (1982). *Athletic injuries to the head, neck, and face*. Philadelphia: Lea & Febiger.

Appendix A: Organizations

Professional

National Football League (NFL)
www.nfl.com

Canadian Football League (CFL)
www.cfl.ca/

National Hockey League (NHL)
www.nhl.com

National Basketball Association (NBA)
www.nba.com

Major League Soccer (MSL)
www.nmlsnet.com/

Collegiate

National Collegiate Athletic Association (NCAA)
www.ncaa.org

Amateur Athletic Union (AAU)
www.aausports.org

Junior Leagues

United States Hockey League (USHL)
www.ushl.com

Canadian Junior A Hockey League
www.cjahl.com/

Other Sources

National Athletic Trainers Association (NATA)
www.nata.org

American College of Sports Medicine (ACSM)
www.acsm.org

International Olympic Committee (IOC)
www.olympic.org/

United States Olympic Committee (USOC)
www.olympic-usa.org

Association for the Advancement of Applied Sport Psychology
www.aaasponline.org/

National Athletic Coaches Association (NHSAC)
www.hscoaches.org/

Coaching Association of Canada
www.coach.ca/

Chapter 22

PSYCHOTHERAPY AND PSYCHOLOGICAL ASPECTS OF RECOVERY FROM BRAIN INJURY

M. Alan J. Finlayson
Independent Practice, Dundas, Ontario, Canada

Psychotherapy and Psychological Aspects of Recovery from Concussion

A major barrier to advances in the field of mild traumatic brain injury (MTBI) assessment and treatment has been the continuous efforts to dichotomize causal factors. At one extreme lies the pathophysiological interpretation of all problems rising following MTBI. In contrast, at the other extreme can be found the attribution of all such problems to psychological mechanisms. Kay et al. (1992) characterized these camps as "believers" and "non-believers". More recently, Hines (1999), in the context of headache pain following trauma, criticized the tendency to seek either organic or psychologic mechanisms as causal explanations of this pain. Instead, he argued for an interactive process. A similar position has been espoused by Ruff (1999) who has argued for consideration of the interaction among symptoms, pre injury risk factors, and their temporal course in determining individually specific therapeutic approaches. In many ways, this present controversy is similar to the historical "nature-nurture" controversy. However, as Anastasi (1958) pointed out, that issue was not a question of either hereditary or environment but rather "how" do these two powerful influences interact to produce a specific situation. It seems timely, nearly half a century later, to adopt a similar strategy for understanding the consequences of MTBI.

Most practicing clinical neuropsychologists recognize that the majority of individuals with concussion or mild traumatic brain injury recover quickly with minimal or conservative interventions. A small minority of individuals sustaining such injury do, however, require ongoing interventions. There is no reason to doubt that a similar pattern of outcomes would be expected following concussion or mild traumatic brain injury arising from sports related trauma.

Intervention issues

Intervention strategies for individuals with MTBI typically address the question "can the post concussion syndrome be treated?" Symptoms comprising the post concussion syndrome (PCS) are generally grouped into those of a physical, cognitive or psychological nature (see Table 22.1). Having then applied distinct linguistic labels to the clusters, it is usually assumed that the symptoms are then unique representatives of that arbitrary classification. With few exceptions, these symptoms are rarely seen as interactive.

It is also important to remember that these symptoms are not diagnostic. Their presence cannot be equated solely with a diagnosis of MTBI. For example, Iverson and McCracken (1997) demonstrated the presence of PCS symptomatology in individuals with chronic pain. In their sample of 170 patients with pain, 81% endorsed three or more symptoms of PCS. While the presence of headache was not reported, the three most common symptoms in this group were disturbed sleep, fatigue, and irritability. It is likely that a similar level of endorsement of such symptoms would be found in other medical populations, particularly in conditions where mind-body questions arise. While there may be a similar frequency of symptom endorsement, LaChapelle and Finlayson (1998) have demonstrated that there are quantifiable differences in the nature of these symptoms. Thus, while these symptoms may represent a generic response to injury, there might well be disease specific differences associated with their manifestation.

It is generally accepted that 80–90% of individuals sustaining concussion or MTBI recover relatively well and return to their usual activities fairly quickly. In contrast, the remaining individuals can have persisting symptomatology. Ruff, Camenzuli and Mueller (1996) have referred to this group as the "miserable minority". Reitan and Wolfson (1999; 2000) have argued that it is possible to differentiate these two groups on neuropsychological

Table 22.1. A common classification of PCS symptoms.

Somatic	Cognitive	Emotional
Headache	Attention	Irritability
Dizziness	Concentration	Depression
Fatigue	Memory	Anxiety
Balance	Processing Speed	
Insomnia		

examination. Those individuals with ongoing clinical symptoms often have neuropsychological profiles similar to those of individuals with known tissue destruction. They further argue that most research subjects are routinely drawn from the much larger, early-recovering population. As those individuals who will likely have ongoing symptoms are, therefore, underrepresented in such samples, conclusions based on those data do not necessarily apply to those individuals with persistent impairment. It would follow that interventions targeting these two populations are also likely to have different components and recovery time frames.

In general, intervention strategies immediately following MTBI have been directed toward the elimination or reduction of the symptoms associated with PCS (Kay, 1993). Such interventions take the form of pharmacological or medical strategies to manage headache, sleep disturbance and other physical problems. Interventions typically conducted by physicians are beyond the scope of this chapter and the interested reader can find summaries of such interventions elsewhere. (e.g., Gualtieri, 1999; Zasler, 2000). For example, a recent outline of general medical approaches to PCS can be found in Neppe, (1999). Recent reviews of post traumatic headache have also been completed (e.g. Horn, 1998; Hines, 1999). Hines (1999) provides a detailed approach to the assessment and management of headache following traumatic brain injury. He places post traumatic headache in the context of acute and chronic pain. In his discussion of this topic, he considers physiological and psychogenic aspects of headache as interactive rather than dichotomous variables. He also presented a detailed classification of post traumatic headache along with general management guidelines and specific pharmacological recommendations. Non-pharmacological guidelines for headache intervention have also been described (Pryse-Phillips et al., 1998). Finally, a recent chapter (McAllister & Flashman, 1999) details medical strategies for dealing with emotional factors, primarily affective disturbance. The major psychological interventions at this level constitute education, reassurance, and support.

Mittenberg and Burton (1994) carried out a survey of practicing neuropsychologists in order to determine the nature of the interventions being carried out with individuals with PCS. Those clinicians responding to the survey identified education, reassurance, psychological support, cognitive reattribution of symptoms, and gradual reactivation to be the interventions associated with better treatment outcome. Consensus or agreement in the use of such procedures may meet the criteria for demonstrating reliability. Unfortunately, the evidence that such interventions are effective or valid is quite limited. Some evidence in support of the role of education has been forthcoming.

Minderhoud, Boelens, Huizenga and Saan (1980) were able to demonstrate a marked reduction in the sequelae of PCS following an intervention based on the provision of information and encouragement. In 1972, Relander, Troupp, and Björkesten allocated 178 patients to either a typical hospital routine or to an active treatment group. The routine group was allowed to leave bed when they wished, received information only when they asked for it, and did not have a consistent physician manage their care. In contrast, the active treatment group were managed by the same physician, seen daily, provided with an explanation of their injuries, and encouraged to get up early and to participate in physiotherapy. While the groups did not differ in length of hospital stay, the active group returned to work much more quickly. At the one year follow up, the two patient groups did not differ in symptom reporting.

In a similar manner, Hinkle, Alves, Rimel and Jane (1986) randomly assigned patients with MTBI to one of three conditions: routine care, information, or information and reassurance. Routine care was described as observation for complications, discharge instructions for return should persistent problems occur, and advice to return to normal activities. The information group received the same care but at discharge was provided with greater information regarding the problems associated with mild head injury. The third group received, in addition, an opportunity to pose questions, and reassurance regarding normal recovery that took the form of a weekly telephone call until symptoms abated. The sample size was 1092 patients representing a typical spectrum of such individuals. The results did not reveal significant difference for number of days before return to work or social function among the three individual groups. However, by combining the treatment groups, a significant difference in return to work and social activity was noted. This difference was five days. As an aside, this study presented interesting data regarding prevention or risk control. The authors identified 62% of their sample as having evidence of blood alcohol; 93% were not wearing a seatbelt; 22% of the motorcyclists were not wearing a helmet; and 58% of the crashes occurred on Friday, Saturday, or Sunday.

More recently, Mittenberg and colleagues (Mittenberg et al., 1996) demonstrated the value of providing a printed manual to patients along with a discussion of the nature of potential symptoms and the provision of techniques for minimizing their impact and strategies for gradual reactivation. Patients in the control group received routine hospital and discharge management that included written instructions regarding return to the clinic if problems persisted and prescribing a period of rest. Fifty-eight patients were randomly assigned to one of the conditions. A six month follow up interview revealed that the treatment group reported fewer symptoms and enjoyed a shorter duration of symptoms relative to the control group. The authors argued that information served to reduce the stress associated with the presence of symptoms and misattribution of etiology.

Paniak, Toller-Lobe, Durant and Nagy (1998) performed a similar investigation. One hundred and eleven patients with MTBI were randomly assigned to a single treatment session or were provided with a more extensive assessment, education and received treatment on an as-needed basis. Follow up was conducted between three and four months following initial assessment. The single session treatment was similar to that offered by Mittenberg and his colleagues in that the patients were provided with an information brochure, reassured regarding their symptoms and received education, reassurance and coping strategies. The extended treatment group had the same intervention but also had a brief neuropsychological examination, physiotherapy consultation and feedback about these findings. Where indicated, treatment was provided through the hospital services. The available data suggest that the patients did not take advantage of the therapeutic opportunities. At the time of follow up (3 to 4 months), the groups showed a similar amount of improvement and did not differ on other symptom or outcome variables. In a follow up study (Paniak, Toller-Lobe, Reynolds, Melnyk & Nagy, 2000) they were able to contact 105 of the clients for a one year follow up. Both groups had maintained the gains shown at 3 months and, again, there was no difference between the groups in outcome variables. The authors also noted that further improvement between three and twelve months was minimal and that patients reported greatest improvement in the first three months. They concluded that brief educational intervention was, at least, as valuable as more intensive treatment for most people surviving MTBI.

Collectively, these investigators have demonstrated the significant, positive role that appropriate education and reassurance can play in reducing the sequelae, commonly associated with PCS. It is important to note that the interventions did not consist merely of diagnosis and glib reassurance that "you will be fine". Providing a label without accompanying education and reassurance has been shown to exacerbate the condition that the diagnosis was intended to reduce (Haynes et al., 1978). In a similar manner, the role of physician attitude toward treatment can be a powerful determinant of patient outcome. Hines (1999) cites Kelly (1983) as demonstrating that only 11 of 76 patients who had been denied treatment or received minimal treatment through their physician returned to work prior to their compensation claim being resolved. On the other hand, 25 of 30 patients who had been "vigorously treated" returned to work within a year of onset and often prior to claim resolution.

Attitudes can influence outcome in a number of ways. In general, many of the clients that I have worked with in a rehabilitation capacity have been coping reasonably well until the onset of trauma or disease. For colleagues with a physical orientation, the adjustment difficulties encountered are often attributed to the presence of the physical injury. This often leads to a focus on the treatment of physical impairments or functional components with the mistaken assumption that the psychological problems will resolve when the injury is "fixed". Another sub-group of clients is composed of those who have minimal or undetectable physical signs. These clients often report that they have been informed that their pain, symptoms, etc. are "all in the head". This often presents a formidable resistance to psychological intervention as they perceive themselves as being sent to "the shrink". At such times, I often share Dr. Rotella's quotation: "Whenever someone introduces me or identifies me as a shrink, I am tempted to correct him. I am not a shrink. I am an enlarger." (Rotella & Cullen, 1995, p. 28). Although humourous, this captures well the concept of growth inherent in most psychological interventions.

However, in rehabilitation, in order to enhance growth, we must also assist in the healing process. Psychotherapy is one tool to achieve this end. However, it is important that the psychologist not become too narrowly focused on just their role in addressing injury related psychological impairments and adjustment problems. Taylor and Taylor (1997) have identified four principle psychological factors that influence the course of rehabilitation. Specifically, they cite confidence, motivation, anxiety and focus as important components of the overall rehabilitation process that promote physical and psychological recovery. Psychological techniques are available to address these factors (Taylor & Taylor, 1997). Positive changes in these dimensions have been shown to increase client compliance and adherence to demanding and often repetitive therapeutic regimes. Assisting the client in goal setting and enabling the client to see both the big picture and the small successes associated with gradual change and recovery can enhance motivation and assist the client to maintain the positive attitude necessary for the attainment of quality rehabilitation. Interventions in these domains provide the psychologist with the opportunity to get out of the office and participate with other professionals in the gym, at home, or in the workplace. It also ensures that not only are individual psychological issues addressed at all stages of rehabilitation but also that psychological knowledge is utilized to enhance recovery in other treatment modalities.

I have often characterized my own intervention strategy as involving two simple components: grief counseling and performance enhancement. First, I often assist clients with the resolution of grief regarding loss. The loss can take the form of abilities, functions, dreams or faith. The second phase then involves skill development and the use of these new skills in the search for their potential and the pursuit of that path. This typically involves a combination of coaching and cognitive behavioral strategies. Many clients have thoughts that "I'm going crazy". Such a skill-based approach can assist in overcoming such fears and offer a positive formulation to the client. By acknowledging clients' pre injury coping ability and, at the same time, pointing out that their life experience had not prepared them for the nature and extent of the emotional adjustment to injury helps to normalize the process. The role of the psychologist can then be identified as helping the client to acquire the necessary coping skills for normal life tasks.

Intervention for persistent symptoms

For some individuals with MTBI (the "silent epidemic"), reassurance is not sufficient and more intensive rehabilitation strategies are required. Richter, Cowan and Kaschalk (1995) proposed a treatment protocol for the management of pain and sleep disorder associated with MTBI. They echoed the point made previously by Uomoto and Esselman (1993) that chronic pain is a frequent comorbidity with MTBI. In fact, they argued that headache is more frequently associated with MTBI than with other levels of brain injury severity. They also reported the presence of other pain (i.e., neck, shoulder and back) also persisted in this group. The protocol of Richter et al. (1995) emphasized patient and family education on issues ranging from medication to concepts of illness behavior with the goal of self control and self management of symptoms. In the presence of sleep disorder, discussion focused upon sleep hygiene procedures and, in more complicated cases, appropriate further investigations and the judicious use of medication. Cognitive behavioral techniques including education, desensitization, and psychological activation were recommended to reduce the psychological factors arising with injury. Gradual physical activation was central to the program. These several techniques were combined in a holistic manner to re-establish mastery for the individual client.

Strategies for assessment and intervention for the cognitive sequelae of MTBI have been recently summarized. Neppe (1999) provides an overview of a comprehensive program to address the evaluation and treatment of the broad range of problems associated with "closed head injury syndrome of transient kind (CHIT)" (p. 421). Individual cognitive domains have also been the subject of recent reviews: attention and concentration (Mateer, 2000); memory and related processes (Raskin, 2000a); and higher level executive problems (Raskin, 2000b). Such approaches to symptom management are becoming increasingly sophisticated and refined based on their experimental validation (e.g., Park & Ingles, 2001).

Recently, reviews of approaches to the management of the psychological symptoms associated with PCS have emerged: depression (Raskin & Stein, 2000); anxiety (Hovland & Raskin, 2000); and irritability (Hovland & Mateer, 2000). In these chapters, the authors present psychological distress in the context of an interaction of premorbid style, specific physical components of the injury, and individual adjustment or coping style. The psychological interventions presented heavily favor approaches that can best be described as falling within the realm of cognitive behavioral interventions.

In my own clinical work with survivors of traumatic brain injury, I have found the cognitive behavioral approach to be productive. It provides a system based or interactive approach to the conceptualization of psychological and behavioral problems that can be readily understood by most clients. Briefly, the model describes how, in response to an internal or external stimulus or threat, physiological responses can be set in motion. These sensations are then perceived as emotions or feelings. With this labeling process, automatic or considered thought processes next come into play, eventually producing a behavioral expression in response to the original stimuli. Each of the elements of the system can influence or modulate the other elements. In a cognitive behavioral approach to problem management, emphasis is placed upon both the investigation and modification of the thought processes and the addition or elimination of skills from the behavioral repertoire of the individual. The nature of assessment and interventions associated with this field are quite varied and have been applied to a number of clinical and life problems (e.g. Dobson, 2001); however, they do share many similar elements.

Table 22.2. Core tasks of psychotherapy.

- Develop Therapeutic Alliance
- Provide Education
- Nurture Hope
- Teach and Develop Coping Skills
- Encourage Practice/Personal Experiments
- Encourage Client to Take Credit for Change
- Conduct Relapse Prevention

Recently, Meichenbaum (2001) has distilled the core tasks of psychotherapy in a way that captures the key elements of a cognitive behavioral approach to intervention (see Table 22.2).

The development of an effective therapeutic alliance is critical to successful psychological intervention. It is essential that the sick person and the healer share a common belief in the nature of the problem and the steps necessary for its resolution. This is similar to the concept of confidence and trust espoused by Taylor and Taylor (1997). In some cases, that trust is inherent in the title or training of the practitioner. The relationship must be very carefully nurtured and fostered and an appropriate bond developed that incorporates and respects the beliefs of the client.

The provision of education can take the form of didactic therapist intervention using patient relevant analogy, slides, plastic models, drawings, or information brochures, depending upon the needs of the particular client. This can also aid in modifying an erroneous belief system if that is contributing to symptom maintenance. I find it particularly helpful to devote time to a discussion of the interaction of physical and psychological variables in maintaining pain and illness behaviors or contributing to increased or decreased patient functioning.

Nurturing hope or increasing motivation (Taylor & Taylor, 1997) is essential to the establishment and attainment of rehabilitation goals. Most clients see through blind optimism but do respond to a realistic appraisal of the problem and can develop a positive focus on rehabilitation progress rather than dwelling on perceived loss.

Central to psychotherapy is the concept of change. Many clients are in treatment because they are trapped in a behavioral pattern not seemingly under their control. Cognitive behavioral interventions can assist the client in understanding and modifying their cognitive processes (i.e. self talk) and questioning their attributions regarding illness. Effort is also devoted to the addition of behavioral skills to their repertoire including relaxation, assertiveness, etc., dependent upon client need. However, these skills are not abstract conceptualizations and it is essential that the client practice the implementation of the new behaviors. This can begin as therapeutic role playing and advance to specific homework assignments. The therapist and client can be assisted in the homework process through the use of client centered workbooks. Examples of such tools for use in the management of anxiety and depression would include (but not be limited to) those developed by Greenberger and Padesky (1995) and Bourne (2000). Examples of similar approaches to anger management include workbooks prepared by Gottlieb (1999) and Potter-Efron and Potter-Efron (1995). These workbooks focus upon the interplay of environmental, biological, behavioral, cognitive and emotional factors as central to client problems. Typically, information is provided to assist the client in understanding this interaction along with techniques and exercises designed to facilitate change. As might be expected, an emphasis is placed upon cognition, particularly thoughts or self talk and attributions.

Not only do these and similar volumes serve as aids for conceptual learning and skill acquisition, but they also foster the development of self control. Examining the evidence underlying beliefs and attributions and acquiring tools for behavioral change facilitates clients' acceptance of responsibility and increases their sense of mastery. This success can then become a powerful reinforcer of skill attainment, the maintenance of hope, and a positive outlook. While therapists may bring extensive training and experience to the therapeutic encounter, therapeutic success is clearly determined by the client's behavior. In other words, good client effort and response lead to good therapy. It is important that clients be frequently reminded of this interaction and appropriately reinforced for their role in change in order to encourage their ownership of the problem and its solution.

Meichenbaum's final therapeutic task is to ensure that the client does not relapse. This is the final phase of stress inoculation training that follows the successful real world application of learned coping skills. It can involve education regarding potential stressors, follow up or "booster" sessions, and strategies designed to ensure the maintenance and generalization of treatment gains.

Finally, although not on the core list of therapeutic tasks, Meichenbaum (2001) also emphasizes the need to assist the client in finding meaning or gaining perspective regarding the traumatic event. Prigatano (1994) has also emphasized the search for meaning in psychotherapy as central to healing of the "wounded soul". While this search for meaning could take the form of clarifying the circumstances of the incident and assigning blame to such factors as error or chance, for some clients, however, trauma in general and concussion in particular can challenge their core beliefs and cause them to question their faith. This will often lead therapy in the direction of religious or spiritual values. Often this is not fully resolved in therapy but the client can be equipped with the tools and motivation to continue this journey beyond the office door. However, if the therapist is anxious about this path, the client will not be able to make that journey. Such clients could be helped to identify a potential spiritual advisor from his/her past or present and encouraged to seek guidance from that individual. Clients without such a religious history could be directed to non-denominational study centers.

Prevention issues

No discussion of treatment strategies would be complete without consideration of the adage that an ounce of prevention is worth a pound of cure. At present, there is no cure for brain injury but there are ways in which its occurrence can be prevented. While strategies to reduce the occurrence of concussion are critical, consideration must also be given to minimizing iatrogenic factors once injury has occurred.

In sport, considerable attention is given to equipment standards and to rules of play or conduct as variables that can be manipulated to reduce or prevent injury. Equipment standards can be applied to personal protective devices or to environmental design. Answers to such questions as the quality of ice or the nature of turf could well effect injury occurrence and outcome. In hockey, for example, the rigidity of the boards or glass could well influence the outcome of player collisions with these structures. The design of helmets, mouth guards, and other protective equipment can also influence the extent of injury. Standards alone, however, will not prevent injury. Manufacturers and facility owners must adhere to these standards to minimize risk to competitors. The players, themselves, must also comply with the appropriate use of protective equipment. Often player attitude is critical. For example, in some sports, it appears to be a mark of honor, among males, to wear a loose fitting helmet. Typically, these same athletes invariably ensure that their protective cup is in place. It is just a matter of priorities. The rules of play of an athletic contest, including competitor conduct, can also be modified to minimize risk of injury to the athlete. Such rules also require appropriate enforcement and player adherence. These factors, however, have multiple determinants. There are other variables associated with athletic contests that may also contribute to the risk of injury. In many professional sports, long distance travel with associated disruption of sleep, frequency of play with associated reduced restoration time and similar factors have yet to be evaluated for their potential role in the production of athletic injury.

The role of immediate and appropriate evaluation has been addressed elsewhere in this volume. Such diagnostic efforts, accompanied by appropriate intervention can certainly reduce the secondary consequences of neurotrauma (secondary brain insults, SBI's). Hypotension has been identified as a major SBI in the determination of outcome following severe brain injury. Chestnut and colleagues (1993) reviewed 717 cases from the Coma Data Bank. In their review, they defined hypotension as SBP < 90 mm Hg. On that basis, they identified the presence of hypotension in 34.6% of their sample and reported that it was associated with 150% increase in patient mortality. They argued that the disruptions of autoregulation associated with neurotrauma limit blood profusion such that, even with adequate oxygenation, ischemia can result with devastating consequences for the patient. Chestnut (1997) strongly advocated that all resuscitation protocols for neurotrauma should include the implementation of efforts to reduce hypotensive insult. The pathophysiology of neurotrauma is identical for all levels of injury (mild to severe), differing only quantitatively. It may well be the case that hypotension associated with hypovolemic shock may also influence outcome following concussion and appropriate monitoring and intervention could reduce the dysfunction associated with MTBI. Unfortunately, the nature and extent of this impact awaits empirical demonstration.

In a similar manner, genetic factors may have a role to play in injury prevention. Genetic makeup has been linked to outcome in brain injury (Jordan, Chapter 6 in this volume; Jordan et al., 1997; Teasdale, Jorgensen, Ripa, Nielsen, & Christensen, 2000; Teasdale, Nicholl, Murray, & Fiddes, 1997). These authors have investigated the manner in which the apolipoprotein E gene can impact on outcome following neurotrauma and they have reported that the APOEε4 allele, when present, is associated with negative outcome. Teasdale et al. (1997) indicated that the presence of this allele was strongly related to poor outcome at six month follow up in a sample of brain injury survivors. In a further investigation, Teasdale et al. (2000) demonstrated that although patients with the APOEε4 allele did not differ in functional severity from a non-carrier group at admission to a brain injury rehabilitation program, there was evidence of a deterioration in their functioning relative to the control group at a one year follow up. Similarly, Jordan et al. (1997) reported that the presence of the APOEε4 allele was associated with higher severity levels of neurological deficits in boxers. The allele was present in all of the members of the most severely impaired group and under represented in the mildly impaired group. While this line of investigation must be considered to be preliminary in nature, it does raise the question of genetic screening for participants in high risk sports as a potential preventative measure.

Finally, the development of return to play guidelines (Cantu & Echemendia, Chapter 26 in this volume) is of critical importance in the avoidance of, or minimization of, the deleterious effect of multiple concussions. This is most critical in the pediatric or adolescent population, a group susceptible to sudden impact syndrome (SIS). SIS can arise when an athlete sustains a second brain injury while still symptomatic from a previous brain injury. The second trauma is thought to precipitate irregularities in, or loss of, autoregulation which then result in a sudden and dramatic increase in intercranial pressure with disastrous consequences. While the incidence of this syndrome is relatively low, SIS has gained prominence due to its often fatal but likely preventable occurrence. Due to the high risk of fatality associated with SIS, many clinicians are adamant that individuals should not engage in contact sports while symptomatic and that a longer delay of return to play following attainment of asymptomatic status is justified. The interested reader is referred to Cantu's recent chapter (1998) for more extensive information on this subject.

Education, reassurance and support may also be invaluable in preventing spousal or partner distress. Clinicians have known for some time that disease or trauma to the brain is problematic not only for the injured person but also for those with whom they interact (Stambrook, Moor, Gill, & Peters, 1994). Partners and families appear to cope reasonably well initially but as problems persist, the burden of care can become intolerable (Chwalisz, 1999; Brooks, 1991). Chwalisz (1999) has suggested that this time gap provides a window of opportunity for the implementation of preventative interventions. Education regarding the nature and extent of injury and a discussion of factors contributing to the development and maintenance of behavioral symptoms should be available to partners and spouses. In addition, coping strategies similar to those described above for individuals living with the consequences of MTBI could also be taught to their partners. Finally, the partner should have an opportunity to practice the newly acquired skills in real life circumstances. Such interventions would be consistent with the stress inoculation training strategy as described by Meichenbaum (1993).

The implementation of preventative measures should be guided by clinical research and not instituted in an arbitrary fashion. The impact of change on injury reduction must be carefully evaluated, a task requiring sufficient data for relevant analyses. Clarke and Jordan (1998) reviewed data that demonstrated a significant reduction in brain injury following the development and implementation of uniform standards for football helmets. They cited similar data demonstrating a reduction in fatal cerebral and spinal injury as a result of the enforcement of the rule change penalizing head first tackling and blocking. The clinical significance of theses changes could only be confirmed because football, by virtue of the number of participants, provided sufficient data to adequately test the experimental hypothesis. Unfortunately, few sports have the requisite number of competitors or the necessary data collection systems to permit similar evaluations.

Sport specific issues

A number of different sports have been reviewed and discussed in this volume and will not be covered in detail in this chapter. However, one central theme in all organized sports is the restoration of function and the minimization of handicap (Finlayson & Garner, 1994). In North America, restoration of productivity, particularly return to work, is emphasized. Rehabilitation of athletes has a similar applied emphasis, specifically return to play. In general, rehabilitation programs tend to take a holistic approach and consider the individual client in the context of personal, family, social, and vocational roles. A similar approach is indicated with athletes although in the case of the professional competitor, the number of stakeholders can become much larger. In addition to athletes and their families, the team has a vested interest. These interests will vary as the health professionals attending to the injured athlete may hold different views and values than might owners and managers or coaches and fellow competitors. In addition, there may well be interests associated with league or union contracts, agents and the players' retinue. Even the press and sports fans will hold an opinion with respect to the injury and its implications. In such an environment, information about an injury and/or treatment may actually become a commodity. The practicing clinician must take great care to ensure that the clinical role is clearly defined (see Chapters 21 and 25, this volume).

In the case of psychologists, there are standards of practice that can be used to guide professional behavior in these circumstances. For example, there are standards that guide the nature of the professional relationship and how that is communicated to the client. It is also clear that multiple relationships must be avoided by clarifying the role of the psychologist and clearly identifying the client and the nature of service to be provided to assist in avoiding such conflict. In the case of third party consultation, the athlete needs to be clearly informed regarding the role of the psychologist, the nature of the professional relationship, the extent and limits of confidentiality, and how any obtained information will be utilized. The youthfulness of professional athletes combined with the paternalistic apprenticeships in some professional sports often leads players to be casual about their rights. It is important that psychologists be sensitive to such developments and ensure that consent is truly informed. Anxiety can arise for the injured athlete due to several factors quite similar to those for the general population of individuals with MTBI. Athletes experiencing concussion often voice uncertainty regarding their health and their career. The very nature of concussion symptoms can be quite alarming and raise anxiety about threats to life or, at least, the quality of life. Similarly, the athlete may wonder if he or she will return to competition or be able to play with the same intensity. The possibility that injury may limit the ability to achieve maximum performance (make the team) can pose a significant economic threat to the athlete as they may well worry about being replaced by someone younger, faster, or stronger. Fear of re-injury and long term effects often worry the athlete. Concussion can also lead to crises of identity. For some weekend warriors and elite competitors, sport participation provides a great deal of ego gratification and is a major part of the person's self concept. Individuals who lack the necessary balance of life activities are at risk for psychological distress when the loss of this critical life role is forced upon them.

In some cases, concussion may contribute to a loss of control. Concussion may have career ending implications for both the optimistic rookie and the seasoned veteran. While one may experience the loss of potential stardom and the other the opportunity to "walk" off the field, both would agree that events did not happen on their terms or as they had been planned. Loss of control may also occur as a challenge to perfectionist attitudes, emotional control tendencies or other personality styles as suggested by Ruff et al. (1996). To that list can be added previous trauma. I have seen a number of clients whose injury related stress appears to be disproportionate to the event. Upon further inquiry, a history of physical, psychological, or sexual abuse is uncovered. The client often reports that these issues had been resolved or were behind them. Instead, it seems that they have been buried in a shallow, well marked grave. The recent injury and associated stress rekindles the early experience. Some clients appear able to separate the two issues and focus on injury related problems. They can then, at a later date, deal with the earlier issues from a position of greater strength. In other cases, it is necessary to assist the client in gaining a perspective on the earlier crisis before they can move on to present issues.

The relatively speedy return of athletes to play has been often cited as the standard against which "lack of effort" or secondary gain in rehabilitation is judged. However, the concept of secondary gain must also be considered in the rehabilitation of sports related injury (Taylor & Taylor, 1997). They point out that the injured athlete may gain benefit from maintaining an injured role if the athlete fears the inability to return to the same high level of performance that was displayed pre injury. They also point out that injury may produce a greater degree of attention than previously received, which would also serve to maintain the sick role. In addition, the opportunity to enjoy reasonable retirement benefits without the demands of intense competition could hold appeal. Also, for some journeymen competitors, it may be easier to live with injury and the thoughts of "I could have made it" rather than face an average or mediocre career.

Final thoughts

Mild traumatic brain injury in general and concussion in athletes in particular, offer a unique testing ground for hypotheses related to the interaction of psychological (mind) and biological (body) variables. For example, on a biochemical level, glucocorticoids are produced in response to both disease and stress (e.g. Maier, Watkins, & Fleshner, 1994). Maier et al. emphasized that not only do psychological factors influence the immune system but also that behavior can be similarly modified by the immune system, itself. Glucocorticoids have also been purported to play a role in the occurrence of human hippocampal atrophy associated with chronic stress (McEwen, 1999). McEwen further suggested that individuals might differ in their stress responsiveness, a factor that may contribute to their increased vulnerability to the consequences of their biochemical response to prolonged stress. That is, a person's inability to cope with stress will result in the maintenance of stress at levels that might produce negative changes in brain chemistry. Back pain, whiplash associated disorder and MTBI, are all body traumas in which stress related factors have been identified as contributing to symptom maintenance. The prevalence of persisting symptomatology in these three conditions is remarkably similar. For example, Fordyce (1988) indicated that roughly 15% of individuals with low back pain failed to make the expected recovery. Barnsley, Lord and Bogduk (1998) reported similar levels of persistent symptomatology in individuals with whiplash associated disorder. In the case of MTBI, Alexander (1995) provided a similar estimate of continuing symptomatology. New work regarding genetically determined constitutional factors as contributors to symptom severity and persistence is emerging (Jordan, this volume). There has been an increased understanding of the role of factors associated with pathophysiology (Hovda, Chapter 4 in this volume) and neuropsychology (Macciocchi & Barth, Chapter 16 in this volume) in the recovery process. When such biological factors are juxtaposed with the role of personality factors (e.g., Ruff et al, 1996) and coping style (e.g., Godfrey, Knight, & Partridge, 1996) as outcome determinants, the potential interactions are staggering. On the other hand, wonderful opportunities and challenges for exploring the mind-body question are presented. The role of psychotherapy and its influence in this system is one such question.

References

Alexander, M.P. (1995). Mild Traumatic Brain Injury: Pathophysiology, Natural History, and Clinical Management. *Neurology, 45,* 1253–1260.

Anastasi, A. (1958). Heredity, environment, and the question "how?". *Psychological Review, 65,* 197–208.

Barnsley, L., Lord, S.M., & Bogduk, N. (1998). The pathophysiology of whiplash. *Spine: Stat of the Art Reviews, 12,* 209–242.

Bourne, E.J. (2000). *The Anxiety & Phobia Workbook* (3rd ed.). Oakland, CA: New Harbinger Publications, Inc.

Brooks, D.N. (1991). The head-injured family. *Journal of Clinical and Experimental Neuropsychology, 13,* 155–188.

Cantu, R.C. (1998) Second-Impact Syndrome. In R.C. Cantu (Ed.), *Clinics in Sports Medicine: Neurologic Athletic Head and Neck Injuries* (pp. 37–44). Toronto: W.B. Saunders Co.

Chesnut, R.M. (1997). Avoidance of hypotension: Conditio sine qua non of successful severe head-injury management. *The Journal of Trauma: Injury, Infection and Critical Care, 42*(5), s4-s9.

Chesnut, R.M., Marshall, L.F., Klauber, M.R., Blunt, B.A., Baldwin, N., Eisenberg, H.M. et al. (1993). The role of secondary brain injury in determining outcome from severe head injury. *The Journal of Trauma, 34,* 216–222.

Chwalisz, K. (1999). The problem of comorbidity in spouses. In N.R. Varney & R.J. Roberts (Eds.), *The Evaluation and Treatment of Mild Traumatic Brain Injury* (pp. 465–481). London: Lawrence Erlbaum Associates.

Clarke, K.S., & Jordan, B.D. (1998). Sports Neuroepidemiology. In B.D. Jordan (Ed.), *Sports Neurology* (2nd ed.). Philadelphia: Lippincott-Raven Publishers.

Dobson, K.S. (2001). *Handbook of Cognitive-Behavioral Therapies.* New York: The Guilford Press.

Finlayson, M.A.J., & Garner, S.H. (1994). Challenges in rehabilitation of individuals with acquired brain injury. In M.A.J. Finlayson & S.H. Garner (Eds.), *Brain Injury Rehabilitation: Clinical Considerations.* Baltimore: Williams & Wilkins.

Fordyce, W.E. (1988). Pain and suffering: A reappraisal. *American Psychologist, 43,* 276–283.

Godfrey, H.P.D., Knight, R.G., & Partridge, F.M. (1996). Emotional adjustment following traumatic brain injury: A stress-appraisal-coping formulation. *Journal of Head Trauma Rehabilitation, 11*(6), 29–40.

Gottlieb, M.W. (1999). *The Angry Self: A Comprehensive Approach to Anger Management.* Phoenix: Zeig, Tucker & Co., Publishers.

Greenberger, D. & Padesky, C.A. (1995). *Mind Over Mood.* New York, NY: The Guilford Press.

Gualtieri, E.T. (1999). The pharmacologic treatment of mild traumatic brain injury. In N.R. Varney & R.J. Roberts (Eds.), *The Evaluation and Treatment of Mild Traumatic Brain Injury* (pp. 411–419). London: Lawrence Erlbaum Associates.

Haynes, R.B., Sackett, D.L., Taylor, D.W., Gibson, E.S., Johnson, A.L. (1978). Increased Absenteeism at Work after Detection and Labeling of Hypertensive Patients. *New England Journal of Medicine, 229*, 741–744.

Hines, M.E. (1999). Posttraumatic headaches. In N.R. Varney & R.J. Roberts (Eds.), *The Evaluation and Treatment of Mild Traumatic Brain Injury* (pp. 375-410). London: Lawrence Erlbaum Associates.

Hinkle, J.L., Alves, W.M., Rimel, R.W., & Jane, J.A. (1986). Restoring social competence in minor head-injury patients. *Journal of Neuroscience Nursing, 18*, 268–271.

Horn, L.J. (1998). Post Concussive Headaches. In G.A. Malanga (Ed.), *Spine: State of the Art Reviews, 12*, 377–393.

Hovland, D. & Mateer,, C.A. (2000). Irritability and anger. In S.A. Raskin & C.A. Mateer (Eds.), *Neuropsychological Management of Mild Traumatic Brain Injury* (pp. 187–201). New York: Oxford University Press.

Hovland, D. & Raskin, S.A. (2000). Anxiety and posttraumatic stress. In S.A. Raskin & C.A. Mateer (Eds.), *Neuropsychological Management of Mild Traumatic Brain Injury* (pp. 171–186). New York: Oxford University Press.

Iverson, G.L., & McCracken, L.M. (1997). 'Postconcussive' symptoms in person with chronic pain. *Brain Injury, 11*, 783–790.

Jordan, B.D., Relkin, N.R., Ravdin, L.D., Jacobs, A.R., Bennett, A., & Gandy, S. (1997). Apolipoprotein E e4 associated with chronic traumatic brain injury in boxing. *Journal of the American Medical Association, 278*, 136–140.

Kay, T. (1993). Neuropsychological Treatment of Mild Traumatic Brain Injury. *Journal of Head Trauma Rehabilitation, 8*(3), 74–85.

Kay, T., Newman, B., Cavallo, M., Ezrachi, O., & Resnick, M. (1992). Toward a neuropsychological model of functional disability after mild traumatic brain injury. *Neuropsychology, 6*, 371–384.

Kelly, R.E. (1983). Post-traumatic headache. In P.J. Vinken, G.W. Bruyn, & H.L. Klawaans (Eds.), *Handbook of Clinical Neurology, 48* (pp. 383–390).

LaChapelle, D.L. & Finlayson, M.A.J. (1998). An evaluation of subjective and objective measures of fatigue in patients with brain injury and healthy controls. *Brain Injury, 12*, 649–659.

Maier, S.F., Watkins, L.R., & Fleshner, M. (1994). Psychoneuroimmunology: The interface between behavior, brain, and immunity. *American Psychologist, 49*, 1004–1017.

Mateer, C.A. (2000). Attention. In S.A. Raskin & C.A. Mateer (Eds.), *Neuropsychological Management of Mild Traumatic Brain Injury* (pp. 73–92). New York: Oxford University Press.

McAllister, T.W., & Flashman, L.A. (1999). Mild brain injury and mood disorders: causal connections, assessment, and treatment. In N.R. Varney & R.J. Roberts (Eds.), *The Evaluation and Treatment of Mild Traumatic Brain Injury* (pp. 347–373). London: Lawrence Erlbaum Associates.

McEwen, B.S. (1999). Stress and hippocampal plasticity. *Annual Review of Neuroscience, 22*, 105–122.

Meichenbaum, D. (1993). The "potential" contributions of cognitive behavior modification to the rehabilitation of individuals with traumatic brain injury. *Seminars in Speech and Language, 14*, 18–30.

Meichenbaum, D. (2001). *Treatment of Individuals with Anger and Aggression.* Waterloo, Ontario: Institute Press.

Minderhoud, J.M., Boelens, M.E.N., Huizenga, J., & Saan, R.G. (1980). Treatment of Minor Head Injuries. *Clinical Neurology, Neurosurgery and Psychiatry, 82, 127–140.*
Mittenberg, W. & Burton, D.E. (1994). A Survey of Treatments for Post concussion Syndrome. *Brain Injury, 8,* 429–437.
Mittenberg, W., Tremont, G., Zielinski, R.E., Fichera, S., & Rayls, R.A. (1996). Cognitive-behavioral prevention of postconcussion syndrome. *Archives of Clinical Neuropsychology, 11,* 139–145.
National Headache Foundation. (1996). *Standards of care for headache diagnosis and treatment as established by the National Headache Foundation.* Chicago: Author.
Neppe, V.M. (1999). Integration of the evaluation and management of the transient closed head injury patient: some directions. In N.R. Varney & R.J. Roberts (Eds.), *The Evaluation and Treatment of Mild Traumatic Brain Injury* (pp. 421–449). London: Lawrence Erlbaum Associates.
Paniak, C., Toller-Lobe, G., Durant, A., & Nagy, J. (1998). A randomized trial of two treatments for mild traumatic brain injury. *Brain Injury, 12,* 1011–1923.
Paniak, C., Toller-Lobe, G., Reynolds,S, Melnyk, A., & Nagy, J. (2000). A randomized trial of two treatments for mild traumatic brain injury: 1 year follow-up. *Brain Injury, 14,* 219–226.
Park, N.W., & Ingles, J.L. (2001). Effectiveness of attention rehabilitation after an acquired brain injury: A meta-analysis. *Neuropsychology, 15,* 199–210.
Potter-Efron, R. & Potter-Efron, P. (1995). *Letting Go of Anger.* Oakland, CA: New Harbinger Publications, Inc.
Prigatano, G.P. (1994). Disordered mind, wounded soul: The emerging role of psychotherapy in rehabilitation after brain injury. *Journal of Head Trauma Rehabilitation, 10*(3), 87–95.
Pryse-Phillips, W.E.N., Boddick, D.W., Edmeads, J.G., Gawel, M.J., Nelson, R.F., Purdy, R.A. et al. (1998). Guidelines for the Non-Pharmacologic Management of Migraine in Clinical Practice. *Canadian Medical Association Journal, 159,* 47–54.
Raskin, S.A. (2000a). Memory. In S.A. Raskin & C.A. Mateer (Eds.), *Neuropsychological Management of Mild Traumatic Brain Injury* (pp. 93–112). New York: Oxford University Press.
Raskin, S.A. (2000b). Executive functions. In S.A. Raskin & C.A. Mateer (Eds.), *Neuropsychological Management of Mild Traumatic Brain Injury* (pp. 113–133). New York: Oxford University Press.
Raskin, S.A. & Stein, P.A. (2000). Depression. In S.A. Raskin & C.A. Mateer (Eds.), *Neuropsychological Management of Mild Traumatic Brain Injury* (pp. 157–170). New York: Oxford University Press.
Reitan, R.M., & Wolfson, D. (1999) The two faces of mild head injury. *Archives of Clinical Neuropsychology, 14,* 191–202.
Reitan, R.M., & Wolfson, D. (2000). *Mild Head Injury: Intellectual, Cognitive, and Emotional Consequences.* Tucson: Neuropsychology Press.
Relander, M., Troupp, H., & Bjorkesten, G. (1972). Controlled trial of treatment fo cerebral concussion. *British Medical Journal, 4,* 777–279.
Richter, K.J., Cowan, D.M., & Kaschalk, S.M. (1995). A Protocol for Managing Pain, Sleep Disorder, and Associated Psychological Sequelae of Presumed Mild Head Injury. *Journal of Head Trauma Rehabilitation 10,* 7–15.
Rotella, B. & Cullen, B. (1995). *Golf Is Not a Game of Perfect.* Toronto: Simon & Schuster.
Ruff, R.M. (1999). Discipline-specific approach versus individual care. In N.R. Varney & R.J. Roberts (Eds.), *The Evaluation and Treatment of Mild Traumatic Brain Injury* (pp. 99–113). London: Lawrence Erlbaum Associates.

Ruff, R.N., Camenzuli, L., & Mueller, J. (1996). Miserable Minority: Emotional Risk Factors that Influence the Outcome of Mild Traumatic Brain Injury. *Brain Injury*, *10*, 551–565.

Stambrook, M., Moor, A.D., Gill, D., & Peters, L.C. (1994). Family adjustment following traumatic brain injury: A system-based, life cycle approach. In M.A.J. Finlayson & S.H. Garner (Eds.), *Brain Injury Rehabilitation: Clinical Considerations*. Baltimore: Williams & Wilkins.

Taylor, J., & Taylor, S. (1997). *Psychological Approaches to Sports Injury Rehabilitation*. Gaithersburg, Maryland: Aspen Publishers, Inc.

Teasdale, G.M., Jorgensen, O.S., Ripa, C., Nielsen, A.S., & Christensen, A.-L. (2000). Apolipoprotein E and subjective symptomatology following brain injury rehabilitation. *Neuropsychological Rehabilitation, 10*, 151–166.

Teasdale, G.M., Nicoll, J.A.R., Murray, G., & Fiddes, M. (1997). Association of apolipoprotein E polymorphism with outcome after head injury. *The Lancet, 350,* 1069–1071.

Uomoto, J.M. & Essleman, B.C. (1993). Trauamtic Brain Injury and Chronic Pain: Differential Types and Rates by Head Injury Severity. *Archives of Physical Medicine and Rehabilitation, 74,* 61–64.

Zasler, N. (2000). Medical aspects. In S.A. Raskin, & C.A. Mateer (Eds.), *Neuropsychological Management of Mild Traumatic Brain Injury* (pp. 23–38). New York: Oxford University Press.

Chapter 23

CULTURAL ASPECTS OF NEUROPSYCHOLOGICAL EVALUATIONS IN SPORTS

Ruben J. Echemendia
Psychological and Neurobehavioral Associates
State College Pennsylvania

The role of linguistic and cultural influences on neurocognitive functioning has often been overlooked in clinical neuropsychology despite evidence suggesting the importance of these variables. Some have argued that neuropsychology has ignored these variables because of the belief that neurocognitive functioning is largely immune to effects of culture. Others have suggested that neuropsychology, as a relatively new science, has had to focus on understanding more "basic" issues (Ardila, Roselli & Puente, 1994). The study of culture presumably occurs as the science matures. Given the increasing maturity of our science and the increasing cultural diversity that is evident in the U.S., a greater focus on cultural factors in neuropsychology has been evident over the last decade.

Sports represent a truly worldwide phenomenon. Anyone who has watched the opening ceremonies of the Olympic Games can't escape an appreciation for the cultural diversity that exists within sports. Indeed, it can be argued that sports have a culture all their own and that this culture may interact with ethnocultural differences in many unknown ways. The impact of culture on neuropsychological variables can be studied in many ways. A cross-cultural perspective can be adopted that examines differences across countries. A related, but distinctly different approach is to examine ethnocultural differences within a given country. Because of space limitations, the focus of this chapter will be to discuss the influences of culture on neuropsychological assessment with athletes in North America.

At the outset, it is important to define some of the variables that will be presented. Culture is a complex, multifaceted concept. Bernal and Gutierrez (1988) have described culture as a "dynamic" process that includes the social transmission of ideas, attitudes, and traits that condition social behavior. Echemendia and his colleagues (Echemendia, Harris, Congett, Diaz & Puente, 1997) suggested that culture has often been inadequately defined within neuropsychology. This has led to confusion between the concept of culture and other variables such as education, language, and socio-economic status. Harris, Echemendia, Ardila and Rosselli (Harris, 2001) discuss the differences between cultural values and cognitive values. Whereas culture dictates what is and is not situationally relevant by providing models for ways of behaving, feeling, thinking and communicating, cognitive values reflect the skills and abilities that are valued by a given society. Harris et al. also remind us that within any given culture there may be multiple cultures and societies, which creates a situation where intracultural variability in cognitive functioning may be as great or greater than cross-cultural differences.

In this chapter, linguistic differences refer to differences that occur in written and spoken language between two groups of people, i.e. when an athlete's language differs from the majority culture (e.g. speaking Czech or French within the U.S.). Ethnic or ethnocultural differences refer to cultural differences that exist between peoples of different ethnic or racial backgrounds within a majority culture. For example, Latinos or Russians within the North America U.S. census data clearly underscore the increasing ethnic diversity within the U.S. In fact, ethnic "minority" groups are now the majority in certain areas, e.g. Los Angeles, Miami-Dade County. Within North America, the athletes involved in sports represent the diversity that exists within our populations. This diversity is much more obvious at the professional level because many professional sports recruit worldwide. For example, soccer is the most widely played sport in the world and foreign-born players represent a sizable proportion of the professional athletes on U.S. teams. Data provided by the National Hockey League Player's Association (NHLPA) indicate that 84% of the NHL players during the 1997–98 season were foreign born. Players were born in the following countries: Canada, USA, Czech Republic, Soviet Union, Sweden, Finland, Russia, Germany, Slovakia, England, Lithuania, Poland, Belarus, Latvia, N. Ireland and the Ukraine. Baseball, often described as America's pastime, is increasingly played at the professional level by athletes from Latin America, South America, and Japan. Many international athletes often view sports as their "ticket" to America and the financial prosperity that is expected to come with professional contracts and endorsement deals.

Although the most visible, the diversity noted above is not restricted to professional sports. Many elite college programs recruit heavily from the international scene. It is not unusual for international students to participate in ice hockey, soccer, tennis, rugby, and baseball, among others. As only one example, the Penn State men's soccer team currently has student-athletes from the U.S., Finland, England, Brazil, Angola, and Ireland.

The Challenges

The cultural diversity that exists within our population presents interesting challenges to the practice of neuropsychology in sports. These challenges include language differences, differences in acculturation, different experiences with medical personnel, and differences in motivation to play sports. For ease of presentation each of these factors will be discussed independently, although they are all clearly interdependent.

Language differences represent the most significant challenge to English-speaking neuropsychologists. At a very basic level there may be significant problems for the neuropsychologist and athlete in simply understanding each other. One needs only to attend the training camp of an NHL team to appreciate the barriers to communication that exist between a U.S. neuropsychologist and a young (usually 18 to 21 year old) foreign-born player who just arrived in the U.S. the morning of training camp. These basic communication barriers are then compounded by the fact that the tests that neuropsychologists use are almost exclusively English-based and generally only have U.S. based norms. In addition to the language differences and the use of English-based tests, there exist differences in acculturation.

Acculturation refers to the process by which a foreign-born individual becomes exposed to and adopts cultural influences from the host culture. For example, the extent to which a player from Argentina becomes more conversant in English, listens to English music, wears U.S. fashions, enjoys North American cuisine, etc. Differences in acculturation often highlight the variability that exists regarding the role of medical personnel across cultures. Americans are accustomed to first-rate medical care that involves many different types of testing, including cognitive testing when needed. Whereas it is commonplace in the U.S. educational and medical system, many foreign-born athletes have not been exposed to any type of standardized testing, particularly when it includes the word "psychology". The experience may be confusing at best, and quite frightening at worse. Since neuropsychological testing in sports usually occurs in the context of a "concussion" program or following head injury, the confusion for players is confounded by the fact that concussions are viewed very differently around the world. For some countries and sports, concussions are just "part of the game" and not much to be alarmed about. For example, there are many European Athletic Trainers in soccer who believe that Americans may be making "much to do about nothing" when it comes to concussions and heading.

Differences in the reasons for emigrating to the U.S. compound the problems with language, psychometric issues, and acculturation that have been discussed above. Some athletes come to the U.S. to play sports at a higher or different level than they can play back home. Some come from relatively comfortable backgrounds with relatively high levels of education and want to be part of a professional league because of their love of the game, financial compensation packages, and the prestige. Still others view sports in the U.S.

as a mechanism for escaping political, economic or religious oppression. For these individuals, coming to the U.S. is more than a chance to play "in the big leagues," it is a chance to dramatically change their lives and the lives of their families. For example, take a young Cuban baseball player who has defected to the U.S. or illegally entered the U.S. borders in the hope of securing a professional contract. It is quite likely that this young man will feel threatened by a set of alien tests that may be perceived to be barriers to his obtaining a contract.

Taken together, these issues of cultural diversity are exceedingly complex and may impact neuropsychological testing in myriad ways. It is often the case that when the complexity of cultural issues is discussed in neuropsychology, the neuropsychologist easily feels overwhelmed and decides that it is better to not take on the challenge. Although the easier route to take, it is unlikely that failure to tackle these issues will move neuropsychology forward into new areas of both science and practice. Sports represent a new and exciting application of neuropsychological science with significant economic implications (Echemendia, Lovell & Barth, 2003). Cultural and linguistic diversity is inherent in sports. If our profession wishes to apply its science and practice to sports, we must accept the challenge of not only "dealing with" cultural issues but also generating novel solutions that can be applied beyond the realm of sports.

The Solutions

Ideally, every foreign-born athlete will be tested in his or her native language by a multicultural neuropsychologist who has an in-depth appreciation for the athlete's subculture, who preferably has played the same sport, at the same level, and uses tests specifically developed for that (sub)culture. All test data would be interpreted using norms derived specifically for that culture (adjusted for age, education, and sex). Unfortunately, reality rarely approximates the ideal and many trade-offs have to be made. The goal is to only make those trade-offs that are absolutely necessary while attempting to maximize the reliability of our approaches and the validity of the interpretations.

The most basic approach to minimizing many of the issues discussed above is to conduct baseline testing of each athlete. As discussed in Chapter 16 in this volume (Macciocchi & Barth), baseline testing allows for the control of many confounding variables. Baseline testing provides the opportunity for intra-individual comparisons and thus the athlete is always used as his or her own control. In this sense, baseline testing can mitigate many of the issues discussed earlier. Since the athlete is generally not compared to others from different cultures, there is lees concern regarding the adequacy of noems. However, baseline testing cannot completely account for the effects of acculturation in the foreign-born athlete. As the athlete spends more time in North America and becomes more accustomed to the U.S. culture, it is likely that his or her neurocognitive test scores will change. If the extent of this change is unknown, then post-injury data that show an improvement from baseline may be erroneously interpreted as a recovery of neurocognitive functioning as opposed to an increase simply due to greater levels of acculturation. In addition developmental or maturational changes that may also be an issue when testing relatively young players (e.g. 18 year olds).

A possible solution to this challenge is to repeat the baseline testing more frequently for foreign-born athletes. There are no empirical data that identify the most appropriate interval for testing. However, one possible approach is to test players new to North America yearly for the first three years that they are in the U.S. Thereafter, they could be tested every three years. Given the issue of maturation discussed above, it would be advantageous to test all players every three years.

Although a player may be tested yearly for their first three years in the U.S., the neuropsychologist is still faced with that young player who does not speak English fluently (if at all). It is at this point that adaptation and flexibility are required. The first issue involves test selection. Tests should be selected that are relatively easy to administer and that do not rely heavily on language processes. Generally, non-verbal tests like the Brief Visuospatial Memory Test or the PSU Cancellation Test are thought to have less variance due to culture than do language-based tests like the Hopkins Verbal Learning Test. One approach that has been used by the NHL Neuropsychological Testing program appears to be successful. The NHL project adjusts the standard battery when testing athletes who are not fluent in English by dropping the two most verbally oriented tests (Verbal Fluency and HVLT). Preliminary data suggest that there generally were no differences between English-speakers and Non-English speakers on this adjusted battery . One interesting difference did occur. There was a significant difference between Eastern European players and all the other players on the SDMT, with athletes from Eastern Europe having lower scores than other athletes. This finding is understandable in light of the difference in the alphanumeric systems of these groups.

Although reliance on performance based tests is one approach to minimizing cultural differences, it is important to underscore that no test is "culture-free" and that the neuropsychologist must be constantly vigilant for culture-based variance in the data. Indeed, Harris and Echemendia (Harris, 2001) recently reported that even among bilinguals, differences exist in performance-based scores as a function of language preference. Using the WAIS-III and WMS-III standardization samples (and oversamples) they found that native Spanish speakers (born outside of the U.S.) who were functionally bilingual and preferred to speak Spanish had significantly lower scores on the perceptual organization and processing speed factors even after adjustments for age, education, sex and ethnicity.

In addition to using each athlete as his or her own control, large-scale projects can generate normative data that can be used for normative comparisons. An ideal situation is that of the NHL where data are being gathered for the population of players, not just a sample. These data will contribute significantly to our understanding of cultural variables in sports neuropsychology.

The performance-based tests noted earlier often lend themselves to non-verbal (pantomime) administrative instructions. For example, the Color Trails Test has an instruction section that is specifically designed for non-verbal instructions. Yet there are some circumstances that do not lend themselves to pantomime (demonstration). For example, symptom reporting cannot be done by pantomime. There are two approaches that can be taken in this situation. The first approach involves translating and culturally adapting a symptom scale into a variety of languages. The processes described by Geisinger (Geisinger, 1994) should be followed in order to assure an adequate adaptation. The gold standard is to provide appropriately adapted tests for each language and culture represented in the sport. Although this standard serves as the ideal, it is beyond practicality in most sports programs at the present time.

The second solution to these language barriers involves the use of translators. Using translators is a highly controversial topic with many excellent points made on either side of the debate. The most salient issue with translators is that a neuropsychologist never fully knows that adequacy of the translation/adaptation unless he or she is fluent in the language. Since translators in sports are often other players, the neuropsychologist is also never sure of the extent to which the translator is attempting to "help" the player and changes his or her answer. For these reasons it is recommended that translators NOT be used to provide extemporaneous translations of neuropsychological tests.

However, there may be some situations in which the use of a translator for non-test data is inevitable. One case involves filling out background questionnaires and symptom checklists that have not been translated/culturally adapted. The other case involves gathering concussion history information from a foreign-born player, or more likely, taking a history from a non-English speaking foreign-born player following a concussion. In this case the use of a translator is all but inevitable. In order to minimize error due to translation it is useful for the neuropsychologist to identify and build a relationship with veteran bilingual team members. These veterans tend to be protective of younger players and are very willing to help out when needed. It is helpful to meet with these senior players, discuss the nature and purpose of the evaluations, and enlist their cooperation in generating well-informed translations/adaptations. This approach has been quite useful in working with foreign-born players in the NHL. Although useful, the neuropsychologist must always be cognizant of that fact that there likely exists a significant proportion of error variance and interpretations of the data should be tempered by these limitations. The use of translators and non-standard test administration should be noted in any written summaries that exist of the testing.

Some neuropsychologists have argued that it is inappropriate to test non-English speaking individuals unless it is done by a bilingual neuropsychologist. Although there may be some merit to this argument in the general patient population, the unique approaches used in sports neuropsychology (e.g. baselines) help to render this argument as less relevant. Further, this argument often ignores practical reality (lack of well-trained bilingual neuropsychologists) and serves to stifle research and training. New clinical research programs in sports neuropsychology generally cannot make all of the cultural adjustments that are ideal. However, over time these adjustments can be made and incorporated into other projects. For example, the NHL project is now generating culturally adapted translations of post-concussion symptom scales into the major languages spoken in the league.

Cultural differences impact the testing situation with respect to demand characteristics and differences in interpersonal styles. Most players being tested for the first time are anxious. This anxiety is usually easily alleviated through education about the testing and rapport created by the neuropsychologist (e.g. using humor, "sports-talk", self-disclosures, etc.). Cultures vary in their emphasis on interpersonal relationships. Some cultures place a heavy emphasis on formality in relationships while others place a strong emphasis on informal, affect-based relationships. For example, Latino cultures place a premium on the notion of "simpatico" and expect a relatively close interpersonal relationship with medical personnel. Trust is established through the development of the relationship. It is very important for the neuropsychologist to become aware of these cultural differences and to keep these differences in mind when evaluating players. This is particularly important when evaluating players following a concussion. A strong word of caution is warranted. Simply having knowledge of a culture, even extensive knowledge of that culture, does not automatically make for a valid neuropsychological evaluation. Keep in mind that, by definition, cultural differences are identified by gross generalizations or stereotypes of each culture. There is often greater heterogeneity within a culture than between cultures. The neuropsychologist must always assess the extent to which the individual athlete differs from the expected cultural norm. As a rule, it is fair to start from the gross generalizations and then examine ways in which the player is different from that norm. This is commonplace in neuropsychology since we strive to understand how an individual differs from a statistical mean.

Lastly, there exists the culture of sports. Most neuropsychologists who work with athletes will tell you that "these people are different" from the standard neuropsychological practice. As a group they tend to be younger and healthier than the groups neuropsychologists usually work with. They are largely competitive, have a tremendous drive to succeed, and are very emotionally invested in their sport. They learn to play with pain, tend to hold a very traditional "macho" role, and view injury as a necessary part of sports. These factors influence testing by themselves but may also interact with ethno-cultural differences in ways that we have yet to begin to explore.

For example, is the "athletic culture" universal or does it vary by country of origin or by sport? Are there "cultural" differences between soccer, ice hockey, rugby, figure skating, etc.? These possibilities create many avenues for exciting research but also serve to keep us mindful of the many influences and sources of variation in our data.

Conclusion

Cultural differences in sports present a new challenge to neuropsychology because of the ethnic, national, and linguistic differences that exist among athletes. The complexity of assessing these athletes may be daunting and the solutions presented in this chapter are not fully satisfying. We face challenges with respect to linguistic differences, inadequate test and norm development, cultural differences related to views of medical personnel, as well as the possibility of an "athletic culture" or sport-specific culture. As a young science, there is more that we do not know than we know. Our task is to build on what we know while being forthright about the limitations of our knowledge. At present we cannot capture or explain a sizable proportion of the variance in our tests that is a function of cultural differences. However, through careful reading of the research literature, constant consultation with each other and other cultural "experts", we can begin to explain more of the variance and become a valuable resource for safely returning an athlete to competition.

References

Ardila, A., Roselli, M. & Puente, A. (1994). *Neuropsychological evaluation of the Spanish speaker*. New York: Plenum Press.

Bernal, G., & Gutierrez, M. (1988). Cubans. In L. Comas-Diaz & E. Griffith (Eds.), *Clinical guidelines in cross cultural mental health* (pp. 233–261). New York: Wiley Interscience.

Echemendia, R.J., Harris, J.G., Congett, S.M., Diaz, L.M., & Puente, A. (1997). Neuropsychological training and practices with hispanics: A national survey. *Clinical Neuropsychologist 11*(3), 229–243.

Echemendia, R.J., Lovell, M. & Barth, J. (2003). Neuropsychological assessment of sport-related mild traumatic brain inury. In G.P. Prigatano & N.H. Pliskin (Eds.). *Clinical Neuropsychology and Cost Outcome Research: A Beginning* (pp. 351–369). New York: Psychology Press.

Geisinger, K. (1994). Cross-cultural normative assessment: Translation and adaptation issues influencing the normative interpretation of assessment instruments. *Psychological Assessment* 6(4), 304–312.

Harris, J., Echemendia, R.J., Ardila, A., & Roselli, M. (2001). Cross-Cultural Cognitive And Neuropsychological Assessment. In H.J.J. Andrews & D. Saklofske (Eds.), *Handbook of Psychoeducational Assessment*. New York: Academic Press.

Harris, J.E., & Echemendia, R.J. (2001). *Testing the ethnoculturally diverse with the WAIS -III and WMS-III*. Paper presented at the annual meeting of the American Psychological Association, San Francisco, CA.

Chapter 24

GENDER ISSUES IN BRAIN INJURY

Jill Brooks
Sports Neuropsychology

Gender-related issues have come to the forefront during the past decade. As a result, research has begun to identify the influence of directly or indirectly sex-based differences (also referred to as sex differences). This chapter explores the importance of identifying the need for research into these differences from biologic, educational, social/cultural and policy perspectives.

Gender and Sex

The terms gender and sex are often used interchangeably. The Institute of Medicine, Committee on Understanding the Biology of Sex and Gender Differences stress the importance of defining both. The committee defines *sex* as "the classification of living things, generally male or female according to their reproductive organs and functions assigned by the chromosomal complement," and *gender* as "the person's self-represent-ation as male or female, or how the person is responded to by social institutions on the basis of the individual's gender presentation. Gender is shaped by environment and experience" (Institute of Medicine, 2001, p. 11). *Sex differences* refer to those differences between males and females that have primarily biological origins. *Gender differences* refer to differences that appear to be expressed in response to social influences. The committee noted, however, that it is impossible to know a priori the causes for particular differences between males and females. The distinction was felt to have merit signifying that society responds to individuals on the basis of their sex *and* gender.

The American Psychological Association (APA) publication manual defines *gender* from a cultural perspective, a term to be used when referring to men and women as social groups. *Sex* is defined from a biologic perspective, to be used when a biologic distinction is prominent (APA, 1994).

Biological and environmental delineations are not always clearly defined; implying that no interaction effect nor overlap can occur. The ability of research to look at sex and gender as part of a single system in which biologic and social elements come together to produce health outcomes has important implications for evaluation and treatment. In this way biological questions can be posed as a result of a scientific approach that examines how factors outside the body are translated into differences between males and females.

The History of Women as Research Subjects

The conjoint study of females and males has not been a well-established convention in scientific practice. Prior to World War II, clinical research was conducted primarily with men. It was assumed that beyond the reproductive system, differences did not exist between men and women at the cellular and molecular levels or these differences were not relevant. There was a general belief among researchers that men and women would not differ significantly in response to treatment in most situations. Males, particularly Caucasian males, were believed to provide the "standard" or "norm." There was a tendency to view females as being "deviant or problematic, even in studying diseases that affect both sexes" (Institute of Medicine, 1994, p. 8). The inclusion of women was felt to introduce additional variables (e.g. hormonal cycles), decreasing the homogeneity of the study population (Institute of Medicine, 1994). Despite the fact that the female hormonal cycle represented a significant confounding variable it was widely believed that men and women were similar enough to treat women with therapies developed solely on the basis of studies performed with men as subjects (Haseltine & Jacobson, 1997). There is still evidence to suggest that viewing the male as the norm remains in the current medical literature (Nicolette, 2000).

Justification for excluding females from clinical studies arose in part from efforts to protect them. Efforts to protect women intensified with the serious adverse events caused by thalidomide and diethylstilbestrol (DES) (Institute of Medicine, 1993, 1994). Despite the fact that thalidomide and DES incidents were not related to women's participation in clinical trials, it fostered an aversion to involving women of childbearing age in drug-related research.

In 1985, the U.S. Public Health Service Task Force on Women's Health Care Issues concluded that the quality of health information available to women and the actual health of women had been compromised by the historical lack of research on women's health care issues (U.S. Public Health Service, 1985). In response, the National Institutes of Health (NIH) issued a new policy in 1986 encouraging inclusion of women in clinical research, justification for the exclusion of women, and evaluation of data for differences by sex. Later investigation by the U.S. General Accounting Office (GAO) (1990) found these guidelines not implemented with regularity, however.

As a result of increasing public and governmental concern, the NIH issued a stronger policy statement on the inclusion of women and minorities in clinical studies and created the Office of Research on Women's Health (ORWH). In 1993, the NIH Revitalization Act (P.L.103-43) was passed authorizing guidelines for inclusion of women and minorities. That same year, the Food and Drug Administration (FDA) lifted its 1977 restrictions on inclusion of women of childbearing years in phase I trials, encouraging analysis of clinical data by sex but not requiring inclusion of both sexes in clinical trials (Merkatz et al., 1993). In 1998, the FDA published the Investigational New Drug Applications and New Drug Applications, allowing the agency to refuse filing of new drug applications not appropriately analyzing safety and efficacy data by sex. In 2000, the GAO reassessed the NIH's progress in conducting research on women's health since the publication of the 1990 GAO report. Significant progress was noted in implementing the policy of inclusion of women in clinical research and treating the policy as a matter of scientific merit in the research review process. The report indicated less progress in encouraging analysis of data by sex (U.S. General Accounting Office, 2000).

Limitations relating to the inclusion of women as human subjects has had an impact on the paucity of data in the area of women with concussions or more severe brain injuries. This, coupled with the idea that male brains represented the "norm" has resulted in limited information on the damaged and/or recovering female brain.

Sex Differences

With respect to sex, humans are generally dimorphic. With few exceptions persons are either chromosomally XX and developmentally female, or chromosomally XY and developmentally male. Gender, by contrast, is represented by a continuum. A person may display characteristics considered more typical of the opposite sex. In addition, an individual's sense of gender may change over the course of the lifespan. Gender identity and gender role can effect individual learning, activities, exposures, and access to experiences and care. Factors relating to sex and gender serve to affect health and can vary greatly across cultures.

Differences in the prevalence and severity of a broad range of diseases, disorders and injuries exist between the sexes. Some of the variations appear to be influenced by physiological differences, such as the role of sex hormones (e.g. cardiovascular disease and osteoporosis), while others appear to be related to experiential and environmental differences (e.g. smoking habits) as a result of occupation or recreational activities.

Examples of sex differences extend beyond the reproductive system and are seen in areas such as immune functioning; with females exhibiting a more aggressive immune response to infectious challenge. Women are also more likely then men to develop autoimmune diseases such as systemic lupus erythematosus. Gonadal hormones markedly affect immune and inflammatory cell responses, although women and men appear to respond similarly to infection.

Sex differences in pain perception have been the subject of significant research and review (Berkeley, 1997a,b; Berkeley & Holdcroft, 1999; Derbyshire, 1997; Fillingim, 2000; Fillingim & Maixner, 1996). Females appear more sensitive than males to nociceptive (potentially or frankly damaging) stimuli (Giamberardino, 2000). In studies of pain threshold and tolerance, female subjects report greater pain at high levels of stimulation (Ellermeir & Westphal, 1995; Mumford & Stanley, 1981; Robin et al., 1987). Gender differences in pain perception can be demonstrated using autonomic indicators of pain (e.g., papillary reactions) beyond voluntary control, suggesting that these differences reflect low-level sensory and/or affective components of pain rather than attitudinal or response bias factors (Ellermeir & Westphal, 1995).

In addition to greater sensitivity to pain, females exhibit a higher frequency of painful disorders. Of particular interest is the higher prevalence of headache in women including migraine with and without aura, chronic stress headache, cluster headache and posttraumatic headache (Berkeley & Holdcroft, 1999; Merskey & Bogduk, 1994; Rutherford, Merritt, & McDonald, 1979). Cartlidge and Shaw (1981) found a significant rate of posttraumatic headache (50% during hospitalization, 36% at discharge, 27% at six months, 18% at one year and 24% at two years post-trauma). Jensen and Nielson (1990) found similar rates of posttraumatic headache, with women being affected more than men (sex ratio of at least 5:1).

In addition to the physiologic aspects of pain, social and environmental factors come into play. In American society a more permissive atmosphere exists for women to acknowledge pain or threat of injury and perceived dysfunction (Taylor et al., 2000). Women tend to seek more and varied forms of health care, making use of these in a more positive, multi-dimensional manner, consequently deriving more relief than men (Affleck et al., 1999; Robinson, Riley, & Myers, 2000; Unruh et al., 1999).

One must caution against applying to individuals the group generality that females are more sensitive to pain. The existence and direction of sex-related differences in pain vary with different situations, such as point in the lifespan, testing paradigm or setting, type or location of pain, subject demographics, reproductive status, genetic profile, treatment utilization behavior and responses to different treatments, the way in which pain is measured (and by whom), and analgesics. Two separate issues emerge: determining what factors underlie what appears to be a generally greater female vulnerability to pain over the lifespan from a biologic perspective versus how being female or male contributes to individual and situational variations in pain and response to treatment (Institute of Medicine, 2001).

Sex differences in response to pain medications have been noted. Human studies suggest that μ-opiod drugs are more effective analgesics in young adult women (Berkeley & Holdcroft, 1999; Gear et al., 1999, Miaskowski, Gear, & Levine, 2000). Males and females use different strategies to reduce pain. Females bring a greater variety of coping strategies and therapies to bear on their pain, including drugs, somatic interventions and situational approaches (Berkeley & Holdcroft, 1999; Robinson et al., 2000). It is possible that females use smaller amounts of μ-opiods as they engage in other forms of effective coping strategies, consequently reducing their need for μ-opiods. It is also possible that males use more μ-opiods as this is the only relief they are able to find. Therefore, efficacy is not simply related to whether the opiod user is male or female, but is also influenced by sociocultural factors.

Sex differences may originate in events that begin in the womb. The fetal environment, especially hormones present during development has been shown to effect later behavioral and cognitive sex differences. Studies have suggested sex differences in brain structure size as the brain develops in children (Giedd et al., 1987; Lange et al., 1997).

Hormonal and physical changes at puberty have implications for sex differences in behavior in early adolescence. Increasing testosterone levels in boys are associated with increasing aggression and social dominance, and changes in estrogen level in girls associated with mood changes (Brooks-Gunn, Graber, & Paikoff, 1994; Buchanan, Eccles, & Becker, 1992; Finklestein et al., 1997; Schaal, Tremblay, Soussignan, & Susman, 1996).

Hormone levels themselves can be changed by behavior. For example, winning an athletic competition has been correlated with an increase in testosterone levels in males (Booth et al., 1989). Hormonal and physical changes occurring during puberty contribute directly and indirectly to differences between adolescent boys and girls.

Throughout the lifespan, there are sex differences in the brain's responsive-ness to sex hormones exerting influence on later behavior, including cognitive functioning. Maccoby and Jacklin (1974) postulated a classification delineating three general cognitive domains demonstrating sex differences: verbal, quantitative and visuospatial abilities. Consensus has emerged relating sex differences to specific patterns of cognitive function. In general, women demonstrate an advantage in verbal abilities, in particular verbal fluency, speech production, decoding language, spelling, perceptual speed and accuracy and fine motor skills. Men show an advantage on tests of spatial abilities, quantitative abilities and gross motor strength (Hampson & Kimura, 1992). Sex differences have been reported on tests of memory, particularly working memory with females exhibiting an advantage in recall of both verbal and nonverbal material including memory for visual information (Halpern, 2000; Hampson & Kimura, 1992).

Sex hormones continue to exert effects later in life. This has been seen with respect to cognitive abilities, especially the relationship between sex hormones in females and verbal skills. Sex hormones affect neural systems in women during their active reproductive and postmenopausal years and appear to enhance performance of skills usually performed better by females, with a decrement in performance noted in performance of skills usually performed better by males (Hampson, 1990a, b; Hampson & Kimura, 1988; McCourt et al., 1997; Moody, 1997).

Hormonal levels in women change during menopause when estrogen levels undergo dramatic decline after cessation of cyclic ovarian function. Animal studies suggest that estrogen positively affects basic neural processes and cognitive functions (McEwen & Alves, 1999). The influence of estrogen on cognitive functions in humans, especially postmenopausal women, has been more difficult to establish. Observational studies and clinical trials with women receiving hormone replacement therapy have been inconsistent (Barrett-Connor, 1998; Haskell, Richardson, & Horowitz, 1997; Rice, Graves, McCurry, & Larson, 1997; Sherwin, 1997; Yaffe, Grady, Pressman, & Cummings, 1998). The inconsistency may reflect differences in the ages of women studied. Several studies have found estrogen to have a positive effect on cognitive function at midlife (Shaywitz et al., 1999; Sherwin, 1997). Studies with older women have demonstrated more varied results, with some showing a positive influence of estrogen on cognitive function (Jacobs et al., 1998; Resnick, Metter, & Zonderman, 1997; Steffens et al., 1999) while others fail to show an effect (Barret-Connor & Kritz-Silverstein, 1993; Matthew, Cauley, Yaffe, & Zmuda, 1999). It may be that the effects of estrogen on cognitive function are observed most strongly when the agent is first introduced, an effect that has been reported in animals (Miranda, Williams, & Einstein, 1999). When effects have been observed they tend to be positive influences on verbal functions, specifically verbal memory and verbal fluency. Yaffe and colleagues (1998) followed postmenopausal women longitudinally; with cognitive functions evaluated at baseline and at six years. Measures of free circulating estrogen revealed that women with the highest levels of hormone were least likely to show signs of cognitive decline.

Shaywitz and colleagues (1998) studied postmenopausal women on and off estrogen replacement therapy. Tasks involving verbal and nonverbal memory were completed utilizing functional MRI (fMRI). The fMRI scans showed a significant influence of estrogen on neural systems for memory, demonstrating that brain plasticity continued into midlife. Berman and colleagues (1997) noted hormonal milieu modulates cognition-related neural activity in humans; directly testing the central nervous system effects of gonadal steroid hormones in young women by measuring regional cerebral blood flow (rCBF) as a marker of local neuronal activity. Control of hormonal state with gonadotropin-releasing hormone (GnRH) agonist leuprolide (Lupron) was coupled with a neuropsychological task targeting the frontal lobes, typically activating prefrontal cortex, inferior parietal lobule and posterior inferolateral temporal gyrus on PET scans. During treatment with Lupron alone (absence of gonadal steroid hormones) there was marked attenuation of the typical activation pattern even though task performance did not change. There was no rCBF increase in the prefrontal cortex. When either progesterone or estrogen was added to the Lupron regimen, there was normalization of the rCBF activation pattern with augmentation of the parietal and temporal foci and return of dorsolateral prefrontal cortex activation. This study demonstrated the first use of a PET activation paradigm to observe hormonal modulation of regional neurophysiological activity in response to cognition.

Fewer studies have focused on the effects of male sex hormones and cognition. Additional studies are needed to examine the possible relationship between male sex hormones and reported male advantages in spatial and quantitative functions. Gron and colleagues (2000) used fMRI to study brain organization during performance of navigational skills. Sex differences were noted in regions of the brain activated, with male brains demonstrating activation of the left hippocampus and females activating the right parietal and right prefrontal cortices. These findings provide a neural basis for observed sex differences in spatial performance.

Sex differences may also influence brain metabolic and plasma catecholamine responses to $\alpha 2$-adrenoceptor blockade. Activation of these receptors on cell bodies in the locus ceruleus reduces the firing rate of central noradrenergic neurons. Activation of presynaptic receptors on noradrenergic nerve endings inhibits neurotransmitter release providing feedback control of the noradrenergic system (Freedman & Aghajanian, 1984; Dennis, L'Heureux, Carter, & Scatton, 1987; van Veldhuizen, Feenstra, Heinsbroek, & Boer, 1993). Responses to $\alpha 2$-adrenoreceptor drugs can be influenced by estrogen concentration. These receptors appear to modulate release of several neurotransmitters implicated in the pathophysiology and treatment of mood and anxiety disorders. Sex differences are noted to occur in the prevalence of each.

Protective Effect of Hormones Following Injury

Emerging evidence suggests that male and female nervous systems respond differently to injury caused by stroke or trauma. Sex differences exist in the pathophysiology and outcome of central nervous system (CNS) insult with the brains of females consistently exhibiting less damage compared to their male counterparts (Roof & Hall, 2000). While some of these findings are believed to be due to female vasculature, relative neuroprotection has been attributed to the effects of gonadal steroid hormones. As a result, the efficacy of potential treatments for CNS injury may differ by sex. The effect of a clinical trial using aspirin for threatened stroke (U.K.-TIA study) showed a significant risk-reduction for men (48%) and no significant effect for women. In a phase-III clinical trial of the 21-aminosteroid antioxidant tirilazad, a sex-dependent effect was also found, with the drug significantly decreasing mortality and improving neurologic recovery 3 months following subarachnoid hemorrhage primarily in men ((Kassell et al., 1996).

The incidence of ischemic stroke is lower in premenopausal women compared to men (Barret-Conner & Bush, 1991; Sivenious et al., 1991; Wenger et al., 1993). The difference has been attributed to several factors including lifestyle, vascular differences (Berry, Wisniewski, Svarz-Bein, & Baez, 1975) direct and indirect effects of estrogen on the blood vessel wall (Miller, 1999; Mendelsohn & Karas, 1994; Farhat, Abi-Younes, & Ramvell, 1996) and other endocrine influences (Grady et al., 1992). Animal studies have indicated that the magnitude of injury following experimental ischemia is gender-linked with mortality and the number of brain lesions significantly higher in male animals following carotid occlusion (Alkayed et al., 1998; Berry et al., 1975; Hall, Pazara, & Linseman, 1991; Zhang, Altura, & Altura, 1998). Hall and colleagues (1991) have shown that the degree of neuronal loss in the cortex and CA1 of the hippocampus tends to be less in female gerbils following ischemic injury.

Circulating gonadal hormones and their effect on the injured CNS are felt to be at the heart of observed sex differences in neuroprotection. This hypothesis has been examined to a greater degree in cerebral ischemia than traumatic brain injury (TBI). The majority of reports suggest that females may be protected due to higher levels of circulating estrogen, although progesterone has been shown to exert protective effects as well. Estrogen's putative effects include preservation of autoregulatory function, an antioxidant effect, reduction of Aβ production and neurotoxicity, reduced excitotoxicity, increased expression of antiapoptotic factor bcl-2 and activation of mitogen activated protein kinase pathways (Roof & Hall, 2000).

One way to test the hypothesis that circulating gonadal hormones are responsible for sex differences in outcome from ischemic or traumatic brain injury is to remove the primary source of these hormones by studying ovariectomized or reproductively senescent females and comparing outcomes with intact females or males. Several studies with rats have indicated that the brains of the ovariectomized females were similar to males following temporary middle cerebral artery occlusion. Increased histopathology, neurologic dysfunction and mortality were noted relative to intact females (Alkayed et al., 1998; Zhang et al., 1998; Wang, Santizo, Braughman, & Pelligrino, 1999). Alkayed and colleagues (2000) found that infarct size following ischemia in reproductively senescent female rats did not differ from males. In essence, loss of circulating female sex hormones eliminated neuroprotection.

Roof and colleagues (1993) measured cerebral edema following cerebral contusion in rats. Normally cycling females exhibited less edema than males, and pseudopregnant females were virtually spared from post-injury edema. The presence of estrogen was not necessary for this effect. It was postulated that progesterone may improve the blood-brain barrier function post-injury either by influencing ion transport via Na+, K+-ATPase (Chaplin, Free, & Goldstein, 1981), by influencing the astroglial-inducer or the endothelial-effector cell components of the blood-brain barrier (Wolff, Laterra, & Goldstein, 1992) or by inhibition of vessel growth associated with leaky blood-brain barrier function following brain injury (Plum, Alvord, & Posner, 1963). A second study by Roof and colleagues (1994) demonstrated that progesterone injections following posttraumatic medial frontal contusive injury reduced edema and were equally effective in female and male rats. Progesterone is postulated to be a free radical scavenger (Betz & Coester, 1990; Olson, Poor, & Beck, 1988) and may act to reduce peroxidative damage. It appears to have a membrane stabilizing effect that reduces damage caused by lipid peroxidation. It may also provide neuroprotection by suppressing neuronal hyperexcitability (Roof & Hall, 2000). Thus, treatment may limit tissue breakdown and edema formation limiting secondary damage and cognitive sequelae.

Differential Injury Rates in Males and Females

Although opportunities for women's participation in sports and organized fitness have increased, little is known about the risks for injuries associated with increased physical activity and exercise for women. Injury incidence and risk factors associated with military training have been more thoroughly studied than in the civilian population (MMWR, March 31, 2000). Many civilian exercise activities have corollaries in military physical training.

Military studies of training-related injuries have identified shared and sex-specific intrinsic risk factors. Most of the injuries identified in basic training have been overuse injuries. Specific injuries (e.g. anterior cruciate ligament tears in the knee) have been found to occur more frequently in females. Studies of military populations suggest that the most important factor associated with injuries involved vigorous weight-bearing aerobic activity and aerobic fitness rather than female sex. Higher levels of exercise or physical activity are risk factors for injury due to increased exposure. To date, studies that compare injury rates between men and women with similar fitness levels have not been conducted in the civilian population (MMWR, March 31, 2000).

Powell and Barber-Foss (1999) reported on the type, frequency and severity of mild traumatic brain injury (MTBI) among ten high school sports activities during a three-year period. Football accounted for the majority of MTBIs (63.4%). Girls' soccer accounted for slightly more injuries than boys (6.2% vs. 5.7%) as did girls' basketball versus boys' basketball (6.2% vs. 4.2%) and softball versus baseball (2.1% vs. 1.2%).

Evidence from the Consumer Product Safety Commission National Electronic Injury Surveillance System (NEISS) database from 1990 to the present demonstrates different concussion injury rates for males and females. In softball and field hockey, a greater number of concussions were reported for females in younger age groups (ages 0–24) while males (ages 25–65 and up) experienced more injuries. This pattern was also noted for concussions associated with gymnastics. Concussions related to volleyball and rollerblading reflected greater injury rates in males for younger ages (0–14) than in females (ages 15–65 and up). A higher incidence of concussions in males were reported at all age levels for lacrosse and basketball (CPSC, 2000). These findings reflect data extrapolated from visits to hospital emergency rooms and most probably correlate with participation rates at the age levels reported.

The National Collegiate Athletic Association (NCAA) has collected data on sport injuries, including concussions utilizing the Injury Surveillance System (ISS) for the past seventeen years. Data collected for the 1999–2000 season reflected different concussion rates for men's and women's soccer games with women sustaining greater rates than men (11% vs. 7%). Data for women's field hockey games revealed a 12% concussion rate while women's basketball surveillance identified that concussions accounted for 10% of all game injuries (as compared with a 6% concussion rate in men's basketball) (NCAA, 2000). Higher concussion rates in female collegiate athletes has not been systematically studied. Speculation about underlying factors range from decreased neck muscle strength, improper technique, sex and gender based differences to issues concerning coaching, safety and rules.

In martial arts, 63% of severe injuries are cerebral concussions (Birrer, 1996). Men experience higher injury and severity rates than women (Zemper & Pieter, 1989). However, Paup and Finley (1994) found that the injury incidence rate for women was double that of men during the first 30 months of training. A Consumer Product Safety Commission study utilizing the NEISS system estimates significantly higher injury rates for males in all age categories, with lowest injury rates and severity for prepubertal sexes (U.S. Consumer Product Safety Commission, 1994). Increased incidence of head trauma has been described in Tae Kwon Do due to kicks. Zemper and Pieter (1989) reported that men sustain more concussions than women and that the dominant injury mechanism in both males and females was receiving a direct blow. The rates and distributions of judo injuries are the same for males and females; 20% of the injuries judged to be serious, the majority of morbidity and mortality related to choke holds, and brain and cervical cord trauma. Protective equipment in martial arts has been shown to significantly reduce injury rate and severity (Koiwai, 1979; Jackson, Earle, & Beamer, 1967).

Carson and colleagues (1999) explored the epidemiology of women's rugby injuries and concluded that the incidence of injuries in women's rugby was comparable with other women's contact and collision sports. Barnes and colleagues (1998) explored the concussion histories of elite male and female soccer players. Headaches, dazing injury and dizziness were the most common symptoms reported. Based on concussion history the authors reported odds of 50% that a male and 22% that a female would sustain a concussion in a 10-year period. Boden and colleagues (1998) looked at potential risks for head injuries, evaluating concussion rates in male and female soccer players. Over a two-season period, 59% of the concussions observed were in males and forty-one percent in females, resulting primarily from contact with another player's head.

Dryden and colleagues ((2000) found that the observed injury rate for women's recreational soccer players was lower than rates reported for male recreational and collegiate players. This observation was thought to be related to several potential factors including the absence of intentional body checking, mandatory facial protection, differences in the nature of the game coupled with body mass, speed and impact as well as gender-specific mechanical differences. Although not a major focus of the study, concussions accounted for the second most common injury to the head and neck area.

Outcome Research Following Traumatic Brain Injury

Gender and sex constitute substantial determinants of brain injury incidence (Kraus, McArthur, & Silberman, 1994). Few studies have provided detailed epidemiologic data on mild traumatic brain injury (TBI). However, studies show a higher incidence of TBI in males (Rimel, Giordani, Barth, Boll, & Jane, 1981; Kraus & Nourjah, 1988; Pentland, Jones, & Roy, 1986). Injury rates are two to three times greater in men than in women. However, higher case fatality rates were noted in women (Klauber, Barrett-Conner, Marshall, & Bowers, 1981; Kraus & Nourjah, 1988). Rates of poor outcomes including death, persistent vegetative state and severe disability were higher for women at 6, 12 and 18 months post-discharge. Most studies have focused on more severe TBI and not concussion, using data available from non-sports related injuries.

Several studies have demonstrated no sex differences in childhood incidence of TBI (Hahn, Fuchs, & Flannery, 1988; Henry, Hauber, & Rice, 1992). No sex differences were reported in older persons (> 65 years of age) (Pentland et al., 1986). However, two studies noted a slightly higher incidence of injury in women over age 75 and under age 5 (Kraus & Nourjah, 1988; Pentland, 1986). Farace and Alves (2000) completed a meta-analysis of sex and gender differences in traumatic brain injury outcome and were struck by the paucity of studies. Only studies reporting results separately for women and men were included. Outcome was worse for women than men for 85% of the variables measured. The authors postulated multiple factors that might influence outcome including: psychosocial factors, symptom reporting greater in females, sex differences in brain function, and/or sex hormones and metabolism impacting treatment effects. More importantly, the authors raised concerns about the potential for gender bias in referral and treatment, the limited data available on TBI outcomes for women and the effect this consequence can have on selection and effectiveness of post-injury treatment for women.

Higher incidence rates of post-concussive symptoms in females have been reported (Edna & Cappelen, 1987; Adler, 1945; Lidvall, 1974; Rutherford, Merritt, & McDonald (1977). Female gender has been noted to be a significant predictor of post-concussive symptoms at one month following mild

TBI (Bazarian, Wong, & Harris, 1999). Groswasser and colleagues (1998) reported that females sustaining TBI have a better predicted functional outcome at discharge from an inpatient rehabilitation program. It was postulated that an explanation resides in the different organization of brain functions in males and females (Kimura, 1987). Pyschosocial factors were believed to influence late outcome while predicted outcome at discharge was more closely linked to biological factors.

The area of traumatic brain injury outcome research remains fertile ground for study and analysis by sex and gender. The sparse amount of research is conflicting, but demonstrates different outcomes for women and men. Issues related to the interaction between biological underpinnings and social and environmental influences remain.

Education, Socialization and Gender Roles

The human brain is a tool for dealing with the social environment. Gender differences are apparent in areas such as communication, education and self-esteem. One of the purposes attributed to language is the transmission of culture. During childhood, children learn to behave the way people of their sex and age are expected to behave in their society. Socialization is the process of adapting one's behavior to that of the other members of one's social category.

Gender stereotypes are cognitive structures that contain the set of beliefs an individual holds concerning the supposed reliable differences between males and females (Cann, 1991). Gender expectations of parents begin to influence the perception of a child from birth with children less than a day old being described by parents in gender-typed terms. Girls have been described as softer, smaller and cuter than boys despite a lack of actual differences in physical size or responsiveness (Rubin, Provenzano, & Luria, 1974). In the cultural realm, contributions by individuals such as anthropologist Margaret Mead contradicted some of the western world's most cherished notions about child-rearing, family relationships and the role of women in society. In *Coming of Age in Samoa*, Mead observed that matrilineal societies allowed women and children greater freedom, producing greater self-respect. Most importantly, she asserted that gender roles were not innate, but culturally determined (Mead, 1928).

Education experiences have proved different for women and men. In 1792, Englishwoman Mary Wollstonecraft published her controversial book *A Vindication of the Rights of Women* in America. To counter the prevailing view that women's subordination was natural and inevitable, she insisted that education shaped character and argued that inequities in the educational system should be changed to make women strong and independent. Emma Willard, one of the first female educators in America, appealed to the New York state legislature in 1818, asking that taxes be allocated for the education of young women. The Troy Female Seminary, opened in September 1821, offering subjects comparable in rigor to the curriculum in the best men's schools. (Lunardini, 1994). In 1885 the American Association of University Women undertook their first study to dispel the myth that higher education was harmful to women's health (AAUW Report, 1992).

Our educational system mirrors our culture, the rules and beliefs of our society. Curriculum delivers the central messages of education and can serve to strengthen or weaken student motivation, effort and development through the presentation of images that students receive about themselves. Sex-role stereotyping is reduced in students whose curriculum portrayed males and females in non-stereotypical roles. Girls are often not expected or encouraged to pursue higher levels in math and science and are less apt to see themselves reflected in the materials they study (The AAUW Report, 1992). According to the AAUW report (1992) *How Schools Shortchange Girls*, not only do girls receive less attention from classroom teachers; teachers do more self-esteem building with boys. The report noted a tendency beginning at the preschool level, for educators to choose classroom activities that appeal to boys' interests and to select presentation formats in which boys excel.

Girls do not emerge from school with the same degree of confidence and self-esteem as boys. In a 1990 AAUW nationwide poll, interviewing 3,000 girls and boys ages 9 to 15, (*Shortchanging Girls, Shortchanging America)*, loss of self-confidence in girls was twice that of boys as girls move from childhood to adolescence. Teachers were noted to receive little or no training in gender equality from schools of education. In a 1993-94 review of articles and studies on girls and K-12 education entitled *Gender Gaps*, the most time spent on gender equity was two hours per semester. One third of education professors spent one hour or less on the topic (AAUW, 1998).

In a study completed by Brooks and colleagues (2000) female student-athletes at the high school level reported different levels of knowledge about concussions. Females tended to feel less informed than males from all potential sources (e.g. coaches, athletic trainers, the media), and reported a greater variety of symptoms, especially headache. Barriers to reporting concussion (to an athletic trainer or team physician) were different for females and males. Females viewed concussion as not being a serious phenomenon, while males were more concerned with not being able to return to play.

Sports and Gender Differences

Several studies have provided evidence of important gender differences in decisions about sports participation (Greendorfer, 1977, 1979, 1987; Greendorfer & Ewing, 1981; Greendorfer & Lewko, 1978). Family plays a crucial role in determining sports participation in children. In families where parents are actively involved in sports, girls and boys are likely to develop sports interests continuing into adulthood. However, at every age level, boys are more likely to be involved in sports than girls (Lewko & Ewing, 1980). Girls were found to garner little encouragement outside the family, unlike boys. In fact, for girls, the number of role models in terms of female coaches and athletic administrators is decreasing (Acosta & Carpenter, 1985).

The stereotype of a successful athlete embodies the qualities of drive, aggressiveness and self-confidence (Tutko, Ogilvie, & Lyon, 1969). These characteristics tend to overlap with the *typical male* (Cann, 1991). Many believe that the female athlete must possess qualities that contradict one of the two important social categories that she occupies (female or athlete). The implication of this contradiction is that the female possesses feminine qualities (so she must not be a very good athlete) or she is to be viewed as masculine (or less feminine). In either case there can be social rejection with a failure to meet either set of expectations (Eitzen & Sage, 1978; Felshin, 1974; Mrozek, 1987). The female athlete must combine two roles; that of female and athlete which can result in role conflict.

Staurowsky (1995) examined gender-based inequity in sport as reflected in the final report of the NCAA Gender Equity Task Force, identifying underlying ideological and structural frameworks in college athletics that supported a gendered division of labor in which male athletes, particularly football and basketball players, were perceived as breadwinners, whereas female athletes were regarded as passive consumers. The argument was made that these economic roles for males and females in sport, give rise to powerful assumptions about the profitability of intercollegiate athletic programs.

Contributions in sports have set the stage for the development of the idea that women could participate and excel at sports. The evolution of sports and physical fitness in America involves two separate histories based on the sex and gender of the participants. Controlling social systems and attitudes toward women have influenced the acceptance and involvement of women in sports, with sports representing a microcosm of the larger social system (Cann, 1991).

The Women's Movement and Public Policy

Warner and Steel (1999) examined the effect of child gender on parent's commitment to gender equality. Results revealed that fathers' and mothers' support for public policies addressing gender equity was greater when parents had daughters only. The finding was stronger for men, suggesting that childrearing might provide a mechanism for social change; the connection of fathers and daughters undermined fathers' commitment to patriarchy. When men have sons only, they exhibit the least support for gender equity public policies.

Betty Friedan (1963) described "the problem that has no name" affecting women in post-World War II America as a vague feeling of discontent persisting despite having what science and popular culture deemed as their most fulfilling roles in life as wives, mothers and homemakers. This "cult of domesticity" might have continued unchallenged if not for the expanded role opportunities for women created by World War II, that were later retracted, resulting in a groundswell of boredom, and loneliness. *The Feminine Mystique* was the first book to discuss issues such as unequal salaries, limited opportunities for women, and women's powerlessness in both family and society.

On July 2, 1964, the U.S. Senate passed the Civil Rights Act of 1964, the most ambitious and far-reaching piece of civil rights legislation to date. Included in the act was Title VII, prohibiting employment discrimination, based on sex or race. The law provided for the establishment of the Equal Employment Opportunity Commission (EEOC), charged with enforcement of Title VII. Sex discrimination provisions were added to Title VII as a ploy to defeat the Civil Rights Act (Lunardini, 1994). An on-going struggle between Michigan Representative Martha Griffiths and the EEOC precipitated the founding of the National Organization of Women in 1966.

In 1972, Title IX of the Education Amendments Act was passed prohibiting sex discrimination in educational programs or activities at any educational institution that receives federal funds. The law prohibited discrimination against women in secondary and post-secondary educational institutions, eliminating quotas on admission of female students to law, medicine and business schools. Title IX required that girls and women have access to the same opportunities as boys and men playing varsity sports. It opened high school and college coaching and athletic management professions to women and allowed them to pursue the educational credentials needed for career interests in sports.

In the year prior to passage of Title IX, only 1 in 27 high school girls participated in varsity sports. By 1998, that figure was 1 in 3, nearly equal to male sports participation at the high school level (1 in 2) (NJSIAA, 2000). According to the National Collegiate Athletic Association (NCAA), only 31,852 females participated in sports during the 1971-72 school year. Five years later, during the 1976-77 school year, one season prior to mandatory compliance with Title IX, that figure more than doubled to 64,375. During the 1998-99 season there were 145,832 female athletes playing on teams sanctioned by the NCAA. The number of male sports participants during the 1971-72 season was 172,447. Male sports participation rose to 201,063 during the 1984-85 season and 211,273 during the 1998-99 season (NCAA, 2000).

In 1987 the NCAA reestablished the Committee on Women's Athletics to study opportunities for women at the institutional, conference and national levels and issues directly affecting women's collegiate athletes. In 1991, Judith Sweet became the first female president of the NCAA, That year, the NCAA surveyed its member institutions on expenditures for women's and men's athletic programs, noting inequities. With publication of that study, the NCAA established the Gender-Equity Task Force, charged with defining gender equity, examining NCAA policies, and recommending a path toward realizing gender equity in intercollegiate athletics (NCAA Gender-Equity Task Force, 2001). In 1994, the U.S. Congress passed the Equity in Athletics Disclosure Act (EADA) requiring coeducational institutions of higher education participating in federal student financial aid programs and sponsors of intercollegiate athletic programs to provide specific information on those programs. However, men continued to receive at least two-thirds of the budget in all divisions except I-AAA. In all divisions granting scholarships, approximately 60% went to males. Male head coaches receive approximately 60% of salary expenditures (NCCA, Gender Equity Report, 1999).

In summary, gender inequities continue to exist at the player-athlete and coaching levels. To date only 20% of high schools and colleges are currently in full compliance with Title IX. Boys continue to receive twice the participation opportunities, scholarship dollars and athletic program benefits (Women's Sports Foundation, 2000). Training, education and sports participation opportunities are affected by lack of compliance with Title IX as are coaching, safety, practice and game schedules. These issues play a significant role in health of the female athlete as well as risk factors for concussive injury and injury in general.

Women were excluded from Olympic participation in ancient times and the inagural modern day Olympics in 1896. In the 1900 Paris games, eleven women, less than 1% of participating athletes, competed in golf, tennis and yachting. Most of the women did not realize their events were part of the official Olympics. The 1996 Olympic Games in Atlanta produced the largest number of American female participants (277) in the history of the 100-year event. In that same year, U.S. women's basketball, soccer and softball teams won Olympic gold medals, marking the first year any country had won gold medals in all three events. In the 12 months following the 1996 Olympics three new professional leagues, two in basketball and one in fast-pitch softball were established. Women participated in 44% of all events in the 2000 Olympics in Sydney, Australia.

The media has played an important role in the presentation and distribution of images of female athletes. More recently, female athletes are portrayed as competent, successful and highly skilled, serving to increase the aspirations of girls and women to participate in sports. Corporations have changed their advertising campaigns from portraying girls and women in stereotypical ways to recognizing girls and women as serious athletes.

Summary and Conclusions

Gender and sex differences reflect an important fundamental variable in human research and should be considered when designing and analyzing basic and clinical research. Differences exist on the biologic, social and cultural levels. Different gonadal hormones at varying levels during the lifespan influence cognitive, emotional and physical attributes, neuro-protection, response to injury and potential outcome. Incidence and severity of traumatic brain injury appear different for males and females.

Sociocultural and environmental differences between females and males exist as well. Boys and girls often receive different messages based on gender roles and expectations from parents, educators, coaches and other role models in life. Significantly fewer role models exist for girls and young women than for their male counterparts. The ways in which boys and girls are educated fosters different perceptions and knowledge about health, injury and risk potentially resulting in different outcomes from the reporting of concussion symptoms to return to play decision-making and utilization of treatment strategies.

Rules for playing sports, protection and training for sports reflect gender differences. In parallel sports, such as men's and women's lacrosse head-gear is a rule for men but not for women (except for the goalie). Although the rules of play reflect differences, the composition of the stick and ball are essentially the same. Safety should reflect gender equity; unintentional and intention injuries occurs in men's and women's sports.

The study of neurologic and neuropsychological sequelae following concussion is in its infancy, with the majority of work focusing on men's sports. Further study of concussion injury rates in various sports, and recovery and treatment outcome responses is necessary and may lead us to designing different types of prevention, education and treatment programs based on sex and gender. It is clear that neuroprotection and hormonal influences reflect significant sex differences. This area of study holds promise for both prevention and treatment in the areas of mild and more severe traumatic brain injury.

The terms *gender* and *sex* have been used loosely and at times, inappropriately in reporting results. Sex and gender impact differences in injury rate and type, and health and illness demonstrating the influence of genetic, biologic and physiologic factors and environmental and experiential factors. Gender and sex reflect environmental and biologic definitions that are not always clearly or completely teased apart. The importance of looking at the interaction between the two cannot be underscored.

Sports participation in the United States was discouraged as inappropriate female activity prior to 1970. Now 55 million women regularly participate in women's sport or fitness (Women's Sports Foundation, 2000). Gender equity is crucial to the achievement of high standards for all students as equity deals with opportunity and outcomes. Girls and boys are not uniform groups, nor are their needs singular. Caucasians should no more be the model for which Hispanics and African Americans are measured than should boys be the model against which girls are measured.

References

Acosta, R.V. & Carpenter, L.J. (1985). Women in athletics: A status report. *Journal of Physical Education, Recreation and Dance, 56,* 30–34.

Adler, A. (1945). Mental symptoms following head injury. *Archives of Neurology, 53,* 34–43.

Affleck, G., Tennen, H., Keefe, K.F., Lefebvre, J.C., Kashikar-Zuck, S., Right, K. et al. (1999). Everyday life with osteoarthritis or rheumatoid arthritis: Independent effects of disease and gender on daily pain, mood, and coping. *Pain, 83,* 601–609.

Alkayed, N.J. Harukuni, I., Kimes, A.S., London, E.D., Traystman, R.J. & Hurn, P.D. (1998). Gender-linked brain injury in experimental stroke. *Stroke, 29,* 159–65.

Alkayed, N.J., Murphy, S.J. Traystman, R. J., Hurn, P.D., & Miller, V.M. (2000). Neuroprotective effects of female gonadal steroids in reproductively senescent female rats. *Stroke, 31,* 161–168.

American Association of University Women Education Foundation & Wellesly College Center for Research on Women. (1992). How schools shortchange girls. Washington, D.C.

American Association of University Women Education Foundation. (1991). Shortchanging girls, shortchanging America. Washington, D.C.

American Association of University Women Education Foundation. (1998). Gender gaps: Where schools still fail our children. Washington, D.C.

American Psychological Association. (1994). Publication Manual (4th ed.). Washington, D.C.

Barnes, B.C., Cooper, L., Kirkendall, D.T., McDermott, T.P. Jordan, B.D. & Garrett, W.E. (1998). Concussion history in elite male and female soccer players. *American Journal of Sports Medicine, 26,* 433–438.

Barrett-Connor, E. (1998). Rethinking estrogen and the brain. *Journal of the American Geriatric Society, 46,* 918–920.

Barrett-Connor, E. & Bush, T.L. (1991). Estrogen and coronary heart disease in women. *Journal of the American Medical Association, 265,* 1861–1867.

Barrett-Connor, E. & Kritz-Silverstein, D. (1993). Estrogen replacement therapy and cognitive function in older women. *Journal of the American Medical Association, 269,* 2637–2641.

Bazarian, J.J., Wong, T., & Harris, M. (1999). Epidemiology and predictors of post-concussion syndrome after minor head injury in an emergency population. *Brain Injury, 13,* 173–189.

Berkeley, K.J. (1997a). Female vulnerability to pain and the strength to deal with it. *Behavioral and Brain Sciences, 20,* 473–479.

Berkeley, K.J. (1997b). Sex differences in pain. *Behavioral and Brain Sciences, 20,* 371–380.

Berkeley, K.J. & Holdcroft, A. (1999). Sex and gender differences in pain. In P.D. Wall & R. Melzack (Eds.), *Textbook of pain* (4th ed.). (pp. 951–965). Edinburgh: Churchill Livingstone.

Berman, K.F., Schmidt, P.J., Rubinow, D.R., Danaceau, M.A., Van Horn, J.D., Esposito, G. et al. (1997). Modulation of cognition-specific cortical activity by gonadal steroids: A positron-emission tomography study on women. *Proceedings of the National Academy of Science, 94,* 8836–8841.

Berry, K., Wisniewski, H.M., Svarz-Bein., L. & Baez, S. (1975). On the relationship of brain vasculature to production of neurological deficit and morphological changes following acute unilateral common carotid artery ligation in gerbils. *Journal of Neurologic Science, 25,* 75–92.

Betz, A.L. & Coester, H.C. (1990). Effects of steroids on edema and sodium uptake of the brain during focal ischemia in rats. *Stroke, 21,* 199–204.

Birrer, R.B. (1996). Trauma epidemiology in the martial arts: The results of an eighteen-year international survey. *Journal of Sports Medicine, 24,* 72–78.

Boden, B.P., Kirkendall, D.T., Garrett, W.E. (1998). Concussion incidence in elite college soccer players. *American Journal of Sports Medicine, 26,* 238–241.

Booth, A.G., Shelley, A., Mazur, A., Tharp, G. & Kittok, R. (1989). Testosterone and winning and losing in human competition. *Hormones and Behavior, 23,* 556–571.

Brooks, J., Ivens, D. & Hammond, J.S. (2001). *Evaluation of attitudes and knowledge about concussions among female high school student-athletes.* Abstract presented at the American College of Sports Medicine Annual Meeting. June 2, 2001. Baltimore, MD.

Brooks-Gunn, J., Graber, J.A. & Paikoff, R.L. (1994). Studying links between hormones and negative affect: Models and measures. *Journal of Research on Adolescence, 4,* 469–486.

Buchanan, C.M., Eccles, J.S. & Becker, J.B. (1992). Are adolescents the victims of raging hormones: Evidence for activational effects of hormones on moods and behavior in adolescence. *Psychological Bulletin, 111,* 62–107.

Cann, A. (1991). Gender expectations and sports participation. In L. Diamont (Ed.), *Psychology of Sports Exercise, and Fitness. Social and Personal Issues* (pp. 186–214). New York: Hemisphere Publishing Corporation.

Carson, J.D., Roberts, M.A., & White, A.L. (1999). The epidemiology of women's rugby injuries. *Clinical Journal of Sports Medicine, 9,* 75–78.

Cartlidge, N.E.F. & Shaw, D.A. (1981). *Head injury.* London: W.B. Saunders Company.

Chaplin, E.R., Free, R.G., & Goldstein, G.W. (1981). Inhibition by steroids of the uptake of potassium by capillaries isolated from rat brain. *Biochemical Pharmacology, 30,* 241–245.

Dennis, T., L'Heureux, R., Carter, C. & Scatton, B. (1987). Presynaptic alpha2-adrenoceptors play a major role in the effects of idazoxan on cortical noradrenoline release (as change measured by in vivo dialysis) in the rat. *Journal of Pharmocologic Experimental Therapy, 241,* 642–649.

Derbyshire, S.W.G. (1997). Sources of variation in assessing male and female responses to pain. *New Ideas in Psychology, 15,* 83–95.

Dryden, D. Francescutti, L.G., Rowe, B.H., Spences, J.C. & Voaklander, D.C. (2000). Epidemiology of women's recreational ice hockey injuries. *Medicine and Science in Sports and Exercise,* 1378–1383.

Edna, T.-H., & Cappelen, J. (1987). Late postconcussional symptoms in traumatic head injury. Analysis of frequency and risk factors. *Acta Neurochhirurgica, 86,* 12–17.

Eitzen, D.S. & Sage, G.H. (1978). *Sociology of American Sport.* Dubuques, IA: W.C. Brown.

Ellermeir, W. & Westphal, W. (1995). Gender differences in pain ratings and pupil reactions to painful pressure stimuli. *Pain, 61,* 435–439.

Farhat, M.Y., Abi-Younes, S., & Ramvell, P.W. (1996). Non-genomic effects of estrogen and the vessel wall. *Biochemical Pharmocology, 51,* 571–576.

Farace, E. & Alves, W.M. (2000). Do women fare worse: A metaanalysis of gender differences in traumatic brain injury outcome. *Journal of Neurosurgery, 93,* 539–545.

Felshin, J. (1974). The social view. In E.W. Geber, J. Felsin, P. Berlin & W. Wyrick (Eds.), *The American woman in sport* (pp. 179-279). Reading, MA: Addison-Wesley.

Fillingim, R.B. (2000). In R.B. Fillingim (Ed.), *Sex, gender and pain.* Seattle: IASP Press.

Fillingim, R.B. & Maixner, W. (1996). Sex-related factors in temporo-mandibular disorders. In R.B. Fillingim (Ed.), *Sex, gender and pain* (pp. 309–325). Seattle: IASP Press.

Finklestein, J.W., Susman, E.J., Chinchilli, V.M., Kunselman, S.J., D'Arcangelo, M.R., Schwab, J., et al. (1997). Estrogen or testosterone increases self-reported aggressive behaviors in hypogonadal adolescents. *Journal of Clinical Endocrinology and Metabolism, 82,* 2433–2438.

Freidan, B. (1963). *The Feminine Mystique.* New York: W.W. Norton & Company, Inc.

Freedman, J.E. & Aghajanian, G.K. (1984). Idazoxan (RX781094) selectively antagonizes alpha2-adrenoceptors on rat central neurons. *European Journal of Pharmocology, 105,* 265–272.

Gear, R.W., Miaskowski, C., Gordon, N.C., Paul, S.M., Heller, P.H. & Levine, J.D. (1999). The kappa opiod nalbuphine produces gender-and-dose-dependent analgesia and antianalgesia in patients with postoperative pain. *Pain, 83,* 339–345.

Giamberardino, M.A. (2000). Sex-related and hormonal modulation of visceral pain. In R. Filligim (Ed.) *Sex, gender and pain* (pp. 135–163). Seattle: IASP Press.

Giedd, J.N., Castellanos, F.X., Rajapakse, J.C., Vaituzis, A.C., & Rapoport, J.L. (1987). Sexual dimorphism of the developing human brain. *Progress in Neuropsychopharmocology and Biological Psychiatry, 21,* 1185–1201.

Grady, D., Rubin, S.M., Petitti, D.B., Fox, C.S., Black, D. & Ettinger, B. (1992). Hormone therapy to prevent disease and prolong life in postmenopausal women. *Annals of Internal Medicine,* 1016–1037.

Greendorfer, S.L. (1977). Role of socializing agents in female sports involvement. *Research Quarterly, 48,* 304–310.

Greendorfer, S.L. (1979). Childhood sport socialization influences of male and female track athletes. *Arena Review, 3,* 39–53.

Greendorfer, S.L. (1987). Gender bias in theoretical perspectives: The case of female socialization into sport. *Psychology of Women Quarterly, 11,* 327–340.

Greendorfer, S.L. & Ewing, M.E. (1981). Race and gender differences in children's socialization into sport. *Research Quarterly for Exercise and Sport, 52,* 301–310.

Greendorfer, S.L. & Lewko, J.H. (1978). Role of family members in sport socialization of children. *Research Quarterly, 49,* 146–152.

Gron, G., Wunderlich, A. P., Spitzer, M, Tomczak, R. & Riepe, M.W. (2000). Brain activation during human navigation: Gender-different neural networks as substrate of performance. *Nature Neuroscience, 3,* 404–408.

Groswasser, Z., Cohen, M. & Keren, O. (1998). Female traumatic brain injury patients recover better than males. *Brain Injury, 12,* 805–808.

Hahn, Y.S., Fuchs, S., Flannery, A.M. (1988). Factors in post-traumatic seizures in children. *Neurosurgery, 22,* 864–867.

Hall, D., Pazara, K.E., & Linseman, K.L. (1991). Sex differences in postischemic neuronal necrosis in gerbels. *Journal of Cerebral Blood Flow and Metabolism, 11,* 292–298.

Halpern, D.F. (2000). *Sex differences in cognitive abilities* (3rd ed.). Mahwah, N.J.: Lawrence Erlbaum Associates.

Hampson, E. (1990). Variations in sex-related cognitive abilities across the menstrual cycle. *Brain and Cognition, 14,* 26–43.

Hampson, E. (1990). Estrogen-related variations in spatial and articulatory-motor skills. *Psychoneuroendocrinology, 15,* 97–111.

Hampson, E. & Kimura, D. (1988). Riciprocal effects of hormonal flucuations on human motor-perceptual-spatial skills. *Behavioral Science, 102,* 456–459.

Hampson, E. & Kimura, D. (1992). Sex differences and hormonal influences on cognitive function in humans. In J.B. Becker, S.M. Breedlove & D. Crews (Eds.), *Behavioral Endocrinology* (pp. 357–398). Cambridge, MA: Cambridge Press.

Haskell, S.G., Richardson, E.D. & Horowitz, R.I. (1997). The effect of estrogen replacement therapy on cognitive function in women: A critical review of the literature. *Journal of Clinical Epidemiology, 50,* 1249–1264.

Haseltine, F.O. & Jacobson, B.G. (Eds.) (1997). *Women's health research: A medical and policy primer.* Washington, D.C.: Health Press International.

Henry, P.C., Hauber, R.P., & Rice, M. (1992). Factors associated with head injury in a pediatric population. *Journal of Neuroscience Nursing, 24,* 311–316.

Institute of Medicine. (1993). *Veterans at risk: The health effects of mustard gas.* E. Lewiste, C.M. Pechura & D.P. Ralls (Eds.) Washington, D.C.: National Academy Press.

Institute of Medicine. (2001). *Exploring the biological contributions to human health. Does sex matter?* T.M. Wizemann & M.-L. Pardu (Eds.) Washington, D.C.: National Academy Press.

Jacobs, D., Tang, M.X., Stern, Y., Sano, M., Marder, K., Bell, K.L., et al. (1998). Cognitive function in nondemented older women who took estrogen after menopause. *Neurology, 50,* 368–373.

Jackson, F., Earle, K.M., & Beamer, Y. (1967). Blunt head injuries incurred by Marine recruits in hand-to-hand combat judo training. *Military Medicine, 132,* 803–808.

Jensen, O.K. & Nielson, F.F. (1990). The influence of sex and pre-traumatic headache on the incidence and severity of headache after head injury. *Cephalalgia, 10,* 285–293.

Kassell, N.F., Haley, E.C., Apperson-Hansen, C., Stat, M., & Alves, W.M. (1996). Randomized, double blind, vehicle-controlled trial of tirilazed mesylate in patients with aneurysmal subacrachnoid hemorrhage: A cooperative study in Europe, Australia and New Zealand. *Journal of Neurosurgery, 84,* 368–373.

Kimura, D. (1987). Are men's and women's brains really different? *Canadian Psychology, 28,* 133–147.

Koiwai, E.K. (1977). Judo. In J. Borozne, C.A. Morehouse, S.F. (Eds.), *Safety in individual sports, monograph 4, sports safety series* (pp. 37–42). Washington, D.C.:American School and Safety Association.

Klauber, M.R., Barrett-Conner, E., Marshall, L.F., & Bowers, S.A., (1981). The epidemiology of head injury. A prospective study of an entire community: San Diego County, CA, 1978. *American Journal of Epidemiology, 113,* 500–509.

Kraus, J.F., McArthur, D.L. & Silberman, T.A. (1994). Epidemiology of mild brain injury. *Seminars in Neurology, 14,* 1–7.

Kraus, J.F. & Nourjah, P. (1988). The epidemiology of mild uncomplicated brain injury. *Journal of Trauma, 28,* 1637–1643.

Lange, N., Fiedd, J.N., Castellanos, F.X., Vaituzis, A.C. & Rapoport, J.L. (1997). Variablitiy of the human brain structure size: Ages 4-20 years. *Psychiatry Research, 74,* 1–12.

Lewko, J.H. & Ewing, M.E. (1980). Sex differences and parental influences in sport involvement in children. *Journal of Sport Psychology, 2,* 62–68.

Lidvall, H.F. (1974). Causes of post-concussional syndrome. *Acta Neurologica Scandanavia [supplement], 56,* 50.

Lunardini, C. (1994). *What every American should know about women's history. 200 events that shaped our destiny.* Holbrook, MA.: Bob Adams, Inc.

Maccoby, E.E., & Jacklin, C.N. (1974). *The psychology of sex differences.* Stanford, CA: Stanford University Press.

Matthews, K., Cauley, J. Yaffe, K., & Zmuda, J.M. (1999). Estrogen replacement therapy and cognitive decline in older community women. *Journal of the American Geriatric Society, 47,* 518–523.

McCourt, M.E., Mark, V.W., Radonovich, K.J., Willison, S.K. & Freeman, P. (1997). The effects of gender, menstrual phase and practice on the perceived location of the midsaggital plane. *Neuropsychologia, 35,* 717–724.

McEwens, B.S. & Alves, S.E. (1999). Estrogen actions in the central nervous system. *Endocrine Reviews, 20,* 279–307.

Mead, M. (1928). *Coming of age in Samoa: A psychological study of primitive youth for western civilization.* N.Y.: American Museum of Natural History.

Mendelsohn, M.E. & Karas, R.H. (1994). Estrogen and the blood vessel wall. *Current Opinions in Cardiology, 9,* 619–626.

Merkatz, R.B., Temple, R., Subel, S., Feiden, K. & Kessler, D.A. (1993). Women in clinical trials of new drugs. A change in Food and Drug Administration policy. The working group on women in clinical trials. *New England Journal of Medicine, 329,* 292–296.

Merskey, H. & Bognuk, N. (1994). Chronic pain. In H. Merskey & N. Bognuk (Eds.) *Classification of chronic pain: Descriptions of chronic pain syndromes and definitions of pain terms (*2nd ed.). Seattle: IASP Press.

Miaskowski, C., Gear, R.W. & Levine, J. D. (2000). Sex-related differences in analgesic responses. In R.B. Fillingim (Ed.), *Sex, gender and pain* (pp. 209–230). Seattle: IASP Press.

Miller, V.M. (1999). Gender and vascular reactivity. *Lupus, 8,* 409–415.

Miranda, P., Williams, C.L. & Einstein, G. (1999). Granule cells in aging rats are sexually dimorphic in their response to estradiol. *Journal of Neuroscience, 19,* 3316–3325.

Moody, M.S. (1997). Changes in scores on the mental rotations test during the menstrual cycle. *Perception and Motor Skills, 84,* 955–961.

Morbidity and Mortality Weekly Report, March 31, 2000/49(RR02). Exercise-related injuries among women: Strategies for prevention from civilian and military studies. (pp. 13-33). Retrived October 15, 2000. from http://www.cdc.gov/epo/mmwr/ preview/mmwrhtml/rr4902a3.htm.

Mrozek, D.J. (1987). The "Amazon" and the American "Lady": Sexual fears of women as athletes. In J.A. Mangan & R.J. Park (Eds.), *From "fair sex" to feminism: Sport and the socialization of women in the industrial and post-industrial eras* (pp. 282–298). London: Frank Cass.

National Collegiate Athletic Association (1999). *Equity in Athletics Disclosure Act. 1997-1998 gender-equity report.* http://www.ncaa.org/ news/1999/199991025/active/3622n01.html

National Collegiate Athletic Association (2000). *The NCAA News: News and features, July, 31, 2000.* Retrieved October 3, 2000 from http:www.ncaa.org/news/20000731/active/ 3716n18.html.

Nicolette, J. (2000). Searching for women's health: A resident's perspective. *Journal of Women's Health and Gender-Based Medicine, 9,* 697–701.

Olson, J.J., Poor, M.M. & Beck, D.W. (1988). Methylprednisolone reduces the bulk flow of water across an in vitro blood-brain barrier. *Brain Research, 439,* 259–265.

Paup, D.C. & Finley, P.L. (1994). A comparison of male and female injury incidence in martial arts training. *Medical Science, Sports and Exercise, 26,* S14.

Pentland, B., Jones, P.A., & Roy, C.W. (1986). Head injury in the elderly. *Age and Ageing, 15,*193–202.

Plum, F., Alvord, E.C., & Posner, J.B. (1963). Effects of steroids on experimental cerebral infarction. *Archives of Neurology, 9,* 571–573.

Powell, J.W. & Barber-Foss, K.D. (1999). Injury patterns in selected high school sports: A review of the 1995-1997 seasons. *Journal of Athletic Training, 34,* 277–284.

Resnick, S., Metter, E.J., & Zonderman, A.B. (1997). Estrogen replacement therapy and longitudinal decline in visual memory. A possible protective effect? *Neurology, 49,* 1491–1497.

Rice, M., Graves, A.B., McCurry, S. & Larson, E.B. (1997). Estrogen replacement therapy and cognitive function in postmenopausal women without dementia. *American Journal of Medicine, 103,* 265–356.

Rimel, R.W., Giordani, B., Barth, J.T., Boll, T.J. & Jane, J.A. (1981). Disability caused by minor head injury. *Neurosurgery, 9,* 221–228.

Robin, O., Vinard, H., Verney-Maury, E. & Saumet, J-L. (1987). Influence of sex and anxiety on pain threshold and tolerance. *Functional Neurology, 2,* 173–179.

Robinson, M.E., Riley III, J.L. & Myers, C.D. (2000). Psychosocial contributions to sex-linked differences in pain responses. In R.B. Filligim (Ed.), *Sex, gender and pain* (pp. 41–68). Seattle: IASP Press.

Roof, R.L., Dudevani, R,. & Stein, D.G. (1993). Progesterone facilitates outcome of brain injury: Progesterone plays a protective role. *Brain Research, 607,* 333–336.

Roof, R.L., Dudevani, R., Braswell, L., & Stein, D.G. (1994). Progesterone facilitates cognitive recovery and reduces secondary neuronal loss caused by cortical contusive injury in male rats. *Experimental Neurology, 129,* 64–69.

Roof, R.L. & Hall, E.D. (2000). Gender differences in acute central nervous system trauma and stroke: Neuroprotective effects of estrogen and progesterone. *Journal of Neurotrauma, 17,* 367–388.

Rubin, J.Z., Provenzano, F.J., & Luria, Z. (1974). The eye of the beholder: Parents' views on sex of newborns. *American Journal of Orthopsychiatry, 44,* 512–519.

Rutherford, W.H., Merritt, J.D., & McDonald, J.R. (1977). Sequelae of concussion caused by minor head injuries. *Lancet, 1,* 1–4.

Rutherford, W.H., Merritt, J.D. & McDonald, J.R. (1979). Symptoms at one year following concussion from minor head injuries. *Injury, 10,* 225–230.

Schaal, B., Tremblay, R.E., Soussignan, R., & Susman, E.J. (1996). Male testosterone linked to high social dominant but low physical aggression in early adolescence. *Journal of the American Academy of Child and Adolescent Psychiatry, 35,* 1322–1300.

Shaywitz, S.E., Shaywitz, B.A., Pugh, K.R., Fulbright, R.K., Constable, R.T. & Menel, W.E. (1998). Functional disruption in the organization of the brain for reading in dyslexia. *Proceedings from the National Academy of Sciences of the United States of America, 95,* 2636–2641.

Shaywitz, S.E., Shaywitz, B.A. Pugh, K.R. Fulbright, R.K., Skudlarski, P., Menel, W.E., et al. (1999). Effect of estrogen on brain activation patterns in postmenopausal women during working memory tasks. *Journal of the American Medical Association, 281,* 1197–1202.

Sherwin, B.B. (1997). Estrogen effects on cognition in menopausal women. *Neurology, 48,* 521–526.

Sivenious, J., Laakso, M., Penttila, I.M., Smets, P., Lowenthal, A., & Riekkinen, P.J. (1991). The European stroke prevention study: Results according to sex. *Neurology, 41,* 1189–1192.

Staurowsky, E.J. (1995). Examining the roots of a gendered division of labor in intercollegiate athletics: Insights into the gender equity debate. *Journal of Sport and Social Issues, 19,* 2844.

Steffens, D., Norton, M., Plassman, B., Tschanz, J.T., Wyse, B.W., Welsh-Bohmer, K.A. et al. (1999). Enhanced cognitive performance with estrogen use in demented community-dwelling women. *Journal of the American Geriatric Society, 47,* 1171–1175.

Tutko, T., Ogilvie, B., & Lyon, L. (1969). *The Athletic Motivational Inventory.* San Jose: Institute for the Study of Athletic Motivation.

Unruh, A.M., Ritchie, J., & Merskey, H. (1999). Does gender affect appraisal of pain and pain coping strategies? *Clinical Journal of Pain, 15,* 31–40.

U.S. Consumer Product Safety Commission (1994). National Injury Electronic Surveillance System (NEISS). Raw data literature search requested.

U.S. Consumer Product Safety Commission. (2000). National Injury Electronic Surveillance System (NEISS). Raw data search literature search requested.

U.S. General Accounting Office. (1990). Problems in implementing policy on women's study populations. National Institutes of Health, *Publication Number: GAO/T-HRD-90-38.* Washington, D. C.: U.S. General Accounting Office.

U.S. General Accounting Office (2000). Women's health: National Institutes of Health has increased its efforts to include women in research. *Publication Number: GAO/HEHS-00-96.* Washington, D.C.: U.S. General Accounting Office.

U.S. Public Health Service (1985). Report of the public health service task force on women's health issues. *Public Health Reports, 100,* 73–106.

Van Veldhuizen, M.J.A., Feenstra, M.G.P., Heinsbroek, R.P.W. & Boer, G.J. (1993). In vivo microdialysisof noradrenaline overflow: Effects of α-adrenorecptor agonists and antqagonists measured by cumulative concentration-response curves. *British Journal of Pharmocology, 109,* 655–660.

Wang, Q., Santizo, R., Braughman, V.L. & Pelligrino, D.A. (1999). Estrogen provides neuroprotection in transient forebrain ischemia through perfusion-independent mechanisms in rats. *Stroke, 30,* 630–637.

Warner, M.S. & Stiel, A.L. (1999). Exercise and female adolescents: Effects on the reproductive and skeletal system. *Journal of the American Medical Women's Association, 54,* 115–120.

Wenger, N.K. (1994). Coronary heart disease in women: Gender differences in diagnostic evaluation. *Journal of the American Medical Women's Association, 49,* 181–185.

Wolff, J.E.A., Laterra, J., & Goldstein, G.W. (1992). Steroid inhibition of neural microvessel morphogenesis in vitro. Receptor mediation & astroglial dependence. *Journal of Neurochemistry, 58,* 1023–1032.

Women's Sports Foundation, (2000). http://www.women'ssportsfoundation. org/templates/res_center/rclib/results_topics2.html

Yaffee, K., Grady, D., Pressman, A., & Cummings, S. (1998). Serum estrogen levels, cognitive performance, and risk of cognitive decline in older community women. *Journal of the American Geriatric Society, 46,* 816–821.

Zhang, A.M., Altura, B.T., & Altura, B.M. (1998). Effects of gender and estrodial treatment on focal brain ischemia. *Brain Research, 784,* 321–324.

Zemper, E.D. & Pieter, W. (1989). Injury rates during the 1988 United States Olympic trials for taekwondo. *British Journal of Sports Medicine, 23,* 161–164.

Chapter 25

ETHICAL ISSUES IN THE EVALUATION OF ATHLETES

Elizabeth S. Parker[1],
Ruben J. Echemendia[2] and
Craig Milhouse[3]
[1]Clinical Professor, Neurology, College of Medicine, University of California, Irvine, Clinical Professor, Psychiatry and Neurology, University of Southern California.
[2]Director, The Psychological Clinic, and Clinical Associate Professor, Department of Psychology, The Pennsylvania State University
[3]Kerlan-Jobe Medical Group, Anaheim, California

Introduction

As a neuropsychologist working in the sports field, what would you do if faced with the following: the team trainer urgently calls you to give test results of a player you have just examined to know if that player will be in the lineup that night? – the head coach demands a copy of your post-concussion test report on one of his star players? – your payment for post-concussion testing requires a copy of your report on a player be sent? – the team physician is relying on your test results to clear a player after a concussion and the test results are ambiguous? - a player who speaks virtually no English is sent for immediate post-concussion testing? The purpose of this chapter is to help the neuropsychologist prepare for these and other situations in order to avoid serious ethical and even legal mishaps.

Sports neuropsychology is a new and growing field. Neuropsychologists must prepare to face a host of ethical questions for which there are no established guidelines (cf Bailes, Lovell & Maroon, 1999). We have addressed some ethical questions in an earlier chapter (Echemendia & Parker, 1999). This chapter is written for the clinical neuropsychologist who is about to embark on a relationship with an athletic team, either collegiate or professional. We shall review some of the points made in our previous chapter and discuss new ethical issues that have come to our attention. We provide some specific recommendations based on our experiences as an opening for further discussions among sports neuropsychologists and their medical colleagues.

As is noted in the Consultation in Sports Organizations chapter, the clinical neuropsychologist can play a variety of different roles with sports teams. For example, there is the neuropsychologist as researcher who is only involved in data collection and analysis, but with no clinical role. Ethical guidelines for the "pure" researcher are not discussed in this chapter but they are very important and the reader is referred to Section 6.0 of the American Psychological Association Ethical Guidelines (1992). Sports neuropsychologists, particularly those in university settings, often find themselves wearing two hats, playing the role of both researcher and clinician. The neuropsychologist may be a member of the faculty conducting research with athletic departments, while also serving as part of student health services providing psychological services to the team. Outside academia and collegiate athletic programs, sports neuropsychologists serve primarily a clinical role, evaluating athletes who have suffered some form of brain injury, typically related to their sport but sometimes related to extracurricular activities such as motor-vehicle accidents.

The focus of this chapter is on issues that arise when the neuropsychologist is part of the sports medicine team taking care of athletes in high-risk team sports such as football, soccer, ice hockey, basketball, baseball and lacrosse. As such, the players typically undergo baseline neuropsychological screening to provide comparative scores in the event of a subsequent concussion. The clinical neuropsychologist is responsible for the collection and interpretation of baseline data as well as neuropsychological assessments following injury.

Why Ethics?

There is a trend for ethical standards to become legally binding. Although ethics are the standards of professional practice that psychologists use as a guide to insure responsible and moral behavior, they can have legal ramifications as well. Ethical guidelines provide the neuropsychologist with set of principles and guidelines to check their professional activities to insure quality control, to prevent complaints of violations to ethical standards, to meet standards for their malpractice coverage, and to guard against legal entanglements. In California, ethics have become a matter of law. In the year 2000, the Laws and Regulations Relating to the Practice of Psychology for psychologists licensed in the state of California incorporated the American Psychological Association code of ethics (Section 2936, Rules of Ethical Conduct). Thus, a person found in violation of the APA Ethical Code can lose their license to practice psychology in California. This may soon affect other states as well.

Every neuropsychologist should familiarize themselves with the APA Ethical Principles and Code of Conduct, whether they are members of APA or not (membership is strongly recommended). They should also be aware of the proposed revisions published in the APA Monitor (2001). We cannot emphasize enough the importance of ethical considerations when participating in a new field. For it is the novelty and the lack of precedent with ethical considerations that increase the risk of inadvertently making a mistake that can have profound ramifications both to the practicing neuropsychologist and to the very parties whom the neuropsychologist is trying to help.

The Setting and The Participants

Most neuropsychologists entering the field of university and professional sports will find themselves in a new culture that could not be more different from the academic environment in which they were educated. Other chapters in this volume address various aspects of the novelty of situations in which the sports neuropsychologist might find him or herself. We shall summarize some issues we find particularly significant in terms of ethical questions and problems that can arise. Neuropsychologists will often find themselves under complex pressures exerted by teams, coaches, trainers, agents and players. Skill, speed and risk are what make many sports exciting, however they create an environment that can result in ethical mistakes for the unprepared clinical neuropsychologist. Neuropsychologists are advised to learn as much as they can about the culture, language, psychology, politics and economics of sports to understand the potential uses and misuses of the neuropsychological evaluation, the resulting report and consultation. The reader is referred to the chapter on Consultation with Sports Organizations for further discussion on this matter, particularly when the neuropsychologist is serving as an organizational consultant, rather than a player examiner.

In universities and colleges, athletic programs are a significant means by which the institutions gain an *esprit de corps*, and promote the institution as a cohesive entity. Athletic programs can generate sizeable incomes for the school. Media coverage of sports adds to the institution's visibility and for many potential students successful athletic teams increase the institution's desirability. Athletic programs can facilitate the educational mission of the school through the generation of increased revenues and scholarships. They can help athletes gain an education that they might not otherwise have had through athletic scholarships. For the athlete, success in collegiate sports can be the necessary step for going on to a lucrative professional career.

At the professional level, the revenue stakes and pressures increase. Indeed, the popular fascination with the economic, political and medical complexities of professional sports is the stuff of Hollywood movies such as Oliver Stone's "Any Given Sunday" and "Jerry McGuire". Both of these movies depict the popular culture and complex pressures brought to bear on the athletes and those who work with them. Sports agents are negotiating extraordinarily high contracts for players. Team owners and management are under pressure to generate revenues through advertising, and merchandising, and this requires successful team performance. The injured, sidelined player can be financially costly, particularly if the player is a star member of the team. Removing a player not only may hurt the team's chances of winning but it can also have significant impact on the player's signing bonuses. The situation becomes even more problematic when a player is taken out of play as the result of a concussion; an injury that cannot be seen directly such as a broken bone can be seen on X-ray or MRI.

In addition to the economic variables influencing contemporary collegiate and professional sports, there are unique and complex psychological variables that may be new to some neuropsychologists. The athlete is very different from the type of "patient" that most neuropsychologists see in hospital, clinical or private practice settings. One important difference is their drive to play their sport and the competitive way they attack neuropsychological tests. There is a considerable literature on malingering or "faking bad" performance on neuropsychological tests in clinical populations. We are not aware of any neuropsychological research on hyperperformance or on "faking good" which may be seen in athletes. Clinical neuropsychologists have little scientific or practical training with people who might have an interest in masking neuropsychological problems while putting themselves in a position to sustain further injury. This is one of the new issues about which neuropsychologists need to be aware when working in the sports field.

Neuropsychologists need to become familiar with the psychology of the athlete to appropriately interpret self-reported symptoms and neuropsychological test results. In this sense, athletes can be viewed as a special population as described in Ethical Standard 2.04 (Use of Assessment in General and with Special Populations). There are, of course, a variety of different subsets of athletes including those with learning disabilities, and in the case of professional hockey and soccer players, those who have limited to nonexistent English-language skills. Athletes accept a certain level of risk as part of their profession. They have to be able to play in spite of aches and pains that might disable a less driven person. They are stoics about physical and mental injuries. This creates many interesting but complex issues for the sports medicine team, particularly in the evaluation of concussions.

Some athletes approach neuropsychological tests as another competitive event. By way of illustration, one of us was testing a professional athlete for baseline assessment. The player was given the Symbol Digit Test and told to work as quickly as he could. He asked how long he had. When he was told he had 90 seconds, he looked at the page and confidently insisted he could complete the entire page of items in 90 seconds, a nearly impossible feat. Furthermore, he wanted to bet the examiner $500 that he could do so. Needless to say the bet was not accepted and the page was not completed, yet the player not only wanted to try it again but he also wanted to wager his $500. This kind of competitiveness and drive is rarely, if ever, seen in traditional hospital or clinical settings.

Another variable to consider is the personality of the neuropsychologist who is attracted to sports neuropsychology and their motivations for becoming involved in this field. Examination and reflection on his or her motivations may help guard against making poor ethical decisions for unhealthy, and often unconscious influences. Certainly there is little money for the direct clinical services the neuropsychologist provides as part of the sports medicine team. And there is no direct relationship between the fame or fortune of a team and the amount of money paid to its medical team. If direct financial rewards are not the motivator, what is? Very often the neuropsychologist is interested in the area of concussions. They may want to help players at risk for sustaining repeated concussions and prevent serious neuropsychological deficits that can ensue. They may be fascinated with the scientific questions raised about brain-behavior relationships surrounding concussions. Another driving force can be the neuropsychologist's love of sports and the sports setting. But neuropsychologists need to be careful about conflicts between the attraction to sports and our professional role. Some neuropsychologists may find that they share many personality characteristics with the athletes and need to guard against fast, pressured decisions that could eventuate in poorly thought out and ethically dubious actions. Other neuropsychologists may be attracted to the "star power" that surrounds successful athletes and athletic teams in this society. These neuropsychologists need to be prepared to stand up to and offer opinions that may be unpopular to the very institutions and athletic stars they admire. This can be a daunting task and there is a need to understand and prepare for such eventualities.

Defining The Role: The Player's Neuropsychologist

Many problems can be avoided by clearly defining the neuropsychologist's role. APA Ethical Standard 1.03 (Professional and Scientific Relationship) states that psychologists must perform their services only in the context of a defined professional or scientific role. In defining their role, neuropsychologists are generally well advised to consider the player as patient and unless specifically and explicitly engaged in a different role, conduct their services with the player's best interests in mind.

The position of the team clinical neuropsychologist can be modeled to some extent on that of the team physician. Often the team physician is hired by the team but their role is to be the treating doctor to the patient/player. The neuropsychologist is typically positioned as consultant to the team physician. When a player sustains a concussion, the team physician is responsible for evaluating the player and obtaining whatever consultations and tests he or she deems necessary to ascertain the best course of treatment for that player. Typically, the team physician is an orthopedist or orthopedic surgeon. They will decide if there needs to be a neurological consultation, neuropsychological assessment, brain scan, and/or EEG workup of the brain-injured player. The neuropsychological assessment can therefore be seen as one part of the overall evaluation of the concussed player.

In defining their role, neuropsychologists must be cautious to avoid multiple relationships that could impair their objectivity, find themselves practicing outside their defined areas of competence and possibly breaching confidentiality. Ethical standard 1.21 (Third-Party Request for Services) mandates that the psychologist clarifies at the outset of the service the nature of their role and the probable uses of their services. Moreover, if there will be limits on confidentiality, the player needs to understand this. In the simplest case, the team physician refers the player to the neuropsychologist, the neuropsychologist explains this to the player and obtains in writing the player's consent to examination and for release of the results to the physician (Ethical standard 4.02, Informed Consent to Therapy).

Informed consent by the player basically gives the neuropsychologist the structure of consultation and confidentiality. In a later section, we will be explaining the importance of cross-consultation. For now, we mention the issue of consulting with other neuropsychologists as this needs the informed consent of the player. In fact the player needs to understand and give his/her consent to each source where their information will be shared, including other neuropsychologists, insurance companies, team trainers, and of course, the team physicians. Ethical standard 5.02 (Maintaining Confidentiality) specifies psychologists' obligation to respect the confidentiality rights of their clients. Moreover, Ethical Standard 5.01 (Discussing Limits of Confidentiality) mandates that the neuropsychologist discuss confidentiality and its limits at the outset of their professional or scientific relationship with the client.

Even when the neuropsychologist explains to the player that the results will be sent to the team physician and discussed with other expert neuropsychological consultants, other parties are likely to become involved. The neuropsychologist is advised to be prepared for this and to prepare specific guidelines for communicating with the team, the trainers, and other parties that may want to know the test results. There is no single solution to these problems. It is critical that guidelines are developed at the outset and the players' consent be obtained to avoid breaching confidentiality and to prevent the neuropsychologist finding themselves with a conflict of interest situation.

Very often, team trainers, who are the medical eyes and ears of the sport medicine team, are under pressure to obtain test results in order to help coaching staff make decisions about whether a player is able to return to play. Teams differ in their approach to the neuropsychologist. Some teams and physicians prefer that the neuropsychologist communicate with both the athletic trainer and the team physician. Other teams prefer that the communication exist solely between the neuropsychologist and the team physician. Whatever the arrangement, the communication protocol must be clear to all parties involved, most importantly, clear to the player and with the player's informed consent.

Neuropsychologists need to be prepared for requests from the player to not discuss their test results with trainers and coaching staff. Failure to follow the agreed upon communication protocol could breach confidentiality (Ethical standard 5.02, Maintaining Confidentiality), and could find the neuropsychologist in the midst of multiple relationships (Ethical standard 1.17) for which potential harm could come to the player.

For example, let's suppose that the agreed upon communication protocol was for the neuropsychologist to discuss the case with the team physician. What harm could come from the neuropsychologist giving their test results to the trainer (Ethical standard 1.14, Avoiding Harm)? In most instances a problem does not exist if the player consented for results to be communicated. But let us take the very real situation where the neuropsychologist tells the test results to the trainer, the trainer tells the coaches and a player is put back into play for a game that same day, without the physician's consent. In this instance, giving the results to the athletic trainer could be seen as conflicting roles between working for the team/trainer and the player/doctor and in violation of the agreed upon protocol. The neuropsychologist might rightly be viewed as undermining the role of the physician and practicing outside the scope of his or her training. (Ethical standard 1.04).

When in Doubt, Consult

APA ethical guidelines are highly specific when it comes to issues of practicing in a new, emerging area of psychology. The very nature of psychology is that it is based on valid and reliable scientific data (see Preamble, para 1). Some aspects of sports concussion testing are based on a body of reliable, scientific data and some are not. The efficacy of the abbreviated screening battery continues to be assessed. Research is lacking on practice effects from repeated testing and how these practice effects influence diagnostic utility of the tests. The issues about learning disabilities and fluency with English as they affect test sensitivity to concussion effects have not been thoroughly examined. The relative sensitivity of self-reported symptom checklists and objective test performance is in need of scientific analysis. This makes it very important for sports neuropsychologists to communicate with one another about their practices, their test selection and their interpretations, basing decisions on current science and clinical practices until a better body of research exists.

Most neuropsychologists know that they should only provide services in the areas in which they have competence, and when they do not, they must seek appropriate training, consultation and supervision (Ethical Standard 1.04, Boundaries of Competence). There are many avenues by which the neuropsychologist can gain competence in the new field of sports neuropsychology. Certainly reading a book such as this one is a good beginning. Other ways include attending professional meetings, reading the scientific literature and most importantly, we suggest, consulting with other colleagues in the field. The clinical neuropsychologist is strongly advised to consult with experienced colleagues about various factors that can limit their interpretations of the test results (Ethical standard 2.05, Interpreting Assessment Results).

Clarify the Purpose of the Exam and the Report

The clinical neuropsychologist will be called upon to examine a player for a variety of reasons. We have already discussed the role in evaluating a player for the effects of a recent concussion to help the team physician make decisions about return to play. There are a couple of additional points we would like to make regarding this type of assessment.

The clinical neuropsychologist who is new to the area of practice is well advised to find out where their reports can end up after they leave their offices (Confidentiality). If the report goes directly to the team physician and remains as confidential records in the team physician's office, confidentiality is maintained. Often, athletes' medical records are maintained adjacent to locker rooms and are accessible by many different individuals. The neuropsychologist needs to be aware that most teams require athletes to sign a waiver of confidentiality of medical records. Unless neuropsychological records are separated, they will find themselves considered under this waiver. Moreover, in professional sports, concussions are considered work-related injuries and in most teams in the United States, payment for post-concussions services may be covered by the team's Workman's Compensation Carrier, who will demand a report for payment and for which the player's separate consent is required.

Another role for the clinical neuropsychologist is in the assessment of a player to provide information about possibly disabling neuropsychological deficits. Here the neuropsychologist must be very careful to clarify whether they are being hired by and reporting to the player, team management, Worker's Compensation Carrier, or a separate Disability Carrier. The neuropsychologist must clarify this first and obtain written consent from the player so that the athlete is fully informed about the potential uses of the examination. Since players are often naïve about such issues, the neuropsychologist is advised to have the player discuss the examination and the consent form with other people they trust such as their agent and/or their family.

Neuropsychologists who have been involved in forensic assessments are experienced in the need to specify their relationships with a client/patient prior to examination. The same model is appropriate for neuropsychological assessment of athletes, however there are new relationships to be considered. For example, in the forensic setting, if the neuropsychologist is hired by defense to perform a court ordered examination of a plaintiff, the neuropsychologist makes the relationships clear to the plaintiff before undertaking the examination. Moreover, written informed consent for the plaintiff is obtained. The neuropsychologist makes clear to him/herself and to the examinee that the neuropsychologist in this instance has been retained by defense counsel and is not in this case working on behalf of the plaintiff/patient. We suggest the same logic be applied to the evaluations of athletes when third parties are involved.

Limitations on Test Validity and Need for Research

Neuropsychological screening batteries are increasingly used in sports neuropsychology. They have the advantage of being brief and providing baseline data against which post-concussion data can be compared. The neuropsychologist, however, must be ever vigilant of the limitations of brief batteries in making clinical decisions. Ethical Standard 2.02 (Competence and Appropriate Use of Assessments and Interventions) states that psychologists need to know the research and appropriate uses of tests they administer. They also must recognize limitations on the certainty of their diagnoses according to Ethical Standard 2.04 (Use of Assessment in General and With Special Populations). Repeated testing can have significant practice effects, which can affect the original diagnostic purpose of the repeated test. As of now, there are limited norms for athletes and none for those with specific language and cultural considerations. Furthermore, a brief battery is not a substitute for a more complete neuropsychological examination. We strongly encourage the sports neuropsychologist to use their judgment and consult with other colleagues about when to supplement a screening battery with additional tests.

Many sports neuropsychologists are facilitating research in the field. One of the stated professional responsibilities of psychologists is to "adapt their methods to the needs of different populations" (Principle C: Professional and Scientific Responsibility). For example, those neuropsychologists that are part of the National Hockey League Testing Program, with the players consent, send baseline and post-concussion test results to a common database where anonymously coded information can be analyzed on a league- wide basis to develop better norms and identify tests most sensitive to the effects concussion. In addition, these data will help identify which tests are best suited to testing athletes whose primary language is other than English, and who may have developing English language skills the longer they stay in the league (Ethical standard 2.04, Use of Assessment in General and with Special Populations).

Ethical Issues Speicifally Related to University Settings

University and college settings present unique opportunities for neuropsychologists while also presenting interesting challenges. Sports-related neuropsychological testing programs in most colleges and universities have largely been developed as research programs. However, the increased popularity of neuropsychological tests and the value of neuropsychological test data in documenting injury severity can often create confusion between the role of the researcher and that of the clinician. What was originally an interesting "study" can easily turn into a full-fledged clinical program.

The shift between a research study and a clinical program requires considerable thought. In research studies, participants are usually volunteers, data are coded anonymously, data remain within the confines of the research team, and data are not usually used to make clinical decisions on-line. In a clinical program, player participation can be required as part of the general medical program for the team, post-injury data (or the interpretation of data) will need to be released to team physicians or athletic trainers, and the neuropsychologist will often be asked to make recommendations for return-to-play. Most likely, the university program will be a hybrid of both approaches: a clinical program whose data are used for research. In any of these programs the best assurance of ethical practice will be a carefully crafted statement regarding the role of the neuropsychologist. The following should be clear to all parties:

What information that will be gathered?
How will the information be gathered?
Who will be gathering the information?
Why is the information being gathered?
How will the data be stored?
Who has access to the data?
How will the information be used (e.g. research database vs. return-to-play)?
What type of information will be disseminated and to whom ?

The difference between baseline data and post injury data needs to be made explicit. For example, in general it is preferable that access to baseline data is limited to the neuropsychologist. Similarly, the neuropsychologist should store all of the data apart from any team records. Conversely, team physicians need post-injury data when return-to-play decisions are being made.

In conclusion, the area of sports neuropsychology is new and exciting. As with any young field, there are many challenges to be faced and pitfalls to be avoided. This is particularly true with respect to ethics. This chapter has attempted to outline some of the issues that we have faced in working with sports teams. We realize that we have only scratched the surface and that our list of "issues" is certainly not exhaustive. However, you will be generally doing well if you remember for whom you are working, clearly define your role to all parties, establish good working relationships with the team physician and team athletic trainers, and as is the case with most questions of ethics – When in doubt, Consult!

References

American Psychological Association. (1992). Ethical principles of psychologists and code of conduct. *American Psychologist, 47*, 1597–1611.

American Psychological Association. (2001). Proposed revisions of ethical principles. Psychology Monitor.

Bailes, J.E., Lovell, M.R., & Maroon, J.C. (1999). *Sport-Related Concussions.* St. Louis, Missouri: Quality Medical Publishing, Inc.

Echemendia, R. & Parker, E.S. (1999). Ethical Issues. In J.E. Bailes, M.R. Lovell, & J.C. Maroon (Eds.) *Sport-Related Concussions* (pp. 157–170). St. Louis, Missouri: Quality Medical Publishing, Inc.

Laws and Regulations Related to the Practice of Psychology. (2000). California Department of Consumer Affairs, Sacramento, California, www.ca.gov/psych.

Chapter 26

RETURN TO PLAY FOLLOWING BRAIN INJURY

Ruben J. Echemendia
Psychological and Neurobehavioral Associates
State College Pennsylvania

Robert C. Cantu
Chief of Neurosurgery Service and Director of Sports Medicine Emerson Hospital
Adjunct Professor of Exercise and Sports Science, University of North Carolina – Chapel Hill

Concussion is derived from the Latin *Concussus*, which means "to shake violently." Initially it was thought to produce only a temporary disturbance of brain function due to neuronal, chemical, or neuroelectrical changes without gross structural change. We now know that structural damage with loss of brain cells does occur with some concussions. In the last several years, the neurobiology of cerebral concussion has been advanced, predominantly in animal studies but also in studies in man. It has become clear that in the minutes to days following concussive brain injury, that brain cells that are not irreversibly destroyed, remain alive, but in a vulnerable state. These cells are particularly vulnerable to minor changes in cerebral blood flow and/or increases in intracranial pressure and especially anoxia. Animal studies have shown that during this period of vulnerability, which may last as long as a week, a minor reduction in cerebral blood flow that would normally be well tolerated, now produces extensive neuronal cell loss (Lee, Lifshitz et al., 1955;

Lifshitz, Pinanong et al., 1955; Jenkins, Marmarou et al., 1986; Jenkins, Moszynski et al., 1989; Sutton, Hovda et al., 1994).

A sobering influence is the realization that the ability to process information may be reduced after a concussion, and the severity and duration of functional impairment may be greater with repeated concussions (Symonds, 1962; Gronwall & Wrightson, 1974; Gronwall & Wrightson, 1975). There are studies that suggest that the damaging effects of the shearing injury to nerve fibers and neurons is proportional to the degree the head is accelerated, and that these changes may be cumulative (Peerless & Rewcastle, 1967; Gennarelli, Seggawa et al., 1982; Schneider, Kennedy et al., 1985). Studies also suggest that once players have sustained an initial cerebral concussion, their chances of incurring a second one are three to six times greater than an athlete who has never sustained a concussion (Gerberich, 1983; Zemper, 1994; Guskiewicz et al., 2000).

The decision of returning an athlete to competition following a cerebral concussion is complex and dynamic. Ideally, a well-thought out decision will return a player to play at the precise moment that the effects of concussion have ended. This minimizes any disruption to the player's career while keeping the player safe from additional injury. A premature RTP can result in catastrophic injury that may terminate the career or the life of the athlete. Unfortunately, today there are no neuroanatomical or physiological measurements that can be used to precisely determine the extent of injury with concussion nor precisely when it has cleared. It is this fact that makes RTP decisions after a concussion such a challenging clinical decision. The focus of this chapter will be to examine those variables that are involved in the RTP decision. Traditional RTP guidelines rely on variables directly related to the concussion (e.g. loss of consciousness, post-traumatic amnesia) and history of concussion (e.g. number of concussions in a season). In this chapter we will first review these models, then propose a data-based revision to the Cantu grading system, and elaborate on a model that recognizes that RTP is a dynamic process that involves numerous types of information (player symptom report, observed symptoms, physical findings, imaging data) from numerous sources (player, family, team). We will discuss how neuropsychological data can be incorporated into the decision-making process and the usefulness of such data.

The Decision Making Process in Context

There are a host of individuals that may be involved in the RTP decision. Although each of these individuals may not be present in every situation, it is usually the case that many of these people will provide input into the process. In most instances, it is the ***team physician*** who holds the ultimate responsibility of when an athlete should be returned to sport. It is the role of the team physician to gather the necessary information, weigh the various sources of information, and ultimately decide whether to clear the player for RTP. Teams vary significantly as to the designation and involvement of the team physician. In some instances the team physician is dedicated to the particular team. He or she travels with the team, knows the players, staff and family. These physicians know the coaches well and have good working relationships with a variety of specialists who they rely on for consultation. In other situations, there may be a group of team physicians that are assigned to various teams (usually the case in Division I sports). These physicians generally do not travel with the team (except for the marquis sports) but they do get to know the players and coaches quite well. Some colleges do not have team physicians and rely on the general student health service or the local hospital. Many high school districts do not have team physicians. Usually, players are treated by their primary care physicians.

Some physicians have a great deal of training and experience in the diagnosis and management of sports-related concussion while many do not. Given the importance and the dynamic nature of the RTP decision it is imperative that physicians charged with the decision-making role seek training and consultation when returning an athlete to sport.

One of the key figures in the sports medicine staff is the *athletic trainer*. The athletic trainer generally knows the players best. They know the quirks and idiosyncrasies of each player and are in a good position to judge whether the player is behaving unusually. Changes in behavior and personality are often early signs that a concussion has occurred. Athletic trainers have been called the "eyes and ears" of the team physician. In most instances, they are the first responders to any incident or injury to a player and must make the judgment of whether a concussion has occurred. In essence, it is the athletic trainer who is making the first RTP decision by either benching a player or deciding that the signs do not warrant removal from play. Arguably, the sideline or on-site decision is the most difficult since the effects of concussion can be quite subtle early on and may actually take hours or days to develop. It is often the case that athletic trainers do not have team physicians to back them up on site.

Similar to the case with physicians, there are many different models that are found with athletic trainers. Some teams have dedicated certified athletic trainers that travel with the teams and attend every practice. Others have trainers that are assigned to teams but do not travel and only occasionally attend practices. In high school, there may be one or two athletic trainers assigned to a school and they generally have hours during which injured athletes are evaluated. Some teams do not use athletic trainers at all.

Since the role of athletic trainers is specific to sports-related injuries, they generally receive training in the assessment and management of concussion. The topic of concussion is often discussed in the professional journals for athletic trainers as well as the annual meeting of the National Athletic Trainers Association.

Each player is part of a team and there are many components of a team that are important to the RTP decision. First and foremost is the *coach*. The coach sets the tone in a team regarding respect and value of the medical staff and ultimately the medical decision. Some coaches may treat the medical staff as an unwelcome nuisance that they must tolerate. Others welcome the medical staff as part of the team and view them as a valuable resource for keeping their players healthy and productive. Although this range of perspectives is true for most sports injuries, it is particularly important in the area of concussion. Since concussions are generally not visible and an athlete may look "fine", a negative attitude from a coach can serve to completely invalidate any education that a team may get regarding concussion. We have heard countless coaches say "He's fine, he just needs to shake it off" or worse "I don't believe in concussions." Conversely, a coach that understands the complexities of concussion can help instill an understanding among players that will lead to more accurate reporting of symptoms and better care for the players.

The coach also plays a very significant role in the detection of concussion. Often, it is the coach who notices that a player has missed a play or is acting "goofy." They then send the player to be evaluated by medical staff. In many sports (particularly high school or youth sports) where medical personnel are not available, it is actually the coach that will make the determination on the field of whether a concussion has occurred. Taken together, these factors point to the vital role that coaches play in the development of an active concussion program. It also strongly suggests the continuing need for education of coaches regarding the signs and symptoms of concussion.

The *team* itself is an important element in the RTP decision. The team may be tempted to exert influence on the medical staff when a star player has been sidelined because of a concussion. This may be more the case when a "big game" is on the horizon as opposed to an insignificant game where a win is almost guaranteed. The *players* are also important. If players understand the importance of concussive injuries they can be quite helpful in identifying those players who "took a hit" and appear to be acting "funny." Players can also be quite helpful in easing the pressure that an athlete might feel for RTP and for providing information as to whether the athlete is continuing to experience symptoms. It is not unusual for a player to deny having symptoms when in fact their roommate reports that they are continuing to have headaches, lethargy, etc.

Families are integral parts of the lives of athletes. Whether it is the professional athlete who is married and has children, or the college athlete who has a boyfriend/girlfriend and a family of origin, or the sophomore in high school's family, these people are all touched by the RTP decision. The wife of a professional athlete may be concerned that her husband will sustain serious debilitating problems if he continues to play after several concussions, or the father of a high school football player who insists that his son should play despite having continuing symptoms from a concussion, or the boyfriend who reports that his girlfriend who sustained a concussion playing lacrosse lied when she told the medical staff that she was "fine."

All these scenarios describe individuals who have a vested interest in the RTP decision. These factors should be understood and taken as data in the RTP decision.

Lastly, there is the *athlete*. The athlete is the person with the most direct interest in the RTP decision. He or she has the most to gain or lose from the decision. Ideally, the athlete would be in agreement with the RTP decision and feels comfortable either returning to play or continuing to sit out. However, there are instances where the athlete is quite apprehensive about returning to play. Knowledge of the athlete is very helpful in this situation. Is this an athlete who tends to minimize or maximize complaints? Returning an apprehensive athlete to play may have negative consequences both psychologically and physically. For example, an ice hockey player who returns to play and is apprehensive about being hit or executing a check may place himself in greater danger of injury than would usually be the case. The opposite situation involved is the athlete who argues that she should RTP following concussion despite continued symptoms or abnormal neuropsychological findings. In both cases, education is critical, as is spending time with the athlete and listening to his or her concerns.

Historical Approaches to the RTP Decision

There is no more challenging problem faced by team physicians, athletic trainers and other medical personnel responsible for the medical care of athletes than the recognition and management of concussion. Indeed, such injuries have captured many headlines in recent years and have spurred studies both within the National Football League and the National Hockey League. When discussing concussion it must be realized that there is no universal agreement on the definition and grading of concussion (Jenkins, Marmarou et al., 1986; Roberts, 1992; Kelly & Rosenberg, 1997). In fact, it has been estimated the there are approximately 14 concussion grading systems that have been published to date (Collins, Lovell et al., 2000). Tables 26.1-3 present the three most widely used systems for grading concussion. As can be seen, the grading

Table 26.1. Cantu grading system for concussion.

GRADE 1.	No LOC; PTA less than 30 minutes
GRADE 2.	LOC less than 5 minutes in duration or PTA lasting longer than 30 minutes but less than 24 hours
GRADE 3.	LOC for more than 5 minutes or PTA for more than 24 hours

Note. LOC = Loss of Consciousness
PTA = Post traumatic amnesia (anterograde/retrograde)

Table 26.2. Colorado Medical Society grading system for concussion.

GRADE 1.	Confusion without amnesia; no LOC
GRADE 2.	Confusion with amnesia; no LOC
GRADE 3.	Any LOC

Note. LOC = Loss of Consciousness

Table 26.3. AAN practice parameter (Kelly & Rosenberg) grading system for concussion

GRADE 1.	Transient confusion; no LOC; PCS or mental status abnormalities on examination resolve in less than fifteen minutes.
GRADE 2.	Transient confusion; no LOC; PCS or mental status abnormalities on examination last more than fifteen minutes.
GRADE 3.	Any LOC, either brief (seconds) or prolonged (minutes).

Note. LOC = Loss of Consciousness
PCS = Post concussion sign/symptoms

systems focus on loss or non loss of consciousness and post traumatic amnesia (PTA) as hallmarks in determining the severity of concussion. Unfortunately, they do not give enough attention to post-concussion symptoms (PCS). Concussions can give rise to a wide variety of symptoms. Any combination of the following signs and symptoms may be encountered: a feeling of being stunned or seeing bright lights, a brief loss of consciousness, lightheadedness, vertigo, loss of balance, headaches, cognitive and memory dysfunction, tinnitus, blurred vision, difficulty concentrating, lethargy, fatigue, personality changes, inability to perform daily activities, sleep disturbance, and motor or sensory symptoms. Players often complain of feeling "hung over" even though they have not been drinking. Table 26.5 presents a list of PCS in a format that has been found to be useful in assessing the player with a concussion.

Whether one has been unconsciousness is an important consideration in assessing concussion. It is generally believed that the degree of brain injury sustained is indicated by the depth and duration of coma (Benson, Gardner et al., 1976; Alexander, 1982; Katz, 1992). But, the coma referred to by these authors is not the seconds to minutes usually seen on the athletic field, but rather hours or days duration. Thus, while not diminishing the importance of being rendered unconsciousness, it appears illogical to grade a concussion that produces PCS lasting months or years as less severe because there was no LOC as compared to the frequent occurrence of athletes being briefly rendered unconsciousness with resolution of all PCS within a few minutes or hours.

Table 26.4. Post concussion signs/symptoms checklist.

(Please check all that apply)

	Initial Symptoms	Symptoms Today
Depression	☐	☐
Dizziness	☐	☐
Drowsiness	☐	☐
Excess sleep	☐	☐
Fatigue	☐	☐
Feel "in fog"	☐	☐
Feel "slowed down"	☐	☐
Headache	☐	☐
Irritability	☐	☐
Memory Problems	☐	☐
Nausea	☐	☐
Nervousness	☐	☐
Numbness/Tingling	☐	☐
Poor Balance	☐	☐
Poor Concentration	☐	☐
Ringing in the ears	☐	☐
Sadness	☐	☐
Sensitive to Light	☐	☐
Sensitivity to Noise	☐	☐
Trouble falling asleep	☐	☐
Vomiting	☐	☐

Presently, there is no universal agreement that PTA is a better or more sensitive predictor of outcome following traumatic brain injury than depth and duration of unconsciousness (Teasdale & Jennett, 1974; Alesandre, Colombo et al., 1983; Stuss, Ginns et al., 1999). However, many do consider the duration of PTA the best indicator of traumatic brain injury severity (Teasdale & Jennett, 1974; Jennett & MacMillan, 1981) and the most dependable marker of outcome prediction (Shores, 1989; Gillingham, 1969; Evans, 1976; Brooks, Aughton et al., 1980; Brooks, Hosie et al., 1986; Bishara, Partridge et al., 1992; Haslam, Batchelor et al., 1994), even in mild cases (Crovitz et al., 1983; Stuss, Ginns et al., 1999).

Although variously described by different investigators, PTA as core ingredients include impaired orientation, i.e., retrograde amnesia and anterograde amnesia (Shores; Levin, O'Donnell et al. 1979; Daniel, Crovitz et al. 1987; Geffen, Encel et al. 1991). Recently, some investigators have suggested that PTA might better be called post traumatic confusional state (Benson, Gardner et al., 1976; Alexander, 1982; Barth, 1989; Katz, 1992). Post-traumatic amnesia may be divided into two types; *retrograde* defined by Cartlidge and Shaw (Cartlidge, 1981) as a "partial or total loss of the ability to recall events that have occurred during the period immediately preceding brain injury." The duration of retrograde amnesia usually progressively decreases.

The second type of post-traumatic amnesia is *anterograde* amnesia, which is a deficit in forming new memory after the accident, which may lead to decreased attention and inaccurate perception. Anterograde memory is frequently the last function to return following recovery from loss of consciousness (Russell, 1932).[1]

In understanding the pathophysiology of PTA, it is important to note that memory and new learning is believed to involve our cerebral cortex as well as subcortical projections. Not only are the hippocampal formations (gyrus dentatus, hippocampus and parahippocampal gyri) involved, but also the diencephalons, especially the medial portions of the dorsomedial and adjacent midline nuclei of the thalamus (Adams, Victor et al., 1997). In addition, frontal lobe lesions may cause alterations in behavior including irritability, aggressiveness and losses of inhibition and judgment. Recent evidence has been presented that the right frontal lobe plays a prominent role in sustained attention (Stuss, Shallice et al., 1995).

The lack of a universal definition or grading scheme for concussion renders the evaluation of epidemiologic data extremely difficult. We have evaluated many athletes who have suffered a concussion. Most of these injuries were mild and did not involve a loss of consciousness, and were associated with post-traumatic amnesia, which was helpful in making the diagnosis, especially in mild cases.

Cantu has developed a practical scheme for grading severity of concussion based on the duration of unconsciousness and/or post-traumatic amnesia, which has worked well on the field and sidelines (Table 26.1). The mildest concussion (Grade I) occurs without LOC and the only neurologic deficit is a brief period of post traumatic confusion and/or PTA, which by definition when present, lasts less than thirty minutes.

With the moderate (Grade II) concussion, there is usually a brief period of unconsciousness, not exceeding five minutes. Less commonly, there is no loss of consciousness but only a protracted period of PTA lasting over thirty minutes but less than twenty-four hours.

Severe (Grade III) concussion occurs with a more protracted period of unconsciousness lasting over five minutes. In the past it was thought that rarely would a grade III concussion occur without a loss of consciousness but with a very protracted period of PTA lasting over twenty-four hours. In reality, prospective studies over the last several years indicate that virtually all Grade III concussions by this guideline; occur because of PTA lasting over twenty-four hours (Erlanger, 2000). A protracted period of unconsciousness

[1] It should be noted that the neuropsychological literature makes a clear distinction between anterograde and retrograde amnesia whereas it is common practice to combine these two types of amnesia as "post-traumatic amnesia" in the fields of neurology and neurosurgery.

Table 26.5. Data-based Cantu grading system for concussion.

GRADE 1. (Mild)	No LOC, PTA; PCSS < 30 minutes
GRADE 2. (Moderate)	LOC < 1 minute or PTA/PCSS > 30 minutes
GRADE 3. (Severe)	LOC = 1 minute or PTA = 24 hrs, PCSS > 7 days

Note. LOC = Loss of Consciousness
PTA = Post traumatic amnesia (anterograde/retrograde)
PCSS = Post concussion sign/symptoms

lasting over five minutes is almost never seen on athletic fields. Most periods of unconsciousness last seconds to a minute. Furthermore, prospective studies over the last ten years have shown a correlation among duration of PCS, PTA and abnormal neuropsychological test data (Erlanger, Feldman et al., 2000). Therefore, a data-based modification of the original Cantu Guidelines is found in Table 26.5.

The Role of Neuropsychology

Neuropsychology is a relative newcomer to the sports medicine arena. Although neuropsychological approaches and instruments have long been used in the assessment of mild traumatic brain injury, it is only recently that neuropsychological data have been used in the RTP decision (see Echemendia & Julian, 2002). Although neuropsychologists may play many different roles in sports medicine, the most common model is that of the neuropsychologist as a consultant to the team physician. In this role, the neuropsychologist conducts baseline and post-injury evaluations and provides recommendations based on the neuropsychological data to the team physician regarding RTP. Generally, the neuropsychologist is not making the RTP decision. As is discussed in Parker and Echemendia (this volume), it is very important for the team and the neuropsychologist to be very clear about the role that the neuropsychologist has undertaken.

As a consultant to the team physician, the neuropsychologist relies on data from tests that assess cognitive functioning. How effective are neuropsychological tests in detecting the subtle neurocognitive changes that often accompany mild concussion? Although relative new, there is a growing body of literature (Echemendia & Julian, 2001) that suggests that neuropsychological tests are able to differentiate concussed athletes from non-injured controls soon after injury. For example, Echemendia, Putukian, Mackin et al. (Echemendia, Putukian et al., 2000) found significant differences between athletes with mTBI and their matched controls as early as 2 hours post-injury.

They found that injured players scored worse at 48 hours post-injury than they did at 2 hours post-injury, whereas the control group's scores *improved* from the 2-hour to the 48-hour post-injury assessment. Also of significance is that although a subjective report of symptoms differentiated the injured from the control group at 2 hours post-injury, symptoms failed to significantly differentiate the groups at 48 hours even though statistically and clinically significant differences were found between the groups on the neuropsychological measures.

Other researchers and clinicians have used neuropsychological techniques to assess football players (Barth, 1989; Olesniewicz, Sallis et al., 1997; Collins, Grindel et al., 1999), soccer players (Abreau, Templer et al., 1990; Tysvaer & Lochen, 1991; Matser, Kessels et al., 1999; Putukian, Echemendia et al., 2000), boxers (McLatchie, Brooks et al., 1987; Murelius & Haglund 1991), race car drivers (Mermis & Barth), basketball players (Putukian & Echemendia, 1996), and Australian Rules football (Cremona-Meteyard & Geffen, 1994). These studies suggest that neuropsychological tests are useful and accurate in identifying neurocognitive deficits following mTBI.

In addition to serving as a consultant to the team physician, the neuropsychologist also serves a vital role in directly assessing and treating the injured athlete. Athletes who experience a concussion are often frightened by their symptoms and have concerns about how these symptoms will affect them in the future. They also may develop feelings of anxiety and depression in addition to conflicts that may arise within a family. The clinical neuropsychologist is well suited to provide counseling for these athletes and their families. Since the neuropsychologist is usually not part of the team structure, athletes often feel that they can talk with the neuropsychologist without fear that their discussions will impact their standing on the team.

A Dynamic Model for Return-To-Play Decision Making

As stated at the outset of this chapter, the RTP decision is a complex interplay of many variables that interact in complex ways – some direct (e.g. medical factors) and some indirect (team issues). Our goal in elucidating this model is to point out the many variables that can, and often should, be considered in the RTP decision. As such, the model is descriptive rather than prescriptive. We are not putting forth a new classification system nor are we offering new RTP guidelines.

The variables in this model have been grouped into Concussion Factors, Medical factors, Player factors, Team Factors, and Extraneous factors for ease of presentation. The model is based on the premise that no RTP decision is ever risk free. Athletes who have sustained a concussion and have recovered from that concussion, are being sent back into an arena where the likelihood of having another concussion is significantly higher than if they had not had a previous concussion (Gerberich, 1983; Zemper, 1994; Guskiewicz, 2000).

In light of this, every RTP decision involves a risk/benefit analysis in which the possible risks are weighed against the possible rewards. The variables outlined below do not have equal weight in the decision-making process; the relative weights will vary depending on the issues at hand for any particular athlete. Figure 26.1 presents the model. As can be seen, each of the variable groupings has a relationship to the RTP decision. Some variables are believed to be highly salient in ANY RTP decision. For example, the medical factors box is connected directly to the RTP box by a bold multi-line arrow, which suggests a very strong relationship between these factors. The medical factors have a direct and critical role in the RTP decision since athletes with positive physical findings, and/or positive radiologic findings, or continuing symptoms should never be returned to play. Similarly, Concussion Factors and Neuropsychological Data have direct effects on RTP, although not as strong as medical factors. In some cases, variable groups have relationships with each other as well as to the RTP decision. Player factors and Team factors are bi-directional and have an indirect (dotted lines) impact on RTP. Player factors also influence Team Factors, Medical Factors, and Concussion Factors. Each of the variable groups will be discussed below.

Medical factors

These factors have the most direct relationship to the RTP decision. Specifically, there is widespread consensus that any positive finding on neuroimaging interpreted to be a result of the concussion should prevent an athlete from returning to play until the pathology has been resolved and the imag-

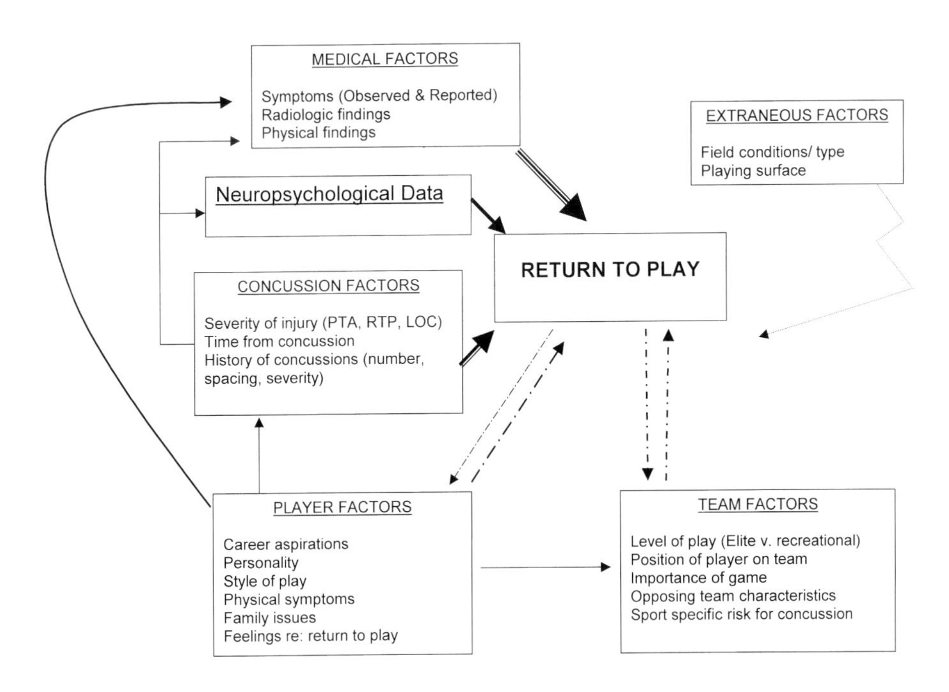

ing returns to normal. It is also the case that if neuroimaging inadvertently discloses structural findings that place the athlete at increased risk of brain injury (e.g. cavum septum pellucidum, arachnoid cyst, hydrocephalus) that RTP may not be appropriate. Players who exhibit any abnormal findings on comprehensive physical/neurological examination should not RTP until the abnormal findings have resolved. Similarly, it is widely observed that any player who reports symptoms or is observed to have symptoms either at rest or during exertion should not return to sport until the symptoms have cleared. However, the absence of reported symptoms should not automatically provide a green light for RTP. The recursive loop between player factors and medical factors suggests that athletes differ significantly in their willingness to accurately report their symptoms. Similarly, personality types may influence whether athletes have a tendency to exaggerate symptoms or, more likely, minimize symptoms. As has been stated earlier, Echemendia et al. (Echemendia, Putukian et al., 2000) demonstrated that symptoms are not as powerful a predictor of injury status as are neuropsychological tests.

Concussion factors

A careful examination of the features of a concussion as well as the player's history with concussions is a vital component of any RTP decision. Although there is substantial disagreement regarding the validity of concussion grading systems and their relationship to RTP, several factors should be examined in any RTP decision. First and foremost is the severity of the injury. The guidelines may be quite useful for those practitioners who do not routinely work with sports-related concussions. An examination of the number of symptoms that a player reports or are observed is important. The more symptoms a player experiences, the greater the likelihood that the concussion is more severe than the report of a single symptom. A thorough assessment of amnesia is indicated. The extent of any retrograde or post-traumatic amnesia should be carefully documented. The greater the period of amnesia, the more severe the concussion is thought to be (see Cantu Data-Based Grading System). It is important to note however that many players do not regain memory for the period of time prior to or following the concussion. Thus, restoration of memory is not necessary for RTP. What is important is that memory has returned to normal (e.g. as assessed through NP testing) and the player is able to learn and recall new information.

Loss of Consciousness has long been held as an indicator of the severity of a concussion. In some of the guidelines in use today (e.g. Colorado Medical Society, AAN), any LOC automatically makes the concussion "severe." This has been a clinically useful and defensible position, particularly in light of the traumatic brain injury data which suggest that the duration of LOC (greater than 15 minutes) is a strong predictor of outcome. However, on the athletic field it is very unusual for periods of unconsciousness to be more than a few seconds to a minute in duration. Recent data (Lovell et al., 1999) suggest that LOC of short duration (e.g. less than 2 minutes) may not be predictive of concussion severity. Also, Erlanger found no significant correlation between Grade III concussion and the duration of PCS or abnormal NP testing. Most clinicians with experience in sports medicine have had the experience of an athlete who experiences a period of LOC for a short period (e.g. 1 minute) who reports no other symptoms. This is in contrast with the athlete with no LOC or PTA but has protracted symptoms following concussion. These clinical and empirical findings suggest that the evaluation of concussion symptoms is not as easily categorized as is suggested by the guidelines. Certainly, the guidelines can serve as useful heuristics in understanding the severity of a player's concussion, but the nature and extent of the symptoms should be examined in relationship to each other, as well as other factors suggested in this model.

A player's history of concussion is also important to examine although there are very few data in the sports domain that directly speak to the effects of multiple concussion. Variables of interest are the total number of concussions in the player's history, their severity, and their temporal sequencing. Concussions that are closely spaced apart are considered to be more serious than those further apart because of the threat of Second Impact Syndrome. The total number of concussions in a player's career is thought to be important because of the cumulative effects of mild brain injuries on the player's long term functioning. There are many highly publicized professional athletes (e.g. Merryl Hoge, Harry Carsons, Pat LaFontainne, Steve Young, Steve Miller, Troy Aikman, Eric Lindros) whose careers were influenced by multiple concussions. In some instances careers were terminated because of problems with PCS, in others, careers were terminated because of the possibility of long-term neurocognitive deficits, while in another there have been suggestions that a career should be terminated for fear of longstanding problems. One study with college athletes has found that players with 2 or more concussions had poorer (Collins, Grindel et al., 1999) baseline neuropsychological test scores than those with less than 2 concussions. The study had a relatively small sample size within one sport and their results await replication. In contrast, Macciocchi et al. (Macciocchi et al., 2001) found that college football players who sustained two concussions did not exhibit significantly more neurocognitive impairment when compared to players with one concussion.

Neuropsychological factors

As discussed earlier, neuropsychological test results are relative new entries into the RTP decision. In some circles, there is unease in using these data to influence the RTP decision because their use in sports is relatively new. However, the body of empirical literature noted above clearly points to the usefulness of NP data and its effectiveness in differentiating injured from non-injured athletes. There are still many questions that remain unanswered. For example, if a player is returned to sport with abnormal neuropsychological findings what are the likely consequences? Or, what level of neuropsychological deficit is necessary to prevent RTP? These are important questions that are currently being examined systematically through empirical studies. It is our recommendation that neuropsychological test data, when available, should be an important component of the RTP decision. Many programs and team physicians have already adopted the perspective that a player should not be returned to play until he or she is judged to have returned to baseline. However, since this is a new area for neuropsychology, it is recommended that only neuropsychologists who have experience with sports-related concussion be consulted about RTP decisions. Neuropsychologists seeking experience in this domain may make use of peer consultation as has been successfully used in the NHL (see Lovell & Echemendia, Chapter 13 in this volume).

Player factors

The player is the central figure in any RTP decision yet very little attention has been focused on player variables in the RTP decision. It was said earlier that the more a team physician or athletic knows the player, the better able they are to determine whether the player is exhibiting personality or behavioral changes following concussion. This information is helpful in deciding whether a concussion has occurred as well as an indication of when the concussion has resolved. The player's personality is also important in how aggressive or passive they play the sport, the extent to which they will either minimize or exaggerate symptoms, how they respond to having had sustained a concussion, and their willingness to follow the advice of medical personnel. Involving the player in the RTP decision may serve a very useful function both in terms of gaining the player's confidence and in gaining acceptance of the decision.

Player skill level and appropriate use of techniques is also important. A player that uses improper technique at a relatively low skill level is more likely to sustain another concussion than a highly skilled player with good technique. It is also important to be aware of the player's goals regarding their career in sports. Some athletes have the skills and the desire to play at a professional level, others do not. There are some that view their athletic careers as "something fun to do" while others view sports as the central and defining feature of their lives. These career aspirations may prove to be useful, albeit indirect, considerations in any RTP cost/benefit analysis. For example, a team physician may be uncertain about returning a player to sport because the data regarding the concussion are unclear. Withholding the athlete who aspires towards a professional career out of an important game may weigh more heavily on the side of RTP than an athlete whose future plans do not involve sports.

An athlete's family is important in the RTP decision for several reasons. Families and friends can be very useful sources of information about how the athlete is functioning and the symptoms they are experiencing. They can also be very useful allies to the sport medicine team by encouraging a supportive atmosphere about the injury and recovery from symptoms. In contrast, families can also be a source of major frustration for the athlete and the medical staff. It is not unusual for a parent to become angry because their child has been removed from competition due to a concussion. Naiveté on the part of the parents regarding the nature and effects of concussion often lead to statements like "my son is tough...let him play" or "come on, she looks fine, let her play." This type of pressure clearly impacts the athlete and his or her relationship with the medical staff.

Team factors

Like the Player Factors discussed above, Team Factors may also have relevance to the RTP decision. The level of play, recreational vs. elite professional, may impact on the RTP decision in very much the same way that a player's career aspirations may be involved. A more conservative stance is sometimes taken with younger individuals or those involved in a less competitive atmosphere. The player's position on the team may also relate to the RTP decision with respect to the probability of sustaining another concussion. For example, it is more likely that a quarterback will sustain a concussion than a center. The importance of the game may also be a consideration in RTP. If there are no clear indications for withholding a player from the game but the team physician wants to err on the side of caution, it is much easier to withhold an athlete from a "lesser" game than a national championship game. Although often overlooked, the characteristics of the opposing team are also important. For example, a star ice hockey player (forward) had a concussion and experienced PCS that lasted 4 days. He was asymptomatic at rest and during exertion for 2 days. Neuropsychological test data were abnormal but returned to baseline. The player feels ready to play. The opposing team is known for their intense physical play and they are known to have a very physical "enforcer" who will likely "go after" the athlete who was injured. Given the possibility (likelihood) of re-injury, would it be prudent to consider holding the player out until the next game and give him more of a chance to rest?

Lastly, it is important to consider the likelihood of sustaining a concussion in any specific sport. Those sports in which the incidence of concussion is high (e.g. Ice Hockey) may warrant an extra degree of caution when compared to those sports where the probability of injury is lower (e.g. baseball).

Extraneous factors

There are many other factors that are not central to the RTP but that some physicians and coaches do consider. For example, if the field conditions are such that it is felt the player may be more at risk for re-injury. In ice hockey, it has been reported that seamless plexiglass produces greater injuries than the traditional glass, prompting many new arenas to retrofit traditional glass.

Returning to Play

We believe it is most important to realize that before an athlete returns to play, he or she:

a. Must be free of all post concussion signs and symptoms at rest.
b. Neurological evaluation is normal.
c. If done, neuropsychological test data must be equal to or exceed baseline.
d. If done, CT or MRI must show no structural lesions placing the athlete at increased risk of head injury.

Once all post-traumatic amnesia symptoms and all post concussion symptoms have cleared and neuropsychological data have returned to baseline, then progressive exertional challenges may be adopted. These challenges (e.g. running, sit ups, push ups, skating) eventually push the athlete to near maximal heart rate. The athlete should remain symptom free throughout the exertional challenge. If the athlete remains symptom free at rest and on exertion, final clearance to return is given.

Career Ending Injuries – When Is It Time To Stop?

The science of sports-related concussions is relatively short while the clinical experience of evaluating and treating concussed athletes is fairly long. We, particularly the senior author, have been consulted on scores of occasions by professional and scholar athletes regarding terminating a career after multiple concussions. This is clearly one of the most difficult decisions in sports medicine. The following views are based on decades of clinical experience, the world's literature, as well as past and current scientific studies.

Although there is no universal consensus on when an athlete should terminate his or her career, there is one area of nearly unanimous agreement. An athlete still symptomatic with PCS at rest or provoked by exertional exercise should not return to contact or collision sport. The disagreement arises around the number of concussions that must be experienced before advising an athlete to refrain from contact or collision sports. Presently, the literature in this area is somewhat conflicting. Macciocchi et al. (2001) found no deterioration on neuropsychological test scores in football players with multiple mild concussions (46), yet articles in Lancet dating back over 25 years did suggest a cumulative effect with multiple concussions.

Experience has taught us that there is no arbitrary number of concussions that would mandate not returning to sport. Some rare individuals sustain one concussion that leaves them with permanent post concussion signs and symptoms or neurological deficits that prohibit their return to contact sports. Others may sustain 10 or even 20 concussions without any apparent permanent sequelae. There are two main changes that should raise red flags about when the multiply concussed athlete should quit playing. The first change regards duration of PCS. Usually, PCS clear in a few days or a week. But, as the athlete's "functional reserve" for sustaining head trauma without cumulative injury is exhausted, the duration of PCS may last months rather than days. This progressively increasing period of symptom duration should be a warning sign that RTP may not be advisable.

The second change is the forces (amount of acceleration to the brain) required to produce PCS. Whereas prior to the "functional reserve" being exhausted, hits producing concussion are usually directly to the head and with obvious violence. As the reserve is lost, concussion may be produced by striking other parts of the body, especially the chest and posterior thorax and only indirectly imparting forces to the head. It is of maximal concern, therefore, when these indirect hits produce post concussion symptoms that last months. This is the scenario when the athlete should be advised not to return to contact/collision sports. It would be permissible for such an athlete (when asymptomatic at rest and exertion) to return to a sport without risk of head trauma such as golf or tennis.

Summary

The goal of this chapter was to review current approaches to RTP and put forth a new model that captures the complexity of the RTP decision. To this end, we first described the lack of consensus in both the definition of concussion and the grading systems that have been used to gauge the severity of concussion. The three most widely used concussion grading systems and return to play guidelines (Cantu, Colorado Medical Society, AAN practice parameters) were discussed. These guidelines differ on the relative weight that is given to LOC, PTA and PCS in assessing the severity of concussion. We argued that the brief LOC that occurs in athletic competition is not likely to be a very good predictor of concussion severity, particularly in relation to PTA and the duration of PCS. A new, data-based reformulation of the Cantu guidelines was presented that places stronger emphasis on the role of PTA and symptom duration.

The role of neuropsychology in the RTP was discussed. Although neuropsychological techniques and tests are relative newcomers to sports medicine, their ability to detect subtle neurocognitive changes following concussion makes them important contributors to the RTP decision. As a consultant to the team physician, the neuropsychologist can serve a vital role in interpreting neuropsychological data and working directly with concussed athletes to deal with any psychological issues that may arise.

Lastly, a model was proposed that captures the complexity and dynamic interplay of the many variables that must be considered in any RTP decision. The model underscores the fact that a well-informed RTP decision will include data from many sources and that no one approach is sufficient by itself. The complexity of the RTP decision and hence the model, highlights the significance of the decision and the field's continued press to make returning to play as safe as possible for the athletes that entrust us with their care.

References

Abreau, F., Templer, Schuyler & Hutchinson. (1990). Neuropsychological assessment of soccer players. *Neuropsychology, 4,* 175–181.
Adams, R.D., Victor, M. & Ropper, A. (1997). *Principles of Neurology.* New York: McGraw-Hill.
Alesandre, A., Colombo, F. et al. (1983). Cognitive outcome and early indices of severity of head injury. *Journal of Neurosurgery, 59,* 751–761.
Alexander, M.P. (1982). Traumatic Brain Injury. In D. Blumer (Ed.), *Psychiatric Aspects of Neurologic Disease* (pp. 219–248). New York: Grune & Stratton.
Barth, J.T., Alves, W., Ryan, T. et al. (1989). Mild Head Injury in Sports. In H. Levin, H. Eisenberg & A. Benton (Eds.), *Mild Head Injury* (pp. 257-275). New York: Oxford University Press.
Benson, D.F., Gardner, H. et al. (1976). Reduplicative paramnesia. *Neurology, 26,* 147–151.
Bishara, S.N., Partridge, F.M. et al. (1992). Post-traumatic amnesia and Glasgow Coma Scale related to outcome in survivors in a consecutive series of patients with severe closed-head injury. *Brain Injury, 6,* 373–380.
Brooks, D.N., Aughton, M.E. et al. (1980). Cognitive sequelae in relationship to early indices of severity of brain damage after severe blunt head injury. *Journal of Neurology, Neurosurgery, and Psychiatry, 43,* 529-534.
Brooks, D.N., Hosie, J. et al. (1986). Cognitive sequelae of severe head injury in relation to Glasgow Outcome Scale. *Journal of Neurology, Neurosurgery, and Psychiatry, 49,* 549–588.
Cartlidge, N.E.F., Shaw, D.A. (1981). *Head Injury.* London: WB Saunders.
Collins, M., Grindel, S. et al. (1999). Relationship between concussion and neuropsychological performance in college football players. *Journal of the American Medical Association, 282,* 964–970.
Collins, M.W., Lovell, M. R. et al. (2000). Current issues in managing sports-related concussion. *Journal of the American Medical Association, 282,* 2283–2285.
Cremona-Meteyard, S.L. & G.M. Geffen (1994). Persistent visuospatial attention deficits following mild head injury in Australian rules football players. *Neuropsychologia, 32*(6), 649–662.
Crovitz, H.F., H. R.W. et al. (1983). Inter-relationships among retrograde amnesia, post-traumatic amnesia and time since head injury: a retrospective study. *Cortex, 19,* 407–412.
Daniel, W.F., Crovitz, H.F. et al. (1987). Neuropsychological aspects of disorientation. *Cortex, 23,* 169–187.
Echemendia, R.J. & Julian L. (2001). Mild traumatic brain injury in sports: neuropsychology's contribution to a developing field. *Neuropsychology Review, 11*(2), 69–88.
Echemendia, R.J., Putukian, M.P. et al. (2000). Neuropsychological test performance prior to and following sports-related mild traumatic brain injury. *Clinical Journal of Sport Medicine, 11,* 23–31.
Erlanger, D. (2000). President Headminder, Inc. *Personal communication.*
Erlanger, D.M., Feldman, D.J. et al. (2000). Development and validation of a web based protocol for management of sports related concussion. Orlando, National Academy of Neuropsychology (President Headminder, Inc.).
Evans, C.D. (1976). Assessment of disability after head injury. *Rheumatology Rehabilitation, 15,* 168.
Geffen, G.M., Encel, J.S. et al. (1991). Stages of recovery during post-traumatic amnesia and subsequent everyday memory deficits. *Neuroreport, 2,* 105–108.
Gennarelli, T.A., Seggawa, H. et al. (1982). Physiological response to angular acceleration of the head. In P.L. Gildenberg (Ed.), *Head Injury: Basic and Clinical Aspects* (pp. 129-140). New York: Raven.

Gerberich, S.G., Priest, J.D., Boen, J.R., Staub, C.P., Maxwell, R.E. (1983). Concussion Incidences and Severity in Secondary School Varsity Football Players. *American Journal of Public Health, 73*, 1370–1375.

Gillingham, F.J. (1969). The importance of rehabilitation. *Injury, 1*, 142.

Gronwall, D. & Wrightson, P. (1974). Delayed recovery of intellectual function after minor head injury. *The Lancet, 2*, 605–609.

Gronwall, D. & Wrightson, P. (1975). Cumulative effect of concussion. *Lancet, 2*, 995–997.

Guskiewicz, K.M., Weaver, N.L., Padua, D.A., Garrett, W.E. Jr. (2000). Epidemiology of concussion in collegiate and high school football players. *American Journal of Sports Medicine, 28*(5), 643–50.

Haslam, C. & Batchelor, J. et al. (1994). Post-coma disturbance and post-traumatic amnesia as nonlinear predictors of cognitive outcome following severe closed head injury: findings from the Westmead Head Injury Project. *Brain Injury*, 519–528.

Jenkins, L.W. & Marmarou, A. et al. (1986). Increased vulnerability of the traumatized brain to early ischemia. A. Unterberg, 273–282.

Jenkins, L. W. & Moszynski, K. et al. (1989). Increased vulnerability of the mildly traumatized brain to cerebral ischemia: The use of controlled secondary ischemia as a research tool to identify common or different mechanisms contributing to mechanical and ischemic brain injury. *Brain Research, 477*, 211–224.

Jennett, B. & MacMillan, R. (1981). Epidemiology of head injury. *British Medical Journal, 282*, 101°104.

Katz, D.I. (1992). Neuropathology and neurobehavioral recovery from closed head injury. *Journal of Head Trauma Rehabilitation, 7*, 1–15.

Kelly, J.P. & Rosenberg J.H. (1997). The diagnosis and management of concussion in sports. *Neurology, 48*, 575–580.

Lee, S. M., Lifshitz, J. et al. (1995). Focal cortical-impact injury produces immediate and persistent deficits in metabolic autoregulation. *Journal of Cerebral blood flow metabolism, 15*, s722 (Abstract).

Lifshitz, J., Pinanong, P. et al. (1955). Regional uncoupling of cerebral blood flow and metabolism in degenerating cortical areas following a lateral cortical contusion. *Journal of Neurotrauma, 12*, 129 (Abstract).

Lovell, M., Iverson, G., Collins, M., McKeag, D. & Maroon, J. (1999). Does loss of consciousness predict neuropsychological decrements after concussion? *Clinical Journal of Sports Medicine, 9*, 193–198.

Macciocchi, S.N., Barth, J.T., Alves, W.A., Littlefield, L., Jane, J.A. & Cantu, R. (2001). Multiple concussions and neuropsychological functioning in college football players. *Journal of Athletic Training, 36*(3), 303–306.

Matser, E., Kessels, A.G. et al. (1999). Neuropsychological impairment in amateur soccer players. *Journal of the American Medical Association, 282*(10), 971–973.

McLatchie, G., Brooks, N. et al. (1987). Clinical neurological examination, neuropsychology, electroencephalography and computed tomographic head scanning in active amateur boxers. *Journal of Neurology, Neurosurgery, and Psychiatry, 50*, 96–99.

Mermis, B. & Barth J. (xxxx) *Neuropsychological screening assessment of "Indy car" drivers.*

Murelius, O. & Haglund Y. (1991). Does Swedish amateur boxing lead to chronic brain damage?A retrospective neuropsychological study. *Acta Neurologica Scandanavia, 83*, 9–13.

Olesniewicz, M.H., Sallis, R.E. et al. (1997). *The neuropsychological changes that occur from head concussions in football at the National Collegiate American*

Association Division Three level. Sports Related Concussion and Nervous System Injuries Conference, Orlando, Florida.
Peerless, S.J. & Rewcastle, N.B. (1967). Shear injuries of the brain. *Canadian Medical Association Journal, 96*(10), 577–582.
Putukian, M. & Echemendia, R.J. (1996). Managing successive minor head injuries – Which tests guide return to play? *Physician and Sportsmedicine, 24*(11), 25–&.
Putukian, M., Echemendia, R.J. et al. (2000). Acute effects of heading in soccer: a prospective neuropsychological evaluation. *Clinical Journal of Sport Medicine, 10*, 104–109.
Roberts, W.O. (1992). Who plays? Who sits? Managing concussion on the sidelines. *Physician Sports Medicine, 20*, 66–76.
Russell, W.R. (1932). Cerebral involvement in head injury: a study based on the examination of two hundred cases. *Brain, 55*, 549.
Schneider, R.C., Kennedy, J.C. et al. (1985). *Sports Injuries*. Baltimore: Williams & Wilkins.
Shores, E. A. (1989). Comparison of the Westmead PA Scale and Glasgow Coma Scale as predictors of neuropsychological outcome following extremely severe blunt head injury. *Journal of Neurology, Neurosurgery & Psychiatry, 52*, 126–127.
Stuss, D., Ginns, M. et al. (1999). The acute period of recovery from tarumatic brain injury: posttraumatic amnesia or posttraumatic confusional state? *Journal of Neurosurgery, 90*, 635–643.
Stuss, D.T., Shallice, T. et al. (1995). A multidisciplinary approach to anterior attentional functions. *Annual New York Academy of Science, 769*, 191–211.
Sutton, R.L., Hovda, D.A. et al. (1994). Metabolic changes following cortical contusion: Relationships to edema and morphological changes. *A Ca Neurochir, 6*, 466–448.
Symonds, C. (1962). Concussion and its sequelae. *Lancet, 1*, 1–5.
Teasdale, G. & Jennett, B. (1974). Assessment of coma and impaired consciousness. A practical scale. *Lancet, 2*, 81–84.
Tysvaer, A.T. & Lochen, E.A. (1991). Soccer Injuries to the Brain. *American Journal of Sports Medicine, 19*, 56-60.
Zemper, E. (1994). Analysis of cerebral frequency with the most commonly used models of football helmets. *Journal of Athletic Training, 29*(1), 44–50.

INDEX